Guide to Surgical Principles and Practice

Dedication to Professor Zawawi

Professor Zawawi was very much involved with the inception and initial preparation work for this book, and his untimely death before its completion was the cause of much sadness among the other contributors. He was a most able surgeon, a stimulating and effective teacher and most fair but thorough examiner. It is much to his credit that the clinical teaching first in the medical schools of Tripoli and secondly of Benghazi was established in such a promising manner. He also successfully encouraged young postgraduate surgical trainees to obtain good clinical experience and further qualifications acceptable on an international level.

The editors and authors are pleased and proud to dedicate this volume to his memory.

For Churchill Livingstone

Publisher: Andrew Stevenson
Editorial Co-ordination: Editorial Resources Unit
Copy Editor: Liz Graham
Design: Design Resources Unit
Sales Promotion Executive: Louise Johnstone

Guide to Surgical Principles and Practice

Edited by

Iain E. Gillespie MD (Hons) MSc FRCS (Edin; Eng; Glas)
Professor of Surgery, University of Manchester; Honorary Consultant to Manchester Royal Infirmary, Manchester, UK

Nasim Ansari MB BS (Cal) FRCS (Eng)
Professor of Surgery and formerly Chairman, Department of Surgery, Jawahar Lal Nehru Medical College, Aligarh Muslim University, Aligarh, India; Visiting Professor of Surgery: Arab Medical University, Benghazi and Al Fateh University, Tripoli, Libya; and Institute of Postgraduate Medical Education and Research, Chandigarh, India

The late **A.R. Zawawi** MB ChB FRCS
Formerly Professor, Garyounis University, Benghazi, Libya

CHURCHILL LIVINGSTONE
EDINBURGH LONDON MADRID MELBOURNE NEW YORK AND TOKYO 1992

CHURCHILL LIVINGSTONE
Medical Division of Longman Group UK Limited

Distributed in the United States of America by Churchill Livingstone Inc., 650 Avenue of the Americas, New York, N.Y. 10011, and by associated companies, branches and representatives throughout the world.

First published 1992

ISBN 0-443-04430-9

British Library Cataloguing in Publication Data
A catalogue record for this book is available from the British Library.

Library of Congress Cataloging in Publication Data
A catalog record for this book is available from the Library of Congress.

Produced by Longman Singapore Publishers (Pte) Ltd
Printed in Singapore

Preface

Although there are already available several surgical textbooks, it has been felt for some time that there is a need for one more, particularly for undergraduates in countries other than the UK and North America who pursue their medical studies in English. Most of the contributors have taught and/or examined in surgery in various countries in the Middle East, the Asian continent, the Far East and Africa and are aware of the patterns of disease and health-care facilities available to medical practitioners in these areas of the world.

The idea of preparing this book came primarily from discussions between the late Professor Zawawi, Professor of Surgery in Tripoli and later in Benghazi, Professor Ansari of the Aligarh Muslim Medical School, India and the late Mr John, of Bath, UK, and several British surgeons. After a preliminary draft covering mainly general surgical topics had been prepared, further additions of more specialist topics were invited from an international team of contributors, and Professor I.E. Gillespie of Manchester University, UK, undertook to collate, revise and edit all the contributions.

It is hoped that this volume, representing a compilation of approaches to the range of clinical problems likely to be encountered by general surgeons, will be of interest and help, especially to those studying surgery in English, though not having this language as their primary one, and that it may also have a wider appeal.

Manchester 1992 I.E.G.

Acknowledgements

I am greatly indebted to Dr Richard Fawcitt for Figures 3.10, 16.4, 42.3, 42.4, 42.5, and 42.10; and to Professor Isherwood for Figure 26.3; and to Mr S. Payne for Figures 38.10 and 38.14.

All of the line drawings and diagrams are the work of Mr Richard Neave, Medical Artist to the University of Manchester Medical School, and the editors and authors are very appreciative of his very high standard of workmanship and artistry.

The entire text, in both its original and revised form was typed most efficiently and patiently by Mrs J. B. Smith, Secretary to the University Department of Surgery at Manchester Royal infirmary and a large debt of gratitude is owed to her for this considerable volume of work most expertly handled.

I.E.G.

Contributors

Nasim Ansari MB BS (Cal.) FRCS (Eng.)
Professor of Surgery and formerly Chairman, Department of Surgery, Jawahar Lal Nehru Medical College, Aligarh Muslim University, Aligarh, India; Visiting Professor of Surgery: Arab Medical University, Benghazi and Al Fateh University, Tripoli, Libya; and Institute of Postgraduate Medical Education and Research, Chandigarh, India

Ahmed Elzawawy MD D.d'Etat (France)
Professor and Head, Department of Radiotherapy, Oncology and Nuclear Medicine, Faculty of Medicine, Suez Canal University, Ismailia, Egypt; Head of Oncology Unit, Port Said General Hospital, Port Said, Egypt

Iain E. Gillespie MD (Hons) MSc FRCS (Edin; Eng; Glas)
Professor of Surgery, University of Manchester; Honorary Consultant to Manchester Royal Infirmary, Manchester, UK

Hossam Hamdy MD
Professor of Surgery, Faculty of Medicine, Suez Canal University, Ismailia, Egypt

The late **H.T. John** MS FRCS
Formerly Consultant Surgeon, The Royal United Hospital, Bath, UK

R.W.G. Johnson MB BS MS FRCS
Consultant Surgeon and Honorary Reader in Surgery, Transplant Unit, Manchester Royal Infirmary, Manchester, UK

F.D. Salama MB BCh FRCS (Eng; Edin) LMSSA
Consultant Thoracic Surgeon, City Hospital, Nottingham, UK

Prakash N. Tandon MS FRCS FAMS FNA
Bhatnagar Fellow, Department of Neurosurgery, Neuroscience Centre, All India Institute of Medical Sciences, New Delhi, India

The late **A.R. Zawawi** MB ChB FRCS
Formerly Professor, Garyounis University, Benghazi, Libya

Contents

1. History of surgery

The practice of surgery, i.e. the care of wounds, fractures and dislocations, is as old as man's history. Attempts to treat diseases by surgical methods must have been a later development. It is perhaps justified to assume that the arts of surgery and magic existed together, the latter overshadowing the former. It is also tempting to think that trephining of the skulls was practised in the belief that evil spirits needed to be allowed to escape from the body through these holes. No doubt some of these holes must have also helped patients suffering from extradural haemorrhage. The trephined skulls found in Peru probably date back to about 8000–10 000 BC, and provide the earliest proof of the practice of surgery.

Civilized men must have taken centuries before they were able to write about their surgical experiences and evolve theories to guide the practice. The existence of two centres of civilization as far back as 6000 years ago is known. One of these was the ancient Egyptian civilization around the Nile Valley in North Africa. The second was in Mesopotamia between the Tigris and Euphrates rivers. The earliest writings which have survived the ravages of time are the famous papyri of Egypt. These are medical treatises written on sheets prepared from papyrus plant during the reign of King Zoser (2980–2900 BC) when Amhotep was his minister. Amhotep was a remarkable man. Besides being regarded as the legendary god of Egyptian medicine, he was also an architect and poet. There are two papyri related to medicine—the Edwin Smith papyrus and Eber's papyrus. The former deals with surgery. In this, not only the care of wounds is described, but there are also a number of case histories which throw light on their clinical understanding. For example, feeble pulse, palsy and loss of hearing are described as complications of wounds of the skull. There are 48 dissertations on surgery in this papyrus.

In Mesopotamia, Babylon (the present Syria–Iraq) was the second centre of civilization in those days. The most interesting document related to surgery in Babylon which is available to us deals with the code of conduct of surgeons. This was prepared during the reign of King Hummurabi (about 2000 BC). The penalty for performing faulty surgery on a prince was chopping off the hands of the surgeon!

At this stage, medical practice was gradually being separated from witchcraft. There then followed an era of great intellectual development—mathematics, philosophy, geometry, geography, logic and astronomy were seen developing with medicine. Two great centres of this development were Greece and India.

GREEK MEDICINE

Greek medicine is rightly considered as the beginning of scientific medicine. The four great teachers of Greece were Socrates, Plato, Aristotle and Hippocrates. It is to Aristotle that the credit of laying the foundation of scientific medicine goes, as he propounded the physiological principles based on the concept of four humours—the blood, the phlegm, the yellow bile and the black bile. But it is Hippocrates (460–370 BC) who is regarded as the father of modern medicine, as he devoted most of his time to the teaching and development of this science. Hippocrates' oath is still accepted as the living bond between a medical student and teacher. Hippocrates described methods of treating fractures and dislocations. His method of reducing anterior dislocation of shoulder was universally employed till very recently, and is still sometimes employed when other methods fail. He taught that wounds should be kept dry after being cleaned with ordinary boiled water or wine. He advocated opposing the skin edges in superficial wounds which, of course, helps in early healing.

The most distinguished disciple of Hippocrates was Galen (AD 131–201) who lived during the second and early third century AD. He was a Greek but spent most of his life in Rome and Alexandria. He was not particularly interested in surgery, but he should be acknowledged as a great teacher of surgeons because of his works on physiology. His book *Experimental Pathology* contributed a great deal to the knowledge of surgeons.

HINDU MEDICINE (2000–500 BC)

While these remarkable developments were taking place in Greece, another centre of civilization was flourishing in India. There is evidence that surgery had developed as an art and was practised in India about this time. The best known surgeon of ancient India was Sushreta. There is some uncertainty about when he lived. The surgical work attributed to him, and which is now available as *Sushreta Sambitha*, was most probably compiled in the seventh century AD, but certainly was originally composed many centuries before Christ. In this, methods of removal of cataracts and bladder stones, incision of abscesses, resection of tumours and extraction of foreign bodies have been described. The Hindus were also the founders of plastic and reconstructive surgery, as women during that period were punished for adultery by amputation of the nose. The Hindu surgeons used to replace them by flaps taken from the cheek (rhinoplasty). There is a description of 20 sharp and 101 blunt surgical instruments. Sushreta was also interested in the study of anatomy and had described methods of preparing bodies for dissection.

ARABIC MEDICINE

At this stage of development Arabs and Muslims entered the arena in the eighth century AD. They not only preserved but developed and spread the teachings of their Greek and Indian predecessors. For 700 years—from the eighth to the 15th century AD—they held the intellectual field, and during this time Arabic remained the language of science in Europe, Africa and the greater part of Asia.

This Arab civilization provided opportunities not only to the Muslim scholars but also to others, particularly the Christians and the Jews. This was remarkable at a time when religious intolerance was widespread in many parts of the world, including Europe.

Among the Muslim authors, Abu Baker Mohamad Ibn Zakaria El Razi stands out as one of the most illustrious personalities. He lived between AD 865 and 965, and his book *El Hawi* was regarded as an encyclopaedia of medicine for many centuries. In this book, basic principles of medical practice were laid down, together with descriptions of diseases and their treatment. Razi is remembered even today because he was the first to describe the differences between smallpox and chickenpox.

Abu Ali El Hussain Ibn Abdullah Ibn Sina belonged to the next generation of physicians. He lived from AD 980–1037. His was a colourful personality, and he was very fond of the good things of life. He was truly a prince of physicians. His claim to fame rests not only on his monumental medical work *El Kanoon*, (known as *Cannon* in Europe), but also on his contributions to philosophy, mathematics, Arabic grammar and astronomy, and he was also a poet. *El Kanoon* was translated into several languages including Latin, and this Latin version served as a reference book of medicine in Europe, as did the original Arabic version in Asia and Africa, continuously for about 600 years after his death. In some parts of the world physicians still follow *El Kanoon.* The book is in five volumes and deals with anatomy, physiology, basic principles of medicine and causation of diseases in general, and includes descriptions of all the then-known diseases, therapeutics and pharmacology. In this book, he asserted that the practice of medicine should be based on the existing concepts of the physical sciences, which principles could not be challenged.

Neither Razi nor Ibn Sina were practising surgeons. They have been mentioned here to emphasize the point that Arab surgical practice had a sound theoretical background, and it was during this time that the concept started developing that surgeons were operating physicians.

Abulkasim Khalaf Ibn Abbas El Zahrawi personified this concept in his life and works (AD 939–1013). He was born in Spain where he practised and taught surgery. His monumental work *El Tasreef* was translated into Latin and many other languages. It is regarded as the first illustrated textbook of surgery, containing more than 200 drawings of medical instruments. It is a remarkably modern textbook in its format. Diseases are described organ-wise. Under each heading there is a description of aetiology, pathology, clinical features, treatment and prognosis. Operative details are included, starting with a description of the positions of the patient and the surgeon. Operations such as tracheostomy, tonsillectomy, thyroidectomy, and procedures for hernia, hydrocele, breast cancer, stones in the urinary tract, hydrocephalus, removal of lymph nodes, abdominal injuries, removal of the dead fetus from the uterus, and many others are included. There are also sections on a number of extra- and intraocular operations, including those for the removal of pannus and decompression for glaucoma.

The book also deals with questions of professional ethics and scientific objectivity: the author frankly discusses cases where he had committed mistakes or where his judgement was proved wrong. His teaching that cancer should only be treated surgically if the part of the body or the organ bearing it can be excised totally is followed even today, with some modifications.

Zahrawi personifies the essential Arab approach to clinical medicine. His opinions were based not only on the teachings of the masters but also on his own observations. Thus, describing tracheostomy, he notes that he became convinced of the possibility of this procedure when he saw a patient who had a neck wound from which air was coming out. He cleaned the wound and treated it expectantly. The patient survived and Zahrawi was convinced that a hole in the trachea was compatible with life, and that in upper respiratory tract obstruction, tracheostomy could be a life-saving measure. He described the operation in terms which sound nearly contemporary.

Discussing the causes of lack of progress in surgery in those days, he observed that one of the important factors was the lack of interest in learning anatomy.

Zahrawi was followed about 100 years later by another illustrious Arab, Abu Marwan Abdul Malik Ibn Zoher (AD 1103–1162). In Europe he is known as Avenzoor. His most famous book was *El Tayeir* which was translated into Latin and was popular in Europe for a long time. He described empyema, pericarditis and otitis media. He is said to be the first to have carried out a hysterectomy. However, probably the most important intellectual contribution of Ibn Zoher was his criticism of some of the teachings of Galen, which was remarkable in those days because of the high esteem in which Galen was held throughout the Islamic world. He espoused the concept of a lesser circulation between the heart and the lungs, suggested by Ibn Nafees in the 13th century, i.e. about 200 years before Harvey.

Jurjani (died AD 1136) was an accomplished ophthalmologist. He is known in Europe as 'Zurrein Dust' (surgeon with golden hands). His book *Nurul Uyun* is a classic of ophthalmology.

No description of Arab surgery would be complete without the mention of Ibn Al Quff, who taught surgery in Sham (the present Jordan, Syria and Iraq). He lived between 1233 and 1286 and left a monumental work of surgery called *Al Umdah Fisanaat Al Jirahah*. In this book, he described the treatment of fractures, removal of cysts, mastectomy, circumcision, phlebotomy, exploration of arteries, and lithotomy. He discussed the merits and demerits of different suture materials. Good post operative care of the patient and attention to mental and physical comfort were emphasized in this work. Many catheters, bladder syringes and different methods of suturing abdominal wounds were also mentioned.

The Arab leadership in science and surgery came to a close towards the 16th century. The main contribution was the establishment of surgery as a definite discipline of medical practice. The scientific outlook, i.e. practice based on theory evolved on the basis of observations, permeates through Arabic surgical work. Besides this basic contribution to the science and art of surgery, they made notable clinical observations and developed new surgical techniques. Examples include catheter drainage of the bladder, drainage of liver abscesses and the opening of perianal abscesses, with awareness of the risk of fistula-in-ano as a consequence of inadequate clearance. The removal of tonsils, nasal polyps and the management of nasopharyngeal tumours by cauterization were reported, and plastic repairs of facial and other defects were also clearly within the surgical repertoire. There is also evidence that the treatment of fractures and dislocations reached a high level of skill, and that the basic methods of controlling haemorrhage were well understood.

EUROPEAN MEDICINE

No significant progress in surgical practice appears to have taken place after the Arabs till the 19th century, when the introduction of general anaesthesia revolutionized the whole practice. At this time, i.e. in the 16th century AD, Europe was slowly emerging from its dark ages. Medical schools were being established at Salerno and Padua in Italy where lectures were given at first in Arabic. Later Latin became the language of science. Gradually intellectual leadership was changing and the Europeans were coming into the front rank.

Ambroise Paré (1510–1590) was perhaps the standard-bearer of surgery in Europe at this time. His famous saying, 'I treat the wounds but God heals them', remains true even today because, in spite of the tremendous progress made in surgery, we do not know anything which can enhance the process of healing by a day, though we know many things which delay it and in modern practice we avoid them as far as possible. Ambroise Paré advocated ligature of bleeding vessels as a method of stopping haemorrhage. He also developed new techniques in the practice of obstetrics and gynaecology.

Andreas Vesalius (1514 –1564) was Ambroise Paré's great contemporary. He was a strong advocate of basing the practice of surgery on a sound knowledge of anatomy. His *De Humani Corporis Fabrica* was a remarkable book on anatomy which remained popular for the next 200 years in Europe. Andreas Vesalius made the teaching of anatomy what it is today.

In the UK, John Hunter (1728–1793) is rightly regarded as the father of modern surgery. Born in Scotland, he lived most of his life in London. He was an anatomist, pathologist, surgeon, physiologist and a most prolific writer. His thirst for scientific truth was unquenchable. He would perform post-mortem examinations whenever possible to establish the cause of death. He collected a large number of diseased organs which he had removed from the dead and arranged these in a museum. Unfortunately, a great part of this collection was destroyed during the Second World War (1939–1945), but quite a few specimens were saved and are now housed in the Hunterian Museum at the Royal College of Surgeons in London. By popularizing post-mortem examination, John Hunter put surgery—and indeed the whole practice of medicine—on a solid foundation, so much so that the science of surgery can be divided into pre- and post-Hunterian eras.

There were two great obstacles to the further growth of surgery. Firstly, operative procedures were usually extremely painful—so much so that many patients would prefer death to this agony. No doubt surgeons would try to minimize the pain by preoperative use of narcotics like opium, cannabis indica, and alcohol. But in spite of these measures, many patients would die of pain during operation.

Secondly, most of the wounds became septic and many patients would die because of postoperative infection. Some would suffer more from these side-effects than from their original illnesses.

Both these obstacles were overcome to a great extent in the 19th century. William Thomas Morton, a dentist of the USA, demonstrated in the presence of many surgeons in 1846 that ether could be effectively used as a general anaesthetic. A year later, in 1847, James Young Simpson, Professor of Obstetrics in Edinburgh, successfully employed chloroform for anaesthesia. Other surgeons claimed success in this field at about the same time, and after this the floodgates of progress were opened. Now the science of anaesthesia has developed into a separate discipline and, thanks to the modern anaesthetist, complicated operations can be safely performed on all parts of the body.

The second problem—the prevention of sepsis—was solved by the efforts of the French bacteriologist Louis Pasteur (1822–1895) and the famous British surgeon Lord Lister (1827–1912).

Louis Pasteur demonstrated that germs were the cause of many diseases. Lister came to the conclusion that if wounds could be kept free of germs, there would be no suppuration. On this assumption, he developed his world-famous antiseptic technique and brought about a revolution in surgery. Now the wounds would not get infected as a rule. Subsequently an aseptic technique of operation was developed by which germs were excluded from the field of operation.

In the years to follow, three other developments gave a further fillip to the progress of surgery. These were the discovery of X-rays, and of antibiotics and the technique of administering fluids, including blood, intravenously.

X-rays were discovered by the German scientist Wilhelm Konrad Roentgen (1845–1923), and first utilized for visualizing the interior of the human body for medical purposes by William Ford Canon (1871–1945). The progress in acquiring accurate detailed imaging of nearly every part of the body by a variety of X-ray techniques, especially using contrast radiography, has been most impressive, and the more recently introduced application of ultrasound, computerized tomography and nuclear magnetic resonance now gives us even greater promise of clinically useful precise anatomical and physiological information.

Ionizing irradiation has also, of course, had its therapeutic applications: teleradiation (the application of radiation from a distance), interstitial radiation (the insertion of radioactive material into the tissues) and isotope therapy have all helped in the management of many disorders, particularly malignant disease.

No doubt Lister's antiseptic technique made operations quite safe as far as post operative wound infection was concerned. But what about the patients who in their bodies harboured germs which could not be eradicated by the application of antiseptics, for example patients suffering from tuberculosis of joints? By Lister's method, it was possible to drain abscesses without the danger of secondary infection of the wound, but the disease in the joint persisted because the germs of tuberculosis continued to flourish. It was therefore necessary to discover measures which would kill the germs inside the body or stop their multiplication. The German scientist Paul Ehrlich (1854–1915) discovered salvarsan, which was effective against syphilis, and in 1932 another German, Gerhard Downach, prepared prontosil rubrum, which was effective against staphylococcal infection. Later on, it was discovered that the effective part of prontosil rubrum was sulphanilamide. The British scientist, Alexander Fleming (1881–1951) discovered penicillin in 1938, and 10 years later Howard Florey of Oxford obtained pure penicillin and demonstrated its effectiveness as an anti-infective agent by its systemic administration. In 1944, streptomycin was discovered by Solomon Wakson and the conquest of tuberculosis began.

The advent of intravenous infusion, which made it possible to replace lost blood, as well as to correct fluid and electrolyte deficiency before, during and after operation, was developed only in the 20th century, and was a further significant advance.

These measures gave such an impetus to the development of surgery that it has long ceased to be one discipline, and has proliferated into ophthalmology, ENT, orthopaedics, cardiothoracic surgery, neurosurgery, urology, gynaecology, plastic surgery and paediatric surgery, besides general surgery. No doubt further subspecialties will be defined with the passage of time.

This progress has been made possible by the development not only of all branches of medicine like anatomy, physiology, pathology, bacteriology, pharmacology, biophysics and biochemistry, but by general and scientific developments in society. It is imperative for a modern surgeon to be familiar with these sciences. The physician of today is a clinical scientist, and a surgeon is an operating physician. The surgeon has inherited this role from the great teachers Hippocrates, Galen, Sushreta, Aviccena, Zahrawi and John Hunter, among others.

2. Preoperative care

Although clearly the main decisions to be made are the diagnosis and the decision to advise surgical treatment, there are many other important aspects to preoperative care. There is first the need to elicit whether there are any other pre-existing medical disorders which may increase the risk of complications from the operation. Some of these may require specific measures to correct or improve the condition and it may therefore be necessary to delay a non-urgent surgical procedure until the prophylactic treatment has had time to work. The presence of any active infection may increase the risk of a surgical wound becoming infected and may be a good reason for postponing an operation.

The risks of fatality and serious postoperative complications are small for most planned elective procedures, but even so it is always wise to weigh up the relative chances of outcome of either operation or leaving the patient alone.

The second main concern of good preoperative care is to communicate to the patient so that he or she clearly understands the objective of the operation, what sort of wound it will entail, and what drains, tubes or other appliances will be expected after the operation. It is even more important to gain his or her confidence and establish a good rapport so that the patient approaches the operation with assurance, and with as little tension as possible. It is also helpful to be aware of any social problems which may influence the speed of postoperative recovery and convalescence.

Although ideally in every patient presenting for even the most minor operation the counsel of perfection is to take an exhaustive personal, family, work and social history and complete a thorough physical examination of all systems, in reality a degree of common-sense judgement has to be used. Clearly the assessment of fitness for surgery is more rapid and straightforward in a fit athletic young man with a simple subcutaneous lipoma, than in a 60-year-old chronic bronchitic with hypertension and a history of a previous myocardial infarction, needing relief from benign prostate urinary outflow obstruction. When operation is urgently required to relieve a life-threatening situation there is, of course, very little time for preoperative preparation, but even here a little delay for one or two rapidly applied remedial measures may make a significant difference to the outcome.

Hopefully, most factors likely to affect risks from an operation should come to light in the initial history-taking and assessment as an outpatient, thus giving time for any additional X-ray, laboratory or other special investigations prior to admission for surgery. If necessary further specialist opinion, e.g. of a consultant anaesthetist, cardiologist, or diabetic physician, may be obtained also as an outpatient, thereby avoiding prolonged inpatient stay prior to the operation. Enquiry should be made as to whether the patient has undergone any previous anaesthetic and, if so, whether any problems were encountered. If so this information can warn the surgeon and anaesthetist to take steps to try and prevent a similar occurrence.

Although the trend is towards not applying investigations—even simple ones—in a routine fashion, a case might be made for performing urine testing for sugar, protein and blood, chest X-ray, and haemoglobin and simple haematological indices in everyone due to have a surgical procedure under general anaesthesia. It might also be argued that, in addition, an electrocardiogram (ECG) should be done in those over the age of 40.

REASONS FOR POSSIBLE POSTPONEMENT OF AN ELECTIVE OPERATION

Where the need for operative treatment is non-urgent, but there is present a condition which is known significantly to increase the risk from operation under general anaesthesia, it will be prudent to delay arrangements for admission to hospital to let treatment or the passage of time lessen that risk. The four main reasons for such a postponement are gross obesity; recent myocardial infarction; arterial hypertension, and active infection in the upper respiratory tract, skin, or an organ opening on to the skin surface.

Obesity

It is well known that obesity greatly increases the risks of wound infection, deep venous thrombosis and pulmonary embolism, respiratory infection and pressure sore, among other problems, and if there is a strong likelihood of the patient making a serious effort to reduce weight it is worth deferring the operation for several weeks or months. Often, however, in spite of good intentions, the patient fails to reduce and it is a matter of judgement whether to delay in the hope of some weight loss, or proceed with the operation immediately, accepting the increased risks, rather than have a further fruitless passage of time.

Recent myocardial infarction

Following a previous myocardial infarction there is always, of course, the risk of a further one, and this risk is particularly high if a surgical operation is performed within the first 6 months of the attack. Therefore, all but the most urgent of operations should be avoided during this period. The question of coronary artery bypass surgery prior to an elective or semi-urgent procedure for other pathology should be considered when there is a history of either a definite earlier myocardial infarction or anginal-type pain.

Arterial hypertension

If systemic hypertension is detected and has either remained undetected or inadequately controlled till the preoperative assessment, then it is worthwhile taking a little time to achieve good control of blood pressure levels—particularly diastolic pressure—before proceeding with the operation, to diminish the chances of a per- or postoperative cerebrovascular occlusion.

Active infection

Obviously when there is an open source of bacterial contamination on or in the patient there is a significant risk that this will lead to infection of the surgical wound, and even a small superficial skin abscess may be dangerous in this regard. It is wise to take whatever steps are necessary to heal any such lesion, e.g. drainage of pus, local occlusive dressings and antibiotics, before the operation.

Infection in the respiratory tract, even a simple cold or sore throat, may flare up into a major serious postoperative pneumonia, and it is very risky to give a general anaesthetic under these circumstances. Although it often seems irksome to the patient to be delayed for a week or two so that even a minor upper respiratory infection is cleared, it is time well spent in greatly reducing the risk of a dangerous postoperative problem.

INDICATIONS FOR FURTHER ASSESSMENT AND PREPARATION

Cardiorespiratory impairment

If in the medical history there is any complaint of chest pain, especially if referred to shoulder or arm, breathlessness, especially on exertion, palpitation and ankle-swelling in the latter part of the day, then in addition to measuring pulse rate and blood pressure a fuller cardiac assessment should be made, looking for any arrhythmias, cardiac enlargement, increase in neck vein pressure, liver enlargement, ankle or sacral oedema and moist respiratory sounds over the lung fields. Certainly an ECG is required, and a cardiologist may advise more elaborate tests of cardiac function and suggest ways of improving any impaired function. Patients with any sign of pre-existing cardiac ischaemia are more likely to develop a myocardial infarction postoperatively than those with healthy hearts, and unless a preoperative baseline ECG recording is available it may be impossible to detect any new changes on the ECG should there be a suggestive clinical picture after the operation.

Breathlessness, of course, may also be due to respiratory insufficiency, and questions about the presence of any cough, wheezing or other breathing difficulty should be asked. If coughing is productive, the volume, colour and consistency of the sputum should be ascertained, and a sample obtained for culture and identification and sensitivity of organisms present. As well as chest X-ray, simple measurements of peak expiratory volume and forced vital capacity may give a good estimate of overall respiratory efficiency, and these may be supplemented by blood–gas analysis and more elaborate tests of respiratory function if there is real concern. If marked bronchitis is present a vigorous course of breathing exercises, bronchodilators, physiotherapy and antibiotics may bring about marked improvement and thereby greatly reduce the chances of postoperative chest difficulties.

It should go without saying that no one should smoke, for numerous important health reasons, but certainly if a patient who smokes needs an operation he or she should be most strongly exhorted to stop immediately. The longer the patient has avoided smoking altogether prior to the operation, the less the risks of severe postoperative chest trouble. Of course, the opportunity should also be taken to discourage the patient from restarting smoking after the operation.

Anaemia

If anaemia is detected it is, of course, first necessary to determine whether it is due to blood loss, deficiency of iron or vitamin B_{12}, or, more rarely, of folic acid. This will require examination of the whole range of haematological indices, and may have to be followed up by other specific tests, e.g. iron-binding capacity, serum folate, Vitamin B_{12} estimations or even marrow biopsy. Where the cause of any anaemia is blood loss or iron deficiency and the operation is non-urgent, it will often be possible to correct the blood picture by the oral administration of an iron supplement preparation. If it is inadvisable to delay the operation blood transfusion may be necessary. Rather than give several units quickly over a short period of time, it may cause less physiological disturbance and allow more time for adaptation, particularly where there is any degree of cardiovascular impairment, if the transfusion is spread over several days, say 1 unit per day.

As a general rule one should be reluctant to take a patient to theatre for a general anaesthetic procedure with a haemoglobin level of less than 10 g/dl.

In addition to causing problems with blood–gas exchange and oxygen carriage, anaemia can impair wound healing and reduce the patient's resistance to infection.

Nutritional state

Patients who are seriously undernourished withstand all types of surgery badly. There is a significantly increased risk of dying after any moderate to major operation, mainly on account of grossly impaired healing of anastomoses, sutured structures, and indeed of wounds in all tissues. Furthermore there is an increased chance of all manner of infections arising and being very difficult to control. The problems of undernutrition are most likely to be encountered either when ordinary surgical disorders occur in populations subjected to famine, or in patients with malignant disease, especially affecting the proximal gastrointestinal tract, or in diseases associated with severe vomiting and /or diarrhoea, malabsorption or fistulas.

Although protein deficiency, reflected in gross muscle wasting and/or reduced serum levels of total protein and albumen to below 3 g/dl, is often the main and most obvious impairment, attention should also be paid to the possibility of generalized or specific vitamin deficiency. A number of indices of malnutrition have been devised in an attempt to quantitate degrees of impairment, but most are either too complicated or not reliable enough for direct day-to-day clinical application. In general patients who have lost more than 10% of their body weight as a result of their illness, or who are unlikely to return to a fully adequate dietary intake for a prolonged period after operation, are in need of additional nutritional support.

Where gross undernutrition is present, preoperative correction is highly desirable and even if only a few days can be spent achieving partial improvement this can be greatly in the patient's interest. Of course the ideal way if possible is to give the food, fluids and supplements orally, or by a thin enteral feeding tube introduced pernasally, but if for example there is oesophageal obstruction, high gastrointestinal fistula, disease affecting the digestion/absorption capacity or grossly impaired appetite, the nutritional requirements may have to be given parenterally, i.e. into a central vein. A meticulous technique is needed in the introduction of the special catheter and strictly aseptic nursing attention is vital, otherwise serious infective complications can arise. Parenteral nutrition is preferably undertaken and supervised by an experienced team rather than by the occasional user.

While it is clear that improving the nutritional state of those with severe deficiency before major surgery is highly effective in reducing risks of postoperative death or morbidity, there is no evidence that a short course of preoperative hyperalimentation confers any benefit on those of normal nutrition, and such action seems only wasteful of both time and money.

Drugs

It is important to know if any patient coming to operation is currently taking any medication, if he or she has recently had a course of drugs, and if he or she has experienced any untoward reaction or sensitivity to previous drugs.

Some obvious examples of drugs which have an important bearing on any operative procedure are given below.

Anticoagulants

Clearly if these can be discontinued this is preferable. If, however, there is good medical reason for continued anticoagulant treatment the dosage may be reduced, or temporary reversal may be achieved over the operative period, and full dosage recommenced once the patient is past the stage of risk from reactive bleeding.

Adrenocorticosteroids

Adrenocorticosteroids may reduce the resistance to infective organisms and delay wound healing. Since in those having steroids chronically over a prolonged period of time there may be impairment of the patient's own adrenal function, it is customary to cover the pre-, per- and early postoperative period with increased doses of corticosteroids to avoid acute hypoadrenal crises occurring at this stressful time.

Immunosuppressive drugs

These also impair the efficiency of the body's defence mechanisms against infection and other potentially harmful agencies, and extra precautions may be required to protect against organisms and other injurious agents.

Furthermore, unusual bacterial, fungal or viral infections may arise in immunosuppressed patients and this should be borne in mind when no response is obtained to conventional antibiotics, or unusual clinical features of infection.

Cytotoxic drugs

These can give rise to similar problems to the immunosuppressive agents.

Prolonged antibiotics

Prolonged antibiotics, by suppressing common organisms, may permit the overgrowth and invasion of tissues by unusual bacteria and fungi.

Other medications, such as digoxin and bronchodilators, if clearly prescribed for good medical reason may have to be continued right across the operative periods. If there is a past history of regular consumption of alcohol, or central nervous system suppressants, e.g. barbiturates, phenothiazines or opiates, the anaesthetist should be informed, as adjustment of dosage of the premedication and anaesthetic agents may well be required. The anaesthetist will also want to know about any antihypertensive drugs being taken, in order to take steps to avoid sudden hypotension during the procedure.

It is extremely important to be aware of any history of reaction to any medication, particularly if there appeared to be a cardiorespiratory reaction. The commonest types of allergy are, of course, skin responses, and when asking about these, one should also remember to enquire about sensitivity to adhesive tape or dressings, so that these can be avoided and alternative drugs or dressings can be made available.

Even if there is no direct history of a reaction to any specific drug, if the patient is known to have hayfever, asthma or another disorder with an allergic basis, there is an increased chance that he or she may display sensitivity to a drug, and this possibility should be kept in mind.

Bleeding disorders

If the patient admits to any prolongation of bleeding from simple cuts and injuries, or following a previous dental extraction or operation, a full screening of coagulation factors is advisable. This should also be done in those with obstructive jaundice, liver disease, or on cytotoxic medication. The occurrence of spontaneous bruising and purpura also requires investigation, and probably the advice of a haematologist.

Screening for sickle-cell trait should be remembered in black people, and the possibility of thalassaemia in patients with anaemia, haemolysis, retarded growth and enlargement of liver and spleen.

Hepatic function

Where there is a clear history of a previous episode of jaundice or other symptoms suggestive of liver damage, or a definite or suspected high intake of alcohol, or when physical signs are in keeping with liver disease, a full range of biochemical indicators of hepatic function, testing for hepatitis B antigen and an estimate of clotting factors should be done.

There is no justification, however, for performing liver function tests routinely on otherwise completely healthy persons with no suggestive symptoms or signs, presenting with straightforward surgical conditions.

The urinary system

Although routine screening of a urine sample for blood, protein and sugar has been advised for all those being admitted for operation, no further urinary investigations are required in the vast majority of surgical patients. If, however, there is a history of previous renal disease, symptoms of increasing bladder outflow obstruction, or evidence of dehydration, sodium retention, oliguria or polyuria or reason to suspect gross fluid disturbance, e.g. in vomiting or diarrhoea, then further indices of renal function are required. These include the volume of urine output per hour, the specific gravity of the urine, and measurement of the serum urea and creatinine levels. If infection is suspected microscopy and culture of the urine are indicated.

In elderly men with some degree of prostatic hyperplasia there may be the risk of acute retention of urine occurring after operation, and if there is much frequency, delay in starting micturition and dribbling there may be a case for dealing with this problem by transurethral resection prior to the planned operation if it is not urgent. In this way distressing postoperative urinary retention may be avoided. On other occasions, if the non-urological procedure is required without delay, bladder catheterization may be advisable as a preoperative measure. This will certainly permit an accurate assessment of the hourly output of urine and assist in the determination of postoperative fluid requirements.

GROUPS OF PATIENTS AT SPECIAL RISK

The elderly

Since the number of elderly people is steadily increasing and the range of surgical procedures has widened, more operations are being performed in this age group. As long as there is no overt evidence of major cardiovascular, renal or respiratory disease there need be no undue hesitation in recommending a surgical procedure which can bring relief and improvement of quality of life. However, the cardiorespiratory reserve in the elderly is naturally reduced and it is easier to push the patient into gross failure by inappropriate management or delay in detection of complications which compromise the reserve. In general, older patients require smaller doses of anaesthetic agents, and some drugs and strong analgesics, particularly opiates, may lead to restlessness and mental confusion. Care is also needed to use the minimal amount of premedication. It is also relatively easy to overload the circulation by the administration of more intravenous fluids than necessary and the rate and volume of these should be most carefully monitored, if necessary by central venous pressure, among other measures.

Many elderly patients will of course have a degree of atherosclerosis, which may or may not have been manifest in previous myocardial or cerebral ischaemic episodes. The risk of infarctions in the postoperative period should be borne in mind.

Finally, since tumours are more frequent in the older age groups, any symptoms suggestive of such a disorder should be followed up by the appropriate investigations.

The obese

Grossly overweight patients are more prone to respiratory complications, wound infection, deep venous thrombosis, skin pressure problems, and myocardial infarcts postoperatively than are those of normal build. If the operation is non-urgent, then ideally it should be postponed until as much of the excess weight as possible has been lost by dietary control. However, many overweight patients fail to adhere to their weight-reducing schedule in spite of all encouragement and exhortation, and then the decision has still to be faced to proceed with the operation with all the risks unchanged after a wasted period of time. It is often a matter of difficult clinical judgement to determine whether there is a realistic chance of delay leading to successful weight reduction or not.

If an operation is undertaken in an obese patient extra attention is needed to turn the patient frequently, to encourage early coughing and breathing exercises and to use prophylactic measures against deep venous thrombosis.

Diabetic patients

Operations on diabetic patients are now commonplace. Firstly this common endocrine disorder is more frequently recognized and easily kept under control, and secondly the condition increases the incidence of infections including abscesses which may need drainage, and of arterial disease which may be amenable to grafting or other arterial procedures. Special consideration should be given in the preoperative preparation, during the operation and also well into the postoperative period until the patient is fully restored to stable control on a usual diet and normal activities.

A combination of factors surrounding the operation will tend to upset blood sugar levels. For example, starvation before the anaesthetic will lower the blood sugar, whereas the stress and anxiety will increase it, via the release of adrenocorticoids and/or adrenaline, as will the presence of infection or gross physical trauma. There is therefore a risk of either hypo- or hyperglycaemia occurring before, during and after operation. Of these two, hypoglycaemia poses the much more serious threat.

In the preoperative evaluation of the diabetic patient particular attention should be paid to examining for any concurrent infection in the chest, mouth or skin. Such an infection may increase the need for insulin and may also flare up after the operation and require specific treatment. If the operation is not urgent it is strongly desirable to eradicate the concurrent infection by appropriate measures. It is also prudent to check the urine for protein, as well as for sugar, since proteinuria may be an early sign of diabetic nephropathy. Renal function should be assessed at least by a measurement of the serum creatinine level. It is also helpful to know the serum potassium concentration, since hypokalaemia can lead to a secondary increase in blood sugar levels, and hyperkalaemia may arise from the sequence of renal damage, leading to reduced release of renin, leading to reduced aldosterone secretion.

Control of the blood sugar

The main objective should be to maintain a level of between 100 and 200 mg/dl, but an increase to even around 400 mg/dl during the peroperative phase is still regarded as safe.

Diabetic patients may be regarded as falling into two main broad categories:

1. Type I: These have a severe deficiency of insulin production; the disorder has usually

appeared at a young age, and they require daily insulin injections.

2. Type II : These are generally older, over the age of 50 and, having only a partial reduction in insulin production from their own pancreatic islets, can usually be controlled either by diet regulation alone, or by a combination of diet and an oral hypoglycaemic agent, e.g. one of the sulphonylureas.

The pre- and peroperative management of these two types is in general different, although the objective, as already noted, is to maintain a blood sugar level not lower than 100 mg/dl and not higher than 200–400 mg/dl. Rapid accurate measurements of blood sugar by means of a simple portable electronic apparatus should be available, and if there is at any time concern about the adequacy of control, there should be no hesitation in having a direct blood sugar estimation made.

The milder type II diabetes. In the majority of these patients it is sufficient to omit the morning dose of the oral hypoglycaemic agent and set up an intravenous infusion of 5% glucose, running it at a rate of 100 ml/h. This should be easily handled by the patient's own reduced output of insulin.

If, however, the preoperative fasting blood sugar is in the 250–400 mg/dl range, it may be wiser to add 5 units of soluble insulin to each litre of 5% glucose, again keeping the infusion rate at 100 ml/h. It is stressed that although such a regime should prove to be adequate for minor, straightforward surgery, where the procedure is prolonged or more major there is no substitute for direct measurement of the sugar levels in samples of blood at intervals throughout the operation and alteration of the insulin or glucose doses accordingly.

Insulin-dependent type I diabetes. These patients will already be on a maintenance routine of either one of the long-acting insulin preparations alone or, more likely, a combination of such a preparation and regular or soluble insulin each day. It is even more important in these diabetics than in type II patients to have readings of fasting blood sugar levels and repeated measurements at intervals throughout the operation, particularly if it is a prolonged procedure.

There are three possible approaches to the pre-, per- and postoperative control:

1. to give the insulin dose subcutaneously;
2. to give a mixture of glucose and insulin by continuous intravenous infusion;
3. to add a separate solution of insulin to a constant-rate intravenous glucose infusion through the same giving set. This technique allows alteration of the insulin delivery without affecting the glucose administration, and therefore provides more precise control in response to repeated monitoring of the blood glucose measurements. It is, however, slightly more complicated and requires very close observation of the delivery rates to ensure that insulin overdosage does not occur, leading to hypoglycaemia.

Subcutaneous insulin dose. The simplest, and still most widely used, method of preparing type I diabetics for surgery is to give on the morning of the operation one-third to one-half their usual dose of both the long-acting and soluble insulin subcutaneously, and to establish an intravenous infusion of 5% glucose (even 10% glucose in the severely diabetic) and continue this, again at a rate of 100 ml/h pre- and peroperatively. Conventionally, the operation is scheduled first on the list or as early as can be arranged, so that the fasting state is not unduly prolonged.

Although this simple approach is often satisfactory for all practical purposes, it should be borne in mind that the absorption of soluble insulin from the subcutaneous site is slow, especially with the patient recumbent and inactive, and maximal effect may not be exerted till 4–6 h after the injection. There may therefore be a possibility of incomplete control of the hyperglycaemia in the first hour or so, and then hypoglycaemia some 4–6 h later.

Simultaneous insulin and glucose infusion. In this method the soluble insulin is added to 5% glucose infusion, which is given at a rate of 100 ml/h. The dose of insulin can be either 5, 10 or 15 units, giving a delivery rate of 0.5, 1 or 1.5 u/h respectively. Very occasionally an even higher dosage may be required. The obvious advantages of this approach are that any problems of delayed absorption are avoided, and that the rate of administration can be quickly adjusted either way according to blood sugar findings.

Separate insulin solution. The third procedure, of having a separate insulin solution being infused directly into the delivery tube leading from the glucose infusion, of course gives even greater control of the doses of insulin and glucose independently. As mentioned, however, it demands much more careful supervision and regulation than the other, simpler methods. If this technique is employed it is strongly recommended that a reliable, accurately calibrated automatic constant-rate pump is used for the insulin infusion.

After the operation, and until the patient is fully conscious, oriented and back on the proper oral intake, he or she must be closely observed for clinical signs suggestive of hypoglycaemia—sweating, restlessness, anxiety, tremor—and this is most likely to occur if one of the long-acting insulins has been given subcutaneously preoperatively, or if a larger than usual amount of insulin has been given intravenously. If hypoglycaemia arises it should be easy to correct by increasing the rate of intravenous glucose and reducing the rate of insulin if this is being given.

Estimations of the insulin requirements based on the levels of glucose in the urine are generally so unreliable in the pre- and postoperative phases, that they should not be used, unless there is no access to blood sugar analysis.

SUMMARY (CHECKLIST) OF PREOPERATIVE QUESTIONS AND ACTION

1. Will the patient likely need blood? — Group and cross-match.
2. Is there a significant risk of postoperative infection (e.g. bowel surgery, biliary operations, ischaemic limb operations)? — Give appropriate prophylactic antibiotics in adequate dosage shortly before and during operation.
3. Are respiratory problems anticipated? — Arrange pre- and postoperative physiotherapy and alert anaesthetist and intensive care unit.
4. Has the patient any known allergies? — Alert all medical and nursing attendants.
5. Is there a past history of any anaesthetic problems? — Warn the anaesthetist.
6. What is the complete list of all medication currently taken as well as within the last year? — Inform anaesthetist and discuss which should be continued, and at what dosage.
7. Is there any evidence of chronic abuse of drugs or alcohol? — Warn the anaesthetist and those who will look after the patient postoperatively.
8. Is there a likelihood of postoperative retention of urine, or will it be desirable to have an accurate measurement of urinary output? — Introduce a self-retaining catheter under sterile conditions into the urinary bladder.
9. Is obstructive jaundice present? — Diuresis from intravenous mannitol may protect the kidneys from damage.
10. Is there a possibility that the sickle-cell trait is present? — Test for it.
11. Is there evidence of gross malnutrition? — If the procedure is non-urgent, consider preoperative correction by enteral or intravenous route.
12. Is a paralytic ileus anticipated after the operation, or is gastric resection planned? — Pass nasogastric tube and ensure its distal end is located in the stomach.
13. Is there any suggestion of bleeding disorder? — Check platelets and clotting factors and give appropriate factors for any deficiencies.
14. Should you take prophylactic measures against deep venous thrombosis? — Certainly this is wise in high-risk groups, e.g. hip surgery, anyone with previous history of deep venous thrombosis or other venous problems, the elderly, those with abdominal malignancy, etc.
15. Will the bowel be opened? — Use measures to empty the bowel of solid matter as far as possible, and give antibiotics effective against colonic organisms, including Gram-negative ones.
16. Is the patient diabetic? — Use the approach outlined above.

3. Postoperative care

Postoperative care may be regarded as falling into three phases: seeing the patient safely and fully recovered from the anaesthetic; keeping a careful watch for signs of any complications, and convalescence and rehabilitation back towards as normal a daily routine as can be achieved.

IMMEDIATE POSTOPERATIVE RECOVERY

It is important for someone with knowledge and experience in dealing with acute support measures to keep the patient under close observation until consciousness returns and the vital signs of pulse, blood pressure and respiration are stable. Ideally the postoperative patient should be nursed by fully trained staff in a recovery room adjacent to the theatre for a sufficient length of time to ensure that it is safe to continue less rigorous monitoring in the ward. The main problems which may arise in this very early phase, and which may need swift intervention by either the anaesthetist or surgeon—hence the desirability of having the recovery room adjacent to the operating theatre—are as follows:

1. Obstructed respiration.
2. Severe bleeding.
3. Sudden cardiac collapse.

Obstructed respiration

The rate of recovery of consciousness after a general anaesthetic varies from patient to patient, and of course will be influenced by the agents given before and during the procedure. A smooth gradual reawakening is assisted by nursing the patient in a quiet semi-darkened room, turned to a semi-prone posture, with the legs flexed and the head and neck comfortably supported in a slightly flexed position. The jaw should be allowed to fall forwards to keep the tongue from falling backwards into the throat, and care must be taken to keep bedclothes or any other material from obstructing the nose or mouth. Until the cough reflex returns and is effective, there is always a risk of inhalation of mucus secretions, or regurgitated oesophageal or gastric contents, with serious consequences, and so any liquids collecting in the mouth or throat will have to be aspirated.

Sudden airway obstruction in the immediate postoperative period, with obvious distress, choking, violent respiratory efforts, suffusion and cyanosis, is usually due to mechanical occlusion by

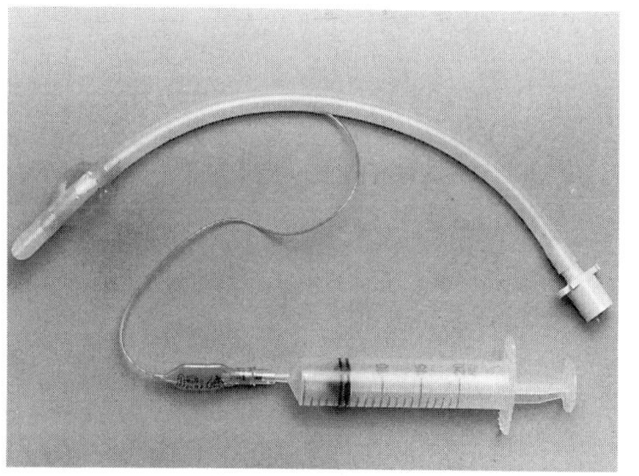

Fig. 3.1 Cuffed endotracheal tube, used for mechanical ventilation. Once the lubricated distal end of the tube has been passed into the trachea, under direct vision via a laryngoscope, enough air is introduced by the syringe to inflate the distal balloon, occluding the lumen and make it airtight. The outer small balloon also inflates to the same pressure, and acts as a guide. If it becomes deflated, the important inner cuff has also deflated.

either the tongue or some liquid or solid material being inhaled. The mouth should be promptly opened, a finger swept into the oral cavity and pharynx to clear any obviously occluding material, and if there is not instant relief of all symptoms and signs, a direct viewing laryngoscope is introduced. This allows inspection and aspiration of any further material, as well as visualization of the larynx. Closure of the larynx by intraluminal substances or spasm of the laryngeal muscles will need endotracheal intubation. Where spasm is present this may require the special expertise of the anaesthetist, and this is therefore one of the reasons for preference for siting the recovery room next to the theatre. Since mechanical ventilation is likely to be required at least for some time, a cuffed endotracheal tube is preferred and should be available (Fig. 3.1).

Severe bleeding

The two main signs to look out for are first, the escape of obviously excessive amounts of fresh blood from either the operation wound or from any drain which has been inserted, and second, the signs of hypovolaemic shock indicating concealed blood loss, i.e. rapid weak pulse and drop in blood pressure. If the bleeding is intra-abdominal there may also be an obvious increase in abdominal girth.

As far as frank bleeding from the wound is concerned this may be from superficial vessels caught up by one or more of the skin stitches, and if so a few minutes of local direct pressure over a sterile pad may control the escape. If this simple manoeuvre is not sufficient then it will be necessary to return the patient to theatre, re-open the wound layer by layer until the site of bleeding is found, and then deal with the vessel either by ligature or by under-running with a suture. Where the bleeding is clearly into a body cavity the patient will need to be re-anaesthetized, the wound re-opened completely and the bleeding vessel rapidly located and dealt with by whatever is the most appropriate technique—clamping and ligation, under-running or, rarely, packing. Rapid transfusion may well also be necessary under these circumstances.

Sudden cardiac collapse

In the immediate postoperative phase the two occurrences to look out for are myocardial infarction and dysrhythmias.

Myocardial infarction

Although the incidence of myocardial infarction directly after non-cardiac operations is very small, the risk certainly increases with the age of the patient, in those having operations for atherosclerotic disease, and in those with a previous history of infarction, other cardiac problems or hypertension. Even a transient period of hypotension or hypoxia during the operation may precipitate the coronary artery occlusion. If a general surgical procedure is required in someone who has had a previous myocardial infarction it is strongly desirable to postpone this till at least 6 months after the heart attack, and even then the risk of a further one in the postoperative phase is around five times that of patients with no such history. If operation is performed in the first 3 months after infarction the chance of another one occurring in the postoperative period is about 25%.

If the patient has sufficiently recovered consciousness then the complaint of sudden chest pain, signs of shock and arrhythmias will alert those monitoring him or her about the possibility of a myocardial infarction. An electrocardiogram (ECG) tracing and measurement of cardiac enzymes, particularly creatine phosphokinase, should be urgently obtained in a blood sample and arrangements made to transfer the patient directly to the intensive care unit.

The infarction, however, may be a silent one, with no dramatic symptoms, and may be recognized only by noting an episode of otherwise unexplained hypotension in the recovery phase. Such an occurrence should also prompt the appropriate measurements, and if the diagnosis is confirmed or strongly suspected, again arrangements should be made for continued close supervision in the intensive care area.

Dysrhythmias

A variety of disorders of the cardiac rhythm can

arise in the early postoperative period. Sometimes these are related to the anaesthetic agents used, e.g. halothane or cyclopropane, etc. and they may also be a consequence of hypoxaemia or electrolyte disturbance, e.g. hypokalaemia or alkalosis. They may also, of course, be associated with myocardial infarction as discussed above.

The commonest variety of dysrhythmia encountered is of supraventricular origin and reverts to normal either spontaneously or when the relevant respiratory or biochemical correction is made. More serious is atrial fibrillation which, if rapid, may require digoxin to assist effective cardiac output, and ventricular dysrhythmias, which may lead to ventricular fibrillation. This is a life-threatening condition which may need the urgent intravenous injection of lignocaine to revert to sinus rhythm and save life.

Cardiac arrest

When there is complete cessation of any detectable heartbeat, unconsciousness and apnoea, the following measures must be swiftly and competently employed. The patient is laid supine on a rigid surface, if necessary the floor, and closed cardiac massage is started. A cuffed endotracheal tube is inserted and manual ventilation begun. If no endotracheal tube is immediately available, mouth-to-mouth respiration is carried out until the tube is obtained. ECG leads are fixed in place and a tracing quickly taken to determine whether asystole or ventricular fibrillation is present. The latter will require attempts to correct back to normal rhythm by electrical defibrillation (Fig. 3.2). Since the patient will rapidly develop acidosis as long as the circulation is at a standstill, intravenous (i.v.) sodium bicarbonate should be given, preferably into an i.v. line which can be used for repeated bolus injection or continuous infusion. As early as practicable blood–gas measurements should be obtained to give a guide to further corrective steps. As a rough guide, probably about 150–200 mmol/ sodium bicarbonate will be required in the first 10 min.

The survival and extent of recovery of brain and other vital organ function depend mainly on the duration of the period of cessation of the blood flow. It is often difficult to decide how long these

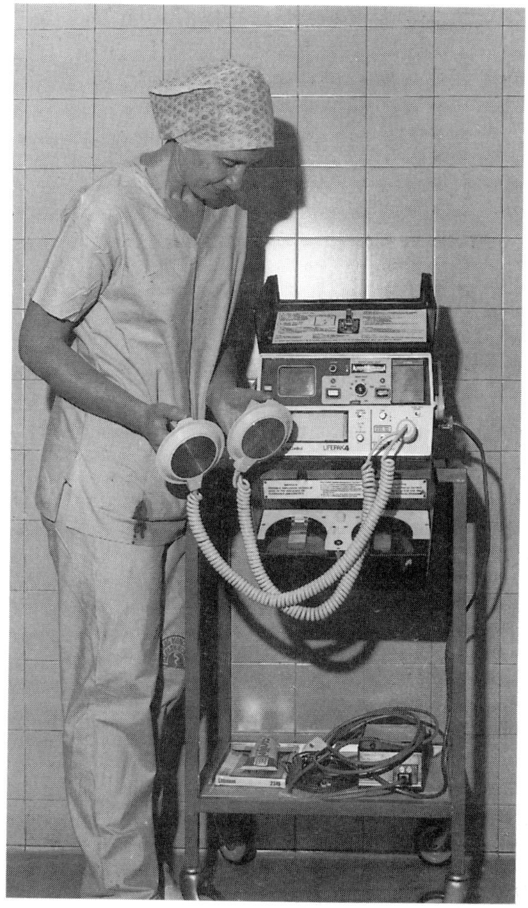

Fig. 3.2 External defibrillator: a very brief, high-voltage, direct current impulse is applied to the heart by placing one of the round electrodes firmly on the skin over the upper sternum and the other in the region of the cardiac apex. It is important from the operator's point of view for the handles to be well insulated. No contact is to be made between any part of the bodies of operator and patient during administration of the electrical impulse.

resuscitative measures should be continued when there is no sign of return of a satisfactory heartbeat and circulation. Once the pupils become widely dilated and fixed, with no response to direct light, irreversible damage to the brain has occurred, and further measures will be fruitless.

MAIN RECOVERY PERIOD IN THE WARD

Once the patient has recovered consciousness and all vital signs are stable he or she should return to the familiar surroundings of the ward, where observations should continue on a regular—though less frequent—basis than in the recovery room. Initially hourly assessment of the patient's general state and comfort plus measurement of pulse, blood pressure, and respiratory rate should be made. Any drains should be checked to ensure that they have not slipped out of position, that they are free to drain whatever material is expected and that the amount of drainage is not greater than anticipated. When a catheter is inserted in the urinary bladder it is important to check that it is draining freely and if a graduated receptacle is used an hourly measurement of output is recorded. The wound dressing should be inspected, but not otherwise disturbed unless there is excess bleeding or discharge, in which case the surgeon should be informed.

Gradually the frequency of these simple observations can be reduced according to the judgement of experienced nursing and medical staff, as the patient's progress continues. However, there continues to be a responsibility on all those involved in the patient's care until he leaves for home, to be on the look-out for any evidence of complications and to take appropriate measures both to prevent them in patients known to be at particular risk, and to treat those which do arise. The main problems to watch for are as follows:

1. Pain control.
2. Care of the wound.
3. Management of drains.
4. Gastric aspiration tubes.
5. Chest problems.
6. Fluid and electrolyte management.
7. Urinary problems.
8. Thromboembolism.
9. Postoperative pyrexia.
10. Psychiatric complications.

Pain control

While some local pain or discomfort is to be expected in the region of any operation wound, it is a common clinical observation that there is a large variation in the amount of wound pain complained of from one patient to the next. Factors such as the amount of anxiety, the patient's expectations, the degree of information the patient has had about what to expect, personality, cultural and social backgrounds can all influence the severity of the complaint. Good medical and nursing practice require that a quietly confident, sympathetic and supportive manner is displayed in explaining clearly and concisely what will be involved in a forthcoming operation, what drains, and tubes, if any, will be used, and giving the reassurance that there are ample means available of dealing with any postoperative needs. Where there is good rapport and attention to clear communication with the patient there is usually little difficulty in coping with postoperative pain, and the amount of analgesic drugs is usually kept to a minimum.

Having made these general points, however, there is no doubt that some operations are followed by more pain than others. Those on the chest, abdomen and major joints are much more painful than those in the head and neck, the soft tissue of the limbs or the abdominal wall. To some extent the amount of pain is related to the length of time, degree of direct operative trauma, retraction, type of incision used, and the presence of any tension in the wound closure. Obviously the pain will be aggravated by contraction of muscles which pull on the wound, e.g. deep breathing and coughing as far as both thoracotomy and abdominal wounds are concerned, and any involuntary muscle spasm across operated joints. In the abdomen transverse and oblique incisions such as subcostal ones have a better reputation than vertical wounds with respect to postoperative comfort.

Analgesic drugs

In nearly every instance some form of analgesic agent is indicated in the immediate postoperative period, and in the case of major procedures in the chest, abdomen, bones or joints one of the potent narcotics is usually preferred. Doses required vary from patient to patient, but the main objective should be to give sufficient to control the pain to an acceptable level. It is well known that from the theoretical point of view these drugs may depress respiration and carry a risk of addiction. However, severe pain is a powerful stimulant to respiration and in previously fit patients who are in great postoperative pain there is little fear of significantly impairing respiration by increasing the amount in order to give satisfactory pain relief. Likewise the chance of such a patient becoming addicted as a result of a few days of necessary medication with these agents is remote. Such considerations should not interfere with the decision to prescribe an adequate dosage of potent analgesia when it is required in the early postoperative period. The most commonly used drugs in this category are morphine, papaveretum (Omnopon), and pethidine. Others which find more occasional use and in general are less satisfactory are diamorphine, methadone, pentazocine, dihydrocodeine and buprenorphine. The latter has the advantage of being suitable for sublingual administration, thus avoiding the discomfort of injection; but the level of analgesia obtained by this sublingual route, although prolonged, is not usually as adequate for postoperative relief as the morphine group or pethidine.

Most patients after major surgery will get good relief from 10 mg morphine intramuscularly. The effect should start to be appreciated within 5–10 min, reach a peak at about 1–2 h and last for 4–6 h. Dosage may be repeated every 3–4 h as long as severe pain is likely. Morphine can also be given intravenously if urgent control is needed: 3–4 mg is diluted in 5 ml physiological saline and the injection is given slowly over 3–5 min. Alternatively 2–3 mg/h can be administered by constant-rate i.v. infusion. However, this requires close expert supervision and is not normally recommended; indeed it is rarely necessary.

An equivalent dose of papaveretum (Omnopon) is 10–15 mg. Although theoretically it has no advantages over morphine, many clinicians seem to prefer it. Pethidine is in general less effective and shorter-acting than morphine, but an intramuscular dose of 100 mg can provide good analgesia after procedures of moderate severity.

When the severity of the pain has lessened, or for relief of the lesser degrees of postoperative pain usually encountered after more superficial procedures, one or other of the milder analgesics may suffice and the oral route is preferred, as long as the patient is permitted to swallow and there is no vomiting. In this clinical situation drugs such as paracetamol, codeine phosphate, pentazocine, mefenamic acid, or even an aspirin preparation (as long as there is no history of gastric disorders) may be useful.

Local analgesia

Several techniques can be employed to render the region of the wound anaesthetic and therefore reduce the amounts of analgesic drugs required, allowing the patient to move, contract the muscles, and in particular breathe deeply and cough more effectively. The procedures are usually undertaken by the anaesthetist before or after the operation (Fig. 3.3).

Regional nerve block. This involves injection of a long-acting local anaesthetic agent, e.g. Marcain, alongside the superficial nerves supplying the area around the incision. A good example of this approach is the intercostal block, in which several injections of a few millilitres of Marcain are made below each of the lower ribs. This can anaesthetize much of the abdominal skin and subcutaneous tissues.

Epidural anaesthesia. A sterile catheter is introduced through the skin of the back into the epidural space and left temporarily in situ. The local anaesthetic can then be introduced at intervals, as required. There is, of course, the slight

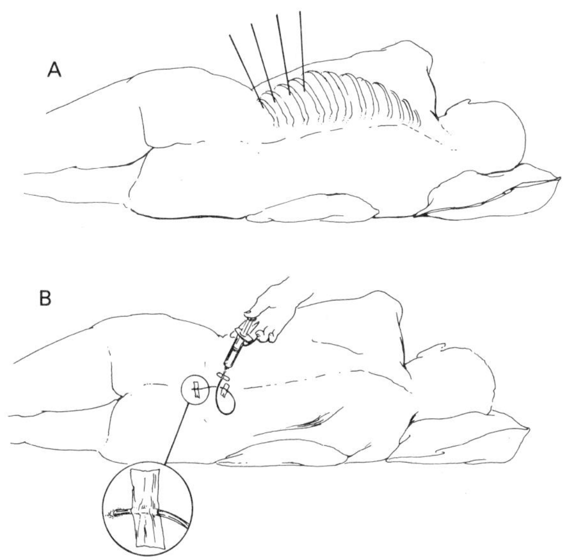

Fig. 3.3 Two ways of achieving regional local anaesthesia in the early postoperative period. (A) infiltration in the region of several subcostal nerves with a long-acting agent, e.g. Marcain, will render abdominal wounds in the affected segments anaesthetic. (B) Epidural anaesthesia—given through an indwelling plastic cannula, the tip of which lies in the epidural space—may be topped up with further small amounts of local anaesthetic as required postoperatively.

risk of introducing infection, as there is with any indwelling catheter. For perineal analgesia block of the cauda equina is often effective.

Care of the wound

Within 2 days a straightforward surgical wound will become completely sealed off from the exterior. The sterile dressing applied immediately at the end of the operation should be left completely undisturbed for at least that time and preferably till day 3 or 4. Any temptation to undo even a corner of the dressing before that should be resisted, as long as there is no leakage around or through it. Should this occur, it is best to remove the dressing with proper sterile conditions, inspect the wound, and if no further interference is necessary, apply a fresh sterile dressing. After 3–4 days the wound can either be left uncovered, or a simple sterile—preferably transparent—dressing applied to prevent irritation by clothes. Swelling beneath the wound may be due to a collection of blood or serous fluid, and if a drain is present this may not be working properly and may need adjustment in position and checking for patency. If there is no drain gentle pressure applied to either side of the wound may cause the fluid to escape through the wound edges. Failing this the removal of one of the sutures or staples may facilitate escape of the material. If necessary adhesive strips may be used to re-seal the wound.

The other main complications to be on the alert for are infection and dehiscence.

Wound infection

This arises because of contamination of the subcutaneous tissues at the time of operation, either from infected material released from a diseased organ or from organs such as the gastrointestinal tract in the patient, or from one of the theatre team. Symptoms of local pain, tenderness and general malaise, and signs such as swelling, redness and tenderness usually develop about the fourth or fifth day and are accompanied by an elevated body temperature. It is important to let any pus out and this is most often easily achieved by removal of one or more skin sutures and gentle parting of that part of the wound. As complete emptying of the material as possible is secured and a sample of the pus sent for culture and antibiotic sensitivity. The gap in the wound is left open to allow the free drainage of any further pus which may form, and an absorbent dressing or drainage bag is applied. As long as the pus has been adequately drained complete healing of the wound should then follow.

Wound dehiscence

This process, which implies separation of all the layers of the wound closure, may occur either as a sudden complete parting of the wound and prolapse of intra-abdominal contents—usually loops of small intestine—or as the sudden or gradual appearance of a swelling below the skin scar, stretching it. A warning sign is the almost invariable leak of a few millilitres of serous or serosanguinous liquid from a part of the skin wound. In both instances return to theatre, general anaesthetic

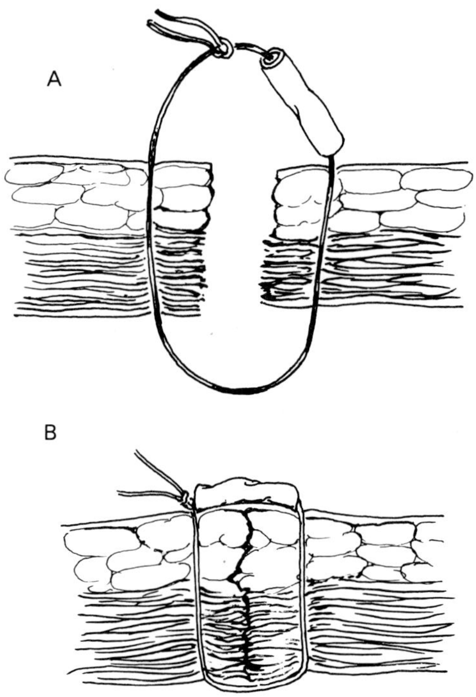

Fig. 3.4 Through-and-through suturing for dehiscence of an abdominal wound. (A) The strong, non-absorbable suture is passed through all layers from skin to peritoneum and out through corresponding layers on the other side. (B) Once the knot has been tied securely a sleeve of rubber or soft plastic minimizes the shearing effect of the suture on the skin.

and re-repair of the entire wound is required. As an emergency measure a pad of sterile packs is applied to any prolapsed organs and a binder wrapped around the abdomen. The second suture is performed with strong non-absorbable stitches passed through all layers from skin to peritoneum, and the reverse on the other side (Fig. 3.4). With such a series of large-bite, evenly spaced deep sutures it is rare for any recurrence of the dehiscence, although there may arise the possibility of an incisional hernia in later months or years.

Suture removal

There is no hard-and-fast rule about when the skin stitches or clips should be removed, but it stands to reason that this should not be until there is good evidence on simple inspection that the edges are closed by new epithelium. Wounds on the face, head and neck, and the hands heal rapidly and it is conventional to remove skin sutures in 4–5 days. The sooner they are removed, the less likely there will be permanent cross-hatch scarring. Abdominal wound stitches need to be left slightly longer, on average around 8–9 days. Wounds on the back of the trunk and in the anterior aspect of the calf take even longer—leaving skin sutures in place for up to 14 days is not unreasonable.

In view of the chances of cross-hatching scars which may persist at the site of the stitches if these are left too long, and the unsightliness this may cause, there has recently been an increasing tendency for some surgeons to remove skin sutures after 3–4 days and replace them with sterile adhesive strips laid across the wound to hold the skin edges in apposition.

Management of drains

Drainage of the operation site is employed either to allow pus to escape from an abscess cavity to prevent the accumulation of fluid, e.g. blood or bile, which might leak after the procedure, or because there is a risk of leakage from an anastomosis or closure of some part of the alimentary tract. It is also virtually routine to drain the pleural cavity after thoracotomy to ensure complete evacuation of any air or blood.

It is always preferable to bring the drain out through a stab wound separate from the main incision. Since the presence of any foreign material, even a tube or other type of drain which has been sterilized and inserted under completely aseptic conditions, leads to the risk of infection along the track, it is desirable also to remove the drain as soon as possible after the risk of further drainage is past. There are, of course, many different types of drain, ranging from simple strips of plain or corrugated rubber or plastic, straight tubes, to closed suction systems (Figs. 3.5 and 3.6). Advantages of the latter are that any fluid is sucked out immediately without the opportunity to accumulate, and there is less risk of infection because of the suction. Another type of drainage is a sump system, which is particularly useful for large intracavitary collections of pus where there might also be the risk of blockage by pieces of particulate matter. In this drain there is a continuous flow of air down through the several holes at the inner end of the tube, being applied on suction to the exterior end. A further alternative is to irrigate a deep abscess cavity at repeated intervals through an indwelling catheter.

While a drain is in place it is important to inspect it several times a day to ensure that it is draining satisfactorily and that it has not changed its position, slipped out or in, or become kinked or otherwise blocked. Some method of fixation is always used to minimize the chances of dislocation, e.g. fixing directly to the skin with one or more stitches plus taping, and in the case of non-tube drains, transfixing with a large safety-pin. These measures are important to avoid the drain dropping out, or, even more seriously, slipping inside the

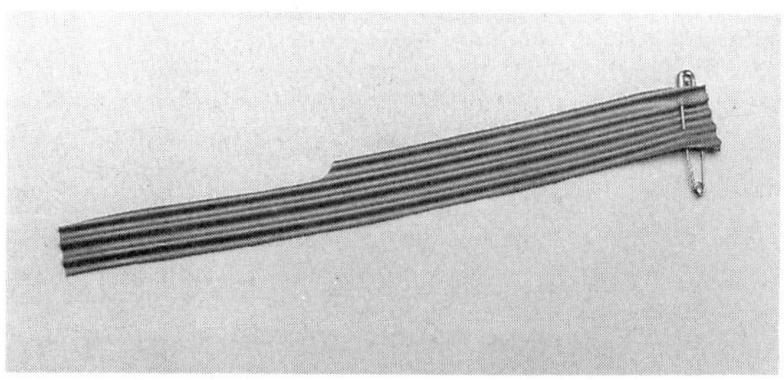

Fig. 3.5 A simple corrugated rubber drain which can be cut to any width and length. A safety-pin is usually attached to its outer end to avoid accidental displacement below the wound surface. Any discharge may flow into either an overlying absorbent dressing or an adhesive collecting bag.

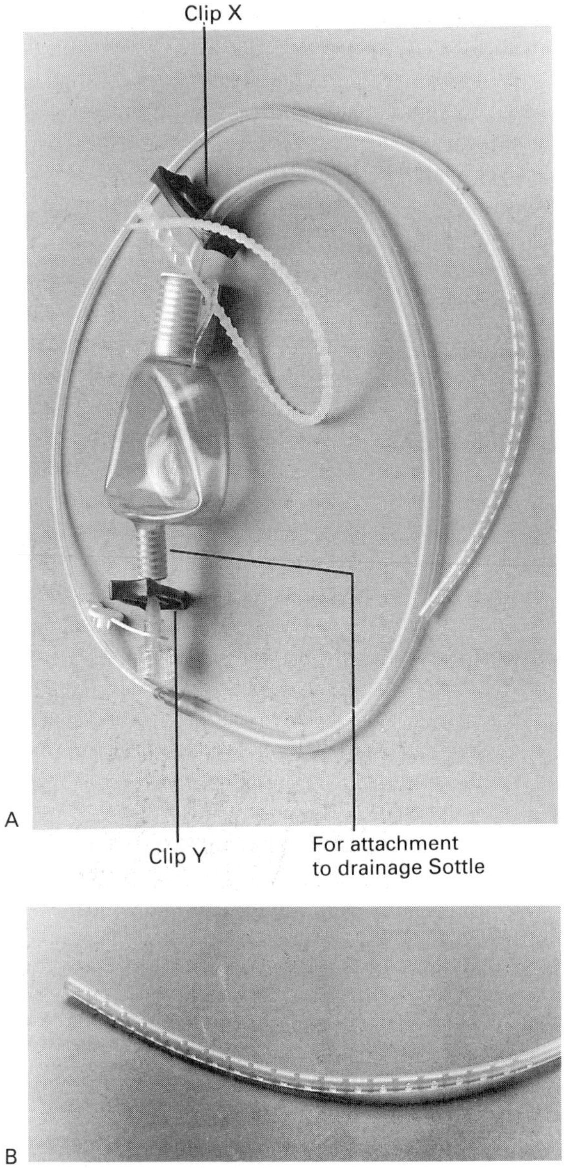

Fig. 3.6 Closed suction drain. (**A**) There are many types; in this simple model, suction is achieved by manual compression of the clear plastic bulb. With the inner multi-perforated end of the tube entirely within the cavity to be drained and an intact segment emerging from a tight, close-fitting stab wound, clip X is closed and Y opened. After compression of the hand-bulb, clip Y is then closed and hand pressure released, thus causing a vacuum in the bulb. Clip X can now be opened to effect suction from the wound end of the tube. As the bag fills up with drained liquid, and the suction lessens, this manoeuvre can be repeated as often as necessary. The outer end of the tube, beyond clip Y, is usually attached to a larger collecting bottle, so that accurate measurement of drainage loss can be made. (**B**) Close-up view of inner multi-perforated end of the tube. This can be shortened by cutting off any unnecessary length of tubing.

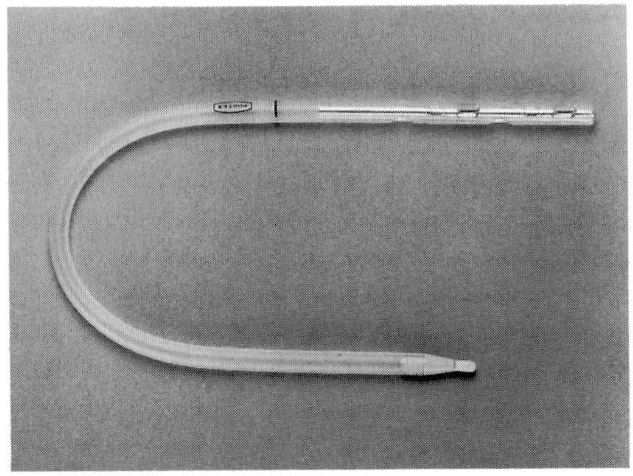

Fig. 3.7 A commonly used pattern of intercostal chest drain. The removable cone-shaped nozzle helps the passage through a very small stab wound in the chosen intercostal space, from the pleural space through to skin surface. This ensures an air-tight snug fit around the tube. The emerging segment is secured to the skin by sutures.

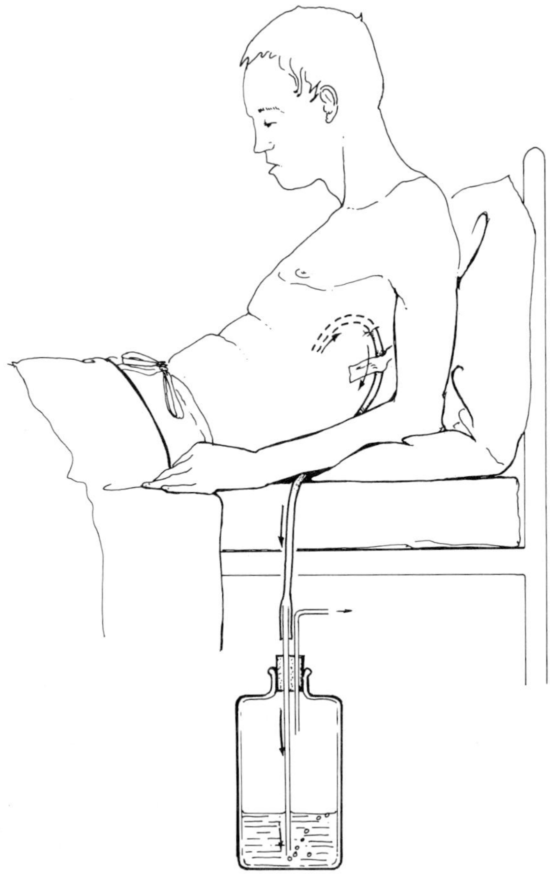

Fig. 3.8 Diagram showing the proper manner of attaching the chest drain to an underwater seal-bottle—see text.

body, and thereby necessitating an exploration to retrieve it.

When it is necessary to redress or handle the drain in any way full sterile precautions are required, and interference should be kept to a minimum. If the amount of discharge is only a few millilitres a simple absorbent-pad dressing is adequate over the drain, but if a greater amount is expected it is better, and easier for nursing, if a plastic adherent drainage bag is applied snugly around the emerging end of the drain. When the drain is finally removed a simple occlusive dressing is applied and sound closure of the small wound can be expected within 1–2 days.

The special points to note in looking after a patient with a chest drain are to ensure at all times that there is no leakage in the tubes leading to the underwater seal-bottle (Fig. 3.7); that the bottle itself is at no time raised up to or above chest level (Fig. 3.8), and that the fluid level within the tube entering the water in the bottle swings up and down freely with each respiratory excursion. The tube emerging from the chest wall must be clamped with a strong forceps when the drainage bottle is being changed, or when any sign of leakage is detected in the system.

Gastric aspiration tubes

Nasogastric tubes are inserted when it is anticipated that there will be delay in gastric emptying after the operation. They are used almost routinely after operations on the oesophagus or stomach, and in major intra-abdominal procedures in which there has been much handling and exposure of the intestine, and therefore a high likelihood of paralytic ileus. Furthermore, if the level of consciousness is likely to be depressed it is often wise to keep the stomach empty and avoid the risk of vomiting, regurgitation and aspiration into the respiratory passages. Since nasogastric tubes cause discomfort to the patient it is unnecessary to insert one for straightforward abdominal procedures, e.g. cholecystectomy or right hemicolectomy, in otherwise fit patients, and if one is used it is desirable to have it removed as soon as the risk of stasis or vomiting has passed. The usual guides to removal are the return of normal sounds on auscultation of the abdomen, and the passage of flatus per rectum.

It is generally sufficient to attach the outer end of the nasogastric tube to a plastic drainage bag by a closed connection, but if there is gross gastric retention or gravity drainage is not fully effective, continuous low-power suction may be applied by means of an electric pump, e.g. a Roberts pump (Fig. 3.9). If drainage ceases abruptly the inner holes in the tube will probably have become blocked either by particulate matter in the stomach or by the gastric mucosa, and it is wise to check the patency and clear any blockage by squeezing a small volume of air down the tube intermittently by means of a hand syringe.

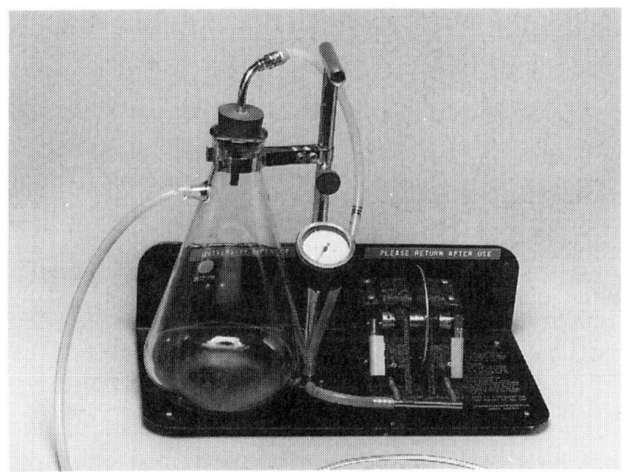

Fig. 3.9 Roberts-type pump for continuous gastric aspiration. The nasogastric tube is connected to the tubing at the left, leading into a large collecting flask. Motorized suction can be regulated and maintained at differing levels by a simple valve.

Chest problems

After operations on either the chest or abdomen several factors may be responsible for impaired efficiency of breathing. First, the general anaesthetic will have suppressed ciliary action in the tracheobronchial tree, and may have made the mucus drier and stickier. Second, the pain in the wound makes the patient reluctant to take any but the smallest of breaths or to cough. Third, potent analgesics, e.g. narcotics, may depress respiration. All of these factors will be of even greater importance in smokers and in those with a previous history of bronchitis, asthma, or other chronic airways disease. The elderly and grossly overweight are also particularly vulnerable to postoperative chest disorders.

The two main complications to arise in this postoperative period are collapse of a segment, lobe, or entire lung, and infection. The latter frequently follows the former.

A number of prophylactic measures to prevent either or both of these complications arising should be part of the routine postoperative nursing care. It is important to ensure that wound pain is adequately controlled, particularly after chest or abdominal exploration, and the patient should be gently but firmly encouraged to take repeated deep breaths and to cough so that any mucus and secretion are expelled. At first reassurance is required that, far from doing any harm to the wounds, these efforts will aid recovery, and it is comforting and helpful if the patient's or attendant's hands lightly support the wound during these actions. If the patient has had practice at what is required, preferably under the guidance of the physiotherapist who will be responsible for postoperative supervision, this often helps. Repeated changes in position in the bed are desirable, and if any degree of collapse is suspected the affected side should be placed uppermost to encourage better expansion. In those with an increased risk of collapse or infection, epidural or regional nerve-block local anaesthesia can be particularly useful in encouraging the patient to co-operate with these moving, breathing and coughing activities. Several simple incentive respirometers are available and may be used to assist in achieving deep enough breathing efforts, but these are not essential, and probably more important are the confident, persuasive and expert attentions of the physiotherapist and other ward attendants.

A further factor which can increase the risk of chest infection and aggravate any existing respiratory problems is pulmonary oedema resulting from excess i.v. fluid administration. This is a particular hazard in the elderly, and great care should always be taken to monitor closely the rate of i.v. fluids and to avoid overload.

Collapse

The warning signs are rapid breathing, tachycardia, some degree of cyanosis, an area of dullness to percussion and decreased breath sounds. X-ray of the chest, if available, will show an area of increased density. Blood–gas analysis reveals a reduction in partial pressure of arterial oxygen.

In the most severe condition where an entire lung is collapsed due to blockage of a main bronchus, the signs and symptoms are dramatic and extreme, with severe breathlessness, dullness and absent sounds in the hemi-thorax and mediastinal shift.

When any degree of collapse has occurred it is a matter of some urgency to dispel the occluding mucus and re-inflate the lung or portion of it. At first irritation of the upper trachea or forcible sudden compression of the chest may be sufficient to shift quite impressive plugs of inspissated secretion. If, however, the various simple manoeuvres are not successful it is necessary to carry out bronchoscopy to identify and suck out the blocking material. It is usual also to give antibiotic cover under these circumstances.

Infection

As already stated, infection most often supervenes in an area of collapsed lung, and the risk of frank pneumonia is increased when there is a history of prior chronic or recurrent infection. Most often it is bronchopneumonia, but particularly when a whole lobe is collapsed lobar pneumonia may arise.

The clinical picture is usually that of pulmonary collapse, described above, plus pyrexia, productive sputum, moist sounds in the chest, and perhaps areas of bronchial breathing. X-ray will show patchy areas of consolidation (Fig. 3.10), or in the case of lobar pneumonia, a uniformly dense lobar shadow and usually an accompanying pleural effusion.

Treatment of postoperative lung infection demands antibiotics in adequate dosage, and continuation of the various measures to counteract collapse. A sample of sputum should be obtained as soon as possible and sent for culture and antibiotic sensitivity. In the meanwhile, ampicillin or cefuroxime can be started and any alteration in the choice of antibiotic can be considered if appropriate when the sensitivity results are known. If, in spite of all efforts to achieve satisfactory ventilation, blood–gases show a persistent hypoxia,

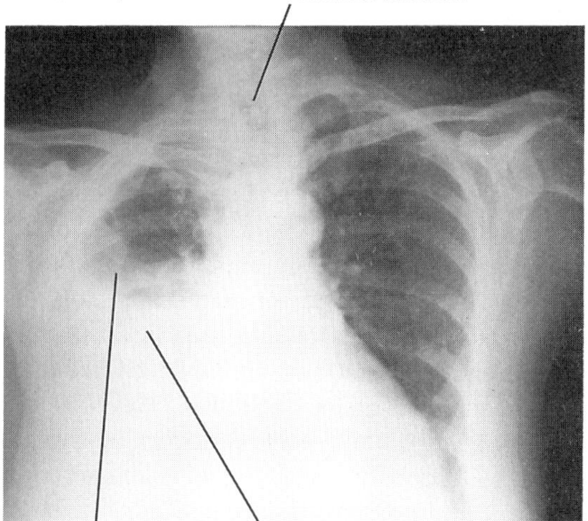

Fig. 3.10 Postoperative chest X-ray showing consolidation of the lower part of the right lung, plus a large pleural effusion. There is slight deviation of the tracheal shadow towards the right, indicating some degree of collapse.

oxygen should be given by facemask and in the most severely affected, mechanical assistance to ventilation may be needed in the intensive care unit.

Fluid and electrolyte management

Most patients having straightforward operations not involving the gastrointestinal tract will be able to resume oral intake of small amounts of water and rapidly return to free fluid intake after about 5 or 6 h and will not require i.v. fluid replacement. However, for those having upper gastrointestinal procedures and when a degree of ileus is expected, intravenous fluids will be required for several days, or at least until there is evidence of return of gut function.

When an infusion is set up full sterile precautions must be used, and any subsequent manipulation after return to the ward also demands an aseptic technique. The giving set should be checked repeatedly to ensure that it is delivering the correct solution at the correct rate, that there is no chance of air entering the vein, and that there is no inflammatory reaction in the skin around the site of entry of the cannula. If a reaction does appear the set should be removed and culture taken of the end of the cannula; if the need for i.v. replacement persists a fresh infusion should be set up under full sterile conditions in another vein, preferably in the other arm.

With regard to the volume and nature of the solutions to be infused, these are discussed more fully in Chapter 7. The objectives are to replace the daily requirements for insensible skin loss plus obligatory urine output; any loss from drains, and gastric aspiration; increased losses if fever is present, or from burns; amounts to balance any pooling of secretions, or sequestration of fluid in oedema or tissue spaces.

The basic daily requirement for a normal-weight, previously healthy adult in a temperate climate is approximately 1500–2500 ml. If it is decided to give a baseline of 2000 ml then it is convenient to make this up of 1500 ml of 5% dextrose and 500 ml of 0.9% saline. To this basic calculation an equal volume of 0.9% saline can be added in respect of loss from drains, tissue fluid, secretions, and burns, as well as an extra allowance of 250 ml 0.9% saline for each 1°C increase in temperature above normal. Theoretically a more balanced physiological solution, e.g. Hartman's, may be preferred to 0.9% saline, but the latter is simpler, cheaper and more readily available and in the vast majority of cases quite satisfactory.

When the i.v. infusion is required for only up to 48 h it will not be necessary to consider giving any added potassium, and indeed since some potassium will be released as a result of the operative trauma, further added ions might be hazardous. It is also unlikely that measurement of the serum electrolyte concentrations will be necessary. However, if more prolonged i.v. administration is needed daily measurements of all fluid intake and output and of serum electrolytes will be required and the question of potassium, other ions and calories will have to be considered.

Urinary problems

Retention of urine

This is a fairly common difficulty immediately postoperatively, particularly after operations in the perineum or pelvis, and in these situations there is nervous reflex inhibition of voiding. Urine retention is also more likely to occur in elderly men who already have a degree of prostatic obstruction to the bladder outflow. The patient should be encouraged to pass water as soon as practicable after operation and once the first voiding has been achieved there is rarely any subsequent difficulty. A quiet, warm, private environment and being allowed to assume a semi-erect position may help to overcome the initial inhibition. Should all simple nursing efforts fail then it will be necessary to introduce a catheter, empty the bladder, and as long as there was not in excess of 1000 ml present, remove the catheter. If the volume exceeds that level it is better to leave an indwelling catheter for continuous drainage and subsequent investigation into the cause of retention.

In a patient who remains unconscious for several hours, restlessness may be due to the discomfort of a full bladder, and catheterization may relieve this completely.

Infection

This may arise in either the upper or lower urinary tract as a postoperative complication, particularly if there has been previous instrumentation, retention, or known infection. Lower tract infection is usually indicated by frequency and dysuria, but upper tract involvement may not be so obvious clinically, and may present mainly as a postoperative pyrexia. Urine culture and sensitivity are taken and appropriate antibiotic treatment given. It is also important to ensure that an adequate urine output is maintained, by full replacement of any fluid deficit.

Renal failure

The main guide to the adequacy of renal function is the volume of urine output, and where there is reason to suspect any degree of renal failure it is desirable to monitor the output each hour. This implies bladder catheterization and continuous collection of the urine in one of the commercially available graduated collection bags. After any major operation there is a reduction in urine production, but a minimum rate of 40 ml/h should be expected, and less than 25 ml/h is frank oliguria.

The commonest reasons for oliguria after operations are periods of hypotension leading to underperfusion of the kidneys, and sepsis. There is also a greater risk in those with previous renal disease and in jaundiced patients.

Knowledge of the specific gravity of the urine is the next most useful guide. If this is high (>1.010), kidney function is reasonable and measures to ensure adequate fluid replacement, maintenance of normal blood pressure and treatment of any sepsis are almost certainly enough to allow good recovery of function. If, on the other hand, the specific gravity is <1.010 and the oliguria persists then frusemide, 20–40 mg should be given i.v. and if only a small response is obtained this dose may be repeated. If no diuresis is forthcoming then the patient will probably have to be managed along the lines of acute renal failure and considered for some form of dialysis.

Thromboembolism

Thrombosis in a segment of the deep veins draining the leg is one of the most serious of postoperative complications because of the risk of a portion of loose clot becoming dislodged, released into the main venous return to the heart, and then in turn causing a pulmonary artery embolism. Fortunately, while postoperative thrombosis is quite common in small veins in the calf, as has been shown by several surveys, only a very small number give rise to life-threatening pulmonary infarction. However, it is wise to take as many precautions as feasible against deep vein thrombosis (DVT). Keeping patients mobile and active right up until the time of immediate preparation for operation; avoidance of any pressure on the muscles of the leg before, during or after the procedure; early active exercises of the legs as soon as the patient recovers from the anaesthetic; early ambulation; the use of graduated compression elastic stockings during operation or mechanically pumping stockings are all measures which can contribute to protection against DVT.

Certain groups of patients are more prone than others to the complications, e.g. the elderly, those with malignant disease, those having hip operations, and those with a previous history of venous disorders. DVT is more likely to follow abdominal pelvic surgery than procedures on the limb or head and neck. There also appears to be an increased risk in women taking a contraceptive pill. In these high-risk groups most surgeons would, in addition to the precautions mentioned above, give small doses of heparin (preferably calcium heparin 5000 u 8–12–hourly, from the time of the premedication till 2–5 days after operation).

While most agree on the use of this form of anticoagulation in the high-risk groups, some surgeons advocate much wider use of prophylactic heparin. There is also some evidence of low molecular weight dextran having a protective effect, though this has not proved so popular.

Whether or not such prophylactic measures have been employed, all patients recovering from operation should be watched for any sign which may suggest the presence of DVT. Warning pointers are any otherwise unexplained increase in temperature, the complaint of pain, even slight, in the calf, or the appearance of any oedematous swelling in the foot or ankle. This latter may be slight, and detectable only in one or more of the web-spaces between the toes. Tenderness in one or more areas of the calf muscles is a highly suggestive sign.

Sometimes the DVT is completely silent, i.e. causes no symptoms or signs, and the first indication of its occurrence is a pulmonary embolus. Indeed, it is a general clinical observation that the most dangerous emboli, which lead to sudden death, are often unheralded by any previous symptoms or signs in the legs or elsewhere.

When the clinical diagnosis of DVT is made it is desirable to confirm the suspicion and locate more precisely the level and extent of thrombosis by ascending venography. The patient is then fully anticoagulinated first with heparin and after 5–7 days transferred on to an oral anticoagulant which will be continued for some months at least.

The more proximal the thrombosis occurs, the greater the risk of fatal embolism and consideration should be given to the insertion of a vena cava filter if it is felt that the risk of dislodged clot is high.

Pulmonary embolism, if small, presents with localized chest pain, often pleuritic in nature, and haemoptysis, which can range from a mild pink tinge of otherwise clear sputum to coughing up frank blood and little else. If large, it causes shock, severe unremitting chest pain, distress and cyanosis. If not rapidly fatal there may very occasionally be the opportunity to remove the occluding embolus surgically under cardiopulmonary bypass.

Postoperative pyrexia

Several causes of a postoperative rise in temperature have already been mentioned. However, since the elevated temperature is often the initial clue to an underlying complication, it may be helpful to summarize the main likely causes of the pyrexia. First, it should be noted that some slight fever is almost invariable after any surgical trauma, and in the majority of patients is of no serious significance. The timing of the pyrexia in relation to the operation is in itself an important guide to the likely cause.

Within the first 48 h a rise in temperature is nearly always due to lung collapse or infection. Beyond the second postoperative day chest causes are less probable and the possibility of urinary tract infection, catheter-related problems or superficial phlebitis of i.v. infusion source should be considered. When it comes to 5–7 days after the operation, infections in the wound or deep inside the operated body cavity become greater likelihoods, and the appropriate physical signs should be sought and investigations arranged. A steadily climbing temperature at this stage often denotes the presence of a deep-seated abscess which will need prompt drainage.

As already noted a rise in temperature—usually a sudden spike—occurring 5–7 days after operation may be the only clue to the presence of a DVT.

Pyrexia arising after the first 7–10 days is rarely a direct consequence of the operative procedure itself, although local abscesses may appear at this stage, especially if the initial inflammatory response had been partially suppressed by antibiotics to which the organisms may not have been completely sensitive.

Psychiatric complications

Although minor emotional or behaviour upset may not uncommonly arise after the physical, metabolic and emotional trauma of an operation, and is usually amenable to reassurance and patient, confident nursing and surgical care, more severe disturbances do occur in a small percentage of cases. Rarely are features apparent in the first 24 h after the operation; they are more likely to be manifest after the second or third day.

Such problems are more likely to be encountered in those with a previous history of psychological problems, in the elderly and those with atherosclerotic impairment of cerebral blood flow, in those having thoracotomy and in particular cardiac operations. Some anaesthetic agents and drugs used for other medical problems or postoperative complications may cause psychotic symptoms, e.g. corticosteroids. Metabolic upsets may also be responsible for changes in affect, and serum electrolytes and blood–gas values should be checked when a psychosis presents otherwise unaccountably in the postoperative period. The presence of deep-seated sepsis can also lead to mental aberration and this possibility should be kept in mind.

Not surprisingly, the intensely active, totally dependent unnatural environment of an intensive care unit, with its mechanical noise, sleep deprivation and multiple tubes and monitoring wires, can induce considerable mental stresses in patients. Disorientation, confusion, restlessness and sensations of unreality are all fairly common. Needless to say, any means of securing peace, adequate sleep, protection against disturbing noise and return to normal ward-care are all desirable to minimize the incidence of these distressing symptoms.

In those addicted to alcohol or narcotic drugs there is a considerable risk of quite dramatic psychiatric disorders appearing after an operation. If those taking care of the patient are aware of this addiction beforehand then they are on the lookout for the problems, but all too often the abuse of either alcohol or drugs has been skilfully kept from the medical and nursing attendants, and indeed often from closest relatives and friends. The appearance of the symptoms after an operation, when for the first time the patient has no access to the material on which he or she has become dependent, may be the first clue to the addiction.

Warning signs may be undue agitation and anxiety and tremors, but these may soon be superseded by wild frantic overactivity, hallucinations, confusion and sometimes fits. It may become difficult to keep any drains, drips or other tubes in place and the patient may pull out stitches, dehisce the wound and in other ways commit self-injury, as well as cause great disturbance to other patients. Attempts at physical restraint may serve only to aggravate the condition and lead to even more violent struggling.

Usually the advice and help of a psychiatrist will be required to deal with both the immediate and long-term problems of the addiction. One temporarily expedient approach is to administer small doses of the drug of addiction and defer the withdrawal therapy until the patient is well recovered from the operation. There is, however, a high chance that as soon as he or she is restored to satisfactory physical health he or she will abscond, to succumb once more to the addiction.

On occasions there is no alternative but to give some form of sedation to calm the patient down during an outburst of these postoperative acute withdrawal symptoms, but care needs to be exercised that respiration is not depressed or hypotension induced. Diazepam or chlordiazepoxide are probably the sedatives of choice for this particular purpose. Dosage may have to be repeated several times over a period of 2–3 days, after which hopefully the worst symptoms will have settled down. In extreme cases the old-fashioned paraldehyde may be given by deep intramuscular injection.

INDICATIONS FOR ADMISSION TO INTENSIVE CARE UNIT

It is sensible to make advance arrangements to admit directly after operation to the intensive care unit those patients undergoing major surgical procedures known to have a risk of vital organ failure. It is also helpful to explain fully to the patient what he or she should expect to find on recovering from the anaesthetic in this particular environment, and a brief visit to the unit before operation is a good idea.

The main reasons for transferring a postoperative patient to the intensive care unit are the need for:

1. Continuous monitoring of cardiac and respiratory function and fluid balance.
2. Support of ventilation by any mechanical means.
3. Management of shock—various causes.
4. Management of severe sepsis.
5. Management of complicated metabolic and biochemical derangements.

4. Wound healing

Healing is a complicated series of physiological events involving cellular and biochemical changes, which lead to the re-establishment of continuity of the tissues after disruption. It is, in many respects, a continuation of the phenomenon of inflammation, and the two are so intermixed that it is very difficult to say where one ends and the other begins.

The essentials of the healing process are similar in all wounds, no matter how and where produced — whether it is a clean surgical incision, a surface wound caused by trauma, a wound in the heart caused by myocardial infarction, or healing of an abscess after the evacuation of pus.

The basic process can best be understood by first considering the healing of a clean surgical wound by first or primary intention. In contradistinction to this, healing by secondary intention is said to occur when the wound margins are wide apart with the loss of intervening tissue.

HEALING OF CLEAN INCISED WOUNDS BY FIRST (PRIMARY) INTENTION

Coagulum formation

Blood shed during an incision clots after the active bleeding stops. A clot is a network of fibrin which contains in its meshes the formed elements of blood, i.e. red and white blood corpuscles. At the same time plasma leaks from the capillaries of the wound margins and floor, and together with the clotted blood, forms a coagulum. This coagulum serves as a scaffold on which further repair takes place. As repair proceeds, the cell debris and other elements of the coagulum are gradually removed by macrophages and leukocytes which act as tissue scavengers (Fig. 4.1). This step is important to prepare the way for the further stages of healing.

Simultaneously, 'H'-like substances are released from the wound margins and a mild inflammatory reaction sets in.

Collagen formation

At the end of the first 24 h, specialized cells called fibroblasts can be recognized in the wound margins. These cells originate from the perivascular areolar tissue, and begin to advance towards the coagulum from the edges, secreting the polypeptide collagen.

The collagen molecule, as seen on electron microscopy, is shaped like a needle, 2800–3000 A in length, 14–15 A in diameter, with a molecular weight of about 300 000–340 000. Many molecules aggregate to form fibrils which exhibit transverse bands at regular intervals of about 640 A. Collagen is argentophil, i.e. it stains black with silver salts.

Collagen fibres at first appear to be laid down in a haphazard manner, but soon they come to lie, by rearrangement, in the line of stress, i.e. perpendicular to the wound margins in an incised wound, thereby binding the edges together.

Collagen formation is a complicated organic process in which, while new fibres are being laid down, older ones continue to be destroyed under the influence of enzymes such as collagenase and protease. The final scar is the result of the forces of remoulding and maturation.

Capillary budding

Coincident with the commencement of fibroblastic activity, the endothelial cells of nearby capillar-

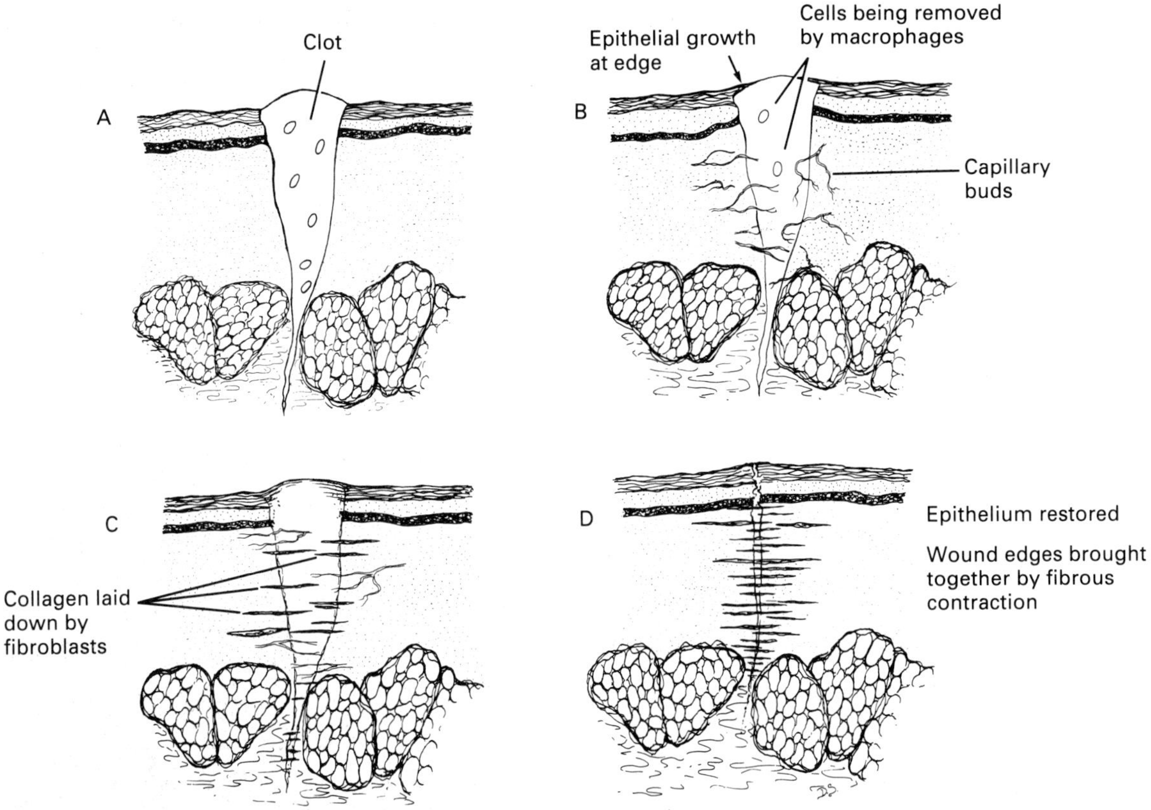

Fig. 4.1 Diagrammatic representation of stages in healing of a clearly incised wound affecting skin and subcutaneous tissues.

ies also become active. These cells sprout out from the vessels nearest the wound margins. Some are derived from the mitotic division of the cells of the capillaries themselves, while others develop from the endothelial lining of larger vessels in the immediate neighbourhood. The solid buds soon become canalized, forming small capillaries which grow into the coagulum, intercommunicating to create a capillary network.

The lymph capillaries also proliferate in a similar way, and at the same rate. The two sets of capillaries, however, do not intercommunicate.

The coagulum, fibroblasts, collagen fibres, and blood and lymph capillary networks are collectively known as granulation tissue. The formation of granulation tissue is fundamental to the healing of all types of wounds in all organs of the body. In closed clean incised wounds the amount of granulation tissue is minimal, and so is the resulting scar.

Wound contraction

While these changes are occurring in the wound, the wound margins contract from all sides and where there is an open wound with loss of surface it is as if a picture frame was getting smaller. It is thought that this contraction occurs due to the contraction activity of specialized cells, called myofibroblasts, in the wound margins. These cells have properties of both fibroblast and smooth muscle cells. Contraction is adversely affected by irradiation and cortisone.

Epithelialization

As the granulation tissue is being formed, epithelium from the wound margins starts to grow, the first evidence of this cellular activity being evident within the first few hours of injury. Cells at or near the wound margins begin to advance towards the coagulum. The cells at the margins show evidence of mitosis, but not the advancing layer of cells covering the coagulum. The cells from the opposite sides meet, and thus a complete epithelial covering is provided over the granulation tissue. The pigmented and cornified layers of skin are absent from this new covering, as are hair follicles, sebaceous and sweat glands.

With the completion of epithelialization over the gap, the first stage of healing is complete.

In the second stage of healing, the young scar undergoes many changes. First, there is a gradual disappearance of cells from the newly formed scar. Some die and undergo autolysis while others actively migrate back into surrounding tissues or fluid from which they originated. Some fibroblasts persist as small fusiform cells, and the new epithelial cells, of course, remain. The capillaries lose their patency and the endothelial cells migrate back to the parent vessels. The vascularity decreases markedly, though some capillaries may persist. The colour of the newly formed scar tissue gradually changes from bright pink to white.

Secondly, the collagen fibres mature, become thicker and firmly bind the wound margins together. Vitamin C is essential for their maturation and wounds do not heal properly during prolonged deprivation of vitamin C. The tensile strength of the wound increases steadily. Once mature scar tissue is formed, there is very little metabolic activity in the scar.

The factor or factors which initiate the process of healing are still unknown, and we cannot enhance the rate of healing, even by a few hours. A number of factors, however, are known to delay the process of healing. These factors are both local and general.

LOCAL FACTORS

Lack of rest of the wounded part

Movement disrupts and disorganizes granulation tissue. Loss of function and pain restrict voluntary movement in the injured area. Adhesions developing around an injured organ also tend to limit movement. Securing adequate rest of the injured part of the body is a basic component of the treatment of wounds, and where the healing process is slow, e.g. in bony fractures, it is usually necessary to achieve complete immobilization, for example by application of a plaster cast.

Infection

This interferes with healing because bacterial toxins tend to destroy the granulation tissue (Fig. 4.2). It is one of the most important factors which may delay healing.

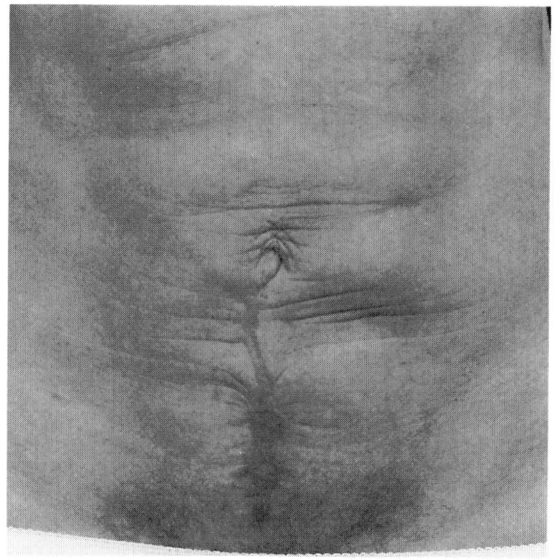

Fig. 4.2 Scar of lower abdominal surgical wound. The line of the wound is deviated and the scar is much broader in its lower half. Both deformities are due to a wound infection and drainage in the postoperative period.

Diminished vascularity

In the injured area reduced blood supply significantly slows down the healing process, as the oxygen and energy sources required for the formation of granulation tissue is lacking in avascular areas. For this reason, wounds in areas with a rich blood supply like the scalp and face heal more quickly than wounds of the trunk or sole of the feet, which are not so rich in blood supply. One way in which local ischaemia may be produced is by suturing under excessive tension.

Local oedema

Excess tissue fluid and any associated impairment of lymph drainage delay the healing process. As inflammation and repair are dynamic processes, requiring rapid turnover of fluids, any interference with the movement of fluid naturally affects the progression of the responses to injury.

Foreign bodies

These may be carriers of bacteria, and thus may delay wound healing indirectly by introducing and prolonging infection. In addition, the more irritant a foreign body is, the more severe and prolonged the resultant inflammation will be, and the more abnormal will be the granulation tissue formation. A large foreign body will, of course, form a physical barrier in the path of the developing granulation tissue. Dead or devitalized tissue, including that damaged by rough handling and retraction, acts as a foreign body, and delays the process of healing.

Clotted blood

Due to improper haemostasis, clotted blood may delay healing as it encourages infection and acts as a foreign body.

GENERAL FACTORS

Nutrition

Hypoproteinaemia, lack of vitamin C and deficiency of certain trace elements are important factors which can delay healing. As the formation of collagen and the multiplication of cells in the granulation tissue are dependent on the availability of sufficient protein, it is obvious that the healing process will be interfered with in conditions of gross hypoproteinaemia. Oedema sometimes results from gross hypoproteinaemia which is an additional factor delaying the process of healing.

As has been mentioned, vitamin C is essential for the maturation of collagen fibres. Ordinarily there is sufficient reserve of the vitamin in the body, so that a few days' deprivation does not interfere with healing. However, in conditions of prolonged deprivation, healing is impaired. Wound repair may also be delayed by deficiency of vitamin A, and of iron and copper. Shortage of zinc, especially in malnourished infants, may reduce the efficiency of some of the enzymes involved in the repair processes.

Metabolic disorders

Healing is impaired in certain metabolic and systemic disorders such as diabetes mellitus, jaundice and uraemia. However, there is no quantitative relationship between the severity of these diseases and the degree of impairment. In diabetes mellitus, probably a number of factors are responsible, such as deranged carbohydrate metabolism at the site of the wound, susceptibility to infection, and poor oxygen perfusion through narrowed blood vessels. In jaundice, fibroblastic activity is impaired, and in uraemia, granulation tissue formation and epithelialization are slow.

OTHER FACTORS

It is still debatable whether cortisol and chemotherapeutic agents given therapeutically delay healing by depressing the formation of new capillaries and the activities of the fibroblasts. However, it has been observed that if cortisol is administered in high doses in the early phases of healing there is some delay. Once the healing process is well established, however, cortisol has little deleterious effect.

Irradiation

As has been mentioned earlier, irradiation adversely affects the contraction activity of the myofibroblasts, and is a factor which may delay healing.

The above description is of the process of healing which occurs in superficial wounds without any significant loss of tissue. In many traumatic wounds, the process is often modified by a number of factors such as loss of tissue, suturing of the wounds and contamination with foreign materials like dust, bacteria, fragments of clothing and other objects.

HEALING OF OPEN WOUNDS AND WOUNDS WITH TISSUE LOSS

If there is loss of tissue, or if there is an area of devitalized tissue, as in deep burns or crush injury, or if a raw area is left after the incision of an abscess, or if a wound is deliberately left unsutured because it is contaminated, healing occurs by secondary intention. Though the essential elements of healing are the same as those in healing by primary intention, there are some differences.

Firstly, contraction of the wound plays an important part in healing by secondary intention, and is mainly responsible for the graded decrease in the size of the wound. In superficial wounds, the effects may be most noticeable in areas where the skin is mobile, e.g. the neck.

Secondly, the process of epithelialization assumes greater importance. As mentioned earlier, the new epidermis so formed in surface wounds is devoid of sweat and sebaceous glands and hair follicles, and is thin because of scanty keratinization. In a large wound epithelialization may not be complete, and in spite of wound contraction a persistent ulcer may be left which requires covering by a skin graft.

Thirdly, healing by secondary intention is likely to be complicated by infection.

Fourthly, the resultant scar formation is greater than in healing by primary intention and so the deformity and disfigurement are greater.

Operative wounds are closed with sutures or clips for a number of reasons. Firstly, the distance to be covered by the developing capillaries, fibroblasts and epithelium is minimized, and consequently the time needed for complete healing is reduced. Secondly, by bringing the edges together the raw surface is covered and the wound is protected from contamination by bacteria, dust and other harmful substances. Thirdly, suturing ensures haemostasis in the sutured edges and other raw areas.

Sutures act as a temporary support for the development of granulation tissue and the formation of a scar which permanently holds the sectioned parts together. Once the scar is formed, the sutures become superfluous and non-absorbable ones may act as irritant foreign bodies. Sutures should, therefore, be inserted with the clear understanding that it is really the tissues betweeen the sutures which heal, and care is necessary in the technique of suturing not to undermine this organic process. For example, too many sutures and suturing under tension may lead to local ischaemia, and thereby delay or interfere with the normal healing process.

These faults should, therefore, be avoided. In mobilizing wound edges prior to suture care should be taken to ensure adequacy of the blood supply of the mobilized parts.

In dealing with contaminated wounds, the basic policy is to convert a dirty wound into a clean one before suturing it. In practice it is often found that wounds, if attended to within a short period after infliction and if antibiotics are used, can be closed by loose sutures with a reasonable expectation of healing, provided this is done after thorough cleaning. Loose suturing provides spaces for the underlying serum or pus to escape without significant interference with the development of granulation tissue.

If the wound is grossly contaminated, it may be left open for a few days to allow the elimination of bacteria and particles by the outpouring of the plasma from the raw surfaces and the formation of clean granulation tissue. It is then closed by loose sutures. This is called delayed primary suturing.

However, if wounds are found to be too contaminated even for delayed primary suturing, they may be left open and allowed to heal entirely by second intention. Alternatively, the raw surface may be covered by a skin graft after clean granulations have formed in the depths of the wound. This converts an open wound into a closed one.

Sutured surgical wounds may be left without a covering dressing. Within minutes of suturing, the wound is covered by a seal of clotted plasma and blood which forms an effective barrier against bacteria and other foreign matter. Although wounds of the face and scalp are usually left without any dressing, incisions elsewhere in the body are conventionally covered with a sterile dry dressing for the comfort of the patient and for protection from trauma caused by friction against the clothes. The dressing is usually not disturbed till the time for suture removal. However, if there is evidence of infection as suggested by seepage through the dressing or local pain, or general signs and symptoms of infection, the dressing should be removed and the wound inspected so that appropriate measures can be taken.

Open wounds on the body surface are usually covered by a dressing to protect them from further trauma and contamination. In some centres, however, no dressing is applied to extensive burns, provided that a satisfactory coagulum has formed over the raw surface, acting as a dressing.

COMPLICATIONS OF HEALING

Complete healing implies the restoration of continuity of the tissue after disruption. Sometimes, however, this process itself causes problems from either a functional or a structural point of view.

Functionally, specialized cells do not regenerate, except those of the liver parenchyma and the epithelial layer of the skin. If the cells of the motor area of the cerebrum are destroyed as a result of injury or disease, the patient will be left with a permanent motor disorder. Similarly, healing in the heart after myocardial infarction is by scar tissue formation, and if the conducting mechanism of the heart muscle is damaged, arrhythmias may be produced.

Tubular organs like the oesophagus, intestine or ureter may become narrow at the site of healing due to strictures caused by the scar tissue.

When healing occurs, divided muscle is replaced by scar tissue, and if this becomes weakened or attenuated it may not be strong enough to keep the underlying organs in their normal place. As a result there may be the dramatic occurrence of wound dehiscence (burst abdomen) in the first few

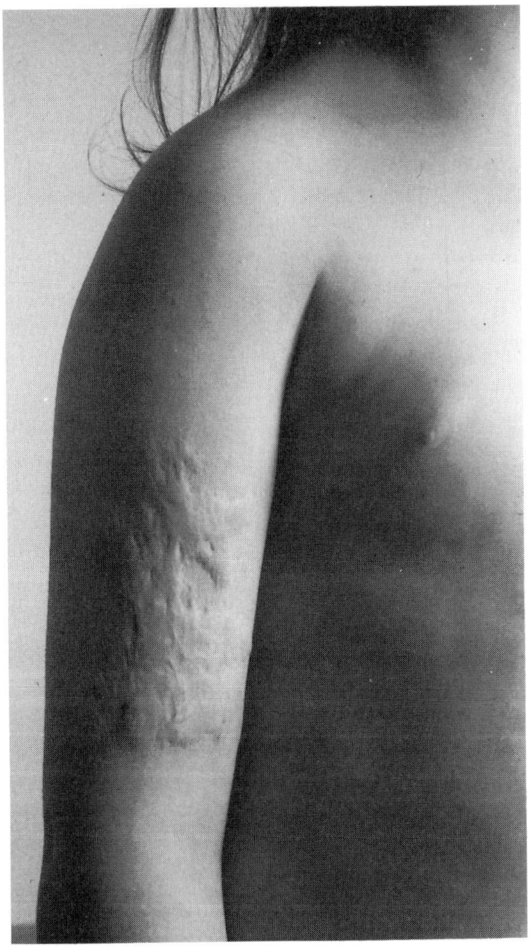

Fig. 4.3 Disfiguring keloid formation at the site of previous vaccinations.

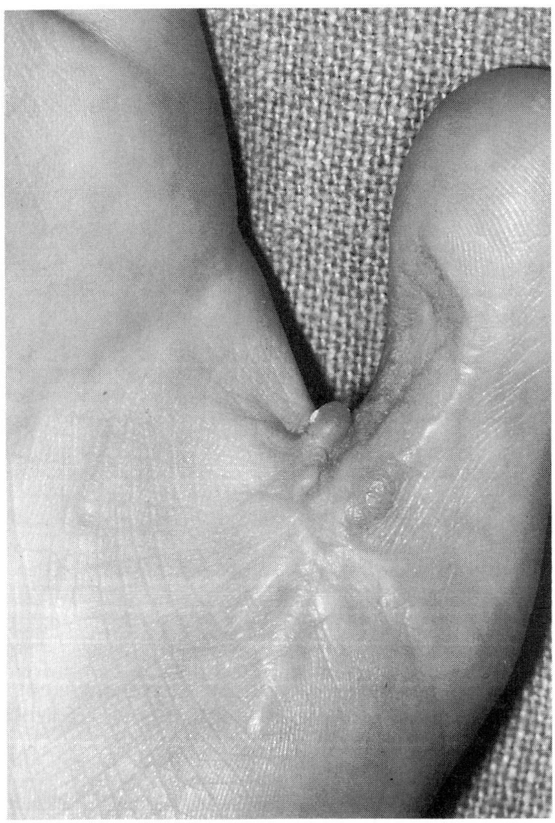

Fig. 4.4 Fibrous contracture across the base of the thumb from healing of a ragged laceration. The contracted scar limits abduction and extension of the thumb.

postoperative days after an abdominal operation, or the later development of an incisional hernia. Most often in such cases there has been further damage to the muscles of the abdominal wall due to infection.

Painful scar

A scar may become painful due to the compression of nerve endings by the surrounding scar tissues, as sometimes occurs in amputation stumps (stump neuroma).

Excessive scarring

The scar may become hypertrophic or it may turn into a keloid (Fig. 4.3) which is a claw-like exuberant projection of fibrous tissue projecting up from the surrounding skin surface. Very occasionally healing remains incomplete and a chronic ulcer develops at the site which may become malignant. This is called Marjolin's ulcer.

Deformities

Contraction of scars may produce ugly deformities, cosmetic disfigurement, and contractures which may limit movements of joints (Fig. 4.4). In managing wounds on the flexor aspects of the body, special care is taken to avoid these complications by proper splintage, resting the inflamed part and by early movements of the joints.

5. Inflammation

Inflammation is the local tissue response to trauma. The traumatic agent may be mechanical, thermal, radiation or chemical, including toxins liberated by infecting organisms.

The classical clinical features of inflammation are swelling, redness, heat, pain and disturbance in the function of the affected part. However, the signs of redness and of increase in temperature of the inflamed part will be found only if it lies near the skin.

In response to the noxious agent some cells are destroyed and others are stimulated to attest their activity. From the damaged and destroyed cells, chemicals including histamine, 5-hydroxytryptamine and kinins are released. These chemical agents act on the arterioles, venules and capillaries of the area causing vasodilatation. They may act not only on the blood vessels of the area directly, but also via axon reflexes, thereby increasing the overall vasodilator activity. As a result of this dual action, the quantity of blood reaching the area increases, and this partly explains the swelling, heat and redness.

As a result of dilatation the capillaries become permeable to plasma. Normally only water and electrolytes pass from the intravascular to the extravascular compartments and vice versa. The net movement depends on the interaction of opposite physical forces, namely hydrostatic and osmotic pressures working in a capillary (Fig. 5.1). At the arteriolar end fluid is forced out because the hydrostatic pressure here is about 32 mmHg, in comparison to the intravascular osmotic pressure of 25 mmHg. At the venous end, the hydrostatic pressure is only 12 mmHg so fluid tends to pass into the vessel at this end. In acute inflammation hydrostatic pressure rises at both the arterial and venous ends so the fluid tends to remain in the extravascular interstitial space.

Chemicals like histamine, serotonin, kinins and some globulin permeability factors liberated at the site of injury alter the permeability of the endothelial lining of the vessels in such a way that plasma proteins also escape into the interstitial spaces. The consequent rise in osmotic pressure outside the capillaries further helps in the escape of plasma into the interstitial spaces.

At the same time, there is some rearrangement of the formed elements of blood in the capillaries (Fig. 5.2). Normally the red and white cells remain in the centre of the lumen, surrounded by plasma. After injury, these cells, especially the white cells, come to lie close to the endothelium, and from here they may migrate into the interstitial space. It is thought that this migration of leukocytes is brought about by a chemical force exerted by the products of tissue damage. This is called chemotaxis.

Increased vascularity and the accumulation of plasma and leukocytes in the interstitial spaces explain the phenomenon of swelling, heat and redness at the site of injury. Pain is due partly to the pressure of extra fluid on sensory nerve endings, and partly to chemical irritation of these nerve endings by the products of tissue damage, especially histamine and 5-hydroxytryptamine.

While these vascular changes are taking place, the reticuloendothelial cells in the injured area also become active. Many of these multiply and become macrophages. These are mainly mononuclear cells, but some multinucleated giant cells may also appear.

The vascular and tissue changes described above

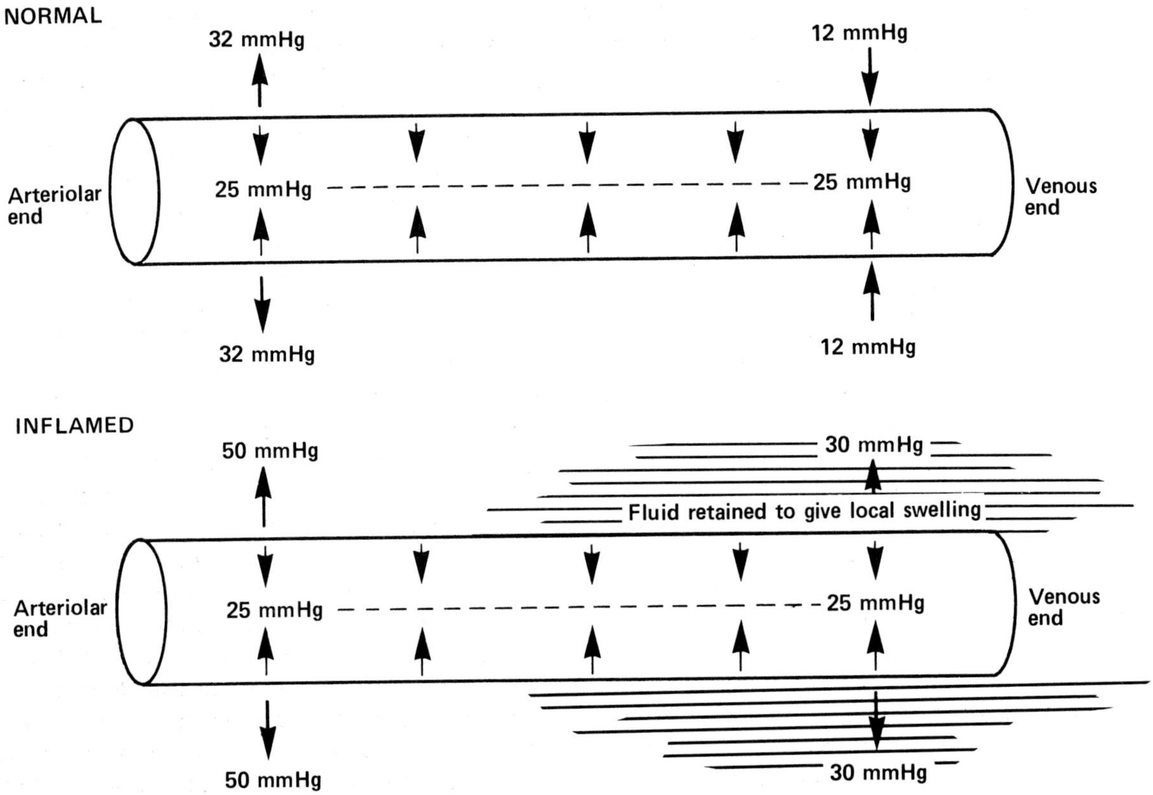

Fig. 5.1 Diagrammatic representation of the various pressures acting across the capillary wall. (**a**) With a more-or-less constant osmotic pressure in the blood plasma and a counteracting hydrostatic pressure which is higher at the arterial end and lower at the venous end, there is normally some movement of fluid out of the vessel at the arteriolar end and return into it at the venous end. (**b**) In acute inflammation an increase in hydrostatic pressure at both arterial and venous ends of the capillary prevents the return of fluid at the venous end, and this contributes to the further accumulation of fluid in the extravascular tissue spaces.

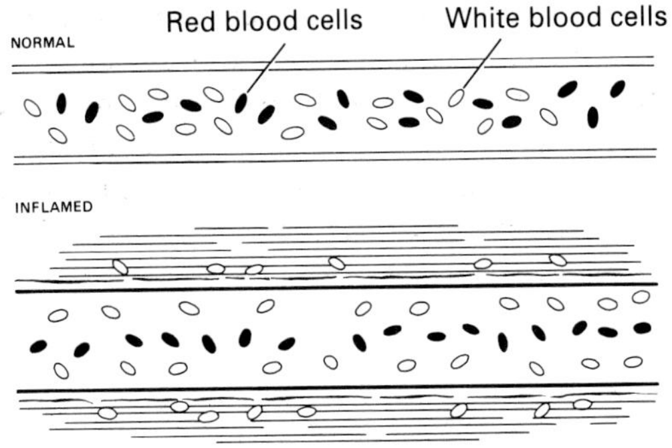

Fig. 5.2 Under normal non-inflamed conditions the cellular elements of the flowing blood are mixed fairly evenly, and tend to travel along the centre of the lumen. In acute inflammation, white blood cells tend to move out into contact with the endothelial lining of the vessel and migrate through this into the perivascular tissue spaces.

constitute the basic elements of inflammation. The purpose of these changes is to localize and counteract the injurious elements. The plasma which leaks into the interstitial space has several beneficial effects. First, it tends to dilute the noxious chemicals causing the injury, and the products of tissue damage. Second, plasma globulins form a coating over bacteria thereby making them more readily phagocytosed by the leukocytes and macrophages. Third, plasma also brings antibodies which may counteract irritating antigens like bacterial toxins. Fourth, fibrinogen becomes converted into fibrin which in turn tends to form a protective wall round the injured area, thereby limiting the spread of harmful substances to the neighbouring tissues. The migration of leukocytes and tissue macrophages helps in the destruction of irritating agents like bacteria and dead cells by phagocytosis.

Inflammation is a dynamic process. It may lead to complete resolution of injury; formation of an abscess; development of chronic inflammatory changes, or, if the inflammatory response fails, necrosis of the part.

In resolution, the inflammatory changes are reversed. The particulate irritating agents, including dead cells, are removed by the leukocytes and tissue macrophages. The leukocytes migrate back into the vessels. The plasma in the interstitial spaces is removed partly by the lymphatics and partly by return to the blood capillaries.

If complete resolution does not occur, and pyogenic organisms are present an abscess,—a localized collection of pus—may develop. It is formed if the irritating agent is strong enough to cause tissue destruction on a considerable scale, but where the process of inflammation has succeeded in localizing its activity by the formation of a firm envelope round the area. The fluid content of the abscess comprises dead cells, mainly leukocytes, bacteria, both live and dead, and tissue fluid, the wall being laid down by fibroblasts in the surrounding tissue.

It is a general surgical principle that when a definite abscess has formed the pus should be evacuated by incision and adequate drainage. The method of approach will vary depending upon the site of the abscess. For superficial ones it is usually a simple matter of incising through the obvious point of maximal fluctuation, providing that no important structures, e.g. nerves, are at risk of damage by the incision. In certain areas, where deep loculated collections of pus are encountered, e.g. ischiorectal abscess, a large skin opening made in cruciate fashion may be needed to ensure complete evacuation. For abscesses located deeply within body cavities exploratory operation may be required to drain the pus and insert an appropriate tube. If the drainage tube is led from the thoracic cavity, e.g. to drain an empyema, it will, of course, require to be connected to an underwater collecting bottle to counteract the subatmospheric pressure in the chest with respiratory movements.

A chronic inflammatory response occurs when the irritating agent is not strong enough to provoke a fully fledged acute inflammatory reaction, or when the site of injury is already diseased and the response to injury is altered. Examples of agents which characteristically lead to a chronic type of inflammation are infection by *Mycobacterium tuberculosis* and *M. leprae*. An example of the effect of a previously damaged site is chronic osteomyelitis in a bone of which the vascularity has already been compromised as a result of acute infection. In this case a dead bone in the area may act as a continuing source of irritation, thereby preventing satisfactory resolution of the inflammatory process. The characteristic of chronic inflammation is a greater proliferation of cells, and less accumulation of fluid in the area. The cells are derived both from blood and the reticuloendothelial system of the area and also from other surrounding tissues. The process is relatively slow to develop as compared to acute inflammation. Blood vessels proliferate as in acute inflammation, but on a lesser scale, and many vessels may also show signs of endarteritis. There is, in addition, a greater deposition of fibrous tissue in and around the affected area. Hence the symptoms of pain and redness and the signs of local heat and tenderness are not so prominent as in an acute inflammatory lesion. Sometimes there is so much proliferation of cells that the swelling becomes very prominent and indeed resembles a tumour. It is then called a granuloma.

6. General response to trauma

Two sets of changes are produced in the body as a result of injury. The first is the obvious local damage and inflammatory response at the site of injury, and the second is a general systemic disorder, involving both neurohumoral and metabolic components.

How a person reacts to injury depends primarily on two factors, namely the nature and severity of the trauma on the one hand, and the physical and mental state of the patient on the other. Factors such as age, general nutritional state of health, and the degree of apprehension and fear at the time of injury can all influence the pattern of reaction. It is common knowledge that young adults can withstand and survive far more serious injuries than the very young and very old. Similarly, a severe wound sustained in combat is often neglected for some time yet overcome, while a similar wound sustained unexpectedly may so unnerve the patient that he or she may die of fright.

Other factors which modify general body response to trauma are the environmental temperature after injury and the treatment the patient receives. Those who are transferred to a warm and comfortable place do better than those left in the cold. Prompt and adequate treatment tilts the balance in favour of the patient.

The changes in response to trauma may be mild, as after minor operations, or may be far reaching as after major operations, multi-organ injuries or severe burns.

ENDOCRINE CHANGES

Adrenomedullary response

Injury, or even the threat of injury, can cause the release of adrenaline and noradrenaline from the adrenal medulla, by impulses conveyed from the central nervous system via the splanchnic branches of the sympathetic trunk. These hormones act on:

1. the heart, causing an increase in the rate and force of contraction;
2. the peripheral and splanchnic vessels, causing arteriolar constriction, thereby increasing peripheral resistance and producing cold extremities and a further elevation in blood pressure;
3. the pupils, which are dilated;
4. the central nervous system, producing quick reactions and sharpened mental awareness;
5. the anal and bladder sphincters, which are contracted.

This is the typical reaction of 'flight or fright', and is usually of short duration.

It is important to note that the adrenal medulla is stimulated also by some anaesthetic agents, and hence this reaction may occur in anaesthetized patients.

In certain situations, the predominant immediate response to pain or fear may be marked slowing of the pulse, fall in blood pressure, coldness, sweating, a sensation of giddiness and even loss of consciousness. These features are indicative of a mainly parasympathetic response.

Major trauma is often accompanied by reduction in blood volume as a result of internal or external haemorrhage, or loss of plasma, as occurs in intensive burns. If the loss of blood or plasma is more than 1200–1500 ml in an adult (or proportionally less in young children), a state of hypovolaemic shock develops leading to mental apathy, cold and clammy skin, rapid and thready pulse, a fall in blood pressure and possibly thirst. If this

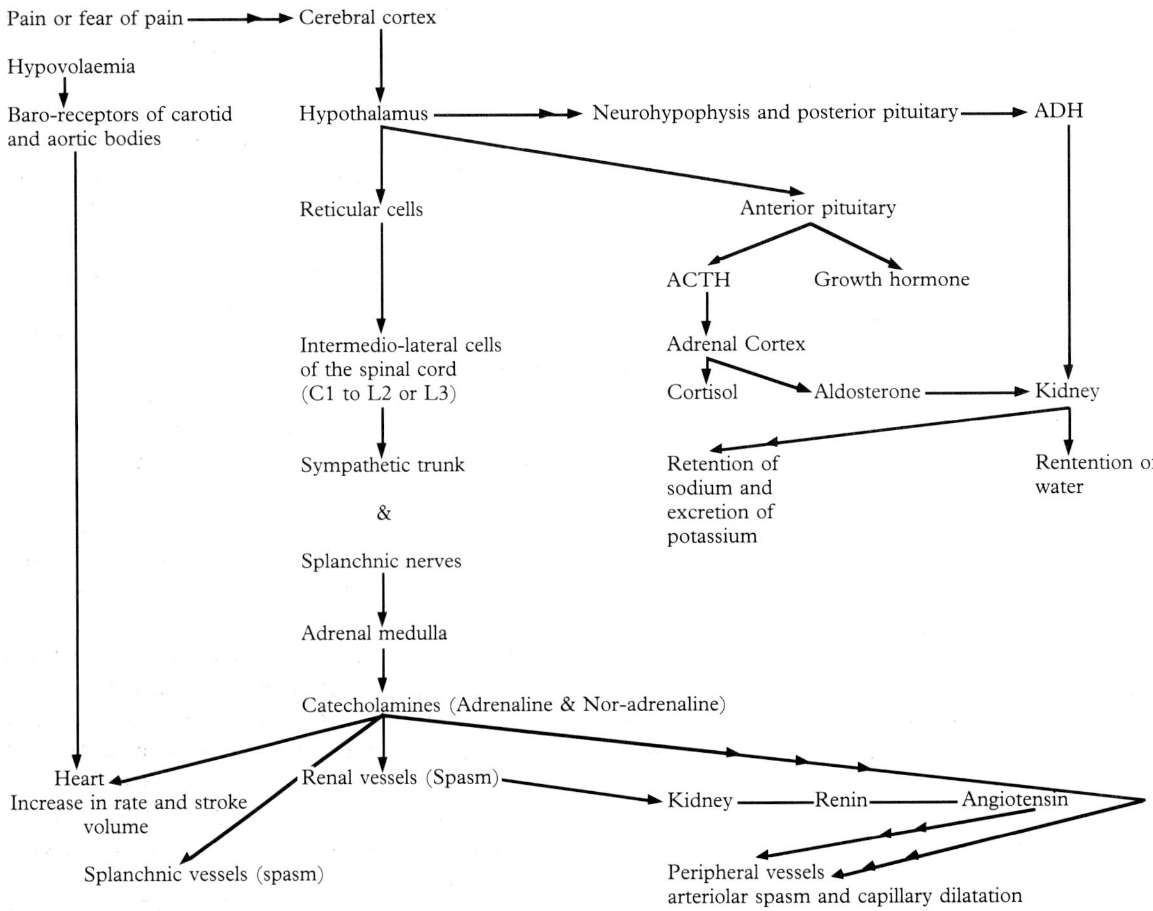

Chart 6.1 General body response to trauma.

state is allowed to continue, hypoxia of the vital centres in the brain, myocardium and kidney may produce irreversible damage. Loss of consciousness and respiratory irregularities indicate that the patient is heading towards this irreversible state and unless urgent measures are taken to correct the hypovolaemia, the patient may succumb to the injuries.

Adrenocortical response

The adrenal cortex is also stimulated to produce cortisol and aldosterone. The stimulation of the former is from adrenocorticotrophic hormone, (ACTH) secretion of the anterior pituitary, while the latter is from the angiotensin renin mechanism (Fig. 6.1). The impulse for the release of ACTH comes to the anterior pituitary from the hypothalamus which in turn is stimulated by hypovolaemia or pain.

Aldosterone affects the metabolism of sodium and potassium. Acting on the kidney tubules, it causes almost complete reabsorption of sodium, which therefore may disappear from the urine. There is also a shift of sodium from the extracellular to the intracellular compartment of the body due to a change in the polarity of cell membranes under the influence of this hormone. Because of this shift, serum sodium measurement may show a fall in level of sodium from the normal 137–147 mmol/l, even though there is an overall bodily retention of sodium. At this stage sodium should

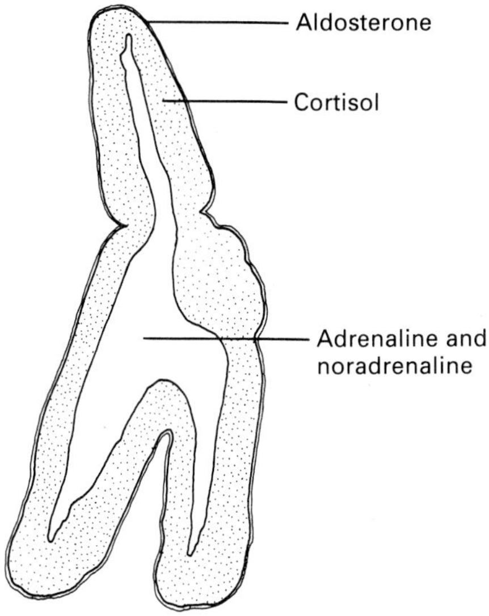

Fig. 6.1 Cross-section of adrenal gland indicating main sources of cortical (aldosterone and cortisol) and medullary hormones (adrenaline and noradrenaline).

not be administered unless there are specific indications, as there is no natural mechanism which can cause the rapid excretion of sodium from the system and prevent undesirable effects of excessive sodium retention, like oedema of the tissues, including the lung.

Potassium metabolism is also altered in a number of ways. It is mainly an intracellular ion in normal health, and it shifts from the intracellular to the extracellular compartment as a result of cellular disintegration at the site of injury and from other non-injured cells under the influence of the released hormones. Its rapid excretion from the plasma into the urine is facilitated by aldosterone. If this loss is prolonged, weakness, drowsiness, nausea and paralytic ileus may develop, and more importantly, cardiac irregularities together with definite electrocardiogram changes may arise. Serum potassium levels may be deceptively normal due to the shift of potassium ions from the intracellular to the extracellular compartment.

Adrenocortical hormones, especially cortisol, appear to play an important role in survival after major accidental trauma or surgical operations. In states of adrenal insufficiency like atrophy of the adrenal cortex due to prolonged therapeutic use of cortisol, or Addison's disease, patients may succumb unless they receive adequate cortisol as soon as possible after the injury or in the case of a planned operation, before, during and after the procedure. It is important to inquire about any previous treatment with adrenocorticosteroids, and in all instances where there is such a medication history, even up to a year previously, patients should be given cortisol preoperatively, during the operation and post-operatively. In an emergency, 100–200 mg cortisol may be given intravenously, as intramuscular cortisol takes about 12–18 h to be effective.

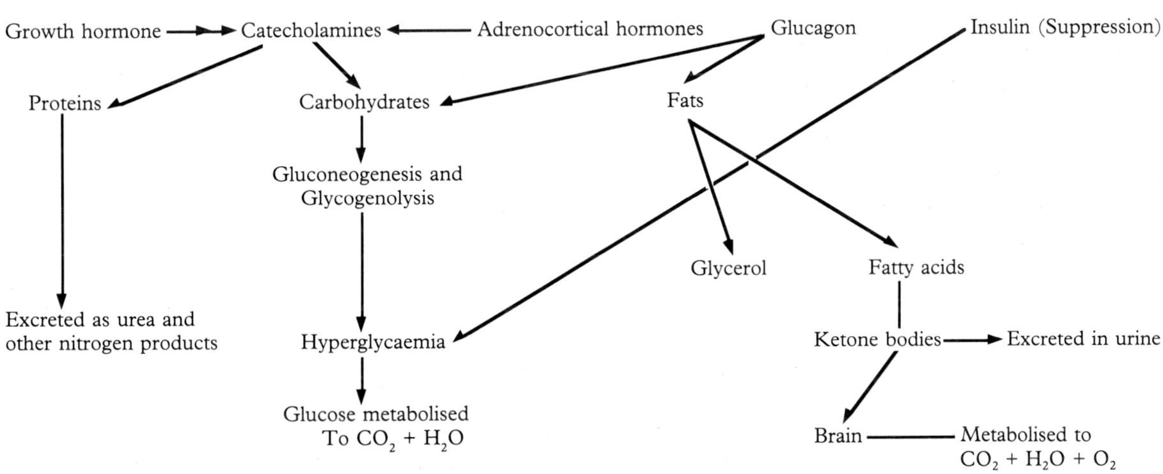

Chart 6.2 Metabolic effects.

The exact mechanism of this life-saving action of cortisol is not known, but it is thought that it may facilitate the action of adrenaline and noradrenaline in the restoration of homeostasis.

Cortisol also plays an important role in the altered metabolism after injury and, as shall be described later, helps in gluconeogenesis and protein catabolism. In this respect, it acts synergistically with glucagon and catecholamines (see Chart 6.2).

Posterior pituitary response

Another result of injury is production of the antidiuretic hormone (ADH) by the neurohypophysis, under the influence of impulses from the hypothalamus (Fig. 6.2). This hormone acts on the distal tubules of the kidneys, causing increased re-absorption of water. As a result the volume of urine passed over a period of 24 h may be reduced from a normal 1.5 l to as little as 600 ml. This oliguria is physiological and is normally seen after all major operations.

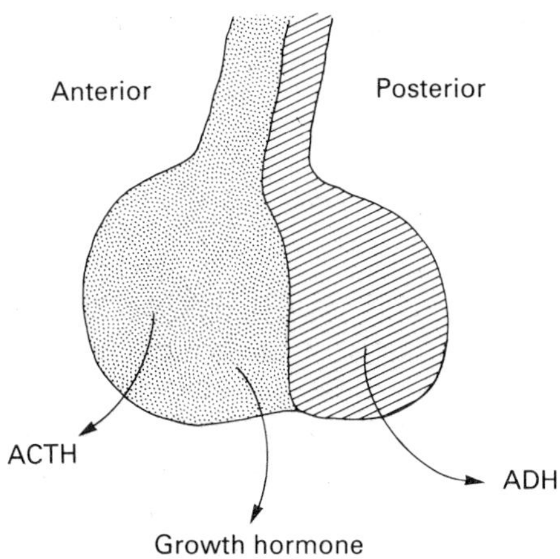

Fig. 6.2 Both anterior pituitary hormones [adrenocorticotrophic hormone (ACTH) and growth hormone] and posterior pituitary antidiuretic hormone (ADH) play a part in the metabolic response.

Growth hormone

Besides ACTH, the anterior pituitary produces growth hormone in response to trauma. This hormone acts synergistically with catecholamines and cortisol to influence carbohydrate, fat and protein metabolism.

Pancreatic hormones

Glucagon and insulin are pancreatic hormones which also take part in the metabolic response to trauma. Their actions are antagonistic to each other and glucagon secretion is increased whereas insulin secretion is suppressed. Glucagon affects carbohydrate and fat metabolism and plays a significant part in the ebb phase of the response to trauma. Insulin secretion is enhanced in the flow or recovery phase.

METABOLIC CHANGES

The metabolic response to trauma occurs in two phases—the ebb or catabolic phase and the flow or anabolic phase (Fig. 6.3). If the patient fails to recover and continues to deteriorate, he or she is said to have passed into the phase of necrobiosis from the ebb phase.

Protein

The metabolism of nitrogen is significantly altered after injury. First, there is loss of appetite so that the intake of proteins is reduced. Partly because of this, and partly because of some esential metabolic changes, the nature of which is not fully understood, the patient consumes his or her own protein and fat for energy. There is a phase of protein catabolism of variable duration which cannot be completely prevented by the administration of protein solutions intravenously. The nitrogen so introduced is utilized only to some extent, but the net result is that nitrogen is excreted in more than normal quantities in the urine.

One gram of nitrogen excreted roughly corresponds to the loss of 1 oz or 28 g of muscle. Normally an adult loses about 10–15 g of nitrogen daily in the urine. The dietary intake adequately replaces this so that the individual remains in proper nitrogen balance. After injury, there is a phase of variable duration in which the patient remains in a negative balance, i.e. the output of nitrogen is invariably higher than intake, no matter how much protein is taken in. The duration and intensity of this phase of negative nitrogen balance depend, among other things, on the severity of the trauma. It lasts for a day or two after mild trauma like that

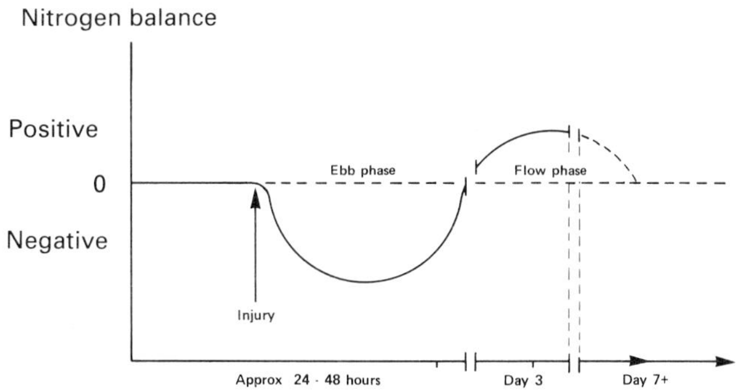

Fig. 6.3 The ebb-and-flow pattern of metabolic changes, with a period of negative nitrogen balance in the first 1–2 days after injury, followed by a (usually longer) period of positive balance. If added complications arise the cycles may continue to alternate.

of an operation on an uncomplicated hernia, with daily loss of around 5 g nitrogen. In severe injuries, like extensive burns or partial gastrectomy, it may last for many days and the daily nitrogen loss may reach 25–30 g. In the presence of sepsis this loss is greater. An interesting feature of this phenomenon is that both the duration and the intensity of the negative nitrogen balance are comparatively less in ill-nourished patients. One explanation is that most of the protein catabolized in the immediate post-traumatic period comes from skeletal muscles, and as in depleted patients there is little muscle protein to spare, the net nitrogen loss is proportionally smaller.

Carbohydrate metabolism

Initially there is a tendency towards hyperglycaemia, due to an increased secretion of glucagon from the pancreas and small intestine, to catecholamines and adrenocortical hormones, and the suppression of insulin under the influence of these hormones. There is both gluconeogenesis and glycogenolysis. However, in prolonged shock and sepsis, there may be hypoglycaemia due to glycogen depletion and glucose utilization at a faster rate than synthesis. Gluconeogenesis may also be defective in these states.

Fat metabolism

Fat metabolism is affected under the influence of catecholamines and glucagon. There is greater breakdown of triglycerides into glycerol and fatty acids. Glycerol is utilized for gluconeogenesis, whereas fatty acids are metabolized to produce ketone bodies and energy. If the period of starvation is prolonged some ketone bodies may be utilized by the brain, and the rest are excreted in the urine.

The flow or anabolic phase

This phase of catabolism is followed by a phase of anabolism in which the patient attains a positive nitrogen balance. He or she starts to gain weight and daily nitrogen loss is a few grams less than intake. During this phase, a high caloric diet is beneficial, and recent evidence suggests that fat may be the preferred calorie source. Moreover, it has been observed that if the illness is prolonged, as in the presence of postoperative sepsis or extensive burns, the rate of recovery is hastened if the patient's energy requirements are fully met, if necessary by hyperalimentation, when carbohydrates, proteins and fats together with vitamins and trace elements are supplied by the intravenous route.

In summary, in the initial catabolic or ebb phase of the response to trauma the main active hormones are ACTH and growth hormone of the anterior pituitary; adrenaline and noradrenaline of the adrenal medulla; ADH of the posterior pituitary;

cortisol and aldosterone of the adrenal cortex and glucagon of the pancreas.

This phase is characterized by:

1. Gluconeogenesis.
2. Glycogenolysis.
3. Hyperglycaemia.
4. Increase in free fatty acids.
5. Protein catabolism.
6. Consequent weight loss.
7. Fluid and sodium retention.
8. Potassium loss.

In uninterrupted recovery this is followed by the anabolic or flow phase, in which insulin plays an important part and helps in:

1. Increased utilization of glucose by the cells.
2. Increased formation of glycogen.
3. Increased synthesis of amino acids and proteins.

In patients whose recovery is not smooth or those who do not recover at all, the ebb phase is followed by necrobiosis which is a continuation of the ebb phase on a greater scale, resulting in an all-round deterioration of condition. This state may be irreversible.

7. Fluid and electrolyte balance

Water, the largest single component of the body, plays an important part in maintaining its normal structure and function. All metabolic activities of the body occur through this medium and an optimum quantity of it is essential for health. Moreover, a proportionate distribution of water and electrolytes in the various systems of the body is essential for proper function. This distribution is disturbed in many diseases, and in turn several important clinical syndromes are produced primarily by upsets in the normal fluid–electrolyte equilibrium.

Water comprises about 60% of body weight in an average man and about 50% in a woman, with a variation of ±15% in both sexes. Extremely obese men and women have 25–30% less water than people of normal weight. In the newborn 75–80% of the body weight is water, but by the time the infant is about 1 year old, the water content is reduced to about 65% and remains at this level throughout childhood (Fig. 7.1).

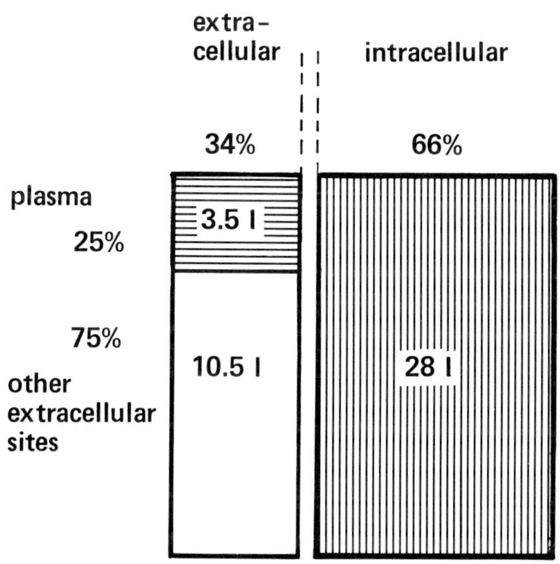

Fig. 7.1 The distribution of water in the various compartments of the body.

About 66% of the total body water is intra-cellular and the remaining 34% is extracellular. Thus, in an average man of 70 kg weight, total body water is about 42 l of which nearly 28 l is intracellular and about 14 l extracellular. The extracellular water is broadly divided into two parts—that in the plasma, 3.5 l which forms about 25% of the extracellular water, the remaining 75% being distributed among the interstitial fluids, dense connective tissue water, inaccessible bone water and the transcellular water, i.e. the water contained in the cerebrospinal fluid, digestive secretions and urine.

The water in the body does not remain static, but there is continuous transfer, on the one hand between the body and the external atmosphere, and on the other, between the various compartments within the body.

In the temperate zones of the world (and probably in winter in the subtropics), the daily intake and output of water in an average man is as shown in Table 7.1.

Inside the body, there are large-scale movements of water. In the first place, there is an exchange of fluid between the vascular and the interstitial compartments. This exchange is mainly determined by the osmotic pressure of the plasma proteins, chiefly albumin, attracting fluid from the interstitial spaces into the vessels, and by the hydrostatic pressure exerted on the capillary wall by the contained fluid tending to move fluid in the opposite

Table 7.1 Daily water intake and output in an average man

Intake		Output	
Beverages	1200 ml	Urine	1500 ml
Water from solid foods	1000 ml	Insensible perspiration and respiration	900 ml
Water from metabolic sources in the body	300 ml	Faeces	100 ml
Total intake	2500 ml	Total output	2500 ml

direction (Fig. 7.2). The average osmotic pressure of plasma proteins is about 25 mmHg. The opposite capillary pressure at the arterial end of the capillary is about 32 mmHg. Fluid therefore tends to leak out through the endothelial lining of the vessels at the arterial end. As the venous end is approached, the capillary pressure decreases to about 12 mmHg. Since this pressure is less than the plasma osmotic pressure fluid therefore tends to be drawn into the venous end. The magnitude of this exchange can be judged from the fact that about three-quarters of the plasma water is exchanged with interstitial fluid every minute.

Moreover, about 170 l of water is excreted by the glomeruli of the kidneys and about 8 l is secreted by the digestive glands every day. Of this total of 178 l, less than 2 l is excreted in the urine and faeces in 24 h; the remaining 176 l is reabsorbed from the kidneys and the alimentary tract.

As far as water loss from the lungs in respiration and through the skin in perspiration is concerned, in a temperate climate there is first an obligatory loss of about 850–1500 ml in 24 h. This insensible loss constitutes the first demand on available water. However, the maximum loss from these routes may reach as high a level as 5% of body weight per hour, i.e. in an average man of about 70 kg, as much as 3.5 l may be lost per hour in very hot weather. There is no significant loss of electrolytes through these routes, except in active loss, i.e. visible sweating, when sodium chloride is lost in addition to water.

ELECTROLYTES

The main cation in the plasma is sodium, whereas potassium, magnesium and calcium are the main intracellular cations. The principal anions in plasma are chloride and bicarbonate, and in the cells phosphate, sulphate and lactate. The relative concentrations of some of these is given below in Table 7.2.

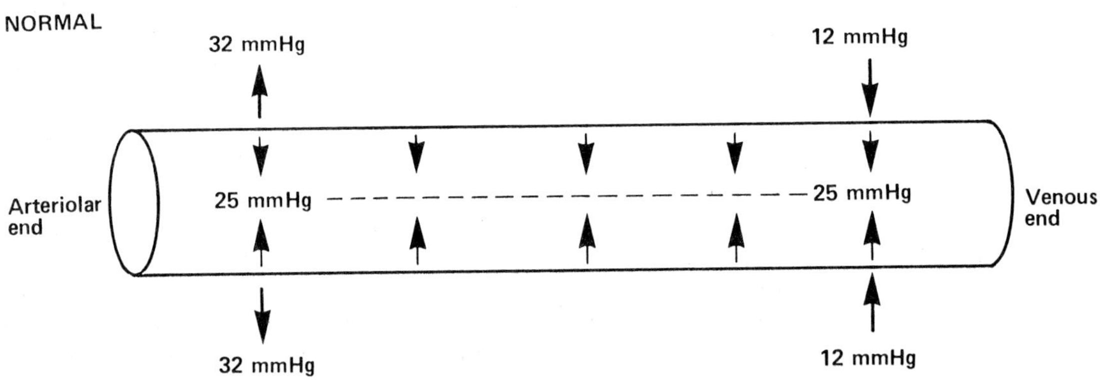

Fig. 7.2 The interplay between hydrostatic and osmotic pressures at the two ends of a capillary, with a net tendency for fluid to move out into the tissue spaces at the arterial end and return into the lumen at the venous end.

Table 7.2 Relative concentrations of some cations and anions

Ions	Extracellular (normal range)	Intracellular (approximate/average)
Sodium	136–148 mmol/1	4 mmol/1
Potassium	3.5–5.0 mmol/1	140 mmol/1
Magnesium	1.5–2.5 mmol/1	15 mmol/1
Chloride	96–105 mmol/1	3 mmol/1
Bicarbonate	25–30 mmol/1	10 mmol/1
Calcium	4.24–5.25 mmol/1	2 mmol/1

Normally an adult ingests about 5–6 g sodium chloride each day and an equivalent amount is excreted in the urine and faeces.

The normal mechanisms regulating fluid and electrolyte balance are disturbed in many conditions of surgical importance. Often the disturbance is of a complex nature, involving both water and electrolytes, but occasionally the deficiency is almost purely one of water.

WATER DEFICIENCY

Pure water shortage can occur if the patient is unable to drink, as in conditions when water is not accessible, or when painful lesions of the mouth or pharynx, or obstructive lesions of the pharynx or oesophagus occur, or in the case of the unconscious patient. Occasionally excessive loss of water may also occur, as in profuse sweating of diabetes insipidus.

In conditions where no water is ingested, only about 300–400 ml is produced daily by cellular metabolism. In comparison, about 850–1500 ml is obligatorily lost by way of respiration and insensible perspiration, and urine continues to be secreted, albeit in small quantities. It has been observed that even in severe water deficit, about 300 ml of urine continues to be secreted daily till the very end. On balance, therefore, there is an absolute shortage of about 700–900 ml of water daily in a bed-ridden patient without any water ingestion. These figures, of course, refer to temperate climates. In a hot and humid climate the loss of water by both respiration and perspiration is considerably more.

Under these circumstances plasma volume and osmotic pressure tend to be maintained at the expense of the fluids in other compartments of the body. As the loss of water tends to lower plasma volume and increase its osmotic pressure, water is withdrawn from the interstitial spaces, causing a rise of osmotic pressure in the interstitial fluid. Fluid is then in turn withdrawn from the cells. Hence the main brunt of pure water deprivation falls on the cells and results in cellular dehydration.

The urinary output is reduced under the influence of the antidiuretic hormone (ADH) of the posterior pituitary and the specific gravity of the urine increases to 1020 or even to 1030. As there is little or no reduction of plasma volume, the haematocrit, haemoglobin and plasma electrolyte values initially remain normal. However, as water deprivation continues, the compensatory mechanisms of the body fail, and hypovolaemia is established, with haemoconcentration and increases in the concentration of serum electrolytes and blood urea. These changes take about 3–4 days to become established.

Clinical features

Thirst develops when there is a deficit of 1–2 l of water. On examination at this stage, the mouth is dry, the tongue is furred and the cheeks are sunken. There is also a decrease in salivation with consequent difficulty in swallowing. The skin becomes dry, loses its normal turgor and elasticity, and the ocular tension is diminished. Systemic blood pressure falls, and the pulse becomes weak and rapid. Laboratory investigation may reveal hypernatraemia. Finally, the patient becomes drowsy, confused and falls into a coma. Death is probably due to general derangement of the body metabolism associated with cellular dehydration.

Unless the clinician is aware of the possibility of dehydration and especially looks for the signs, the diagnosis may not be made and the condition is overlooked. This can be avoided if an accurate input and output fluid chart is maintained; if arrangements are made to weigh the patient, and any change in weight is recorded—loss of weight over a short period of time is a reliable indication of dehydration, and if the volume and specific gravity of the urine are regularly checked.

Management

Pure water deprivation is treated by the oral administration of water, or if for any reason this is not possible, by the intravenous administration of 5% dextrose.

COMBINED WATER AND ELECTROLYTE LOSS

In surgical patients combined loss of water and electrolytes is more common than pure water depletion. It commonly occurs as a result of vomiting, diarrhoea, intestinal obstruction, fistulae, burns or frank haemorrhage. Specific electrolyte deficiency may also occur when there is a diminished intake of salt, as in the treatment of cardiac failure, or in parenteral therapy when glucose solutions are given which make good the water deficit but leave the salt deficit uncorrected.

In combined water and salt deficiency, there is no significant difference in the osmotic pressure in the vascular, interstitial and cellular compartments of the body. Hence, movement from the cellular to the extracellular compartment is not rapid, and plasma volume tends to be maintained at the expense of interstitial fluid. Important factors in the movement of fluid from the interstitial spaces into the vascular network are some lowering of venous pressure allowing the plasma osmotic pressure to draw fluid into the venous end of the capillaries, and at the arterial end a reduction in hydrostatic pressure, so that a lesser quantity of fluid is forced out into the interstitial spaces. These processes help to maintain the plasma volume for some time. But in severe depletion the plasma volume falls, resulting in diminished venous return to the heart, lowering of the cardiac output, fall in blood pressure, hypoxia of the vital centres, and finally death.

Clinical features

In the early stages, the patient is lethargic, with a dry tongue and inelastic skin. The cheeks are sunken and ocular tension is low. Later on, there is postural giddiness and fainting with mental changes such as apathy, stupor, confusion and delusions. There may be muscular rigidity and spasticity, and fits. As the depletion worsens, blood pressure tends to fall. In severe cases, vomiting may develop which further aggravates the problem. Thirst is usually absent except in the early stages of frank haemorrhage.

In the fully established state, the haemoglobin, packed-cell volume, plasma proteins and blood urea levels are all raised. The plasma sodium and chloride concentrations tend to remain normal for some time, but eventually fall. The volume and specific gravity of the urine remain normal at first, but sodium and chloride are either absent or present in very low concentration. As the condition deteriorates, the specific gravity of the urine steadily rises and its quantity is diminished.

There is no single test which gives an accurate estimation of fluid deficit, but if clinical signs of dehydration are obvious, the deficit amounts to about 6% of the body weight, i.e. in an average man of about 70 kg, about 4.2 l. A simple but relatively crude laboratory test to establish the diagnosis of salt and water deficiency is the estimation of chloride levels in the urine. For this purpose 10 drops of urine are mixed with one drop of potassium chromate and a 2.9% solution of silver nitrate is added drop by drop. The end point is reached when the colour of the solution changes from yellow to brown. The number of drops of silver nitrate necessary to bring about this change approximately indicates the number of grams of chloride per litre of urine.

The clinical picture given above indicates severe deficiency of both water and sodium ions. Where there is a more profound selective deficiency of sodium there may be the added signs of raised intracranial pressure, e.g. a rise in systolic blood pressure, and this should be kept in mind when interpreting blood pressure readings.

Management

Salt and water deficiency states are treated primarily by the intravenous administration of adequate quantities of physiological saline.

HYPOKALAEMIA

There are many conditions in which there is either loss of potassium along with other electrolytes, or where the biochemical disturbance is mainly caused by a potassium deficit alone. In conditions such as prolonged diarrhoea or faecal fistula, there is a combined deficiency of both potassium and sodium. If this is corrected by giving normal saline or any other potassium-free fluid, potassium deficiency may then dominate the pathological and clinical picture.

Other disorders are characterized by potassium deficit accompanied by either normal or raised sodium concentrations, e.g. in primary aldosteronism or in patients treated with mineralocorticoids. These patients lose more potassium in their urine under the influence of the steroids than do normal individuals. In such cases, if the intake of potassium is restricted, the features of potassium deficiency may appear. In uncontrolled diabetes mellitus intracellular potassium migrates to the extracellular fluid compartment and some of it may be lost in the urine in excess of the normal loss. When these patients are treated with insulin, potassium migrates back into the cells and the level of plasma potassium falls, sometimes giving rise to features of potassium deficiency.

In acute potassium shortage, there is some degree of shift of potassium from the cells, but the cellular membrane selectively holds back potassium, so that the deficit remains mainly extracellular. In chronic cases, however, loss occurs from both the cells and extracellular spaces but the former has more serious consequences. Muscle cells losing potassium take up sodium and hydrogen ions from the extracellular fluid in a ratio of 2 : 1 and the hydrogen ion deficiency in the extracellular fluid may be serious enough to lead to alkalosis.

Clinical features

Potassium deficit interferes with muscular activity at neuromuscular level and cardiac, smooth and voluntary muscles are all affected. In the heart, the deficiency leads to tachycardia and extrasystoles, and in severe cases, the cardiac muscle dilates and heart failure ensues. Smooth muscles become hypotonic, which may lead to paralytic ileus and abdominal distension. Voluntary muscles also lose their tonicity so that varying degrees of paresis or paralysis develop, which if prolonged and severe may lead to respiratory paralysis and death.

The diagnosis of potassium deficiency is made on the basis of history, clinical examination, electrocardiogram (ECG) and laboratory findings. Since it is a predominantly intracellular ion, considerable body depletion can occur over a period of time without a significant effect on the serum concentration.

Management

Prevention

It is a good general rule that patients who are maintained on parenteral fluids for more than 48 h will need potassium chloride 20–40 mmol dissolved in 1 l of physiological saline in 24 h, provided the urinary output is adequate.

Treatment

Deficiency of potassium is corrected by the administration of potassium salts, preferably orally, but in more urgent circumstances by the intravenous route. The response to treatment should be monitored by clinical observations, ECG recordings and estimations of plasma potassium concentration.

CALCIUM DEFICIENCY

Calcium deficiency is rare in surgical disorders but is occasionally seen in hypoparathyroidism, severe pancreatitis, renal failure and crush injuries. Approximately half the calcium circulating in the serum is free ionized Ca^{++}, the other half being bound to albumin. Alkalaemia decreases the ionized calcium concentration. The clinical features of calcium deficit are well known—numbness and tingling sensations, hyperactive tendon reflexes, positive Chvostek's sign, carpopedal spasm, tetany and, rarely, convulsions.

Management

When hypocalcaemia is first detected it is wise to check the blood pH, for if alkalaemia is present, correcting this may bring about a substantial return of calcium concentration towards normal. In acute pancreatitis a major factor may be protein loss, with a depressed serum albumin concentration, and restoring this may correct the calcium level. Acute true calcium deficiency can be corrected by the intravenous administration of calcium gluconate or chloride, e.g. 10 ml of 10% solution. Chronic deficiency is treated by oral calcium supplements and vitamin D, plus perhaps aluminium hydroxide to bind intestinal phosphate and reduce calcium loss.

MAGNESIUM DEFICIENCY

Magnesium deficiency can occur in starvation, malabsorption disorders, prolonged diarrhoea, vomiting or fistulous discharges and in patients maintained on prolonged intravenous therapy with magnesium-free fluid. The clinical picture is similar to that of calcium deficiency. The diagnosis of magnesium deficit is made on clinical grounds and is best corrected by adding magnesium sulphate or chloride to the intravenous fluid.

OVERLOADING WITH WATER AND ELECTROLYTES

In surgical practice, overloading with sodium and water can be avoided if the neck veins are kept under close observation. Engorgement of these veins and a rise in central venous pressure are early warnings that pulmonary oedema may develop; if not treated promptly and properly, this may lead to death.

The condition is treated by withholding parenteral fluids and the administration of diuretics.

HYPERKALAEMIA

Hyperkalaemia may develop in severe trauma, burns, crush injuries, renal failure or where there is increased catabolism. It may also arise from Addison's disease or acute haemolysis. Renal insufficiency alone, including high-output failure, may give rise to hyperkalaemia, and usually some degree of impaired renal function accompanies these other listed causes of hyperkalaemia.

Clinical features

The clinical picture is that of bradycardia, cardiac irregularities, heart block and eventually cardiac arrest in diastole. Initially the patient may become listless and complain of tingling and numbness in the extremities and may become confused. Early ECG changes include peaking of the T waves, widening of the QRS complex and depression of the ST segment. Later the QRS widens greatly and the T waves disappear.

As a preventive measure, it is a good rule to avoid administering potassium to patients whose urinary output is not adequate.

The first approach to correcting established hyperkalaemia should be the intravenous administration of 100 ml of 5% dextrose with 20 u of soluble insulin added. This will cause a shift of some of the potassium ions from the extracellular to intracellular space. A second measure is to correct any acidosis by intravenous sodium bicarbonate. Thirdly, as a means of specifically counteracting the cardiac effects, an infusion of calcium gluconate may block the toxic action of the potassium.

If the hyperkalaemia is a manifestation of renal failure, peritoneal or haemodialysis may be required and the patient may prove to be a candidate for renal transplantation.

HYPERMAGNESAEMIA

This is very rare in surgical practice. It is only encountered in patients with severe renal disease.

HYPERCALCAEMIA

This rare disorder is seen in hyperparathyroidism and in cancer with bony metastases.

Clinical features

The symptoms are usually vague and are lassitude, weakness, weight loss, anorexia, nausea and vomiting. If the condition is allowed to worsen the patient may become comatose and die.

Management

If the hypercalcaemia is due to hyperparathyroidism, the sooner the patient has surgical removal of the adenoma or hyperplastic glands the better. Hypercalcaemia due to other causes is treated by measures which dilute the serum calcium levels and increase renal loss of calcium. Intravenous physiological saline will increase the volume of the extracellular fluid and therefore reduce the calcium concentration. It should also increase the urine flow and calcium loss from the kidney. This latter may also be assisted by frusemide or intravenous sodium sulphate.

8. Acid–base regulation

The reaction of the blood is slightly alkaline, and the body mechanisms are so tuned to work best at this level. Wide deviations from this slight alkalinity, either towards greater alkalinity or towards acidity, are dangerous and indeed can be fatal. In health various factors act to alter the reaction. For example, there is a fairly constant output of acid from cellular activity, and in vigorous physical exercise lactic acid is produced in the tissues as a result of relative hypoxia. There is thus a tendency towards the acidification of the blood.

In many diseases the acid–base balance may be disturbed, and in general clinical practice acidosis—deviation of the blood towards acidity—is more likely to be encountered than alkalosis—deviation towards greater alkalinity. Examples of the former are obstructive airways disorders, leading to impaired gas diffusion in the lungs and consequent retention of carbon dioxide, and loss of the predominantly alkaline secretions from the lower gastrointestinal tract in profuse diarrhoea, intestinal obstruction or fistula. Alkalosis may arise, e.g. in pyloric stenosis, with the repeated vomiting of large quantities of hydrochloric acid in the gastric secretion.

The body has several mechanisms which act to correct any deviation of the pH from its normal level of 7.4. The first and most rapid to come into play are the buffer systems which are present in both the plasma and tissue fluids and also intracellularly, e.g. in the red blood cells. Secondary lines of defence are the lungs and the kidneys (Fig. 8.1).

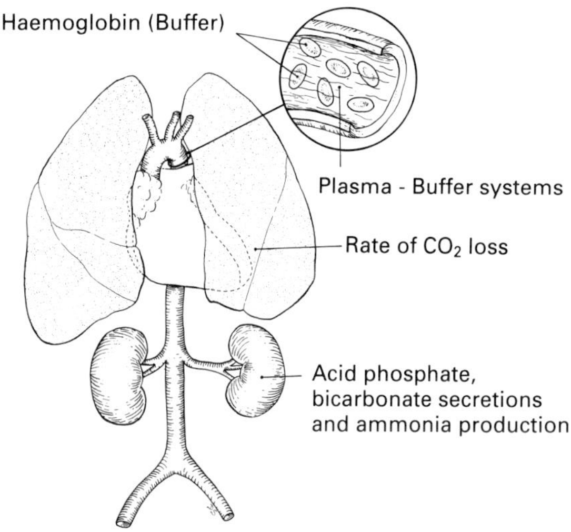

Fig. 8.1 Summary of the main mechanisms contributing to the maintenance of a relatively constant pH in body fluids in the blood, the lungs and the kidneys.

An aqueous solution dissociates into H^+ and OH^- ions. It is acid if there is an excess of H^+ ions; conversely, if there is an excess of OH^- ions, the solution is alkaline. Water is neutral, i.e. it contains an equal number of H^+ and OH^- ions: 1 g equivalent of H^+ ions is present in 10 000 000 l of water. This is written as $[H^+] = 10^{-7}$. If the concentration of H^+ ions becomes 10 times greater, i.e. if 1 g equivalent of H^+ ions is present in 1 000 000 l, it is written as $[H^+] = 10^{-6}$. In a neutral aqueous solution, the concentration of H^+ and OH^- ions is the same, so that in water $[OH^-]$ is also equal to 10^{-7}. This notion is expressed in the form of pH, which is the negative value of the power to the base 10 of the hydrogen ion concentration. In alkaline solution the pH is more than 7, signifying that the number of H^+ ions is less and their dilution is greater. In an acid solution on the other hand, the pH is less than 7, as the number of H^+ ions is more and their dilution is less. The lesser the pH, the less is the dilution of H^+ ions.

BUFFER SYSTEMS

There are several pairs of buffers in the blood, each pair consisting of a weak acid and its sodium or potassium salt. Any excess of acid in the system tends to be neutralized by weak alkalis present in the blood. Similarly any excess of alkali in the system tends to be neutralized by the weak acids of the blood.

Plasma

In the plasma, the main buffers are carbonic acid ($H \cdot HCO_3$) and its sodium salt, sodium bicarbonate ($NaHCO_3$). Other weaker buffers are protein and its salt, i.e. sodium proteinate; sodium dihydrogen phosphate (NaH_2PO_4) and disodium hydrogen phosphate (Na_2HPO_4).

In conditions where an excess of acid is produced in the body, as in violent exercise, the extra acid—in this case lactic acid—is neutralized thus:

$$\underset{\text{(Lactic acid)}}{H \cdot L \cdot} + NaHCO_3 \longrightarrow \underset{\text{(Sodium lactate)}}{NaL} + H \cdot HCO_3$$

$H \cdot HCO_3$ is a much weaker acid than lactic acid: it does not dissociate as rapidly and completely into H and HCO_3 ions as does lactic acid into H and lactate ions. The number of H ions liberated is therefore much smaller than would have been the case in the absence of $NaHCO_3$. Hence the presence of $NaHCO_3$ tends to make it difficult for any acid stronger than $H \cdot HCO_3$ to exist freely in the plasma. So efficient is this buffering mechanism that the pH of the blood is directly related to the ratio of $NaHCO_3$ to $H \cdot HCO_3$, so that

$$pH = pK + \log \frac{[B \cdot HCO_3]}{[H \cdot HCO_3]}$$

where pK is a constant of a value of 6.1 and $B \cdot HCo_3$ represents any bicarbonate, including $Na \cdot HCO_3$.

The normal values are

$$\begin{aligned} pH &= 6.1 + \log 60/3 \\ &= 6.1 + \log 20, \text{ and since} \\ \log 20 &= 1.3, \\ \text{therefore } pH &= 6.1 + 1.3 \\ &= 7.4 \end{aligned}$$

In conditions in which this bicarbonate– carbonic acid mechanism does not prove adequate, other buffers such as NaH_2PO_4 and Na_2HPO_4 come into action, the former acting as a weak acid and the latter as a weak alkali. If there is an excess of OH^- ions in the body, more Na_2HPO_4 is formed, releasing H ions to neutralize the reaction. Thus taking a hypothetical case, $Na \cdot OH + Na \cdot H_2PO_4 \longrightarrow H \cdot OH$ (water) $+ Na_2HPO_4$. There is a corresponding decrease in the quantity of NaH_2PO_4 but the pH of blood tends to remain the same as before the entry of $Na \cdot OH$. Protein and sodium proteinate act in a similar way.

Red blood cells

In the red blood cells the main buffer system is haemoglobin and its potassium salt, potassium haemoglobinate. When there is an increased production of CO_2 in the body, it is converted into H_2CO_3 in the red blood cells; the interaction of $CO_2 + H_2O \longrightarrow H \cdot HCO_3$ is facilitated by the enzyme carbonic acid anhydrase. Only small quantities of H_2CO_3 remain in the plasma, as it contains no carbonic acid anhydrase.

$H \cdot HCO_3$ in the red blood corpuscles reacts with the potassium salt of haemoglobin in the equation:

$$H \cdot HCO_3 + K \cdot Hb. \longrightarrow K \cdot HCO_3 + H \cdot Hb \cdot$$

The $K \cdot HCO_3$ dissociates into K^+ and HCO_3^- ions. The HCO_3^- then migrates to the plasma and in its place chloride ions enter the red blood cells. This process is called the chloride shift. In the plasma, the ratio of $B \cdot HCO_3$ and $H \cdot HCO_3$ tends to be re-established, i.e. it tends to be the same as it was before the influx of the excess CO_2. The conversion of $K \cdot Hb \cdot$ into $H \cdot Hb \cdot$ in the red blood cells does not greatly alter the reaction inside the cells as $H \cdot Hb \cdot$ is an even weaker acid than $H \cdot HCO_3$.

Kidney

While the buffering systems act as a first line of defence in maintaining acid-base equilibrium in the body, the kidneys form the second line of defence. During normal metabolism, fats, carbohydrates, and proteins are metabolized to produce CO_2 and H_2O which combine together to form

H_2CO_3, i.e. an excess of acid. Other acids, like lactic acid and sulphuric acid are also formed during metabolism. The main task of the body in this respect appears to be to get rid of the excess of H^+ ions and to preserve as much base, i.e. Na^+ and K^+ ions, as possible. This differential process is carried out in the kidneys where Na_2HPO_4 is converted into NaH_2PO_4:

$$H{\cdot}HCO_3 + Na_2HPO_4 \longrightarrow \underset{\text{(excreted)}}{Na{\cdot}H_2PO_4} + \underset{\text{(absorbed)}}{Na{\cdot}HCO_3}$$

This serves the dual purpose of getting rid of H ions and preserving sodium in the body. The normal ratio of $NaH_2PO_4 : Na_2HPO_4$ in the blood is 1:4 whereas in the urine it can be as high as 50:1.

The kidneys excrete H ions in other ways also. Na·C1 in the urinary tubules reacts with H_2CO_3 to form HC1 and $NaHCO_3$. The $NaHCO_3$ is absorbed back into the blood, thereby increasing the bicarbonate reserve of the body. HC1 is a very strong acid, and may therefore disturb the equilibrium dangerously. This is prevented by the renal tubule cells producing ammonia (NH_3) which combines with HC1 to produce NH_4C1, which is neutral and is excreted in the urine. By this method, sodium and bicarbonate ions are preserved in the system, and H ions are excreted.

In the tubular urine, $NaHCO_3$ dissociates into Na^+ and HCO_3^- ions, while in the cells of the tubules H_2CO_3 dissociates into H^+ and HCO_3^- ions. The H^+ ions migrate to the renal tubules where they combine with HCO_3^- to form H_2CO_3 which is excreted, and sodium migrates into the cells of the tubules and there combines with HCO_3^- ions to form $NaHCO_3$, which is absorbed into the blood. In this way the body further conserves sodium and bicarbonate ions and gets rid of H^+ ions whenever there is an excess of acid in the system. These actions are influenced by carbonic acid anhydrase at the tubule cell level, and drugs which block the action of this enzyme cause a loss of sodium (and water) from the body.

Lungs

In the lungs CO_2 is given up by the blood by a process which is the reverse of that taking place elsewhere in the body, i.e. chloride migrates back to the plasma from the red blood cell and HCO_3^- migrates to the red blood cell from plasma. In the red blood cells $H{\cdot}HCO_3$ is formed, and again splits into CO_2 and H_2O:

$$\underset{\text{(carbonic acid anhydrase)}}{H_2CO_3 \longrightarrow H_2O + CO_2}$$

CO_2 diffuses out into the alveolar air and is exhaled. As the CO_2 is removed, the concentration of $B{\cdot}HCO_3$ relative to $H{\cdot}HCO_3$ increases. Whenever there is an excess of acid, more CO_2 is lost by rapid breathing and conversely, when there is an excess of alkali, breathing is depressed and less CO_2 is lost. Breathing is regulated mainly by chemoreceptor mechanisms both in the respiratory centres in the brain and in the aortic and carotid bodies.

CLINICALLY SIGNIFICANT ACID–BASE DISTURBANCES

Acidosis due to excessive production of acid, as in diabetes mellitus or in shock, is described as metabolic acidosis, whereas that due to poor diffusion of gases in the lungs leading to retention of CO_2 as may occur in some pulmonary diseases, is called respiratory acidosis.

Alkalosis due to excessive loss of carbon dioxide through rapid ventilation may occur for example in artificial or assisted respiration in anaesthesia. This is called respiratory alkalosis. Metabolic alkalosis is seen in conditions of excessive loss of acid, as occurs in repeated vomiting due to pyloric stenosis.

ACIDOSIS

Clinical features

In acidosis which, as has been stated, is more commonly encountered, there are nervous, cardiovascular and respiratory manifestations.

Nervous system

There is often mental confusion and sluggish responses from the patient and indeed he or she may become unconscious. The respiratory and cardiovascular centres are depressed.

Table 8.1 Various causes of acidosis and alkalosis

Respiratory	
Acidosis	*Alkalosis*
Retention of CO_2 in the blood	Excessive loss of CO_2
Obstruction of the air passages (e.g. by vomitus, blood, secretions)	Increased rate and/or depth of respiration in anaesthesia with assisted ventilation
Inadequate ventilation 1. In respiratory arrest; 2. During anaesthesia; 3. In respiratory depression from drugs, e.g. morphine	Hysterical overbreathing Hyperventilation because of severe pain Rapid ascent to high altitude
Inadequate diffusion of gases 1. Pulmonary infection (pneumonia) 2. Emphysema 3. Pulmonary oedema	
Metabolic	
Vigorous exercise	Repeated vomiting in pyloric stenosis
Shock—cardiac arrest	Excess loss of acid urine, from certain diuretics
Prolonged severe diarrhoea	Excess ingestion of alkalis
Intestinal fistula	
Diabetis mellitus	
Poisoning with methyl alcohol or salicylates	
Renal failure	
Starvation	

Cardiovascular system

The force of contraction of cardiac muscle is depressed, and there is therefore a fall in stroke volume. This effect may be masked for some time by the release of catecholamines which have an opposite effect, but in prolonged acidosis the depressant effect on the cardiac muscle becomes more apparent.

The peripheral circulation becomes sluggish, partly due to the depression of the vasomotor centre in the brain, and partly due to a direct inhibitory effect of the acidosis on the myocardium, and the smooth muscle of the arterioles.

As a result of these effects there is hypotension, with warm extremities as the peripheral blood vessels are dilated. This hypotension responds poorly or not at all to the administration of catecholamines.

Respiratory system

Initially the respiratory centre is stimulated and therefore the rate and depth of respiration are increased. If the acidosis is prolonged, however, the respiration becomes gasping and finally stops altogether.

Management

Removal of the cause of the acidosis is clearly the most important part of treatment, but in addition sodium bicarbonate solution may be required to be given by intravenous infusion. The quantity is determined by the severity of the condition. There should be no hesitation in adding up to 50 ml of 7.5% sodium bicarbonate solution to 500 ml of physiological saline or 5% dextrose in a patient with confirmed evidence of frank acidosis.

ALKALOSIS

In alkalosis most often there is dizziness, nausea, blurring of vision, excessive fatigue and consciousness may be blurred. This may be partly due to an increase in cerebral vascular resistance as a result of the fall in carbon dioxide. In the circulatory system cutaneous vasoconstriction occurs and sluggish blood flow to the extremities may cause peripheral cyanosis, associated with stagnant hypoxia.

Hyperventilation causes a shift of the oxygen dissociation curve to the left, and therefore less oxygen is available for tissue perfusion at a given partial pressure.

At high altitudes, after some time equilibrium develops as more base is excreted in the urine so that the ratio of bicarbonate and carbon dioxide is restored to normal and the pH returns to normal.

Metabolic alkalosis is nearly always associated with dehydration, as in vomiting due to pyloric stenosis, and correction of the dehydration plus surgical relief of the stenosis may be all that is necessary to restore the normal pH of the blood.

9. Tumours

A tumour is a mass of cells which proliferate without the control on growth normally exercised in the body, and which serve no useful purpose.

No age is immune from the development of tumours and they can arise in virtually all tissues. A few examples are given in Table 9.1.

Table 9.1 Tumours arising at different ages

Age	Tumour
Newborn	Sacrococcygeal teratoma
Infants	Wilms tumour of kidney
Adolescents	Bone cancers
Young women	Fibroadenoma of breast
Middle-aged	Carcinoma of stomach and of cervix uteri
Elderly	Carcinoma of lung and of prostate

There are two types of tumours—benign and malignant. It is to the latter that the term cancer (= crab) has been given, because of the resemblance of a malignant tumour in an organ such as the breast to a crab with claws.

There are many differences between benign and malignant tumours:

1. A benign tumour grows for a period and then remains stationary for long periods or throughout life, or expands locally very slowly. A malignant tumour, on the other hand, continues to grow if not removed or checked by other methods. There are examples of malignant tumours which have been experimentally transplanted from mice to mice since 1900, a period during which many generations of mice have lived and died, with the tumour continuing to grow in each new host.
2. A malignant tumour kills the patient if it remains untreated, even though it may be situated in a so-called non-vital part of the body like a toe. A benign tumour does not kill unless it is in such a site that either by its anatomical situation it brings about dangerous changes in the body function, for example an intracranial tumour, or physiologically it produces dangerous effects in the body such as a hormone-producing tumour of the adrenal gland.
3. A benign tumour, while growing, exerts pressure on the surrounding tissues and displaces them—a process called expansion. The tissues in the immediate neighbourhood of the tumour usually form an envelope round it, called its capsule. Malignant tumours spread by infiltrating and destroying the surrounding structures and these tumours usually do not possess a capsule.
4. Benign tumours remain confined locally and do not spread beyond the site of origin. Malignant tumours do not remain so confined and spread to distant parts of the body. The process is called metastasis, or secondary spread. Thus fibroadenoma of breast, a benign tumour, remains confined to the breast, while carcinoma of that organ often gives rise to secondary deposits in the bones and liver, and elsewhere.
5. Benign tumours do not usually ulcerate, whereas malignant tumours do so readily, for example epithelioma of skin, carcinoma of rectum and cancer of the cervix uteri.
6. A benign tumour does not recur if completely removed, while the hallmark of malignancy is recurrence, either locally or at a distance.

This may be for two reasons:

a. Removal may be incomplete so that malignant cells may be left behind either at the site of the original tumour or at a distance. For a varying period, these residual cells may remain under the influence of the ill-understood processes of growth control, but sooner or later growth control is ovewhelmed and the malignant cells proliferate again to give rise to fresh deposits of tumour.
b. In spite of the complete local removal of a malignant tumour, a new tumour of the same pattern arises because the factors which gave rise to the original one continue to operate.

7. Microscopically, malignant tumours fail to reproduce faithfully the parent tissue. For example, in adenocarcinoma, the glandular pattern is distorted. On the other hand, in benign tumours, the parent tissue may be more or less clearly reproduced.
8. Histologically, the hallmarks of malignancy are mitosis and the appearance of atypical cells. These features are absent in benign tumours.

It must, however, be remembered that these are somewhat variable features, and all the characteristic features may not be present in all benign or malignant tumours. For example, innocent tumours of the brain are not encapsulated and may kill though they may be benign; adenoma of the parotid gland is not malignant, though it tends to recur after local excision, and it also has certain microscopic features which do not represent the parent tissue.

All malignant tumours do not behave in the same way and cancer is clearly not one disease but many. Each cancer has its own peculiar features and differs from others not only in clinical presentation and pathological appearance but also in response to various forms of treatment.

AETIOLOGY

At the present stage of knowledge, it is thought that a tumour occurs because of the liberation of a group of cells from the growth-restraining influences in the body. Probably some genetic change occurs in the cells, and the normal structure of the ribonucleic acid (RNA), the deoxyribonucleic acid (DNA) and the nucleoproteins may be so distorted that the cell becomes autonomous and parasitic on the normal tissues of the body. The precise nature of these changes has not yet been discovered. It is, however, clear that three factors have to be considered; first, the changes in the structure and functions of the cells, which make them autonomous and which can be transmitted to the daughter cells; second, the external agents, which have been found either experimentally or on clinical grounds to be causally associated with the cellular changes resulting in malignancy, and third, the normal growth control mechanisms of the body which fail in respect of the cells which assume malignant characteristics. Thus, the study of causation of cancer has to be carried out on cellular, environmental, and general physiological levels. At the moment, our understanding of these problems is incomplete. However, some clinical states are known which precede the development of frank malignancy and a few substances have been found to cause cancer experimentally and clinically. For example:

1. There are some inherited conditions which predispose to cancer formation. Familial adenomatous polyposis of the colon is an inherited disorder transmitted through a dominant gene by both parents to both sexes. It has been found that many of these patients develop cancer after the age of 20.
2. Certain congenital conditions, e.g. undescended testis, predispose to malignancy.
3. Simple benign tumours occasionally become malignant, e.g. fibromyoma of the uterus.
4. Chronic mechanical or chemical irritation may cause changes in epithelium so that it becomes the seat of whitish discoloration, called leukoplakia. (Figs 9.1 and 9.2). The condition may develop in the cheek due to ill fitting dentures or from tobacco-chewing. It is a premalignant condition. If the causative irritation is removed, the condition may disappear. On the other hand, if the irritation persists, cancer may develop in the area of leukoplakia. It is not known at which stage of leukoplakia the process becomes irreversible.
5. Some chemicals used in industry have been found to be associated with the development of

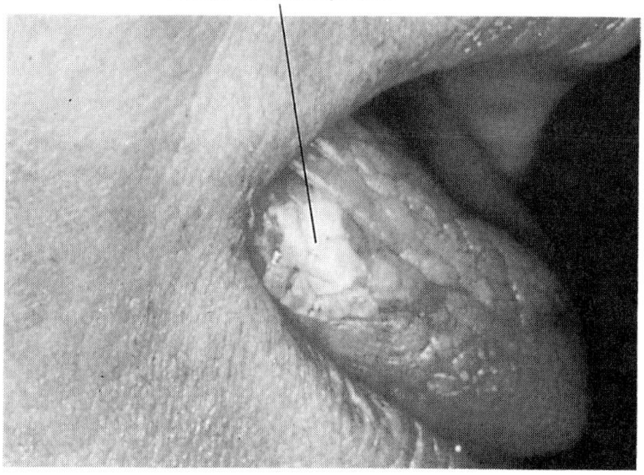

Fig. 9.1 A small localized patch of leukoplakia on the edge of the tongue.

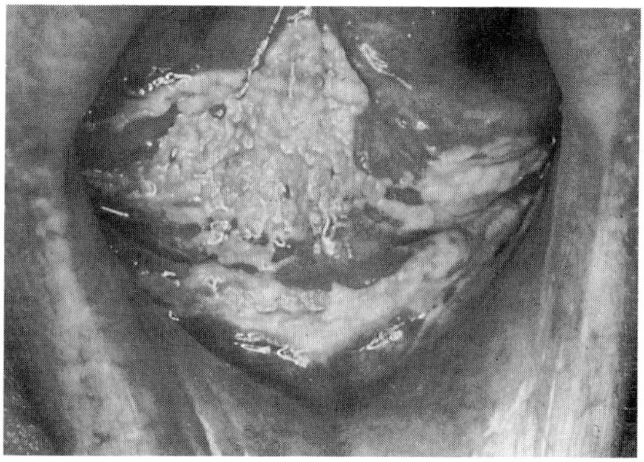

Fig. 9.2 A more extensive area of leukoplakia involving most of the undersurface of the tongue and lower gum.

certain types of cancer. Carcinoma of the bladder is more common in workers in industries in which some chemicals, such as ß-naphthylamine, α-naphthylamine, benzidine and auramine, are used. Two hundred years ago, Percival Pott observed that carcinoma of the scrotum was an occupational hazard in chimney-sweeps in England. More recently, it has been observed that carcinoma of the bronchus is far more common among heavy cigarette smokers than among non-smokers.

6. Radiation has long been recognized as a potent carcinogen, and exposure to the ultra violet rays from the sun is believed to be a causative factor in carcinoma of the skin among white people exposed to strong sunlight in areas such as Australia.

At the present stage of our knowledge, all that can be said is that the above mentioned factors, among others, play an important part in the development of some cancers. They probably prepare a favourable ground for malignancy to occur. The final trigger mechanism, however, is still unknown.

METHODS OF SPREAD

Different tumours spread in different ways:

1. Direct infiltration of the surrounding tissues is the commonest mode of spread. This has two important clinical implications. First, clinical signs of fixation suggest malignancy. Second, treatment is affected, in that fixation determines the operability of the tumour, and defines the scope of the surgical procedure. For example, if a cancer of the oesophagus is fixed to the arch of the aorta, it is clearly inoperable. On the other hand, if the tumour is fixed to the pericardium, the surgeon may remove the tumour with the involved part of the pericardium. Some tumours, e.g. rodent ulcer, spread mainly by local infiltration with little or no evidence of other modes of spread.
2. Lymphatic spread is common in the majority of carcinomas which arise from epithelial tissue but is less common in malignant tumours of the connective tissues (sarcomas). The tumour cells invade the lumen of the lymph vessels and sometimes grow in the lumen as a column till they reach the regional lymph node. Here, the tumour cells may proliferate and destroy the glandular tissue, giving rise to palpable, enlarged nodes. This is called spread by permeation. Another way of spread of cancer along the lymphatics is by way of embolism, in which case malignant cells gain access to the lumen of the lymph vessels and these are carried by the lymph current to the regional or distant nodes where they are arrested and give rise to secondary deposits.

   Lymphatic spread is also of diagnostic and therapeutic importance. For example, a tumour of the stomach with enlarged nodes in the supraclavicular region is most likely to be a carcinoma with secondary deposits. Similarly, a tumour of the breast with enlarged lymph nodes in the axilla is most likely a carcinoma. In planning treatment, the tumour and the involved lymph nodes must both be considered.

However, the enlargement of lymph nodes in association with malignant tumours may not always be due solely to direct invasion by the malignant cells, but may in part be due to an immune response. It follows, therefore, that palpably enlarged lymph nodes in the region draining the site of a tumour may on occasions represent a defensive reaction against the malignancy, and removal or destruction of these nodes may reduce the defensive response.

3. Spread by the blood stream is a common feature of many malignant tumours. The majority of malignant cells entering the blood stream are probably destroyed, but some may survive and give rise to secondary deposits in distant organs such as bone, liver and lung. Some cancers are more liable to form secondary deposits in a particular organ than others, e.g. bones become secondarily involved more commonly in cancers of the breast, thyroid, kidney and prostate, whereas secondary deposits from cancers of the intestine are less common in bones but more common in the liver.
4. Cancer also spreads through normal anatomical passages and spaces, such as the bronchi, peritoneal cavity and the pleural cavity. A classical example is the development of secondary deposits on the ovaries in cancer of the stomach. It is believed that cancer cells infiltrate the serosa of the stomach and from there are shed in the peritoneal cavity to form deposits on the ovaries (Krukenberg tumours).

In clinical practice, an attempt can be made to stage malignant disease, taking into consideration the local characteristics of the tumour, its size and the degree of infiltration, together with the involvement of the regional lymph nodes and the presence or absence of distant metastasis. This is the basis of the TNM classification: T stands for the tumour, N for the regional lymph nodes and M for distant metastasis. Thus, a small tumour of the breast less than 2 cm in diameter, which is confined to the breast tissue, without involvement of the regional lymph nodes and without any metastasis can be graded as $T_1N_0M_0$. This method of classification can be applied to many types of malignant tumours, as a help in the assesment of various methods of treament.

Tumours have also been classified histologically on the basis of the degree of deviation from the normal cells of the tissue of origin. Thus, according to one classification (Broder's), cancers are divided into four grades:

Grade I–Not more than 25% cells lacking differentiation.
Grade II–25–50% cells are atypical.
Grade III–50–75% cells are atypical.
Grade IV–More than 75% cells are atypical.

SARCOMAS

Sarcomas generally appear in young people, are more rapidly growing as compared to carcinomas, and mainly spread by local infiltration and by blood-borne metastasis. Some sarcomas develop in pre-existing benign tumours. A classical example is sarcomatous change in a uterine fibroid.

The commoner sarcomas are:
1. Fibrosarcoma.
2. Osteogenic sarcoma.
3. Ewing's sarcoma of bone.
4. Chondrosarcoma.
5. Lymphosarcoma.
6. Synovioma.

CARCINOMA

Most carcinomas arise either from the squamous epithelium or from the epithelium of glandular structures. The former are squamous cell carcinomas and the latter adenocarcinomas.

Squamous cell carcinomas are the commonest cancers of the skin, mouth (including tongue), oesophagus, bronchus and anal canal. They spread by local infiltration and by the lymphatics. Blood-borne metastasis is usually a late feature. Most of these tumours respond favourably to irradiation.

Adenocarcinomas develop in the stomach, intestines, breast, kidney and prostate. Generally, they are not radiosensitive.

Carcinomas of the bladder, ureter and pelvis of

the kidney are called transitional cell carcinoma as they arise from transitional epithelium.

BENIGN TUMOURS

The common non-malignant tumours are lipoma, fibroma, papilloma, adenoma, myoma, chondroma and neuroma.

Angiomas are tumours of the blood and lymph vessels. However, they are probably better regarded as congenital malformations rather than true tumours.

Clinical management

A provisional diagnosis of cancer is made on the basis of history and clinical examination. Once the suspicion is raised it is nearly always possible to obtain material for direct histological confirmation, and this is most desirable in order to plan the best approach to treatment.

In superficial cancers, like epitheliomas of the skin, the next step is to biopsy the lesion. If the lesion is small and can be excised without causing irreparable damage either cosmetically or functionally, it is excised in toto and submitted for pathological examination. This is called excisional biopsy. If the tumour has been removed completely, this constitutes the definitive treatment also.

In larger lesions, a small piece is removed from the lesion and submitted for histological examination. The peripheral part of the lesion is preferred because the central portion may be necrotic and more difficult to diagnose under the microscope. Moreover, the periphery of the tumour may also reveal the reaction of surrounding tissues to the tumour.

For the diagnosis of deep-seated tumours, e.g. in bone, stomach, lung or kidney, special investigations such as endoscopy, cytology, radiology, scanning procedures and needle biopsy are usually required.

The following are a few examples:

1. A plain X-ray may show typical radiological appearances of bone tumours such as the 'sun-ray' appearance in osteogenic sarcoma (Fig. 9.3).
2. Intravenous pyelography may show distortion of the calyces in carcinoma of kidney.
3. Bronchoscopy may reveal cancer of the bronchus from which a confirmatory biopsy can be taken.
4. Ultrasonic examination may reveal deep-seated tumours in the abdomen, pelvis, or adrenal gland.
5. A radioactive iodine uptake test may show a 'cold nodule' in a multi-nodular goitre, which is a strong pointer towards malignancy of the thyroid gland.
6. Computerized tomography may outline brain tumours.

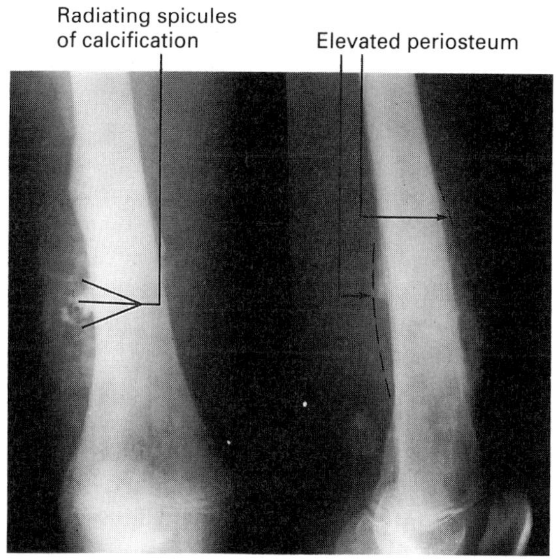

Fig. 9.3 Osteogenic sarcoma. X-ray shows the periosteum of the lower end of the femur; at the site of the tumour it is elevated from its normal site, and abnormal calcification has been laid down by the malignant cells, in a more-or-less radiating fashion.

On the basis of these and other investigations, an exact diagnosis can be made in the vast majority of cases. Rarely, diagnostic surgical exploration like laparotomy is required to establish the diagnosis.

TREATMENT

Nearly 1000 years ago, Zahrawi taught that cancer should be treated surgically only if the limb or the organ bearing it could be completely removed; otherwise it was best not to operate on it. This teaching is still followed, and during the last 100 years, radical operations have been devised with the aim of removing the tumour, plus also a healthy margin of the tissue all round, together with the regional lymph nodes. Radical mastectomy, block dissection of the neck and total gastrectomy are examples of some of these extensive procedures.

Unfortunately, however, this increasingly aggressive surgical approach has generally not been rewarded by greater cure rates and, as one might expect, has also been accompanied by greater risks of mortality and morbidity. In many fields of cancer treatment there has therefore been a swing away from the very radical surgical excision approach. The failure to achieve cure by extensive operations is almost certainly on account of two main factors: first, by the time many tumours are large enough to cause symptoms and lead to diagnosis, there are likely to be microscopic deposits disseminated beyond the accessible operative field, and second, in the case of some tumours the field of potential malignant change may be wide or generalized rather than a local one.

Surgery

Surgery is, however, still the main form of treatment for many malignant diseases. The principal aim is to remove all the diseased lesion which can be seen or felt together with a margin of healthy tissue all round. It is usual to remove the regional lymph nodes together with the diseased part in one block, wherever this is feasible. However, as has been noted, the role of lymph nodes in the disease process is under review and with the acknowledgement that enlargement of the lymph nodes may sometimes indicate part of an immunological tissue response to the tumour, the attitude towards the removal of regional lymph nodes is, therefore, changing.

If it is found impossible to remove the growth at operation, the surgeon may carry out procedures which, although they will not cure, will diminish the functional disabilities of the patient. For example, in a case of obstructive jaundice due to obstruction of the common bile duct by a carcinoma of head of the pancreas, the obstruction may be bypassed by an anastomosis between the gallbladder and a loop of jejunum. These procedures are called palliative in contradistinction to curative ones.

Radiotherapy

As has been mentioned, radiotherapy is capable of destroying certain malignant tissue, especially arising from squamous epithelium. Its action brings about such changes in the cellular structure of the malignant cells that either these are destroyed directly or are rendered incapable of reproducing further cancer cells. Doses of radiation are so calculated that only the abnormal cells are affected and normal body cells are not harmed.

Radiation can be given in three forms:

1. *Teleradiation*—in this method the radiation is delivered by a source placed at distances from the tumour. Relatively low voltage (under 100 kV) may be used for surface lesions like epithelioma and rodent ulcer; medium voltage (between 100 and 200 kV) for deeper tissues like those of breast, larynx and pharynx, and supervoltage (2 000 000 eV or more) for deep seated lesions.
2. *Interstitial radiation* involves the insertion of radioactive material like radium directly into the tissues. Some cancers, like those of the anterior third of the tongue, can be treated by this method.
3. *Radioactive isotopes* like iodine 131 are administered systemically in the treatment of certain thyroid cancers which are able to take up iodine selectively, like normal thyroid tissue.

Chemotherapy

Chemotherapy is a method of treatment with chemicals which destroy the malignant cells without causing any significant damage to the normal cells of the body. One great advantage of this form of therapy over radiation is that being systemic, even those microscopic deposits of malignant tissue which cannot be seen may be destroyed. A number of chemotherapeutic agents are already available, and newer compounds are regularly being developed. The following are some of the drugs in current use.

Alkylating agents

These are so-called because these compounds act by substituting an alkyl radical $R\text{-}CH_2\text{-}CH_{2+}\text{-}H$ for

H atoms of organic compounds like nucleic acid of DNA. These alkylating agents therefore act by disrupting the malignant cell metabolism. The following drugs are included in this group:

1. Nitrogen mustard.
2. Thiotepa.
3. Chlorambucil.
4. Cyclophosphamide.
5. Phenylalanine mustard.

These are also called radiomimetic drugs.

Antimetabolites

Antimetabolites act by inhibiting the enzymes of nucleic acid.
This group includes:

1. Methotrexate.
2. 5-Fluorouracil.
3. Hydroxyurea.
4. Cytosine arabinoside.

Antibiotics

Antibiotics are natural products derived from some fungi. They act on the substrate of cellular enzymes. They form static compounds with DNA and RNA, thereby interfering with the metabolism of malignant cells.
The following are included in this group:

1. Actinomycin D.
2. Mithramycin.
3. Adriamycin.

A few malignant tumours are to some extent influenced by hormones, notably from either the sex organs or adrenal gland, and drugs which increase or suppress these hormones may be helpful in controlling these tumours.

Often the best response to chemotherapy results from the use of more than one agent given either together or in sequence, and the standard approach to chemotherapy in many tumours is a combination of drugs of different action.

Examples of tumours in which chemotherapy has produced encouraging results are trophoblastic tumours of the uterus, Wilm's renal tumour, neuroblastoma and carcinoma of the prostate.

Immunotherapy

Immunotherapy is still in an experimental stage. The basic concept is that cancer cells are different from the normal cells of the patient and may therefore be antigenic. On the one hand, attempts are being made to develop antibodies against malignant cells as an active immune process, and on the other trials are being made using antibodies passively introduced into the patient. There is also some evidence that non-specific antibodies like BCG may be beneficial in augmenting resistance against neoplastic cells.

Combined therapy

While real advances have been made in the control of a number of malignant tumours, unfortunately many are still incurable and much of our effort is rightly concerned simply to prolong useful life and to relieve or minimize unpleasant symptoms.

These are the aims of the palliative surgical procedures so often performed, e.g. bypassing an obstruction, division of nerves conducting pain from the affected area, or excising bulky fungating tumour masses locally even in the presence of distant spread.

Radiotherapy or chemotherapy is also sometimes useful for this purpose. Severe pain due to bone secondaries is often controlled by deep X-ray therapy. Finally, powerful analgesics and sedatives are at hand to minimize suffering.

It is an important part of the training of a surgeon to acquire skill in the use of all these methods of treatment of cancer in collaboration with colleagues in the fields of radiotherapy, haematology, immunology, chemotherapy and psychology.

10. Principles of cancer treatment

The treatment of cancer may be surgery, radiotherapy, chemotherapy or a combination of two or all of these. Hormonal therapy and immunotherapy may also play a part in the treatment.

The overall plan of treatment in the individual patient must often be the product of a multidisciplinary approach involving the pathologist, the surgeon, a radiotherapist and a medical oncologist.

The plan of treatment may be radical, with the objective of cure; it may be aimed simply at the control of the disease; it may be limited to palliative measures to relieve distressing symptoms, or there may be no active treatment at all.

Careful investigation and definition of the stage of the disease and the tumour–host relationship in the individual patient will allow the most rational and effective therapeutic management of that patient.

The treatment of cancer is directed not only towards the tumour but also towards the patient. Attention to communication with the patient and relatives will ensure that morale is kept to the maximum. The patient should be encouraged to ask questions which must be answered expertly by an experienced member of the staff.

Involvement of family doctors, physicians and even psychiatrists (if needed) in specific parts of cancer management should be encouraged. Nurses, experts in nutrition and social workers all have their important roles to play, and they can often offer much help to the cancer patient.

Knowledge of the principles of cancer treatment is of value for all practitioners who may encounter patients with malignant disease, as well as for oncology specialists. It is worth emphasizing that the ideal way to defeat cancer is to prevent it, or at least to detect it early.

SURGERY OF CANCER

Surgery is the oldest approach to the treatment of malignant diseases, and is still regarded as the most successful method of treatment when the tumour is localized and resectable. However, malignant diseases are not truly localized in more than 60% of cases, so that only about one-third of patients can be cured by surgical excision alone.

The roles of surgery in cancer management are summarized here.

Diagnostic surgery

Surgical procedures are used to obtain specimens for histopathological diagnosis. This may involve a simple operation like excision biopsy of a small skin lesion, or a more major procedure like staging laparotomy in Hodgkin's disease. The various methods commonly used are:

1. *Needle aspiration biopsy.* A core of tissue is removed with a biopsy needle.
2. *Punch biopsy.* Small fragments are removed with forceps during endoscopic examination, for example in cases of lesion of the urinary bladder, oesophagus, stomach, colon or rectum.
3. *Incisional biopsy.* A small segment of the tumour, e.g. of skin or the oral cavity, is excised. The incisional site must be chosen carefully and preferably at the edge of the lesion to include a portion of the normal adjacent tissue as well as the tumour.
4. *Excisional biopsy.* Ideally all biopsies should be excisional, i.e. removal of the whole lesion, but this is not always possible. Excisional biopsy is employed in cases like small lesions of the skin

or breast, enlarged lymph nodes or metastatic nodules.

5. *Surgical exploration.* In certain cases, surgical exploration is needed to evaluate the extent of the disease, as in the case of a staging laparotomy in Hodgkin's disease. Sometimes re-exploration (second-look) is required to evaluate the effectiveness of other therapy, e.g. in cases of ovarian tumours.

Radical curative surgery

Radical local excision

Local excision of the tumour with an adequate margin of normal surrounding tissue is done when the tumour appears to be quite localized, e.g. basal cell carcinoma of the skin, and selected cases of small superficial rectal tumours. The surgeon's knife must pass through healthy tissues and the tract of any previous biopsy should be excised completely.

Radical monobloc excision

The tumour is excised en bloc along with the local draining lymph nodes and the intervening tissues, e.g. radical mastectomy for carcinoma of the breast, or abdominoperineal excision of carcinoma of the rectum.

Extended radical resection

Extensive procedures such as pelvic exenteration and hind-quarter amputation are employed when there is wide local infiltration without evident distant metastasis.

Palliative surgery

Palliative tumour resection or debulking of tumour mass

Local resection of an advanced tumour may relieve the patient of some distress, e.g. from fungating or ulcerated tumours. Reduction of the tumour bulk may give a better chance for other types of treatment such as radiotherapy and chemotherapy to be effective.

Excision of metastasis

This may sometimes be justified in selected cases when the primary tumour has been removed or is well controlled, and especially when the metastasis appears to be a solitary one, as occasionally arises in primary renal carcinoma, and for certain brain metastases.

Relief of obstruction

A tracheostomy for laryngeal obstruction, e.g. by carcinoma of the thyroid, may avert rapid death from asphyxia. A colostomy for lower bowel obstruction may relieve the distressing symptoms. A bypass operation for internal hydrocephalus caused by cerebral tumour may provide rapid relief of severe headache, nausea and vomiting.

Arterial ligation

This may be used either to stop bleeding, as in the ligation of the external carotid in cases of tumours of upper aerodigestive tract, or ligation of the hepatic artery to shrink metastatic deposits in the liver.

Palliative neurosurgical procedures

Cordotomy or posterior rhizotomy may be indicated in certain cases to relieve intractable pain.

Surgical procedures for hormonal ablation

Ovariectomy, adrenalectomy and hypophysectomy are examples of palliative ablative hormonal therapy, formerly used more frequently in attempts to control tumours which showed some degree of hormone dependence, especially carcinoma of the breast.

Plastic and reconstructive surgery

Plastic surgical procedures, sometimes quite extensive ones, may be required following radical excision of oral or head and neck tumours, and there is a resurgence of interest in early or immediate reconstruction of the breast after mastectomy.

Role of surgery in prevention

This includes the prophylactic excision of known premalignant disease, e.g. colectomy in familial polyposis coli, or removal of leukoplakia in the oral cavity.

BASIC PRINCIPLES OF RADIOTHERAPY

The science of oncology is concerned with the study of neoplastic diseases, and radiotherapy is one of its component branches, being concerned with the treatment of lesions—almost exclusively malignant ones—by means of ionizing radiations.

All the sources of radiation used in radiotherapy have the common property of producing ionization within the tissues. In practice, the ionizing radiations used are either electromagnetic or corpuscular.

1. *Electromagnetic radiation.* Both X-rays and gamma rays are electromagnetic waves with neither mass nor charge; they are photons. X-rays are produced by striking a target by moving electrons in X-ray machines. The movement of electrons is accelerated in betatrons or linear accelerators to produce X-rays of high energy. Gamma radiations are emitted during the decay of radioactive isotopes, e.g. radium, cobalt 60, caesium and iridium.
2. *Corpuscular radiations.* These include mainly beta particles, e.g. neutrons and protons, and also alpha particles and pimesons.

   Beta particles (which are electrons) are emitted during the decay of radioactive isotopes. Electrons are also produced in betatrons and linear accelerators.

Radiobiological basis

Not all details of the modes of action of ionizing radiations on living tissues are known. However, most of the effects are likely to be due to radiochemical phenomena. The main target of action is the nucleus, and in particular the DNA. Ionizing radiations cause rupture of one or both strands of DNA and modify the bases—adenine, cytosine, guanine and thymine. As a result the cell loses its ability to reproduce itself. Radiation also causes thrombosis and endarteritis obliterans, with subsequent ischaemia and tissue damage.

Therapeutic ratio, radiosensitivity and radiocurability

The difference in sensitivity between malignant and normal tissues is referred to as the therapeutic ratio.

Since the aim of radiotherapy is to increase the damage to malignant tissues and avoid, or at least decrease, the damage to normal tissues, many techniques have been developed to improve the therapeutic ratio. Fractionation of treatment over a period of time, for example 4–6 weeks, will allow some recovery of exposed cells after each dose, and this recovery is likely to be greater for normal cells than for the malignant ones. Hyperfractionation, which means multiple small doses of irradiation per day; the use of hyperbaric oxygen; radiosensitizers (such as metronidazole and misonid-zole); hyperthermia and the application of high-linear-energy transfer radiations as neutrons, protons and pimesons are all methods which increase the radioresponsiveness and improve the therapeutic ratio.

Radiosensitivity is the sensitivity of that particular type of tissue to irradiation, and one of the most important factors influencing this, as far as malignant cells is concerned, is the histological type of the tumour. Squamous carcinoma, anaplastic tumours, embryonic tumours and lymphomas are regarded as relatively radiosensitive tumours, whereas adenocarcinomas are less sensitive to radiotherapy. Soft-tissue sarcomas, osteosarcoma and melanomas are largely radioresistant tumours, within the range of therapeutic dosage.

For normal tissues, embryonic tissues, gonads, lymphocytes, and bone marrow are sensitive to the effects of irradiation, whereas connective tissues, bone and muscles are relatively radioresistant within the range of doses normally used in radiotherapy.

The unit of absorbed dose is the gray (Gy): each gray represents the absorption of 1 joule (unit of energy) per kilogram of tissues. The gray is equal to 100 rad.

In general, curative doses for malignant lesions vary from 50 to 70 Gy, delivered usually over 5–7 weeks. The dose is generally less in Hodgkin's disease and seminoma, and for palliative treatment.

Modes of application of radiation therapy

There are two main modes—external and internal.

External irradiation

The beam of irradiation is directed from an external source at tissue volumes in the body. The energy of radiation beams of similar type determines its depth of penetration into tissues. For superficial lesions where little penetration is required beams of low energy are enough, but for deeply situated lesions high energy is needed (Fig. 10.1).

Granz ray machines. Their energy is about 10–40 kV; they produce rays of little penetration and are therefore used in the treatment of very superficial non-malignant skin lesions.

Superficial X-ray machines (contact therapy). These can produce rays within the range of 50–140 kV and are used to treat superficial malignant skin lesions such as squamous cell carcinoma and basal cell carcinoma.

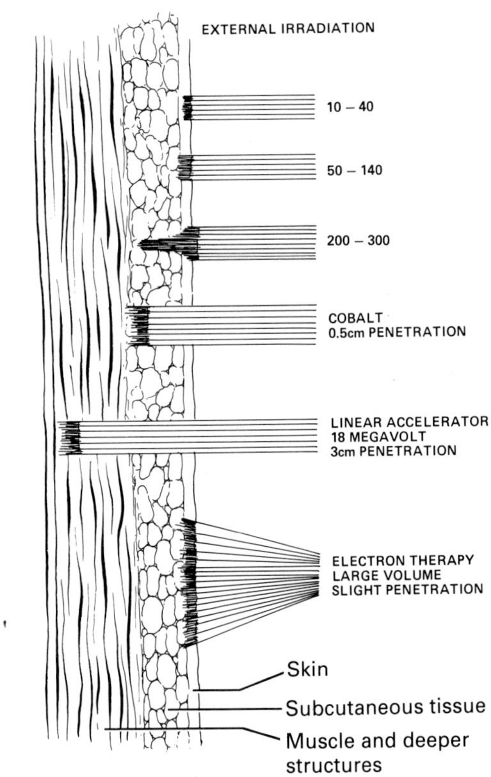

Fig. 10.1 Pattern of penetration from different strengths and sources of external irradiation.

Deep X-ray machines (orthovoltage). These give rays with an energy range of 200–300 kV. For many years they were the standard equipment in radiotherapy departments, but have now been largely replaced by megavoltage equipment which produces rays of higher energy. Deep X-ray therapy is still used in the treatment of lesions situated close to the skin.

Cobalt machines. These produce gamma rays with an average energy output of 1.25 mV (million volts). Radioactive cobalt is contained within a lead shield in the head of the machine. The radioactive cobalt source has to be changed about every 5 years.

Linear accelerators. These produce X-rays of high energy (megavoltage rays). Some models produce electron beams of therapeutic use in addition to X-rays.

Advantages of using megavoltage rays

1. The skin-sparing effect: in deep X-ray therapy (200–300 kV), the maximum dose is received on the skin surface, so the skin reaction is usually of severe nature up to radiation burns. Using megavoltage rays, the maximum dose is received at some distance below the skin surface; the distance varies according to the energy used. With cobalt therapy this distance is about 0.5 cm, while in the case of a linear accelarator producing rays with an energy of 18 mV, the distance is about 3 cm, so that the risk of radiation damage to the skin is reduced to a large extent.
2. There is less bone absorption, and therefore the incidence of radio bone necrosis is diminished.
3. A more sharply collimated beam is obtained, with less penumbra outside the field. This is a particularly marked feature in the case of the linear accelerator, the advantage being that hazards to vital organs close to the field of irradiation can be reduced.

Electron therapy. Electrons are produced by betatrons or linear accelerators. The penetration in tissues is generally very slight, depending on the energy of the electrons. This form of treatment is used for skin lesions with volumes larger than can be conveniently treated by contact X-ray therapy.

Other. There are other types of external beams which are not widely used at present, such as neutron therapy, proton therapy and pimesons.

Internal irradiation (brachytherapy)

Radioactive elements such as radium, caesium or iridium are inserted directly into the tissue (interstitial brachytherapy) or into body cavities (intra-cavitary brachytherapy; Fig. 10.2).

In addition, some isotopes may be used as colloid suspensions or as soluble compounds introduced into body cavities, or given by systemic injection. An example of intracavitary use is in the treatment of malignant pleural effusions, and of systemic use is the selective absorption by tumour tissue after intravenous injection of iodine 131 in cancer of the thyroid.

Interstitial brachytherapy. Implantation of radium or iridium for the time calculated to deliver the desired dosage (usually a few days) is employed in the treatment of many lesions. There are different techniques of implantation, including the use of plastic tubes, hypodermic needles and various patterns of applicators, e.g. for tumours of the tongue and floor of the mouth.

In the conservative treatment of breast cancer brachytherapy may be employed as an alternative to cobalt or electron therapy, to deliver a booster dose to the tumour bed after tumorectomy and megavoltage irradiation of the breast.

Other tumours which may be suitable for this

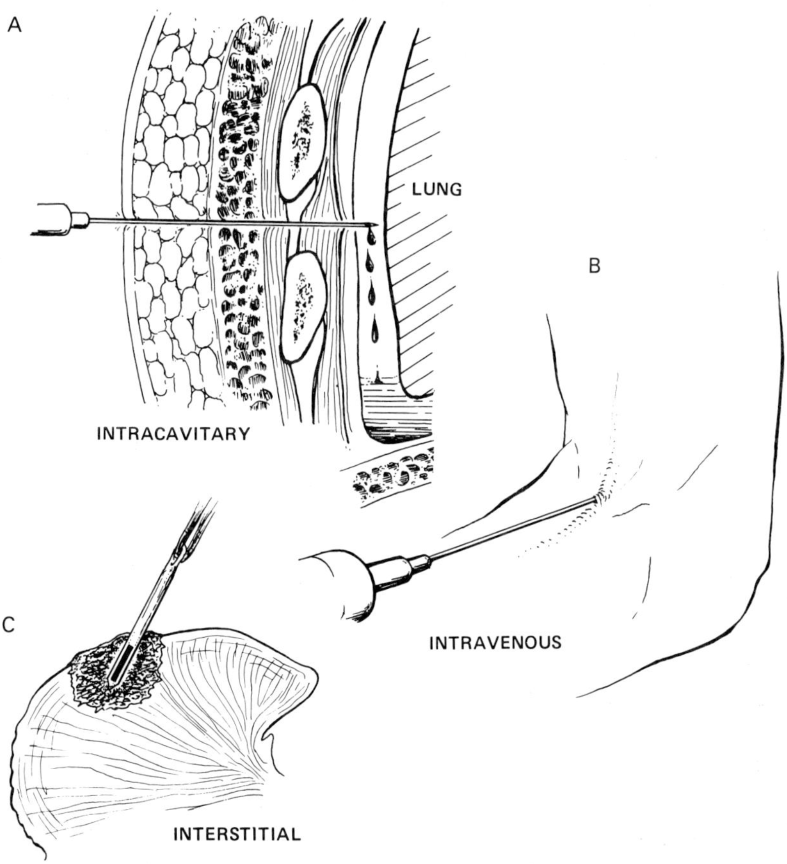

Fig. 10.2 Internal irradiation may be delivered by giving radioactive isotopes (**A**) by instilling the isotope in solution into a body cavity, e.g. the pleural cavity; (**B**) intravenously, when selective uptake by the target tissue follows, e.g. iodine for thyroid tumours, or (**C**) interstitially, by implanting needles or capsules containing the isotope directly into the malignant tissue.

form of treatment include squamous and basal cell carcinoma of the skin, tumours of the penis and urethra, selected cases of small urinary bladder tumours, especially epidermoid carcinoma, and certain anorectal tumours. Carcinoma of the prostate is sometimes managed by the permanent introduction of radioactive gold grains into the malignant tissue.

Intracavitary brachytherapy. A good example is the insertion, for a calculated time period, of a radioactive radium or caesium source in cancer of the cervix or uterine body. This may be used as either preoperative brachytherapy or in combination with external irradiation.

Indications for radiotherapy in the management of cancer

Radiotherapy is used with the intention of cure in clinical circumstances where the tumour can be included in a reasonable volume, e.g. stages I and II of cancer of the cervix; stages I and II of cancer of the larynx; tumours of the anterior two-thirds of tongue, and floor of the mouth; stages I–III Hodgkin's disease and non-Hodgkin's lymphoma, and squamous and basal cell carcinoma of the skin.

Radiotherapy should be preferred when it offers a high chance of local eradication, or the same rate as surgical excision, but with a lower morbidity or better functional results.

Preoperative irradiation may be used to reduce the tumour volume so that surgical excision becomes easier. Sometimes it may convert an inoperable tumour to an operable one. It may also reduce the probability of dissemination of viable cancer cells during the operation.

Postoperative irradiation is indicated in cases where it has not been possible completely to remove the malignant tissue surgically because of its local extension, adhesions, etc. Postoperative radiotherapy can also reduce the risk of local or regional recurrence, for example following mastectomy in cases of cancer of the breast.

Palliative radiotherapy is used in incurable cancer patients who have localized manifestations that can be relieved (even partially) by radiotherapy. It is employed, for example, to relieve the pain arising from bony metastases, or to relieve dyspnoea in mediastinal compression due to a malignancy. Urgent radiotherapy may be required to relieve spinal cord compression. In general, the dose used in palliation is about half to two-thirds of the dose used for curative treatment but in certain circumstances, the required dose may be as great as the curative dose.

In addition to its applications in the treatment of malignancy, radiotherapy may also be beneficial for some benign disorders, e.g. keloid formation, cutaneous warts, angiomas, and to suppress glandular function in subacute parotitis and in subacute thyroiditis.

Side-effects of radiotherapy

The reactions of any tissue to radiation usually occur when it is within the irradiated field, and rarely by diffused rays. The reactions in rapidly renewing cells, e.g. in skin or intestinal mucosa, will appear early—within days—and will usually also heal in a short time, while radiation reactions in other tissues, e.g. the brain, may not become manifest for months or years.

Within the range of curative doses, 60–70 Gy delivered in 6–7 weeks, skin reaction first becomes evident between 2 and 3 weeks from the beginning of treatment, as erythema and then as dry desquamation and finally as moist desquamation. These reactions reach their height at the end of treatment, and usually subside within 1 month of treatment.

Depilation may occur during the third week. Following low doses it is usually reversible, but may be permanent after high doses. Skin reactions should be managed from the start of radiation therapy; the irradiated skin is kept dry, and patients are advised to avoid irritant soaps, antiseptics, perfumes and exposure to direct sunlight. If moist desquamation develops, the local application of aqueous gentian violet or aqueous eosin 1% is recommended. Steroid ointment is especially useful for lesions near the eye.

Reactions in other epithelial tissues include:

1. discomfort and soreness of buccal cavity, with perhaps superadded monilial infection, for which alkaline mouthwashes or antimonilial agents, e.g. mycostatin, may be required;
2. dysphagia from damage to the pharynx and

larynx, for which preprandial local anaesthetics may be helpful;

3. diarrhoea resulting from mucous reactions of the bowel—this is often ameliorated by non-specific antidiarrhoeal agents such as codeine phosphate or loperamide;
4. dysuria from bladder mucosal reactions—in which case a satisfactory urine output should be maintained by sufficient oral intake of fluids; an appropriate antibiotic will be required if frank infection also occurs.

The salivary glands are affected by direct exposure to radiation therapy, and aberration of taste and dryness of mouth are common resulting complaints. These may persist for a year or so and then gradually regress, but with high doses they may remain permanently. Radiation affecting the gums can predispose to dental caries. Any diseased tooth should be extracted before radiation is applied to the mouth.

The radiation sickness syndrome, with its manifestations of nausea, vomiting, and general lassitude, is more marked when a large volume of tissue is irradiated, and especially when the upper abdomen is included within the radiation field.

The haemopoietic tissues are particularly susceptible to the effects of radiation, but a serious fall in the number of circulating leukocytes, platelets and red blood cells rarely occurs unless a large volume of bone marrow is irradiated.

The lens of the eye is very sensitive to irradiation, and cataract formation is seen following even small doses.

The ovaries are also particularly affected by exposure to irradiation, and doses of between 5 and 15 Gy lead to the disappearance of oestrogen production, the cessation of menstruation, and therefore an artificial menopause. In males, complete sterility without impotence is a side-effect of testicular irradiation. Androgen levels and secondary sexual characteristics, however, remain unaffected.

Finally, radiation can produce a teratogenic and an oncogenic effect (radiocancer) in some tissues, with a prolonged latent period of about 10–25 years before the signs become manifest.

Table 10.1 Classification of commonly used chemotherapeutic agents by derivation and/or mechanism of action

Alkylating agents	*Antibiotics*
BiCNU (one of the nitrosoureas)	Actinomycin D (Cosmegen Lyovac)
Busulphan (Myleran, Misulban)	Doxorubicin hydrochloride (Adriablastine, Adriamycin)
Lomustine, (CCNU, Belustine, one of the nitrosoureas)	Bleomycin (Blenoxane)
Chlorambucil (Leukeran)	Daunomycin (Daunorubicin)
Cyclophosphamide (Endoxana, Cytoxan)	Mithramycin (Mithracin)
DTIC (Decarbazine, Deticene)	Mitomycin (Mitomycin C Kyowa)
Mechlorethamine (nitrogen mustard)	
Melphalan (Alkeran)	*Alkaloids*
Thiotepa	Vinblastine (Velban, Velbe)
	Vincristine (Oncovin)
	Vindesine (Eldisine)
Antimetabolites or structural analogues	VM 26
Folic acid antimetabolites	VP 16123 (Vepzide)
Methotrexate (Amethopterin)	*Miscellaneous*
Purine antimetabolites	L-Asparaginase
Allopurinol (Zyloric)	Cisplatinum
Azathiaprine (Imuran)	Glucocorticoids
6-Mercaptopurine (Puri-Nethol)	Hydroxyurea (Hydrea)
Pyrimidine antimetabolites	Procarbazine (Matulane, Natulan)
Cytosine arabinoside (Cytosar, cytarabine)	
5-Fluorouracil (fluorouracil)	

CANCER CHEMOTHERAPY

Plant extracts and chemicals were used empirically in the treatment of cancer by the ancient Egyptians, the Chinese, the Greeks and the Romans. In the 19th century Billroth used arsenic in the treatment of lymphomas. Only in the last four decades, however, has chemotherapy developed on a proper scientific basis.

Classification of cancer chemotherapeutic agents

The commonly employed method of classifying cancer chemotherapeutic agents is based on either the source of the drug or its general mechanism of action (Tables 10.1 and 10.2). The groups most commonly used are described below.

Alkylating agents

These are highly reactive compounds characterized by alkyl side-chains which form covalent bonds with nucleophilic groups within the cell. This chemical union leads to defects in intracellular metabolism and hence cell death may result.

Antimetabolites or structural analogues

These agents interfere with normal cellular metabolism either by inhibiting specific enzymatic steps or by being substituted for normal metabolites, thereby resulting in end-products which prevent cell division.

Antibiotics

These agents are natural products of various bacterial and fungal species, and they interfere with

Table 10.2 Dosage and toxicity of cancer chemotherapeutic agents when used as single agent

Chemotherapeutic agents	Usual adult dosage	Toxicity
Alkylating agents		
BiCNU	100 mg/m^2 per day i.v. for 2 days every 6 weeks	Nausea, vomiting Leukopenia and thrombocytopenia Rarely, hepatic and renal toxicity
Busulphan (Myleran)	2–8 mg/m^2 per day orally	Delayed bone marrow depression Cutaneous pigmentation (occasionally) Amenorrhoea Rarely, pulmonary fibrosis
Lomustine (CCNU)	120 mg/m^2 orally every 6 weeks	Nausea and vomiting Leukopenia and thrombocytopenia Rarely, hepatic toxicity
Chlorambucil (Leukeran)	3–4 mg/m^2 per day orally then the dose is adjusted according to the tolerance	Bone marrow depression
Cyclophosphamide	300 mg/m^2 per day i.v. (or i.m.) for 4 days every 3–4 weeks or 1000 mg/m^2 i.v. single dose every 3 weeks *or* orally 100 mg/m^2 for 10 days every 3–4 weeks	Nausea and vomiting Bone marrow depression Alopecia Haemorrhagic cystitis Immunosuppression
DTIC (Decarbazine)	200 mg/m^2 per day i.v. for 5 days every 3–4 weeks	Nausea and vomiting Bone marrow depression
Mechlorethamine	6–10 mg/m^2 per day i.v.	Nausea and vomiting Bone marrow depression Local corrosive action

Table 10.2 *(Continued)*

Chemotherapeutic agents	Usual adult dosage	Toxicity
Melphalan	2 mg/m² per day orally for 4–7 days every 2-4 weeks	Occasionally nausea and vomiting Bone marrow depression Acute leukaemia may develop in about 5% of patients receiving prolonged therapy
Thiotepa	5 mg/m² per day i.v. (or i.m.) for 4 days every 3–4 weeks *or* 10 mg/m² intrapleural or intraperitoneal	Bone marrow depression even by the intrapleural and intraperitoneal routes
Antimetabolites		
Methotrexate	40–60 mg/m² per day i.v. every week *or* 20–25 mg i.m. twice weekly *or* 2.5–5 mg/day orally for 6–7 days *or* 15 mg intrathecally weekly or every other week for 4 doses	Bone marrow depression Mycotic infection of buccal cavity Hepatic toxicity Neurotoxicity Renal toxicity (antidote: folinic acid)
Allopurinol (supportive agent for prevention or relief of hyperuricaemia)	300–500 mg/day orally	It may enhance the effect and toxicity of mercaptopurine when used in combination
6-Mercaptopurine	60–100 mg/m² per day orally	Bone marrow depression Hepatotoxicity Immunosuppression, particularly when used with methotrexate
Cytosine arabinoside	100 mg/m² per day for 5 days given by continuous i.v. infusion or in divided doses s.c. or i.v. every 8 h *or* 300 mg/m² per day given by continuous i.v. infusion every 4 days *or* may be given intrathecally	Nausea and vomiting Bone marrow depression
5-Fluorouracil	500 mg/m² per day i.v. for 3–5 days every 3–4 weeks	Nausea and vomiting Bone narrow depression Stomatitis Gastrointestinal ulceration Alopecia
Antibiotics		
Actinomycin D	0.3–0.5 mg/m² per day i.v. for 5 days every 10–15 days	Nausea and vomiting Stomatitis Gastrointestinal upset Bone marrow depression Alopecia
Doxuribicin hydrochloride (Adriamycin)	40–60 mg/m² per day i.v. every 3–4 weeks to a maximum total dose of 500–550 mg	Nausea and vomiting Cardiotoxicity Local corrosive action Alopecia Bone marrow depression
Bleomycin	10–15 mg/m² per day i.v. or i.m. every 2–3 weeks to a maximum total dose of 200–250 mg	Allergic reactions Hypotension Fever Dermatitis Pulmonary fibrosis

Table 10.2 *(Continued)*

Chemotherapeutic agents	Usual adult dosage	Toxicity
Daunomycin	20-30 mg/m^2 per day i.v. for 2–3 days every 7 or 15 days *or* 20 mg/ m^2 per day for 2 days every 4 weeks	Fever Nausea and vomiting Red urine (not haematuria) Local corrosive action Stomatitis Cardiotoxicity Bone marrow depression Alopecia
Mitomycin	6–10 mg/m^2 per day i.v. every week *or* 2–5 mg/m^2 per day i.v. for 5 days every 3 weeks *or* 20 mg/m^2 per day i.v. every 6 weeks	Nausea Local corrosive action Gastrointestinal upset Bone marrow depression
Alkaloids		
Vinblastine	5 mg/m^2 per day every week or 10 mg/m^2 per day every 15 days	Nausea and vomiting Local corrosive action Alopecia Bone marrow depression Loss of reflexes
Vincristine	1–1.5 mg/m^2 per day every week (maximum 2 mg weekly) *or* 1.5 mg/m^2 per day every 3–4 weeks	Arreflexia Muscle weakness Peripheral neuritis Convulsions Paralytic ileus Alopecia Local corrosive action
VM 26 VP 16123	100 mg/m^2 per day i.v. every 2–3 weeks *or* 50 mg/m^2 per day i.v. for 4 days every 2–3 weeks	Gastrointestinal upset Bone marrow depression
Miscellaneous		
L-Asparaginase	200 mg i.u./kg per day i.v. or i.m. daily for 2–4 weeks	Allergic reactions Fever Hepatotoxicity Pancreatitis
Cisplatinum	50–75 mg/m^2 per day i.v. every 3–4 weeks	Nausea and vomiting Nephrotoxicity Ototoxicity Neurotoxicity Bone marrow depression
Hydroxyurea	1-2 g/m^2 daily, orally *or* 3–6 g/m^2 per day orally every 3 days	Nausea and vomiting Bone marrow depression
Procarbazine (Matulane)	100–150 mg/m^2 per day orally or i.v. for 14 days	Nausea and vomiting Bone marrow depression Abdominal pain Mental depression Skin rashes

cellular metabolism in different ways, some by binding to nucleic acids, e.g. adriamycin and actinomycin D, and others by disruption of DNA, e.g. bleomycin.

Alkaloids

This group is composed of extracts from plants. Vincristine and vinblastine are derived from the periwinkle plant (Vinca rosa). The main site of their action is at the metaphase of mitosis, most probably by their toxic effect on the microtubules of the mitotic spindles.

Miscellaneous

This heterogeneous group includes drugs that do not fit any of the above categories. Among them, listed in Table 10.1, are glucocorticoids, which seem to have a non-specific effect on some tumours, and are often used in combination chemotherapy, particularly of leukaemia and lymphomas.

Cell cycle, kinetics and chemotherapy

A replicating cell begins its life sequence at the end of mitosis (M). Then it passes through different phases, G_1, S and G_2 and then it starts another mitotic event (Fig. 10.3).

The G_1 phase is the period during which many cells express their particular differentiated functions and most cells can be recognized under the microscope.

The S phase is the period during which the cells synthesize DNA and double their chromosomal complement: at the end of this phase there will be 92 chromosomes.

The G_2 phase is the period during which the biochemical preparations for mitosis are done.

The M phase is subdivided to prophase, metaphase, anaphase and telophase. During this period, the cell divides to yield two daughter cells.

After mitosis (M) there is normally a resting phase, G_0, and cells are regarded as out of cycle. Under certain circumstances, however, they may be brought back to the G_1 of the cell cycle.

The growth fraction is the fraction of cells that are in cycle (proliferating cells).

Most chemotherapeutic agents affect specifically proliferating cells (cells in cycle) and they are classified as cell cycle-specific agents. Some agents affect only proliferating cells in a certain phase and they are classed as phase-specific agents. As examples, vincristine and vinblastine affect cells in the M phase, whereas cytosine arabinoside acts at the S phase.

There are a few drugs that can affect both resting and dividing cells and these are classed as cell cycle-non-specific agents. Mechlorethamine is an example of this group.

The growth of a tumour follows gompertzian kinetics, i.e. when the number of cells is plotted on a logarithmic scale against time on a linear scale, the increase in tumour cells will initially be a straight line because the tumour has a short doubling time (Fig. 10.4). After a period of time the increase in growth will tend to level out.

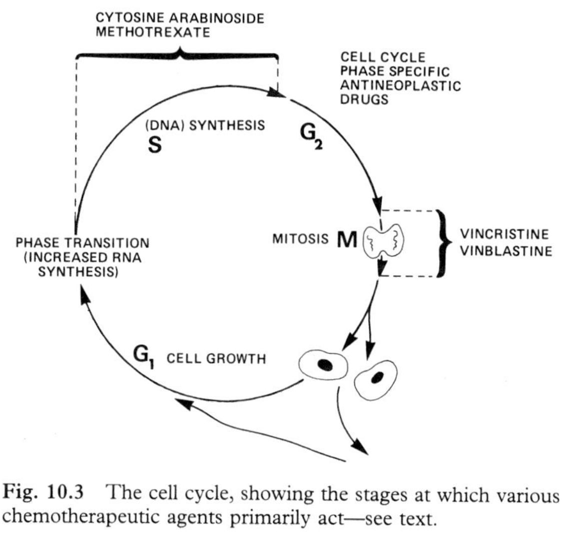

Fig. 10.3 The cell cycle, showing the stages at which various chemotherapeutic agents primarily act—see text.

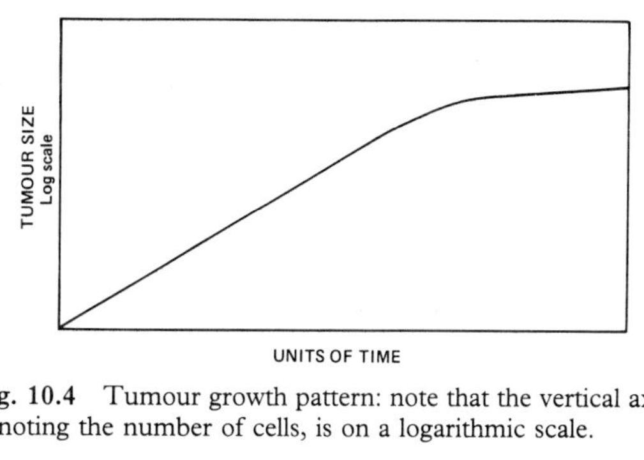

Fig. 10.4 Tumour growth pattern: note that the vertical axis, denoting the number of cells, is on a logarithmic scale.

Thus, the smaller the tumour mass, the greater is the fraction of cells that are in a growth cycle and therefore vulnerable to chemotherapeutic agents. In addition, when the tumour is large some areas may outstrip their vascular supply so that the permeation of chemotherapeutic agents to the malignant cells may be less efficient than in smaller tumours. Debulking of big tumours by surgery or by radiotherapy may therefore increase the efficacy of chemotherapy.

A tumour of 1 ml contains about 10^9 cells. Below this number of cells, the tumour mass is unlikely to be detected clinically, yet it is during this period that chemotherapy is likely to be most effective.

Single-agent and combination chemotherapy

Although at first chemotherapeutic agents were administered singly, it is now usual practice to give several as a schedule of combination chemotherapy, and this approach has several advantages:

1. A decrease in the incidence of side-effects by using drugs with different mechanisms of action.
2. An increase in the effectiveness of chemotherapy by using drugs with synergistic effects.
3. A decrease in the likelihood of resistance to chemotherapy arising.

Combination chemotherapy is usually given every 3–4 weeks to allow bone marrow recovery between courses of treatment.

Routes of administration of chemotherapy

1. *Systemic.* Most commonly used is the intravenous route, either by a bolus injection or by continuous infusion. Less commonly used are the intramuscular route, e.g for methotrexate or bleomycin, and the subcutaneous route, e.g. for cytosine arabinoside for acute myelocytic leukaemia. The oral route is convenient for the administration of some drugs, e.g. melphalan, cyclophosphamide, procarbazine and nitrosoureas.
2. *Intracavitary.* In cases of malignant pleural effusions and malignant ascites, intracavitary instillation of nitrosoureas, bleomycin or thiotepa can be used.
3. *Intrathecal.* Occasionally methotrexate is given by this route in acute leukaemia.
4. *Intra-arterial infusion.* This may be used in an effort to kill tumour cells selectively within the infusion field with much fewer systemic effects.

Indications for chemotherapy

Chemotherapy has the objective of possible cure in certain patients with testicular tumours, lymphomas, choriocarcinoma and acute leukaemia (Table 10.3).

Palliation may be achieved by chemotherapy in certain advanced disseminated tumours; relief is obtained from distressing symptoms in addition to prolongation of survival, e.g. in advanced Hodgkin's disease, non-Hodgkin's lymphoma, multiple myeloma, breast cancer, ovarian tumours, endometrial carcinoma, acute leukaemia, Ewing sarcoma and soft-tissue sarcoma.

Common side-effects of chemotherapy

Gastrointestinal and mucosal problems

Some of the agents used in cancer therapy may cause anorexia, nausea, vomiting and/or diarrhoea (Table 10.4). In many the symptoms may be controlled by reassurance and the administration of drugs such as prochlorperazine and metoclopramide for vomiting and codeine phosphate or loperamide for diarrhoea. However, where these symptoms persist or increase in severity, they are problems due to the effect of the drugs on the rapidly dividing epithelial cells of the mucosa wall of the gastrointestinal tract, and consideration has to be given to withdrawal of the agent or agents. If drug treatment is later reintroduced, it should be done so cautiously.

Oral infection with monilial organisms is fairly common during chemotherapy, and usually responds to local nystatin.

Myelosuppression, immunosuppression and infection

With few exceptions (e.g. vincristine and bleomycin), chemotherapeutic agents are myelosuppressive, and leukopenia and thrombocytopenia are quite common and vary in severity. Drug-induced

Table 10.3 Malignancies responsive to chemotherapy

Disease	Examples of the current treatment of choice	Other valuable agents
Acute lymphocytic leukaemia	*Induction*: vincristine plus prednisone *Maintenance*: Methotrexate, 6-mercaptopurine, cyclophosphamide	L-Asparaginase, adriamycin, daunomycin, VM 26, BiCNU, allopurinol (supportive agent)
Acute myelocytic leukaemia	Daunomycin, cytosine arabinoside and thioguanine or adriamycin, cytosine arabinoside plus prednisone and allopurinol (supportive agent)	Methotrexate, 6-mercaptopurine, allopurinol (supportive agent)
Chronic myelocytic leukaemia	Busulphan (Myleran)	Vincristine, melphalan, 6-mercaptopurine, cytosine arabinoside, hydroxyurea, allopurinol (supportive agent)
Chronic lymphocytic leukaemia	Chlorambucil (Leukeran)	Vincristine, adriamycin, allopurinol (supportive agent)
Hodgkin's disease	MOPP: mechlorethamine, vincristine (Oncovin), procarbazine and prednisone	ABVD: adriamycin, bleomycin vinblastine and DTIC-Pomustine, VM 26
Non-Hodgkin's lymphoma	COP: cyclophosphamide, vincristine and prednisone *or* CHOP: cyclophosphamide, adriamycin, vincristine, and prednisone	VEB: VM 26, cyclophosphamide, lomustine (Belustine) and prednisone VP 16 Methotrexate
Multiple myeloma	Melphalan plus prednisone	Melphalan, cyclophosphamide and prednisone Cyclophosphamide, vincristine, procarbazine and prednisone
Squamous cell carcinoma of head and neck	MEV: methotrexate, cyclophosphamide (Endoxana) and vincristine ABEC: adriamycin, bleomycin, cyclophosphamide (Endoxana), Cisplatinum	Hydroxyurea, fluorouracil
Squamous cell carcinoma of lung	Bleomycin plus cisplatinum, cyclophosphamide, methotrexate and lomustine CAPEC: cisplatinum, adriamycin, lomustine (Belustine), vindesine (Eldisine) and cyclophosphamide (Endoxana)	VP 16123
Adenocarcinoma of lung	Cyclophosphamide, adriamycin plus fluorouracil	Mitomycin
Small cell lung cancer	VAME: VP 16123, adriamycin, methotrexate and cyclophosphamide	Bleomycin, lomustine, procarbazine and vincristine
Breast carcinoma	CMF: cyclophosphamide, methotrexate and fluorouracil Adriamycin, vincristine, cyclophosphamide and fluorouracil ± (chemotherapy)	Mitomycin, methotrexate and VM 26 Prednisone

Table 10.3 *(Continued)*

Disease	Examples of the current treatment of choice	Other valuable agents
Gastrointestinal adenocarcinoma	FAM: fluorouracil, adriamycin and mitomycin FAV: fluorouracil, adriamycin and vincristine	Hydroxyurea, lomustine.
Carcinoid tumour	Adriamycin and cyclophosphamide	Actinomycin D
Ovarian carcinoma	Adriamycin, cyclophosphamide, cisplatinum CAF: cyclophosphamide, adriamycin and fluorouracil CMF: cyclophosphamide, methotrexate, fluorouracil	Melphalan, bleomycin, vincristine, thiotepa, hexamethylmelamine, lomushine, chlorambucil, progestins
Carcinoma of cervix	ABC: adriamycin, bleomycin and cisplatinum Methotrexate, vincristine and cisplatinum	Cyclophosphamide, lomustine, chlorambucil, mitomycin, fluorouracil
Carcinoma of prostate	Oestrogens	Cisplatinum, adriamycin, fluorouracil, cyclophosphamide, prednisone, progestins
Testicular carcinoma	Bleomycin, vinblastine, and cisplatinum ± actinomycin D	Methotrexate, cyclophosphamide, adriamycin, mithramycin, chlorambucil, VP 16123
Insulinoma	Streptozocin	Adriamycin, fluorouracil, mitomycin
Choriocarcinoma	Methotrexate alone Methotrexate, vincristine, Methotrexate, vincristine and actinomycin D Vincristine, bleomycin, cisplatinum	Chlorambucil adriamycin, vinblastine, 6-mercaptopurine
Hypernephroma	Progestins	Hydroxyurea, VM 26, lomustine, prednisone, androgens
Osteosarcoma	Adriamycin, vincristine, methotrexate (with citrovorum factor), cyclophosphamide	Decarbazine, melphalan
Ewing sarcoma	Adriamycin, actinomycin D, vincristine, cyclophosphamide	Methotrexate, procarbazine
Soft-tissue sarcoma	Adriamycin, vincristine, Cyclophosphamide, DTIC Lomustine, vindesine, cisplatinum Methotrexate in high doses with citrovorum factor	Methotrexate, vinblastine, actinomycin D
Melanoma	DTIC and vincristine	Vinblastine, cisplatinum, lomustine, mitomycin, actinomycin D, adriamycin
Wilm's tumour	Actinomycin D, vincristine, adriamycin	Methotrexate, cyclophosphamide

Table 10.3 *(Continued)*

Disease	Examples of the current treatment of choice	Other valuable agents
Neuroblastoma	Adriamycin, vincristine, cyclophosphamide	Actinomycin D, cisplatinum
Carcinoma of adrenal	Mitotan	Adriamycin
Transitional cell carcinoma of urinary bladder	Adriamycin, vincristine, VM 26, fluorouracil Intravesical thiotepa for superficial lesions	Mitomycin C, cisplatinum
Glioblastoma	Lomustine, VM 26 Glucocorticoids	Procarbazine

Table 10.4 Side-effects of chemotherapy

Common	*Less common*
Nausea	Drug-induced anaemia
Vomiting	Hyperpigmentation
Diarrhoea	Allergic complications
Oral infection	Skin rashes
Leukopenia	Hypotension
Thrombocytopenia	Bronchospasm
Unusual infections	Hepatotoxicity
Alopecia	Nephrotoxicity
	Haemorrhagic cystitis
	Pulmonary fibrosis

anaemia is less common. The peripheral blood count should be monitored in all patients receiving these agents. In general, treatment is withdrawn if moderate or severe leukopenia or thrombocytopenia occurs, and reintroduced when adequate levels of leukocytes and platelets are regained. Profound leukopenia requires isolation of the patient in a sterile environment and prophylactic administration of antibiotics. Severe thrombocytopenia should be treated with infusion of platelet concentrates to minimize the chances of bleeding.

An important recent advance in the management of acute leukaemia is the use of bone marrow transplant after the total ablation of leukaemic marrow by radiotherapy or chemotherapy.

Chemotherapy may suppress both humoral and cellular immunity, but myelosuppression and immunosuppression should not always be attributed to the chemotherapy. The patient with widespread malignant disease may have suppression of the bone marrow and immune system from the malignant process itself. Infection may therefore arise as a result of either the cancer or the treatment. Cancer patients are also particularly susceptible to unusual infections such as *Pneumocystis carinii* and toxoplasmosis.

A further possible complication of prolonged immunosuppression or genetic damage caused by chemotherapeutic agents is the increased risk of a second cancer. This is more likely when the chemotherapy is also associated with radiotherapy.

Complications at the injection site

Most of the chemotherapeutic agents administered by the intravenous route are irritants and they may cause phlebitis. Extravasation may produce local pain, pruritis, erythema and, if the reaction is severe, ulceration and sloughing.

Alopecia

This distressing effect, which is commoner with some agents, e.g. cyclophosphamide, than with others, is due to depression of hair follicle growth cells. It is important to inform patients about the possibility of this occurring, and to reassure them that it is usually temporary.

Germinal cells and fetus

Partial or complete infertility of women and oligospermia and azoospermia can occur in men from cytotoxic agents. Chemotherapy must be avoided in pregnancy, especially in the first trimester, as it may cause fetal abnormalities.

Less frequent side-effects

Skin reactions

Cytotoxic drugs, like many others, can cause various types of skin rashes. Hyperpigmentation may appear after prolonged administration of busulphan or bleomycin.

Allergic complications

Hypersensitivity reactions to chemotherapy are usually manifested as skin rashes. Anaphylactoid reactions with hypotension and bronchospasm may occasionally occur.

Hepatic function

Hepatic toxicity is an occasional side-effect of many chemotherapeutic agents, e.g. methotrexate and antimetabolites. Liver function monitoring is recommended to detect early hepatic damage.

Renal and urinary bladder complications

The agent most commonly producing nephrotoxicity is cisplatinum. Cyclophosphamide may produce haemorrhagic cystitis.

Pulmonary disorders

Busulphan and bleomycin can cause serious pulmonary fibrosis. Interstitial pneumonitis is occasionally seen with methotrexate.

Cardiac complications

Adriamycin can cause a cardiomyopathy manifested as tachycardia and electrocardiogram changes.

Nervous system side-effects

Confusion, ataxia, irritability, coma or other signs and symptoms may arise with certain agents, and these are indications to discontinue the use of the drug. Motor and sensory neuropathies can be produced by several agents, notably vinca alkaloids.

Metabolic alterations

A wasting syndrome with hyperpigmentation resembling Addison's disease, but without the biochemical abnormalities, may be caused by busulphan. Hyperuricaemia is an early complication due to increased breakdown of host and tumour cells during chemotherapy, notably in acute leukaemia and lymphoma. Prophylactic administration of allopurinol and good hydration are required in these cases. Severe hyperuricaemia can cause serious uric acid nephropathy.

Hypercalcaemia is an unusual complication, except in cases when large segments of bone are involved, notably in breast cancer; it can usually be controlled by saline diuresis, frusemide and corticosteroid therapy.

HORMONAL THERAPY OF MALIGNANT TUMOURS

Hormonal therapy is usually used either as an adjuvant agent in a treatment schedule aimed at cure, or as a palliative treatment for advanced tumours.

The use of hormones in cancer therapy has been largely empirical, but was clearly initially introduced because some tumours arise in tissue which normally comes under the influence of certain hormones, e.g. the breast. On the other hand, tumours such as hypernephroma which do not have any obvious endocrine basis may yet exhibit a response to progesterone therapy.

The commonest tumours in which hormonal therapy is used are cancer of the breast, prostate, endometrium and renal cell. Corticosteroids are also often used in lymphomas, leukaemias and other tumours.

Hormonal therapy of breast cancer

The use of hormonal therapy in breast cancer became far less empirical after the detection of hormone receptors in breast cancer tissue. However, even when oestrogen receptors are present, as many as 40% of these patients may still not respond to hormonal therapy. The presence of other receptors such as for progesterone or glucocorticoids may increase the response predictability, but routine assays of these receptors are not widely applied as yet.

Additive hormonal therapy

Oestrogens. Ethinyloestradiol and diethylstilboestrol are the most commonly used oestrogens by the oral route. They are prescribed usually for menopausal females. Side-effects include mainly salt and water retention, which may aggravate congestive heart failure or hypertension, and an increased risk of clotting disorders—an important consideration in patients with a history of thromboembolic diseases. Other problems which may arise include hypercalcaemia, endometrial hyperplasia, nausea and vomiting, especially in the first 2 weeks of oral therapy.

Antioestrogens. Tamoxifen is the most commonly used antioestrogen in hormonal therapy of breast cancer. It gives regression in about 60% of postmenopausal patients having positive receptors, but it still gives a response in about 20–30% cases of negative receptors. Lesions in soft tissue such as the breast itself and the skin are more responsive than deposits in bone.

The usual dose of tamoxifen varies from 20 to 40 mg, and this is usually divided into two oral daily doses. Tamoxifen is generally well tolerated, with relatively uncommon side-effects such as hot flushes, nausea, mild leukopenia and thrombocytopenia, skin rashes and vaginal bleeding. About 10% of cases may elicit a hypercalcaemia, as seen also in oestrogen and androgen therapy.

Tamoxifen may stimulate biosynthesis of cytosalic receptors of progesterone, so that the sequential alternative administration of tamoxifen and progestins may be of value.

Progestins. The most commonly used preparations are megestrol acetate, medroxyprogesterone acetate and hydoxyprogesterone caproate. A response to progestins is observed in 20–45% of unselected menopausal patients with metastases, especially with soft-tissue lesions. The response is less frequent with bone and visceral metastasis. The treatment is in general well tolerated and the side-effects are uncommon but may include nausea and vomiting, salt and water retention, vaginal bleeding and occasionally hypercalcaemia.

Androgens. The most commonly used preparations are fluoxymesterone, testosterone propionate, dromostanolone propionate and testolactone.

Androgens are prescribed in both premenopausal and postmenopausal metastatic cases, especially with bone metastases, whereas cases with visceral and soft-tissue metastases respond to a lesser extent. The side-effects include nausea, vomiting, fluid retention and increased libido. The virilizing effects (acne, hirsutism, change of voice and body musculization) vary from one patient to another.

Glucocorticoids. The commonly used preparations are prednisone and dexamethasone. Administration of 10–40 mg prednisone daily usually gives a response in 10–15% of advanced metastatic cases but the detection of glucocorticoid receptors in the breast may improve the selection of cases for glucocorticoids therapy.

Ablative therapy

Ovariectomy

Surgical removal of both ovaries is often followed by a rapid response in premenopausal metastatic cases. Irradiation of the ovaries can achieve similar results and may be less traumatic, but its effect is less rapid than surgical castration. The dose required for ovarian ablation by irradiation is about 12 Gy delivered in 3–5 days by cobalt machine or linear accelerator.

Adrenalectomy

Surgical adrenalectomy has been used more frequently in the past as a palliative treatment for metastatic breast cancer. However, it is a major surgical operation, carrying high risks of mortality and morbidity, in patients who are often already ill and with a poor prognosis and is now difficult to justify.

Medical adrenalectomy, by the use of aminoglutethimide, inhibits the synthesis of oestrogens both in the adrenal glands and in the peripheral tissues. To counteract the consequent hypersecretion of adrenocorticotrophic hormone it is necessary to combine the aminoglutethimide with either dexamethasone or hydrocortisone. The latter is better as aminoglutethimide enhances the hepatic metabolism of dexamethasone. The most effective dose of aminoglutethimide seems to be 1000 mg/day accompanied by 40 mg/day hydrocortisone. If troublesome side-effects develop, e.g. nausea, dizziness, vertigo, lethargy or ataxia, the dose of aminoglutethimide may be reduced to 750 mg/day or less. After long-term therapy, thyroid-stimulating hormone is suppressed, so that thyroid hormone replacement is required.

A response to aminoglutethimide is seen in 25–40% of metastatic cases with positive hormonal receptors or who have previously responded to other hormonal therapy.

Hypophysectomy

Surgical hypophysectomy or ablation of the pituitary gland by the implantation of radioactive yttrium 90 has been used in the past, mostly for bone metastasis resistant to all other types of treatment. These procedures are now almost completely abandoned.

Endometrial carcinoma

Progestins are commonly used in the treatment of both locally recurrent and metastatic endometrial carcinoma. The response rate is about 40%. The action of the progestin may be directly on the endometrial tissues. The agents commonly used are the same as those used for cancer of the breast.

Prostatic carcinoma

Suppression of androgens either by orchiectomy or by oestrogen therapy is used as palliative treatment in patients with metastatic prostatic carcinoma.

Bilateral orchiectomy may cause psychic, social and emotional consequences, even in elderly patients. Oestrogen therapy is not free from complications, as it increases thromboembolic risk, and may lead to gynaecomastia, accumulation of fat in a feminine distribution, salt and water retention, hepatic toxicity, hypercalcaemia and unpleasant gastrointestinal manifestations such as nausea and vomiting.

Diethylstilboestrol and diethyl dioxystilbene are the commonly used oestrogenic agents. Diethylstilboestrol is given orally, the dose range being variable but preferably below 5 mg/day to decrease the risk of cadiovascular complications. Diethyl dioxystilbene diphosphate is given by intravenous injection and may be preferred where there is some degree of obstruction to urinary outflow.

Renal cell carcinoma (hypernephroma)

No apparent relation exists between renal carcinomas and the production or effects of endogenous or exogenous hormones. However, progestins appear to inhibit the growth of some hypernephromas. The response rate in advanced cases is about 20%. It may improve the quality of life and reduce bone pain due to metastases but its effect on overall survival rate seems to be insignificant.

Leukaemia and lymphoma

Glucocorticosteroids are used in combination with other chemotherapeutic agents in the management of Hodgkin's disease, non-Hodgkin's lymphoma and acute and chronic leukaemias.

IMMUNOTHERAPY OF CANCER

It has been observed that cancer patients develop humoral antibodies and cell-mediated immune reactions against the antigens of their neoplastic disease. The objective of immunotherapy is to enhance these immunological reactions on the assumption that the normal immunological defence has been unable to deal with the growing tumour. At present, the use of immunotherapy is of limited value. It does not replace the standard treatment of cancer and when it is used it should be after eradication of the tumour or at least after reduction of the tumour burden by other modalities of treatment. However, immunotherapy holds exciting promise for the future.

Methods of immunotherapy

Active immunotherapy

Specific. The use of irradiated tumour cells has been tried in acute myeloid leukaemia and in melanoma with some promising results. A cell-free, non-antigenic extract from the cellular response transfer factor has been employed in advanced carcinoma and melanoma, but its value is still not established.

Non-specific. BCG and Corynebacterium parvum vaccines are the most widely used forms of immunotherapy. Encouraging results have been reported in acute lymphoblastic, acute and chronic myeloblastic leukaemia, malignant melanoma and some other tumours.

Other forms of active non-specific immunotherapy have been used, e.g. levamisole, thymosine, poly A, poly U and interferon. However, their real values are still not established.

Passive immunotherapy

This consists of the administration of an antiserum prepared specifically against the tumour. This, however, may be dangerous as it may enhance the tumour growth by blocking the effective action of the lymphoid cells.

Adoptive immunotherapy

This implies the administration of foreign immunologically competent cells such as lymphoid cells. The only practical application of this approach currently being explored is in the case of bone marrow transplantation in acute leukaemia.

Local immunotherapy

The local injection of vaccines such as BCG directly into the tumour may reduce its size.

NUTRITION AND CANCER PATIENTS

Nutritional abnormalities are frequently observed in cancer patients. These abnormalities usually correlate with the stage of the disease and may become corrected with the successful control of the cancer. The malnutrition may cause the early death of the patient, even in the absence of damage to a vital organ by the malignant tissue.

Many factors may contribute to the decreased intake of food, and impaired digestion/absorption. Appetite may be diminished as a result of fear and other emotional problems about the disease. Anorexia, nausea, vomiting and diarrhoea may be side-effects from treatment by irradiation or chemotherapy.

Tumours of the gastrointestinal tract may cause dysphagia, obstruction, malabsorption, or excess loss from diarrhoea or fistula. Super-added infection may increase the metabolic and nutritional requirements.

Nutritional therapy may completely or at least partly correct the malnutrition in a certain percentage of patients, and thereby prolong survival. When the nutritional state is improved before or with radiotherapy and chemotherapy, this often strengthens the patient's resistance against side-effects from the treatment.

The ideal is to maintain feeding by the alimentary tract when this is intact. In certain cases feeding by nasogastric tube or gastrostomy is necessary. When there is bowel obstruction or severe malabsorption, total parenteral nutrition may be indicated.

11. Infection

Infection is the invasion of the body by pathogenic organisms, and the harmful local and general effects that this invasion produces. Three groups of organisms can cause infection—bacteria, viruses and fungi.

It must be emphasized that the mere presence of the pathogens in the body does not constitute infection. Many potentially dangerous organisms, e.g. tetanus bacilli, clostridia and *Escherichia coli,* may be present within organs of the body without producing harmful effects. It is only under certain circumstances that these bacteria can gain access to tissues and cause frank infection.

There are always two parties involved in the process—the pathogenic microbes and the patient. Infection cannot occur without the presence of pathogens, but some disturbance in the physiological state of the patient is necessary for the disease to develop.

Normally, there are inbuilt defence mechanisms in all living things which prevent the pathogens from producing harmful effects. These mechanisms have evolved so that survival in an atmosphere infested with organisms is possible. Our knowledge of these defences is incomplete, though many of the factors involved are understood. These range from reflexes which physically remove irritants from the body, such as scratching, coughing, sneezing and phagocytosis of organisms by the white blood cells, to the complex production of antibodies and other mechanisms of the immune system.

Factors which generally reduce the resistance of an individual to infection may be general or local.

General factors

These include congenital defects of gammaglobulin formation, hypoproteinaemia, diabetes mellitus and malignancy.

Local factors

Among the local factors are ischaemia, tissue damage, stagnation of visceral contents and haematoma formation.

The capacity of the microbes to cause disease depends upon:

1. transmissibility—the ability to move from one victim to another;
2. infectivity—the ability to break through the defences of the victim;
3. virulence—the capacity to cause damage to the host.

Pathogenic organisms liberate poisons which may cause damage to the host both locally and at a distance. These poisons or toxins are of two types—exotoxins and endotoxins. The former are produced and released by living pathogens, whereas endotoxins are harmful chemical substances contained within the microbes and are only released on their destruction. *Staphylococcus aureus, Streptococcus haemolyticus* and diphtheria bacilli are examples of the more important pathogens which liberate exotoxins. Gonococci, on the other hand, liberate endotoxins, while pneumococci produce both exo- and endotoxins.

Infection manifests itself in several ways.

Local

Locally a lesion may develop at the site of entry of the pathogens into the body. An inflammatory response is set up, which may or may not completely resolve. If resolution does not occur, an abscess, cellulitis or ulceration may develop, depending on the nature of the organism, the degree of the inflammatory response and the amount of local tissue damage.

Blood stream invasion

Microbes may invade the blood stream causing bacteraemia or septicaemia. The former signifies only the presence of organisms in blood and may be quite harmless, whereas septicaemia implies proliferation of the organisms in the blood and is an illness which may be very grave indeed.

Distant toxic effects

Harmful effects may be produced at a distance from the site of entry of the organisms by the liberation of toxins, as in tetanus.

Distant localized lesions

In this situation after initial invasion, at the site of which there may or may not have been a clinically detectable inflammatory reaction, a lesion is produced at a distance either by microbes travelling along lymphatic channels, as for example in tuberculosis of cervical lymph nodes, or by the invading organisms entering the blood stream and producing a lesion where they are deposited by the circulating blood, as in perinephric abscess or osteomyelitis.

There are two types of infections—specific and non-specific. In specific infections, one particular type of organism produces a specific lesion, which cannot be produced by any other organism. Tuberculous infection, tetanus and syphilis are examples. In non-specific infections, a number of organisms are capable of producing the same pattern of response, e.g. in appendicitis and osteomyelitis.

The important specific infections are described elsewhere, and this section is devoted to non-specific infections.

NON-SPECIFIC INFECTIONS

Non-specific infection may be acute or chronic.

Acute infections

In acute infection, an inflammatory process develops locally, and if the balance is in favour of the body defence against the pathogens, this acute inflammation subsides in a short time. This is probably a frequent occurrence.

However, if the toxins liberated by the bacteria are strong enough to cause considerable damage of the tissues and a number of cells, notably the leukocytes and monocytes mobilized to counteract the infection, a liquid collection of plasma, dead and living organisms and the dead cells is formed and is surrounded by an area of granulation tissue. This is an abscess, and the liquid content is pus.

Abscess

Pathogenesis. An abscess may develop in a number of ways. It may form as a result of direct implantation of bacteria at the site, as occurs for example in an injection abscess when pathogens enter the body with the prick of an unsterilized needle. Blood-borne infection may cause an abscess in any part of the body, and infection conveyed along the lymphatics may cause an abscess in the regional lymph node. The commonest organisms causing abscesses are staphylococcus and *E. coli*.

An abscess declares its presence by both local and general symptoms and signs. Locally, if the abscess is superficial, a painful tender, red, hot and possibly throbbing swelling develops, and fluctuation may be elicited if the tenderness is not so great as to prevent the appropriate examination. General features are malaise, anorexia, fever and tachycardia. A specific substance, pyrexin, produced at the site of the abscess probably acts on the temperature-regulating mechanism in the hypothalamus to produce the fever. Another substance, leukocidin, is also produced and in turn acts on the bone marrow to stimulate leukocytosis.

In deep-seated abscesses, like those in the brain, pelvis, or subdiaphragmatic region, pain may be absent, and the general rather than local clinical features are more prominent. In some locations, fluctuation may be difficult to elicit, partly because of depth, and partly because of the tension within the abscess, e.g. in some abscesses of the breast, the parotid gland, and the ischiorectal fossa.

Occasionally an abscess may resolve spontaneously. The products of inflammation are absorbed, as evidenced by decrease not only in the size of the swelling, but also in the intensity of signs and symptoms. Another uncommon outcome is the change of an acute abscess into a chronic one, the swelling persisting as a non-tender mass after the signs and symptoms of acute inflammation subside.

If left to itself, an abscess usually bursts, and until it does so or until the pus is evacuated surgically, signs and symptoms of acute infection, both local and general, persist. An undrained deep-seated abscess can pose a real threat to life from rupture into body cavities, toxaemia and vital organ failure.

Diagnosis. Usually, a diagnosis can be made on clinical grounds alone. Sometimes, however, special investigations are required to detect or to follow the progress of a deep-seated abscess. Needle aspiration is the simplest method of establishing a diagnosis whenever practicable. A plain X-ray may be sufficient to locate a paravertebral or subdiaphragmatic abscess or thoracic empyema. Ultrasonography has the merit of being a non-invasive and harmless technique and is often the most useful procedure both to locate and to follow the progress of a deep-seated abscess. Computerized tomography scanning is the most widely used and accurate method for the localization of a brain abscess. Radioactive isotopes are occasionally employed to localize some deep-seated lesions like those in the liver.

Evacuation of the pus is the treatment of an abscess, irrespective of the site or the organ involved. It is usually carried out through the most dependent part of the abscess cavity in such a way that all necrotic material and pus can escape. Appropriate antibiotics are usually also given, but antibiotics alone do not cure an abscess. Once pus is formed the pathogens in the middle of the cavity do not come in contact with systemic antibiotics. Moreover, the toxic chemicals in the abscess responsible for the fever, malaise and anorexia remain unaffected by these drugs, which are most effective only early in the cellular stage of infection.

Cellulitis. In between complete resolution and abscess formation, there are intermediate grades of inflammation, for example, infection of the subcutaneous tissue may not always result in abscess formation but may cause more diffuse inflammation, called cellulitis (Fig. 11.1). Here an area of tender red, hot swelling develops without the formation of pus. This pattern of response is more common in infection by certain types of bacteria, especially streptococci.

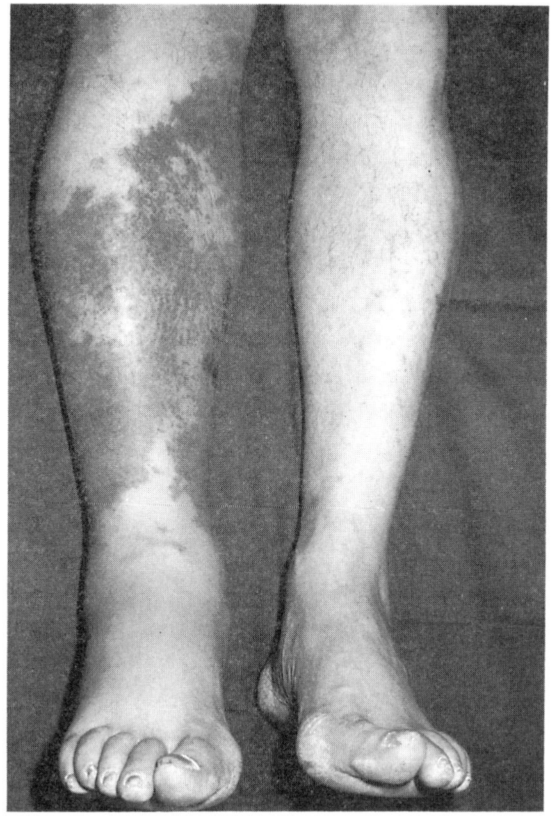

Fig. 11.1 Cellulitis from streptococcal infection in the right leg. There are widespread irregular patches of red inflammatory reaction in the skin, but these areas are not raised up from the skin surface. There is gross oedematous swelling of the lower leg, in contrast to the normal left leg.

Carbuncle (Figs 11.2 and 11.3). A carbuncle is a multi-loculated suppurative lesion of the subcutaneous tissue, mostly caused by staphylococcal infection. The most common site is in the nape of the neck, and many patients are diabetic. The skin of the involved part is red and shiny, and a slough forms in the centre, discharging thick pus. Around this area of central necrosis there may be many other openings.

Treatment consists of local drainage, improvement of the general health of the patient, and administration of an appropriate antibiotic selected on the basis of culture and sensitivity tests on

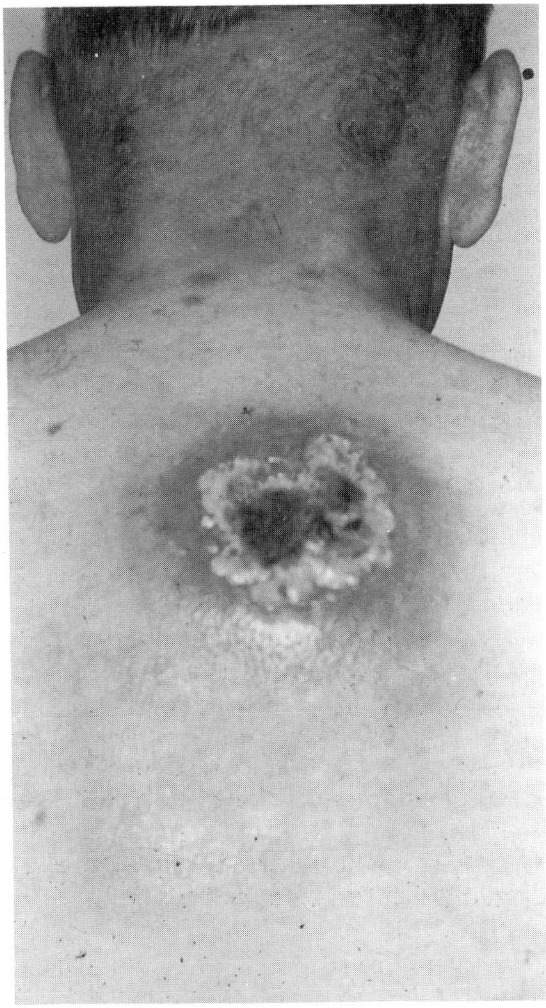

Fig. 11.2 Carbuncle. Usual site. Marked swelling involving a considerable area of subcutaneous tissue, and a large ulcer.

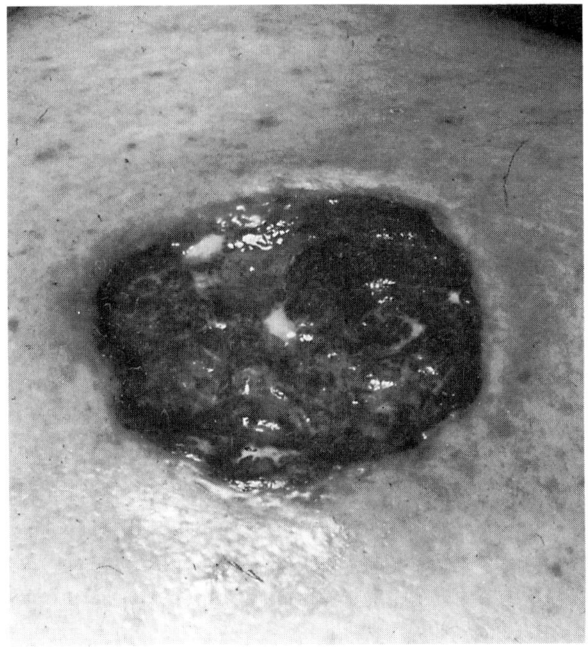

Fig. 11.3 Close-up of carbuncle at a later healing phase. There is little surrounding swelling, and islands of granulation tissue, with residual small pockets of pus. New skin is beginning to grow in from the edges.

samples of the pus. Usually one of the penicillins is found to be most effective.

Wound infection. Infection of surgical wounds has been a problem ever since the beginning of surgical practice. The acceptance of the antiseptic doctrine of Lister helped in reducing wound infection, and the introduction of antibiotics was a further signal advance. However, the hope that wound infection would be completely eliminated has not been fulfilled. Infection of clean wounds still occurs, though much less frequently. If organisms could be completely excluded from a surgical wound, infection would be prevented. This is the basic principle of the aseptic technique of surgery.

Sources of infection. The sources of infection of surgical wounds may be:

1. The patient.
2. The surgeon and team working in the operating theatre.
3. Instruments and materials used in the operation.
4. The environment of the operating theatre.
5. The environment and the occupants of surgical wards.

The patient. The source of infection may be a focus in the body of the patient, e.g. dental sepsis, septic tonsils, pneumonitis, an abscess or cellulitis, and no elective surgical procedures should be carried out on patients suffering from any such infective conditions if possible. Routinely, a wide area of the skin around the operation site is cleaned with antiseptic lotions just before starting the surgical procedure to eliminate any potential pathogenic organisms which may lie on the skin surface. In operating on the large intestine, an attempt is also made to reduce the number of pathogens to a minimum by preoperative preparation of the bowel by colonic wash-outs and administration of appropriate antibiotics.

The surgeon and team. As another possible source of infection is the surgeon and members of the team, all who are directly involved with the operation put on sterilized gowns and gloves after washing their hands and forearms in running water and bactericidal solution for a period of several minutes, and wear masks to minimize the bombardment of bacteria from their mouths and noses during talking, coughing and breathing. No member of the team known to be suffering from any infection is allowed into the operating theatre. Regular bacteriological tests are carried out to ensure that no member of the operating team is suffering from any infection.

Surgical instruments. The patient is completely covered with sterilized sheets. All the instruments used in the operation are sterilized beforehand.

Theatre environment. Disturbance of air in the theatre is reduced to a minimum by prohibiting unnecessary movements and talking. Ideally there should be a constant movement of air under positive pressure into the theatre so that invisible dust does not drop on the wounds. These measures are taken because there is good evidence that contamination of clean wounds by pathogens occurs primarily in the operating theatre.

During the operation, a minimum amount of trauma is inflicted. Tissues are handled and retracted gently by the surgical team and sharp dissection is carried out as far as possible to minimize tissue damage. In securing haemostasis, care is taken not to jeopardize the vascularity of the wound. The basic philosophy of operative surgery is to cause as little physiological and anatomical disturbance as possible.

Haematoma formation is avoided, as both the dead tissue and clotted blood form an ideal medium for the multiplication of organisms.

Too many sutures and suturing under tension are avoided to minimize pressure necrosis of the enclosed tissues and the production of foreign body reaction to the sutures.

Ward environment. In the wards, infection of clean, surgical wounds should not occur unless the wound surface is damaged or the patient develops a focus of infection elsewhere. To prevent this, the ward is kept free, as far as possible, from dust, and all nursing attention to wounds should be performed under careful sterile conditions. Patients with septic wounds should be isolated to diminish the chances of cross-infection to others with clean wounds.

If these principles are always followed, the rate of infection can be greatly reduced.

12. Tuberculosis

Tuberculosis is a specific infective disease caused by *Mycobacterium tuberculosis*. A hundred years ago, it was a very common disease with a high morbidity and mortality. With the general increase in the standard of living and social hygiene throughout the world, and thanks to the campaign of active immunization against the disease, the incidence of tuberculosis has sharply declined, so much so that in many parts of the world it has become a rarity. Nevertheless, it is still common among people living in poorer countries of the world.

Both sexes are equally susceptible, and no age is exempt from risk of infection. Very young children, especially those under the age of 2 years, and similarly the very old are very susceptible, and unless this is kept in mind, the condition may remain undiagnosed in areas where tuberculosis is still common.

Two types of *M. tuberculosis* are pathogenic to man—human and bovine, the former being more common in clinical practice.

Pathology

Tuberculosis can affect most organs of the body, but those most commonly affected are the lymphatic system, lungs, pleurae, pericardium, intestine, bones and joints, meninges, epididymis, kidneys and bladder. Occasionally the disease spreads widely throughout the body and is then called miliary tuberculosis.

Mode of infection

M. tuberculosis gains access to the body by way of inhalation, ingestion or inoculation.

Inhalation. This is by far the commonest mode of infection. Tubercle bacilli coughed out by a patient suffering from active pulmonary tuberculosis may be inhaled by others. This form of infection is called droplet infection. Alternatively, dust on which the bacilli have settled may be inhaled, the capsule of the bacilli having kept them alive during periods of dryness.

Infection. Infected milk causes infection by ingestion. Infected sputum may also be swallowed and may give rise to tuberculosis of the intestine.

Inoculation. On rare occasions, accidental inoculation with pathogens may occur in those handling infected material. Doctors, nurses, pathology technicians and laboratory assistants, as well as butchers dealing with infected carcases are especially at risk.

Factors influencing tuberculosis infection

Development of the disease is greatly influenced by the state of resistance or hypersensitivity of the host, by the number of invading bacteria, and their rate of multiplication in the body. The protein of the tubercle bacillus evokes a cell-mediated allergic response (delayed sensitivity), and this reaction indicates either present or past infection which may have been overt or subclinical. The presence of this delayed hypersensitivity may be demonstrated by a positive response to the intradermal injection of purified protein derivative (PPD). An acquired relative degree of immunity to tuberculosis, which is also cell-mediated, works by a mechanism closely similar to, but not identical with delayed hypersensitivity. For those showing a negative response to PPD, active immunization with BCG is usually recommended. In the previously uninfected, the primary lesion in the disease is a small nodule which is called a tubercle. Microscopically it consists of a necrotic centre surrounded by a zone of endothelioid cells and lymphocytes. A few giant cells formed by the fusion of a number of endothelioid cells may also be present. Tubercle bacilli may continue to live in the endothelial and giant cells for a long time. The outermost layer of a tubercle is formed by fibrin laid down by fibroblasts. No toxin has been isolated from tubercle bacilli, and it is thought that the necrosis is the result of an antigen antibody reaction between the bacilli and the host tissue. The necrosis in a tuberculous lesion is called caseation, as the necrotic material resembles cheese in consistency and colour.

The subsequent course of a primary lesion may be any of the following:

1. The bacilli may be completely destroyed, and the lesion may heal by fibrosis. Later on, it may become calcified or even ossified.
2. The bacilli may remain alive but inactive in the lesion. If the resistance of the host decreases, reactivation of the bacilli may occur, and the disease may be kindled again. This is known as endogenous reinfection.
3. The disease may progress locally, producing an ulcerocavernous lesion. The fibrous envelope in these cases either does not develop adequately or breaks down. The caseous material may become liquified, and discharge into a body cavity or passage, e.g. the bronchus, leaving behind a cavity (Fig. 12.1).
4. The infection may spread by lymphatics: this is the most common mode of spread. Examples are the spread of infection from the tonsils to the cervical lymph nodes (Fig. 12.2), or from the lungs to the tracheobronchial lymph nodes, or from the intestine to the mesenteric nodes. Further spread from the lymph nodes may also extend by direct involvement of neighbouring structures, or via efferent lymph vessels to other nodes, or via the thoracic duct into the venous side of the circulation.
5. The infection may spread directly along anatomical routes, e.g. a lesion in the lung may spread to other parts of the same lung or to the opposite lung.
6. Tubercle bacilli may enter the blood stream, either directly by erosion of a blood vessel, or

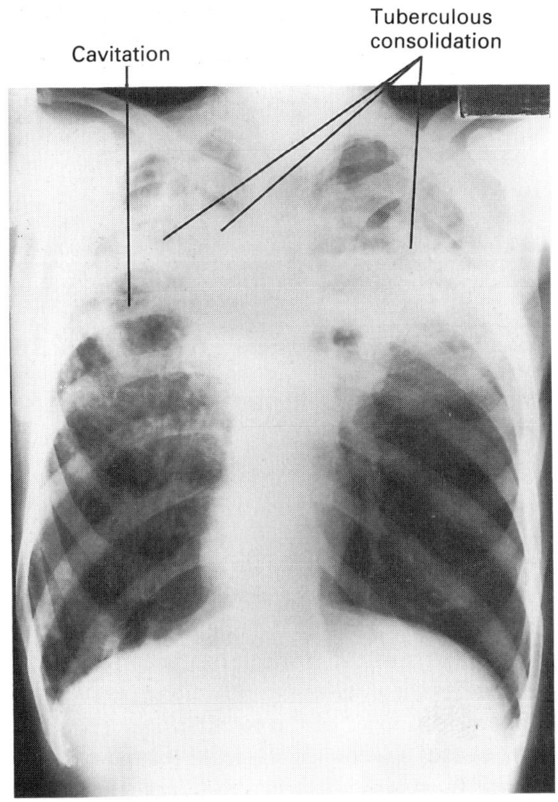

Fig. 12.1 Bilateral tuberculous consolidation in the upper lung lobes. Cavitation has occurred in the right upper zone.

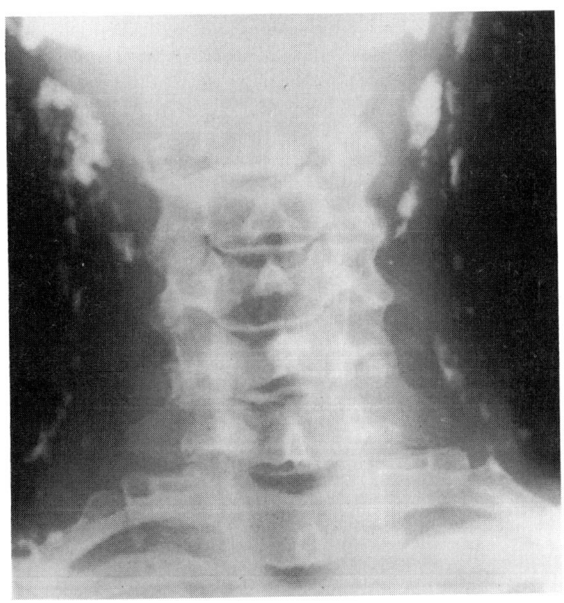

Fig. 12.2 Calcification in tuberculous cervical lymph nodes shown on straight X-ray of the neck. The number of nodes involved is much more extensive than is usually encountered.

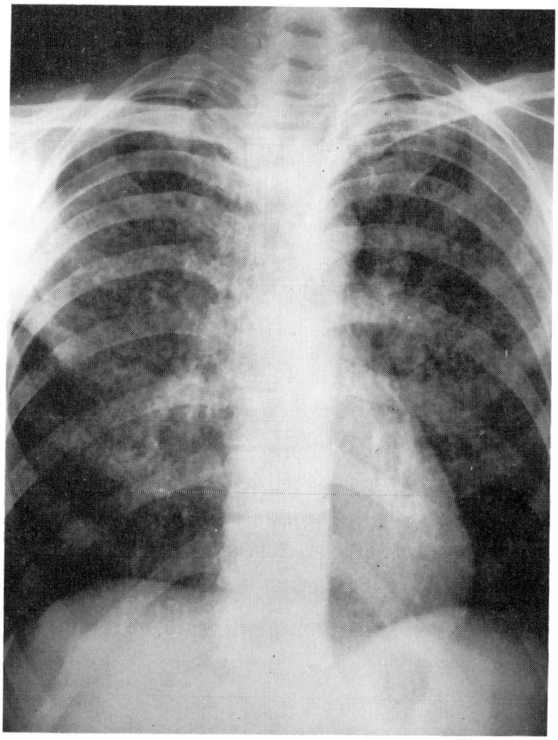

Fig. 12.3 Miliary tuberculosis: numerous blood-borne deposits of tubercle bacilli causing scattered patches of disease throughout both lungs.

by the discharge of infected lymph into the venous side of circulation from the thoracic duct. This may cause a focus of the disease at a distance, e.g. the kidney or a bone. Miliary tuberculosis is a manifestation of the same process (Fig. 12.3).

Clinical features

Tuberculosis is a systemic disorder with signs and symptoms which are both general and local. The latter depend upon the organ involved and are discussed in the relevant chapters. General clinical features are malaise, anorexia, night sweats, loss of weight, and a raised erythrocyte sedimentation rate. A positive skin reaction to tuberculin is usually demonstrated, except sometimes in the presence of an overwhelming primary infection.

The diagnosis is made on the basis of a history of contact with a known tuberculosis patient, the clinical features and investigations, including erythrocyte sedimentation rate, X-ray, and confirmed by identification of the bacilli in cultures of pus, sputum or other excreta. Repeated sampling or animal inoculation may be required to secure positive isolation and identification.

Management

Prophylaxis

The disease has been controlled to a great extent in many countries by a general rise in economic, social and hygienic standards, as well as by the adoption of mass immunization with BCG, an attenuated form of tubercle bacilli. These bacilli are non-pathogenic but are antigenic, and produce active immunity against the disease.

Treatment

The general measures in active treatment include a period of rest in the active stage of the disease, with plenty of fresh air and sunshine. A good diet with an adequate supply of nutriments and vitamins goes a long way towards improving the patient's resistance to the disease. However, the most important part of the treatment is by antituberculous drugs. Streptomycin, para-aminosalicylic acid, isonicotinic acid hydrazide, rifampicin and ethambutol are the commonest drugs in current use. No drug is used singly, as the bacteria acquire resistance against individual drugs very soon. A combination of two or three antibiotics is used, and continued for several months.

With early diagnosis and the success of antibiotic therapy, the indications for surgical treatment are steadily decreasing. The main surgical procedures required are obtaining of biopsy material, aspiration of abscesses, decompression of the spine, relief of intestinal obstruction, operations for painful joints, pericardiectomy for the relief of constrictive pericarditis, and decortication of the lung.

13. Tetanus

Tetanus is a specific infection caused by a Gram-positive bacillus, *Clostridium tetani,* which bears a terminal spore. The spores are resistant to heat and to chemicals. Ordinary bacteria are killed when heated to 55–60°C for about 30 min, but the spores of more resistant strains of tetanus are only killed by exposure to 100°C for at least 3 h. The organism is anaerobic in that it does not flourish in the presence of free oxygen, and it is normally present in bovine and human intestine. These characteristics have practical importance.

The bacilli produce powerful exotoxins, the most important being tetanospasmin, which increases the excitability of the anterior horn cells of the spinal cord and their homologues in the medulla oblongata and pons. The toxin also interferes with the acetylcholine–cholinesterase relationship at the motor end-plates in the voluntary muscles, thereby prolonging the action of acetylcholine which is responsible for muscle fibre contraction.

The bacilli do not cause any harm while in the intestine, but occasionally produce disease when they invade wounds. As the organism is anaerobic, the wounds which do not have free access to oxygen or which are heavily infected with aerobic organisms (which use up most of the oxygen) are more liable to provide favourable conditions for the bacilli to flourish and produce disease. Thus, puncture wounds and wounds sustained in fields rich in human and bovine excreta are more liable to become the starting point of tetanus. The raw umbilicus of the newborn provides fertile ground for the bacteria. Foreign bodies contaminated with the bacilli introduced into the body—occasionally even surgical catgut—may cause the disease.

From the site of inoculation liberated exotoxins, e.g. tetanospasmin, travel along the motor nerves of the area to the central nervous system, where they are fixed to the anterior horn cells of the spinal cord and the brainstem. Toxin is also fixed to the motor end-plates of the voluntary muscles by diffusion through the blood stream. Another toxin, tetanolysin, causes haemolysis of the red blood corpuscles.

The incubation period varies between 48 h and 21 days, and occasionally more—sometimes even months or years.

Clinical features

Usually the first symptom is stiffness of the jaw, sometimes accompanied or followed by difficulty in swallowing. Later, pain in the neck, back and abdomen appears. These are early symptoms which should at once arouse the suspicion of the clinician, before the generalized and painful convulsions begin and the diagnosis becomes clear. The patient remains conscious and appears to have a sardonic smile in spite of great pain, due to spasm of the facial muscles. In general, since the extensor groups of trunk muscles are more powerful than the flexors, in extreme cases the patient's occiput touches his or her heels (Fig. 13.1). This condition is called opisthotonus. In this state, groups of muscles such as rectus abdominis or the psoas major may rupture. Spasms of the muscles of respiration and larynx may interfere with respiration and cyanosis may develop. The patient remains conscious till the end.

Complications

Complications which develop during the illness include myocarditis, producing signs of cardiovas-

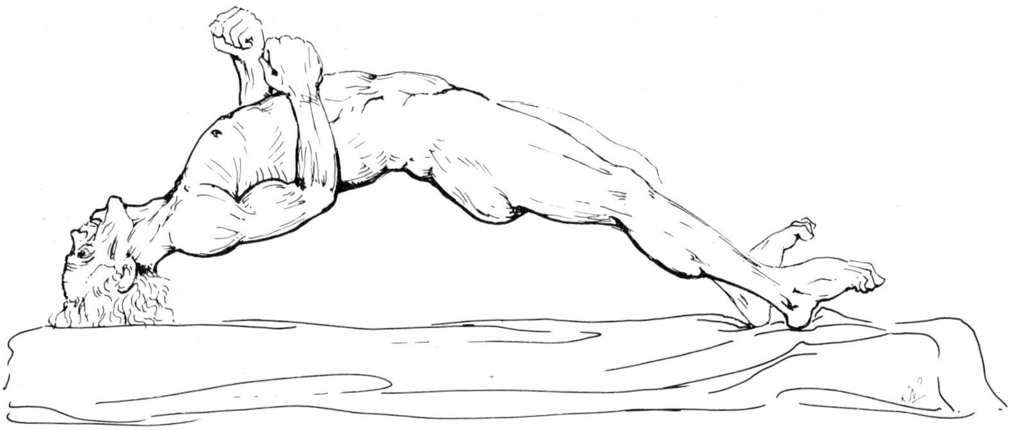

Fig. 13.1 The position of opisthotonus. All muscles go into violent spasm and the position, with only occiput and heels supporting the arched body, with flexed elbows and clasped fists, is the result of the more powerful groups of muscles predominating over the less powerful groups.

cular failure, and damage to brain or spinal cord leading to paralysis. The exact mechanism of these developments is not known.

Cause of death

The mortality of tetanus is high; death usually occurs from exhaustion, respiratory failure and myocarditis.

Management

Prophylaxis

Active immunization. The disease can be completely prevented if the entire population is actively immunized against it. This can best be done by giving triple antigen to babies. This vaccine protects them from diphtheria, whooping cough and tetanus. Three injections should be given at monthly intervals from the age of 3 months, with a further booster dose at the age of starting school.

Patients at risk who have not received triple antigen can be actively immunized by tetanus toxoid. Three doses of 0.5 ml by intramuscular injection are given at a 6-week and 9-month intervals. The toxoid is generally safe and a booster dose is recommended at 5 yearly intervals, or after sustaining a wound in circumstances which may favour tetanus infection.

Passive immunization. Opinions differ about the use of antitetanus serum (ATS), which contains specific antibodies against tetanus toxins, as a prophylactic measure. At present, in many centres a dose of 1500 u is given intramuscularly, although some advocate a much higher dose, i.e. 100 u/kg body weight.

Opposition to the administration of ATS prophylactically rests on two points. Firstly, there is a real danger of a serious serum reaction, including anaphylactic shock, developing in sensitive patients, with possibly even a fatal outcome. Secondly, after receiving the serum, which is usually raised from horses, the patient may develop antibodies against the serum so that subsequently if active treatment for tetanus is required, the administered ATS may be rapidly destroyed, and the disease may not be controlled.

More recently human antitetanus globulin has been developed, known as ATG. It is thought to be far more effective than ATS. The dose is 250–500 u by intramuscular injection.

In all patients, immunized or otherwise, the best protection against tetanus is the thorough toilet of any wound which must include removal of all foreign bodies and devitalized tissue. This is combined with the administration of a full course of penicillin or other suitable antibiotic.

Treatment of active disease

In the treatment of established tetanus, patients

can be divided into three groups—mild, moderate and severe.

Those who only suffer from neck and jaw spasm, in whom generalized convulsions are infrequent, and who do not suffer from difficulty in swallowing, are regarded as mild. Patients who have difficulty in swallowing and have frequent convulsions are considered moderately affected, whereas those who have in addition respiratory difficulty are considered to be severe cases.

All patients with tetanus require specialized nursing in isolated, dark, quiet rooms as the slightest stimulus of sound, light or touch may spark off generalized convulsions.

Mild. In mild cases, sedatives are given. A good combination is to give promazine hydrochloride 100–200 mg and amylobarbitone 200 mg by intramuscular injection at 6-hourly intervals. In addition penicillin and streptomycin should be given in full doses as well as ATG in a dose of 250–500 μ, by the intramuscular route. If ATG is not available, ATS is substituted in the effective dose of 1 000 000 μ, half by intravenous route and the rest intramuscularly.

Moderate. In moderate cases, in addition to the above measures, intravenous narcotics such as pentothal sodium in appropriate doses are employed to control convulsions. As these patients remain under the effect of the narcotics, nourishment should be maintained by a nasogastric tube. Tracheal intubation may be performed in order to aspirate the bronchial tree.

Severe. In severe cases, in addition to the above measures, muscle relaxants are given and positive pressure respiration is instituted. Muscle relaxants such as gallamine, pancuronium or tubocurarine may be given, at first intravenously and then intramuscularly. These patients remain paralysed but conscious and so must be treated with great care.

The prognosis depends on the interval between onset of the disease and the development of generalized convulsions. If this is less than 48 h the patient usually does not survive.

14. Gas gangrene

Gangrene is the death of a part of the body. In contradistinction to necrosis, in which only one constituent tissue of the part dies, in gangrene all tissues of the part die.

Gangrene is conventionally described as either dry or moist. Dry gangrene is due to the gradual obliteration of the blood supply of the part leading to mummification of the tissues. In moist gangrene there is fluid in the tissues allowing multiplication of the infecting organisms and putrefaction.

Gas gangrene belongs to the category of moist gangrene. It is a specific infection caused by gas-producing organisms. These microbes, like those of tetanus, belong to the clostridia group of anaerobic, Gram-positive bacilli which are normally present in human and animal excreta. They are biochemically active, some acting upon carbohydrates, e.g. *Clostridium welchi (perfringens), C. oedematiens (novyi)* and *C. septicum* which are therefore classified as saccharolytic, and others acting upon proteins, e.g. *C. sporogenes* and *C. histolyticum* which are designated proteolytic.

These bacteria liberate a number of toxins: aggressin which discourages leukocyte attraction; fibrinolysin and spreading factor which interfere with fibrin formation and hence allow the infection to spread; haemolysin which causes haemolysis and may cause anaemia and/or jaundice; suprarenal toxin which suppresses the activity of the adrenal glands.

Mode of infection

Lacerated deep wounds with extensive muscle damage, such as war wounds, and those in the neighbourhood of the anus, are most likely to become the starting point of gas gangrene infection. Aerobic organisms such as streptococci, staphylococci or *Escherichia coli* may first colonize the wound and in their metabolism use up all the oxygen in the area, thus creating favourable conditions for anaerobic activity. Organic acids produced by saccharolytic activity accumulate between the muscle fibres and their sheaths, thereby disrupting the blood supply to the fibres, which may then undergo ischaemic and coagulative necrosis. Proteolytic organisms then attack the dead muscle protein with the production of hydrogen sulphide (H_2S) and ammoniacal bodies. The H_2S acts on the iron of muscle haemoglobin, changing the bright red colour of the muscle fibres first to a dark red then to greenish yellow and finally black. The ammoniacal substances neutralize the organic acids produced by the saccharolytic group and thereby nullify the restraining effects of an acid medium on the bacterial activity and help in the spread of the disease.

Clinical features and diagnosis

The type of wound and the circumstances of injury likely to lead to gas gangrene should arouse suspicion if such a patient complains of pain in the wound which goes on increasing without any apparent reason. The wound should at once be opened and examined. In the presence of gas gangrene, the affected part is swollen and there is oedema of the surrounding skin. The wound appears to be under tension and often there is a brownish discharge with a 'mousy' odour. Palpation demonstrates crepitation and X-ray of the part confirms the presence of air bubbles in the soft

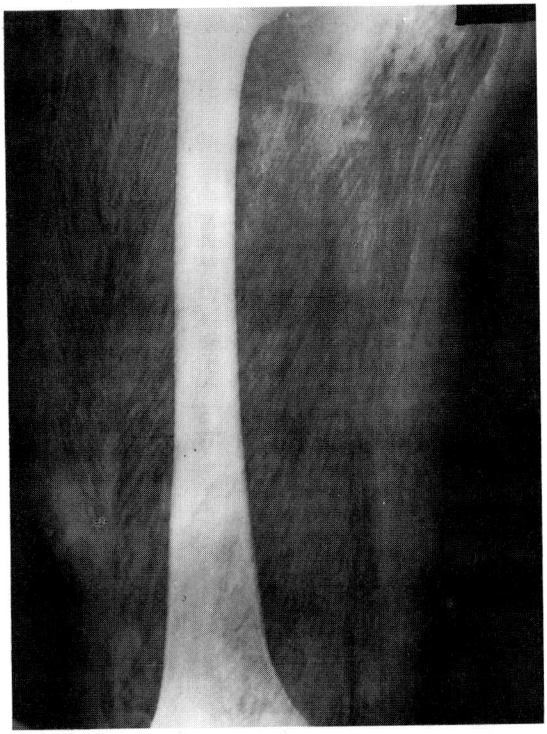

Fig. 14.1 X-ray of thigh showing extensive permeation of linear translucent gas shadows in gas gangrene, which has spread through all the muscle planes.

tissues (Fig. 14.1). The pulse becomes rapid and there is a slight rise in temperature. However, in severe cases the temperature may become subnormal and the blood pressure may fall due to circulatory failure. Mentally the patient usually remains alert and death may come suddenly.

In the differential diagnosis, it should be remembered that crepitations can sometimes be detected soon after an operation if a small quantity of air has been allowed to collect in the subcutaneous tissues and not been expelled before wound closure.

Management

During the last 40 years, the disease has largely been brought under control and very few cases are now encountered. This is mainly because the general principles of wound toilet have been accepted throughout the world.

All foreign bodies are removed, if necessary under anaesthesia, and all dead tissue is excised. The deep fascia, if penetrated, is widely opened so that there is free access of oxygen to the deeper tissues and the muscles are free from tension. The wound is then irrigated with hydrogen peroxide to make extra oxygen available to the damaged tissues. In many cases, it is advantageous to delay skin suture for a few days so that infection can be controlled. Systemic antibiotic therapy is started preferably even before the wound toilet.

Anti-gas gangrene serum (AGS) used to be employed in all severely injured cases. Now it is seldom used, as it has been found that with proper wound toilet and systemic antibiotics it is rarely necessary.

In established cases the wound should be widely opened and all dead tissue removed. There should be no hesitation in amputating the gangrenous part. Penicillin is specific against the gas gangrene organisms. Three ampoules of polyvalent AGS serum should be given intravenously and shock treated by intravenous fluids. Analgesics are prescribed for pain. Exposure to hyperbaric oxygen may be considered, although the evidence for its usefulness remains uncertain.

15. Schistosomiasis (Bilharziasis)

INTRODUCTION

Schistosomes are trematode blood flukes that infect about 200 million persons in the world, and have been known to exist in Egypt since the Pharonic era.

The disease is contracted usually in childhood and early adult life, with the appearance of its complications in adults commonly between 20 and 40 years of age.

Schistosomiasis is endemic in Africa (the Nile valley and Central Africa), South-East Asia and South America (Brazil).

The damaging effect on the health of the population, mainly during the productive phase of life, leads to a reduction in economic productivity of the countries where the disease is endemic.

There are different species, but all have a similar life-cycle and they only differ in their geographic distribution and main target organ.

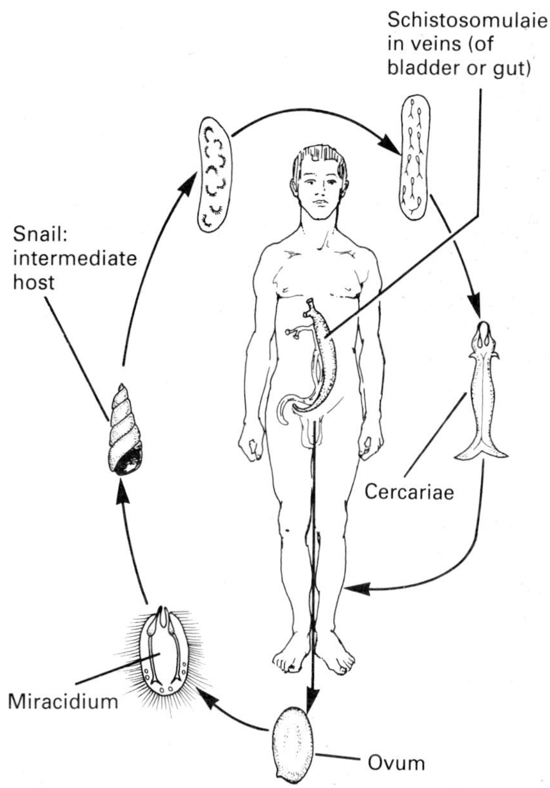

Fig. 15.1 Life-cycle of schistosomes. Ova excreted in human urine or faeces are taken up by the appropriate species of snail where proliferation into cercariae occurs. Cercariae which are freely mobile, penetrate the skin of other humans, usually when the lower legs are exposed to contaminated water.

LIFE-CYCLE

Acquisition of the disease depends on human contact with fresh water containing the necessary ingredients, namely suitable snails (the intermediate hosts) and human excreta from infected persons (Fig. 15.1).

Each schistosome ovum gaining access to water in the faeces or urine of an infected human releases a single miracidium which infects a particular snail. In the case of *Schistosoma haematobium* the snails are of the genus *Bulinus*, while snail species of the genera *Biomphalaria* and *Oncomelania* act as intermediate hosts for *S. mansoni* and *S. japonicum* respectively. The miracidium develops in the intermediate host to form numerous cercariae, which in turn are released into water and infect the human host by penetrating the skin, after which they are called schistosomulae. The latter migrate via the blood stream through the lungs and heart and come to rest in the vascular plexuses where they develop into adult worms. The development in humans takes from 6 to 12 weeks.

Male and female worms lie together, in copulo, in the veins of the vesical plexus in the case of *S. haematobium* infection, and in the tributaries of the inferior and superior mesenteric veins in *S. mansoni* and *S. japonicum* infection.

Eggs of *S. mansoni* and *S. japonicum*, having been produced by the female, breach the wall of the appropriate blood vessel and pass into the lumen of the gut to be discharged in the faeces. Ova of *S. haematobium* reach the bladder and are passed in the urine. The passage of live ova in faeces or urine into snail-infested water completes the life-cycle.

GENERAL PATHOLOGY

The fundamental pathological lesions of bilharziasis are the same for the different species.

The penetration of the cercariae produces an allergic reaction which disappears in a few days. Adult worms do not produce lesions but dead worms produce allergic inflammatory reactions manifested by necrosis of the vascular wall and surrounding tissues and a dense infiltrate of eosinophils, neutrophils and macrophages.

The main factor in the development of the different important pathological changes and complications of schistosomiasis is the presence of ova, whether alive or dead. Their deposition in the liver, colon, bladder and ureter produces an immunological reaction to antigens secreted by the living egg.

This response brings about the development of a granulomatous lesion. Macrophages and a small number of lymphocytes and plasma cells collect around the ova and form small nodules (bilharziomata) or a diffuse tissue reaction. At a later stage, the cellular infiltrate diminishes while fibroblasts proliferate and new capillaries form. Subsequently fibrosis of this lesion will occur. The extent of damage to the tissues is correlated to the intensity and duration of egg production by fertile worm pairs.

The clinical manifestations of schistosomiasis are related to the gastrointestinal tract, the urinary tract, or both.

GASTROINTESTINAL SCHISTOSOMIASIS

Although schistosomal lesions may occur in any part of the alimentary tract, only the liver and colon are of surgical significance.

The acute phase

Soon after infection with the parasite, the patient presents with diarrhoea and lower abdominal pain from the colonic lesion. This is usually the only complaint at this phase, and the diagnosis depends mainly on stool examination and rectal mucosal biopsy, showing the characteristic *S. mansoni* ova in the rectal mucosa.

The chronic phase

Hepatosplenic schistosomiasis

The essential pathology in the liver is a periportal cellular infiltration excited by the presence of the parasite, its products and ova. This is followed by fibrosis. The liver parenchyma initially remains intact, differentiating it from other types of cirrhosis. Portal involvement shows two varieties—fine or coarse—depending on whether the smaller or larger tracts are involved. As a consequence of both the action of the parasite toxins and back-pressure in the portal vein, the spleen undergoes a progressive proliferative congestive enlargement. The haemodynamic changes are characteristic of periportal fibrosis leading to presinusoidal portal hypertension. This in turn leads to enlargement of the portosystemic collaterals, the most important and dangerous being at the lower end of the oesophagus, where varices may form. Satisfactory liver function is usually preserved for a long time in pure schistosomal hepatic fibrosis. The development of hepatitis in patients with bilharzial hepatic fibrosis is not uncommon, and will lead to a mixed type of bilharzial hepatic fibrosis and post hepatic cirrhosis.

Clinical presentation

The surgeon faces the disease either in a patient who bleeds from the varices (haematemesis and melaena) or in a patient with a splenomegaly with or without ascites.

The bleeder

The most serious complication of hepatic schistosomiasis is the development of oesophageal varices which rupture leading to life-threatening haematemesis and melaena.

The splenomegalic

The presentation is usually in the form of a complaint of a mass in the left side of the abdomen due to the enlarged spleen which may reach very large dimensions. It often causes a dragging pain, abdominal discomfort, abdominal swelling from the ascites and dyspeptic manifestations. The liver is usually also enlarged, firm in consistency, with a sharp border, although in very advanced cases the liver may shrink due to extensive fibrosis. Other manifestations commonly seen in cirrhotic patients such as caput medusa and spider naevi are not common in bilharziasis. Different mechanisms contribute to the formation of the ascites, e.g. portal venous hypertension, retention of sodium and water, hypoalbuminaemia and disparity between lymph production and clearance.

Diagnosis

If a patient from an endemic area presents with haematemesis, and the examination elicits a palpable liver and spleen, the most likely diagnosis will be oesophageal varices till proved otherwise. Endoscopic confirmation of the source of bleeding is desirable, though endoscopy during the bleed may be difficult and needs experience. If possible, it is better performed early and immediately after the attack of bleeding has stopped. Liver functions are usually not seriously affected in the early phase, but are affected immediately after the bleeding attack, in mixed bilharzial and post hepatic cirrhosis, and in the advanced stages of hepatic schistosomiasis.

Treatment

The following drugs are used in the medical treatment of schistosomiasis (Table 15.1).

Bleeding varices

The management of the initial stages of bleeding varices is the same as that of the non-bilharzial patient. It is usually possible to control the bleeding in 70–80% of patients by a variety of non-operative measures. Some stop spontaneously, requiring only intravenous blood transfusion to make good the loss; others may respond to intravenous infusion of vasopressin, and if these measures do not succeed, local compression by the Sengstaken–Blakemore tube (Ch.31) may be required. In those in whom all such measures fail or are not available and bleeding continues or recurs after initial cessation, urgent operation may be needed. However, as can be imagined, there is a

Table 15.1 Drugs used in the treatment of schistosomiasis.

Species	Drug	Total dose (mg/kg body weight)	Regimen
S. haematobium	Metriphonate	22.5–30	Single doses of 7.5–10 mg/kg body weight administered every other week x 3
S. mansoni			
Americas and Caribbean	Oxamniquine	15	Single dose
	Praziquantel	40	Single dose
Africa and Middle East	Oxamniquine	60	15 mg/kg body weight twice per day for 2 days
	Praziquantel	40	Single dose
S. japonicum	Praziquantel	60	20 mg/kg body weight every 4 h

high risk of mortality from surgical intervention in this situation on account of the effects of hypovolaemia and hypoxia on vital organs, coagulation defects associated with massive blood loss and transfusion, and impaired liver and renal function.

The surgical techniques used in the treament of other causes of portal hypertension and oesophageal varices are also used in bilharziasis. Of the non-shunt procedures, splenectomy and devascularization (Hassab operation) is commonly used in the Middle East and Africa (Fig. 15.2). The operation involves splenectomy combined with ligation of the left gastric vessels and of the vessels along the upper two-thirds of the greater curvature, lesser curvature and lower part of the oesophagus. It is claimed that the operation reduces the portal pressure and disconnects the portoazygous link.

The operation has gained popularity in many countries affected by this disease, as it is a relatively simpler procedure than the various shunts, and appears to carry less operative mortality risk. However, recurrence of the bleeding varices varies in different series from 15 to 30%.

Oesophageal transection using the stapler has been used recently in the surgery of bleeding varices (see Ch. 31). It is a simple procedure, but its effects may not be permanent and it is expensive, particularly for developing countries. Endoscopic injection sclerotherapy is being increasingly used in non-bilharzial varices and may be considered in patients with recurrence of bleeding from varices and in those who are unfit for surgery. If the popularity of this approach increases further in to the control of bleeding in other populations of oesophageal varices it may be necessary to review its role in bilharzial varices.

In patients with splenomegaly but without bleeding varices, surgery is not indicated, except if the spleen is huge and accompanied by marked hypersplenism, in which case splenectomy is advised. It is better to combine the splenectomy with a prophylactic decongestion procedure aimed at prevention of further bleeding.

TREATMENT OF ASCITES

The treatment is mainly by correction of any hypoalbuminaemia and diuretics. Repeated paracentesis may be needed in the management of

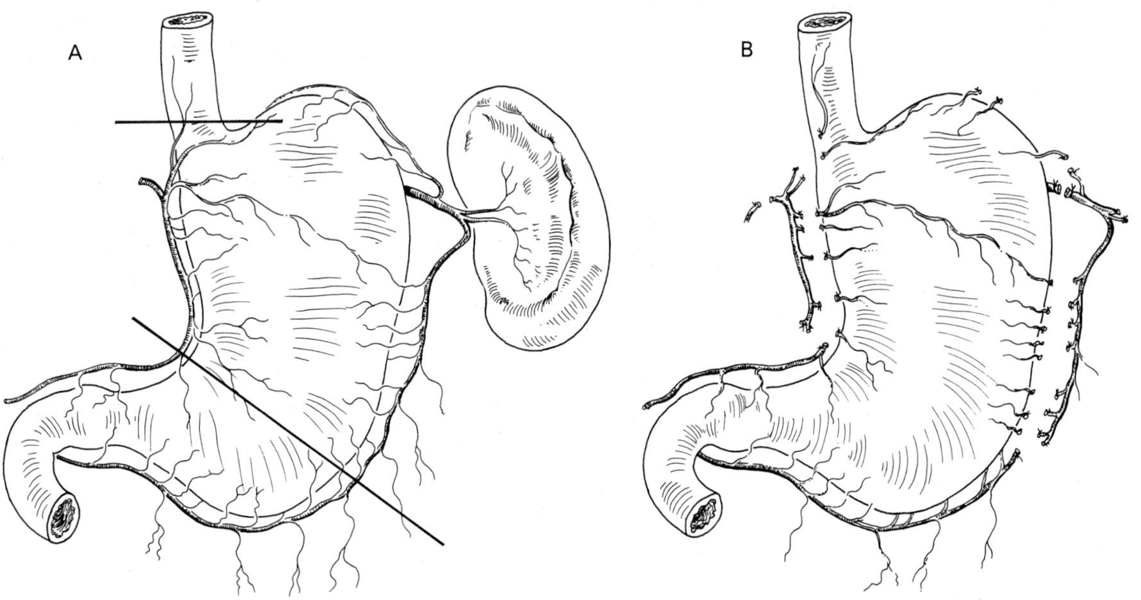

Fig. 15.2 The Hassab operation for bleeding varices in schistosomiasis. Splenectomy is accompanied by division of the left gastric vessels and devascularization of the proximal stomach. The limits of the devascularization are marked in (A); (B) represents the completion of the operation, with the spleen removed, and the various blood vessels supplying both the lesser and greater curvature aspects of the proximal stomach have been divided and ligated.

particularly tense ascites. Surgical measures have little to offer. Anastomosing the proximal end of the external jugular vein to the side of the thoracic duct has been tried with limited success.

Colorectal schistosomiasis

The lesions are produced mainly from infestation with *S. mansoni* or *S. japonicum*. The descending colon, sigmoid and rectum are the main sites affected. The pathological lesions are either diffuse or localized. The patient with colonic schistosomiasis presents with dysenteric symptoms, bleeding per rectum and the passage of large amounts of mucus. The loss may be great enough to lead to hypoproteinaemia, anaemia and loss of weight. A mass (bilharzial mass) may be felt in the lower abdomen.

Diagnosis

Stool analysis and mucosal biopsy are usually positive for *S. mansoni*. Barium enema may show multiple filling defects due to bilharzial polyps affecting a long segment of the left colon. This is important in the differentiation from carcinoma of the left colon, which is commonly annular in type and affects a shorter segment than the bilharzial. Sigmoidoscopy and biopsy of the polyps may be needed for confirmation of the diagnosis.

Treatment

Improvement of the general condition of the patient is important, if necessary by blood transfusion and albumin infusions. Repeated courses of antibilharzial drugs (Table 15.1) may lead to a dramatic improvement in the mild and some moderately severe cases, and even to the disappearance of the small bilharzial masses. Surgery is indicated when there is no response to medical treatment, but resection of the affected colon is not an easy operation, due to the extensive pericolic inflammation and fibrosis. A proximal defunctioning colostomy as a first stage is preferable. Over the following 3–6 months lesions may disappear or at least diminish in size. Colectomy in the presence of the colostomy will then be safer and easier.

UROGENITAL SCHISTOSOMIASIS

Ovideposition in urogenital tissues (particularly the bladder, ureters and seminal vesicles) induces either diffuse chronic inflammatory cellular accumulation or multiple circumoval granulomatous reaction — 'pseudotubercles'. Depending on the duration of lesions, some degree of fibrosis usually exists, and may lead to mechanical complications. The pathological findings vary with the involved organ, intensity and duration of infection and immunological status. One or more of the following pathological states may be found in the urinary bladder:

1. Congestion.
2. Mucosal ulceration.
3. Multiple small, raised, greyish-white pseudotubercles—bilharziomata.
4. Sandy patches: yellow-brown mucosal streaks due to accumulations of calcified eggs, with or without fibrosis and inflammation.
5. Mucosal polyps: an exuberant inflammatory reaction with thickened distorted epithelium and hyperplastic glands, in which ova are usually found.
6. Cysts (e.g. cystitis cystica and glandularis): these may also be found in non-schistosomal cases; they are probably related to chronic irritation.
7. Leukoplakia: denoting patchy white mucosal thickening (microscopically it represents hyperkeratotic urothelial metaplasia to squamous type).
8. Subsequently the effect of healing by fibrosis, e.g. contracted bladder or bladder neck obstruction.
9. Bladder cancer: more common in males of young age: in 40–75% it is squamous cell carcinoma, the remainder being of transitional cell or adenocarcinoma.

Clinical presentation

The acute phase

This is characterized by terminal haematuria and burning micturition due to localized or diffuse cellular reaction in the bladder (cystitis, urethritis). Seminal vesiculitis and prostatitis may lead to haemospermia. The testes are rarely involved, but the scrotum may be affected in heavy infestations, leading to sinus formation. The female genital tract is rarely affected.

The chronic phase

All the late presentations of bilharziasis are mainly due to fibrosis at different levels in the urinary tract, cicatrization of the urethra, bladder neck, bladder wall or lower end of the ureters. The patient will usually present with hydroureter and hydronephrosis, commonly complicated by secondary infections and stone formation. Dysuria and renal colic are the main symptoms.

Schistosomiasis and bladder cancer. As a result of the chronic irritation, squamous metaplasia may occur and become the seat of frank squamous cell carcinoma. This type of cancer is common in areas endemic with bilharziasis and it usually affects young males. The prognosis is bad on account of the aggressive nature of this type of cancer.

Diagnosis

In the acute phase simple urine examination will usually reveal the presence of ova. Plain X-ray may show calcification in the wall of the bladder, and sometimes the ureters and the presence of stones. Intravenous pyelogram will demonstrate ureteric strictures and the degree of hydronephrosis. It may also reveal cancer of the bladder as an irregular filling defect in the bladder. Cystoscopy is indicated whenever any suspected bladder ulcer or other lesion is noted, and appropriate biopsies are taken from any suspect area.

Treatment

The acute phase is treated by full dosage of the appropriate antibilharzial drugs (Table 15.1). In the chronic phase treatment is usually directed to the sequelae of obstructive uropathy, stones, bladder lesions (ulcer, polyp) and carcinoma of the bladder, using conventional procedures.

16. Hydatid disease

Hydatid disease is a chronic infection caused by a parasite, *Echinococcus granulosus*. The parasite has two sets of hosts; a definitive and an intermediate. The definitive host is the dog, whereas humans, cattle and sheep are the intermediate hosts (Fig. 16.1). The adult worm is small, about 3–6 mm long, and lives in the dog's intestine. The ova of the worm are shed with the dog's excreta and the soil is contaminated. The intermediate hosts are infected by ingestion of food, including grass, contaminated with the ova. Once ingested, the ova develop into the larval stage, which is known as

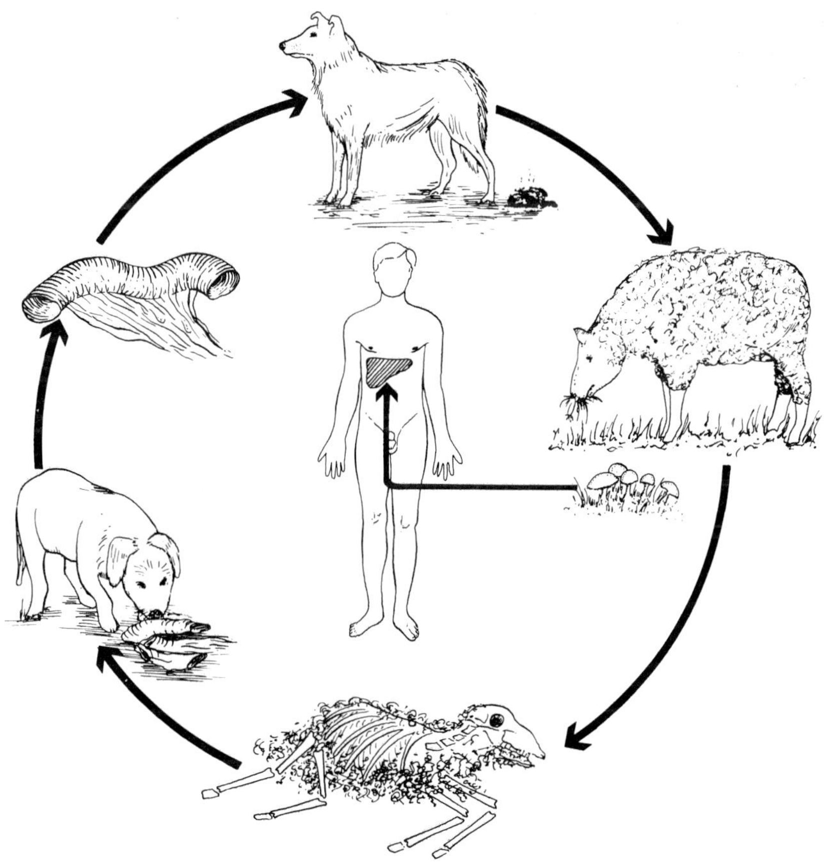

Fig. 16.1 Hydatid disease cycle: the *Echinococcus granulosus* is excreted in the faeces of an infested dog and contaminated grass is eaten by sheep; dogs eating the sheep carcase may then become further infested. Humans are infested by eating contaminated food or water.

hydatid cyst in the tissues of the intermediate host. Infected offal is eaten by the definitive host and thus the life-cycle of the parasite is completed.

The ova ingested by the intermediate host enter the blood stream through a radicle of the portal vein from the gastrointestinal tract. In about two-thirds of cases, the ova settle to form hydatid cysts in the liver. The lungs are the second most common site, and other organs which may be affected are the brain, bones and kidneys, though no organ is immune from the disease.

The cyst contains a clear watery fluid which is albumin-free and its lining consists of three layers (Fig. 16.2). The outermost adventitial layer comprises fibrous tissue and compressed parenchyma from the host organ. The middle layer or laminated membrane consists of hyaline material which is secreted by the innermost lining of the cyst, the germinal layer. This latter is a single layer of epithelium which secretes the hydatid fluid internally and the hyaline substance forming the laminated membrane externally. The cells of the germinal layer multiply in the form of vesicles called brood capsules, from the lining of which a collection of cells, the scolex, grow into the vesicle. The future worm develops from these scolices in the definitive host after ingestion of the infected offal.

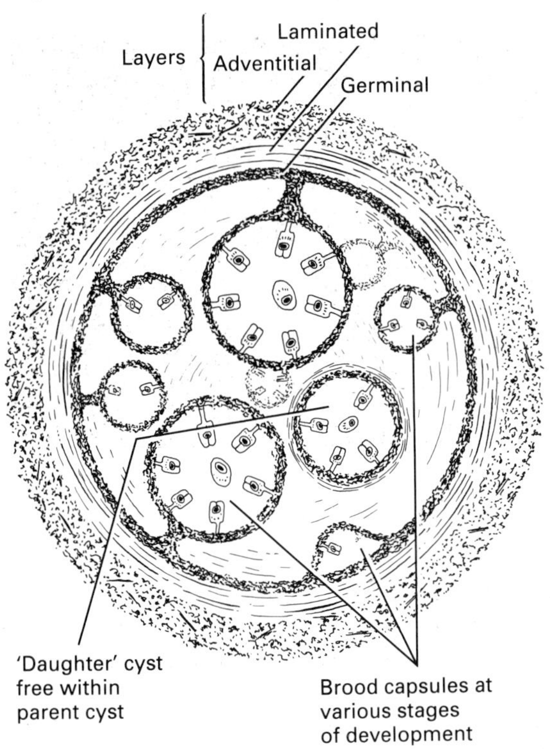

Fig. 16.2 Diagrammatic cross-section of a hydatid cyst, showing the three main layers of the wall and daughter cysts at varying degrees of development.

There are no specific pathognomonic signs and symptoms of hydatid disease. An intra–abdominal mass with discomfort is the main complaint when it arises in the liver. On examination a mass of varying size may be felt, either inseparable from the liver or in a pedunculated form.

Complications of cysts are rupture, infection and calcification. If the cyst ruptures into the peritoneal cavity, either by external trauma or during operation, the patient may go into anaphylactic shock and die. If the patient recovers, daughter cysts may develop extensively within the abdomen and may so interfere with the functions of the viscera as to have a fatal outcome.

Occasionally a cyst may rupture into the biliary passages and daughter cysts may give rise to obstructive jaundice by occluding the common hepatic or common bile duct.

If suppuration occurs the clinical picture is similar to that of a liver abscess. If calcification occurs, a mottled or uniformly dense shadow is seen on X-ray (Fig. 16.3). Accurate location and delineation can be achieved by computerized tomography scan (Fig. 16.4).

When a cyst develops in the lung, the main complaint may be cough and dyspnoea, with or without expectoration. Occasionally the cyst may rupture into a bronchus, and if the patient is not able to cough out the contents, there is a real danger of death from suffocation.

Diagnostic tests

A positive intradermal sensitivity reaction with hydatid fluid is found in the majority of cases. This is Casoni's test. A complement fixation test has also been devised, but it is more complicated. The finding of an eosinophilia on blood examination is supportive of the diagnosis.

Treatment

Treatment of hydatid disease is surgical. The cyst is removed with the utmost care to avoid spillage of the contents of the cyst. For large cysts it is often better to aspirate its contents and fill the cyst

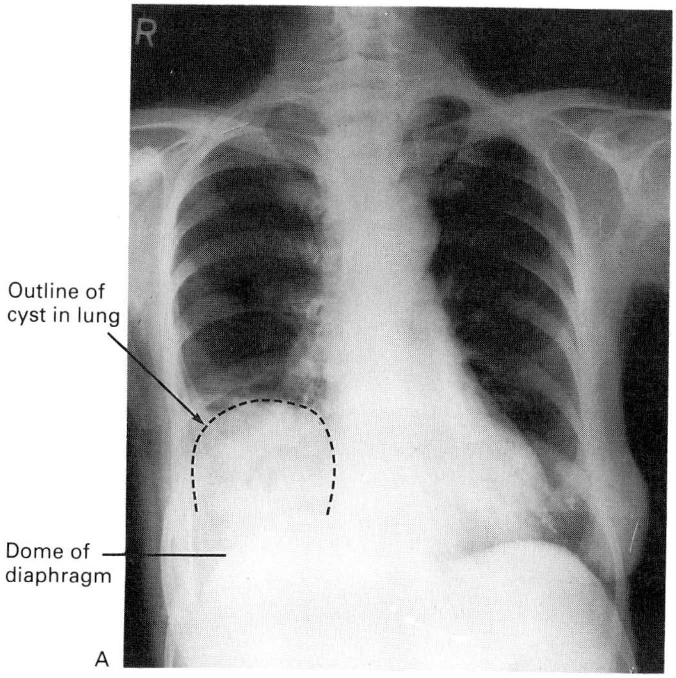

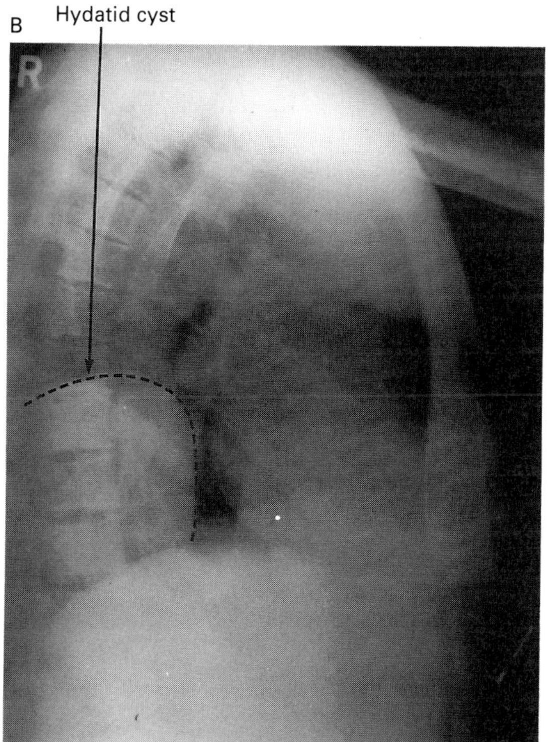

Fig. 16.3 Large hydatid cyst of right lung showing a rounded opaque shadow on chest X-ray. (**A**) Anteroposterior view; (**B**) lateral view.

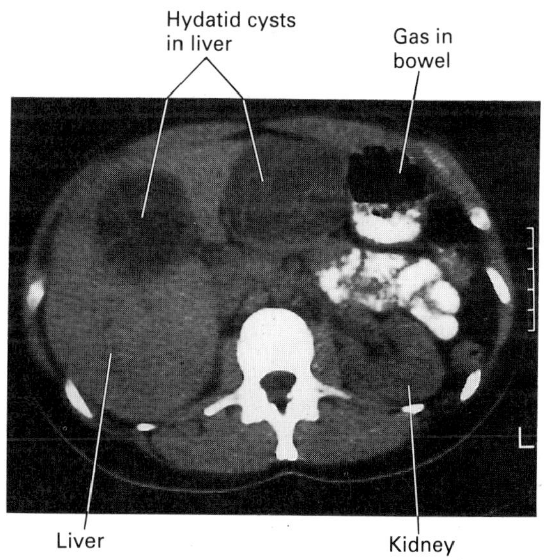

Fig. 16.4 Demonstration of two hydatid cysts by computerized tomography scan.

with hydrogen peroxide. Previously, formalin was used for this purpose. This will kill the parasite and the daughter cysts. The hydrogen peroxide or formalin is then aspirated and the cyst removed by gently separating the laminated membrane from the adventitia.

In the lung, it is sometimes safer to carry out segmental resection or lobectomy.

17. Leprosy

Leprosy (Hansen's disease) is a specific infectious disease caused by *Mycobacterium leprae,* an acid-fast bacillus with some resemblances to *M. tuberculosis.*

Both leprosy and tuberculosis were quite common in Europe a few hundred years ago, but today are rare in that part of the world. This fall in incidence is almost certainly due to the higher social development resulting in increased host-resistance of the population. However, leprosy is still seen among the poorer people of under-developed regions of the world.

Like *M. tuberculosis, M. leprae* is a pathogen of low virulence, and the lesions produced by it are almost always chronic in type.

Although the exact mode of infection is not known with certainty, it is believed that it is most commonly transmitted by inhaling dust contaminated with the nasal secretions of a leprosy patient. Intimate contact over a prolonged period is usually necessary for infection to occur.

The incubation period varies from a few weeks to a few years, but is most commonly between 2 and 4 years.

The main brunt of the attack falls on the skin, the upper respiratory tract and on cutaneous and other peripheral nerves, though almost any organ of the body may be affected.

No toxin has been isolated as yet, and the mechanism of disease production is not known.

Two types of lesions are seen: tuberculoid and lepromatous.

Tuberculoid lesion

The tuberculoid variety is seen in patients with high resistance. In this condition, granulation tissue infiltrates certain nerves, and this is accompanied by the destruction of the nerve fibres. The most commonly affected nerves are the ulnar, median, posterior tibial and lateral popliteal and, less commonly, the radial and facial nerves. Motor disturbances are manifest by paralysis of muscles supplied by the involved nerve, and sensory effects include the development of anaesthetic skin patches, trophic ulcers and ultimately destruction of the affected part.

Lepromatous lesion

In the lepromatous type, granulomatous lesions develop in the skin, mucous membrane and other tissues.

Leprosy is a crippling disorder with a social stigma which is mostly unjustified as the disease is curable and cannot be transmitted by casual or accidental contact. However, the deformities produced in the face, hands and feet often make the patient a social outcast (Fig. 17.1). If the facial nerve is affected paralysis of the levator palpebrae superioris may prevent closure of the eye, so that corneal ulceration may develop, leading to blindness. Lesions developing on the face may cause such distortion as to give the so-called leonine facies, with multiple pendulous granulomas, loss of a part of the eyebrow, deep lines forming on the face, and collapse of the bridge of the nose.

When the ulnar nerve is affected the lesion usually occurs near the elbow, where gross thickening may be easily felt. A patch of anaesthesia on the medial side of the ventral aspect of the palm may result. Some degree of claw-like deformity of the hand, hollowing of the intermetacarpal spaces, and weakness of gripping between thumb and index finger will be demonstrated, in view of the impaired

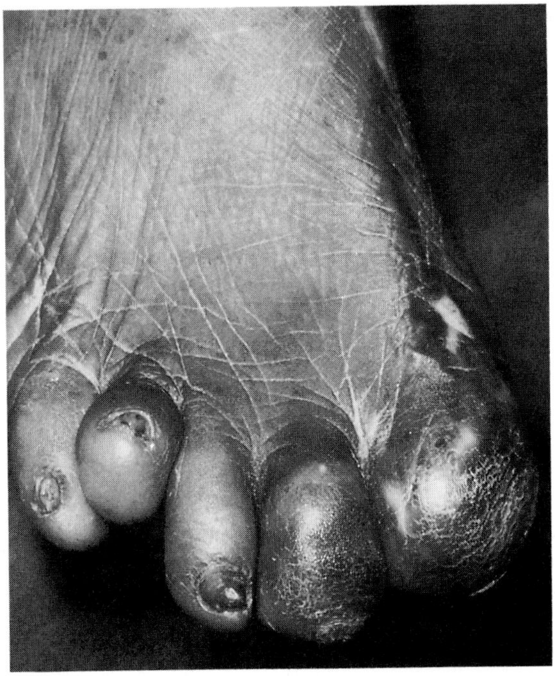

Fig. 17.1 Leprosy affecting the foot: Loss of distal segments of the first and second toes.

supply to many of the intrinsic muscles of the forearm and hand.

In median nerve involvement at the wrist joint, the patient is unable to abduct the thumb completely due to paralysis of the abductor pollicis brevis (pen-touching test). In lesions at the level of the elbow joint, the patient is unable to flex the interphalangeal joints of the index finger because of the paralysis of both the long flexors of the fingers.

If the radial nerve is affected in the upper arm, there will be wrist drop. In lesions in the forearm beyond the point at which the posterior interosseous nerve arises, there will be no muscular weakness, but there may be a patch of anaesthesia on the dorsum of the hand.

In the lower limb, the posterior tibial and lateral popliteal nerves are most commonly involved. If the former, there may be clawing of the toes and if the latter foot drop may develop on account of paralysis of the extensors.

Diagnosis

This is established on the basis of history, physical findings and the microscopic demonstration of intracellular acid-fast lepra bacilli in the scrapings of involved skin or nasal excretion or biopsy specimens of lesions.

Management

There is no doubt that increasing standards of living and improved social hygiene have gone a long way in developing such an immunity among the people of advanced countries that the disease has nearly ceased to exist in Europe and North America, where it was not so rare even until the last century. It still poses a problem of great magnitude in some parts of Africa, Asia and Latin America.

Attempts are being made to develop a vaccine against leprosy. At the moment trials with BCG are being undertaken, but no uniformly successful policy has yet been evolved.

Treatment

Leprosy is a curable disease. In the active stages, it is treated with Dapsone, a sulphone preparation, in a dose of 10 mg/kg/week for 3–5 years or even more. Rifampicin is also effective, especially if given in combination with Dapsone.

Surgical treatment may be necessary to correct deformities, or to make these cosmetically and functionally more acceptable. Surgical procedures such as skin-grafting, tendon transplant, reconstruction of the nose or amputation are performed under cover of anti-leprosy antibiotics. With more experience in this field, the scope of surgical intervention in correcting the deformities is increasing.

18. Burns

Burning by heat, chemicals, electricity or radiation causes coagulative necrosis of tissues. Damage produced by moist heat is called a scald. There are certain differences in the pattern of damage produced by the different agents but there are many features which are common to all from the pathological, clinical and treatment points of view. These common features shall be considered in this chapter.

Pathology

The effects of a burn are local and general, and depend on the extent of the area damaged and on the depth of the tissue involved. In young adults a burn involving more than 10% of the body surface is considered severe because of the general effects produced by trauma of this gravity, and if more than 50% of the body surface is involved, survival is at risk. Old persons do not stand trauma well, and in those over the age of 80 a burn involving only 10% of the surface area may constitute a lethal injury.

For the purpose of estimation of the surface area of the body, 'the rule of nine' is generally useful in adults, and 'the rule of six' in children (Fig. 18.1). According to the rule of nine, the surface area as a percentage of total area is estimated as follows:

Head and neck	9%
Each upper limb	9%
Each lower limb	18%
Front of the trunk	18%
Back of the trunk	18%
Perineum including genitalia	1%

The rule of six is as follows:

Head and neck	12%
Each upper limb	6%
Each lower limb	12%
Front of the trunk	24%
Back of the trunk	24%

Local effects

Two degrees of burns are recognized—superficial and deep. In superficial burns only the epidermal layer is damaged or destroyed, while in deep burns, in addition to the whole thickness of the skin, deeper structures such as subcutaneous tissue, muscle, vessels and nerves, and even bone may be involved.

In superficial burns (Fig. 18.2), apart from the actual epidermal cells, minute blood and lymph vessels are also damaged; the dead tissue acts as an irritant giving rise to an inflammatory response in the area, and plasma pours out from the capillaries in response to the irritant. The fluid may collect under the dead tissue in the form of blisters or, where the epithelium is completely destroyed, pour out on to the raw surface. The quantity of fluid lost depends on the extent of the surface area involved.

In deep burns, relatively bigger vessels may be affected. Some of these vessels may be damaged and in these and neighbouring vessels blood may clot. Plasma loss occurs here also, into the affected tissues. The localized patch of dead tissue, called an eschar, remains adherent and is surrounded by oedematous and inflamed tissue. The eschar gradually separates from the underlying parts during the next few weeks, leaving an open ulcer. Between the eschar and the granulation tissue of the under-

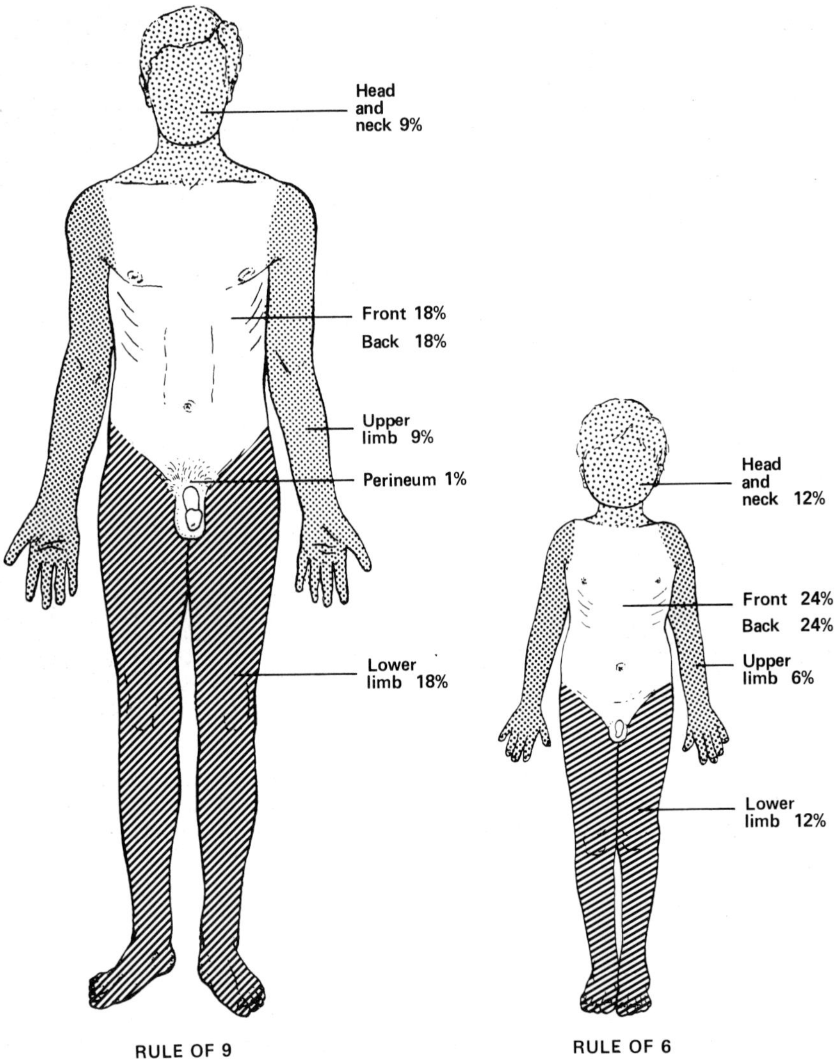

Fig. 18.1 Diagrammatic representation of the guidelines for assessing the area of surface burnt: the rule of nine for adults and the rule of six for children.

lying ulcer, an exudate rich in leukocytes collects. This exudate may become pus as secondary infection usually follows. The time of separation of the eschar from the underlying tissues depends to some extent on the depth of the burn and may take some weeks.

Separation of the eschar leaves a granulating surface which, if left to itself, can only heal by a marginal growth of epithelium towards the centre of the wound. During the process of healing, varying degrees of fibrosis occur, which may result in crippling and ugly contractures (Fig. 18.3).

GENERAL EFFECTS

Reference has already been made to the outpouring of plasma from the capillaries of the damaged area in extensive burns. This shift of plasma from the vascular to the extravascular compartment may assume such proportions that hypovolaemia may result with diminished cardiac output, hypotension and shock. If the condition is not treated promptly, the resulting hypoxia may cause permanent damage to the vital centres and death.

After an interval of about 36–48 h, the capillar-

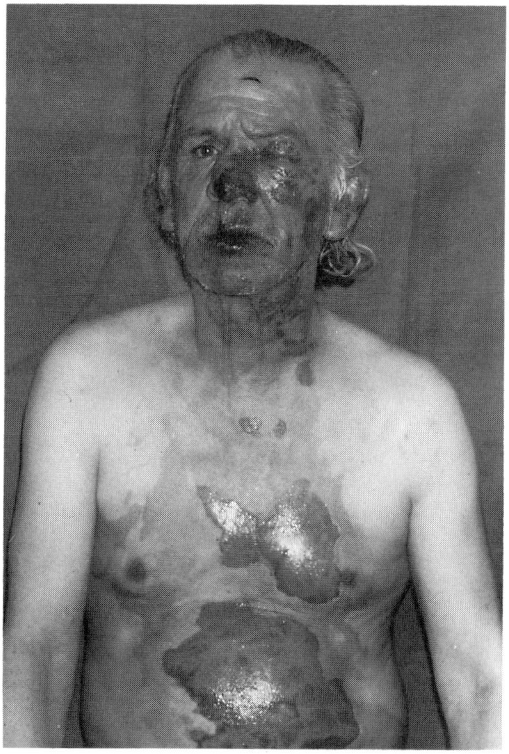

Fig. 18.2 Combination of mostly superficial, plus a few smaller areas of deep burns, on the face and trunk. Oedematous swelling has temporarily closed the left eyelid. These were treated primarily by exposure to encourage rapid drying of the superficial burns, and thereby reduce further fluid loss and establish a seal against bacterial contamination.

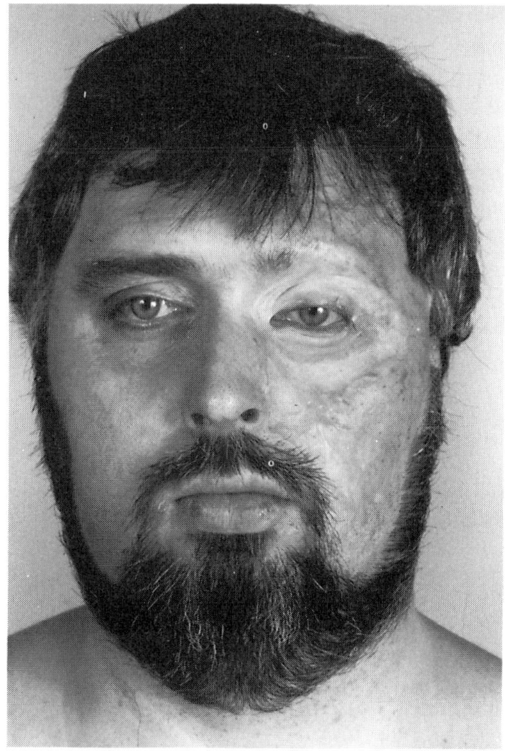

Fig. 18.3 End-result of a healed burn on the left side of the face. Contraction of the fibrous tissue has led to some tightening of the skin. The damaged outer part of the eyebrow will not regrow. There is slight narrowing of the left palpebral fissure.

ies in the burnt area either recover their normal permeability or become thrombosed. The tendency of the fluid to escape from the vessels is then diminished and the oedema fluid starts to be reabsorbed. This fact should always be kept in mind in planning treatment.

All burns are sterile to start with, but very soon infection supervenes as the raw surface and the damaged tissue offer a rich medium for bacterial growth. Infection not only interferes with the process of healing but may also produce toxaemia with its systemic effects.

Anaemia is another general effect in extensive burns. Two types are recognized — primary and secondary.

The former is mainly caused by the destruction of blood in the area of burn, but there are other factors. It is thought that the red blood cells are in some way damaged so that their lifespan is reduced. Moreover, it is quite likely that a haemolytic agent is produced from the damaged tissues and this may be a contributory factor.

Secondary anaemia starts during the phase of negative nitrogen balance of the body, which always occurs in the wake of any extensive trauma. The anaemia, however, continues after the return to a positive nitrogen balance, particularly if infection is present. A contributory factor is probably the non-availability of protein for the synthesis of haemoglobin, as the demand for protein increases after injury. This anaemia is not helped by iron therapy and blood transfusions, perhaps repeated, are usually necessary to correct it.

Other systemic disturbances which may occur from time to time are haematuria, stress gastroduodenal ulceration and haematemesis. Although the mechanism of their production is obscure, their occurrence usually has a grave significance. The mucous membrane of the mouth and upper respiratory tract may be damaged by hot fumes, both chemically and thermally, and produce varying degrees of pneumonitis. The lower respiratory passages may suffer chemical injuries from carbon monoxide in the smoke and from fumes.

Death occurs in the early post burn period due to hypovolaemia and shock. Later mortality is due to toxaemia and consequent myocardial or renal damage or both.

Clinical features

Clinically, superficial burns are more painful than deep ones since in the latter the sensory nerves are destroyed. Oedema of the glottis, bronchial spasm and pulmonary oedema are manifestations of injury of the respiratory system.

Management

Local care

The basic problems in the local care are the prevention and control of infection, and the restoration of normal function of the part as far as possible.

Shortly after the burn, a coagulum forms over the burnt surface, acting as sterile dressing. The main aim of treatment is to protect it from trauma. This can often be done simply by properly arranging the bedclothes. No dressing is necessary to protect the wound from infection, but may be needed to protect the coagulum from trauma and in certain situations, to make the patient more comfortable.

If a dressing is thought to be necessary, for example in some circumferential burns of the trunk or the limbs, a satisfactory method is as follows:

1. An antibiotic cream is smeared evenly over the burnt surface.
2. A layer of cotton is applied.
3. This is covered with absorbent cotton wool, held in position by bandages or strapping. If necessary further layers of cotton wool or other material may be added to absorb excess exudate or protect the bedclothes.

The dressing may be changed and the wound re-examined at intervals of a few days.

Alternatively, superficial burns may be covered with a transparent film, e.g. Opsite, which has the properties of excluding the micro-organisms while maintaining moisture vapour permeability.

Deep burns of the hands and feet can be encased in plastic bags with facilities for irrigation with antiseptic lotions. This arrangement enables the patient to continue active exercises.

To minimize or control infection systemic antibiotics are routinely employed, usually penicillin or broad-spectrum antibiotics. Later on these may be changed according to the culture and sensitivity report on swabs taken from the burned area.

Systemic antibiotics are also important in combating infection when the respiratory tract has been exposed to fumes or direct thermal injury. Assessment of the degree of the injury may require fibreoptic bronchoscopy, as X-ray films may not accurately reflect the state of health of the lungs. Bronchial aspirations are taken for culture and sensitivity test for monitoring antibiotic therapy.

It has been observed that as full-thickness burns are relatively avascular, systemically administered antibiotics are unlikely to be effective in preventing bacterial growth in and on the surface of the slough or eschar. Topical application of antibiotic, e.g. silver sulphadiazine or neomycin, is therefore perhaps more likely to check bacterial growth in this situation.

In a deep burn, if the eschar does not separate within 3–4 weeks, it may be better to excise it under anaesthesia. Unless the eschar separates, any pus underneath it cannot be evacuated and wound healing will be delayed.

After the eschar or slough is separated, the raw surface may be covered with a skin autograft. In some cases, especially where there is a small localized deep burn, it may be preferable to carry out excision and skin grafting as an immediate procedure after the injury, if the patient is considered fit for anaesthesia.

Skin homografts obtained from cadavers are used in some centres to cover the burnt area until separation of the eschar, by which time the granulating area is ready for autografting. The homograft, or even heterograft, not only protects the granulating surface meantime from infection, but also minimizes the fluid and electrolyte loss from the raw area.

In treating burns of the flexor surfaces, splints are sometimes helpful in preventing contractures. When treating burns on the front of the neck, nursing the patient with the neck extended discourages extreme contracture of the neck.

GENERAL MEASURES

It is generally agreed that any adult sustaining a burn of more than 10% of body surface area will require intravenous administration of fluids. The quality and quantity of fluid to be infused depend upon a number of factors, notably the surface area of the burn, the depth of the involved tissue, and the general condition of the patient. In general, the larger and more superficial burns will lose much more than the smaller, deeper ones.

One simple guide for estimating the fluid requirement is Wallace's formula, according to which in the first 48 h an adult patient needs 220 ml of fluid per 1% of body surface burnt. This is over and above the daily fluid requirements. In superficial burns, half of this fluid is given in the form of electrolyte solutions and the rest in the form of plasma. In deep burns, the total quantity is divided into seven parts. Three parts are given in the form of electrolyte solutions, three parts in the form of plasma and the remaining one part in the form of blood. As for the speed of administration, it is recommended that of the total quantity of fluid required, one-third is given in the first 8 h, one-third between 8 and 24 h and the remaining third between 24 and 48 h.

Wallace has also estimated fluid requirements per 1% of body surface burnt in 48 h in different ages (Table 18.1). It is, however, emphasized that the table is only a general guide, and each patient has to be assessed individually to assess the adequacy of restoration of circulating blood volume. Regular measurements of pulse, blood pressure, haemoglobin and haematocrit are required, and if any concern arises a central venous line should be inserted to monitor progress towards sufficient fluid replacement.

Table 18.1 Fluid requirement per 1% body surface burnt according to age (Wallace AB 1951 The Lancet, p 501)

	Birth to 3 months	3–6 months	6–9 months	9 months to 1 year	1–2 years	2–3 years	3–4 years	4–5 years	5–6 years	6–7 years	7–8 years
Electrolyte solution and plasma	7 ml	10 ml	12 ml	13 ml	15 ml	21 ml	24 ml	27 ml	31 ml	35 ml	40 ml
	8–9 years	9–10 years	10–11 years	11–12 years	12–13 years	13–14 years	14–15 years	15–16 years	16–17 years	17–18 years	Adult
Electrolyte solution and plasma.	44 ml	46 ml	51 ml	56 ml	62 ml	67 ml	78 ml	88 ml	96 ml	104 ml	110 ml

19. Skin and subcutaneous tissues

The basic structure of the skin is that of an outer portion of layers of keratin-producing cells—the epidermis—and an inner component of looser connective tissue, including fat, collagen, elastic tissue, blood vessels, lymphatics and nerves—the dermis (Fig. 19.1). The interface between these two is wavy, with upward protrusions of dermal papillae interlocking with downward extending fingers of epidermis (rete pegs).

The epidermal cells are continuously renewed by the very basal layer of the epidermis and although most cells as they mature and work to the surface produce keratin, others produce melanin, which may in turn be passed along processes of these cells into neighbouring ones.

Although the thickness of the skin varies from one part of the body to another, being thickest of all on the soles of the feet and palms of the hands

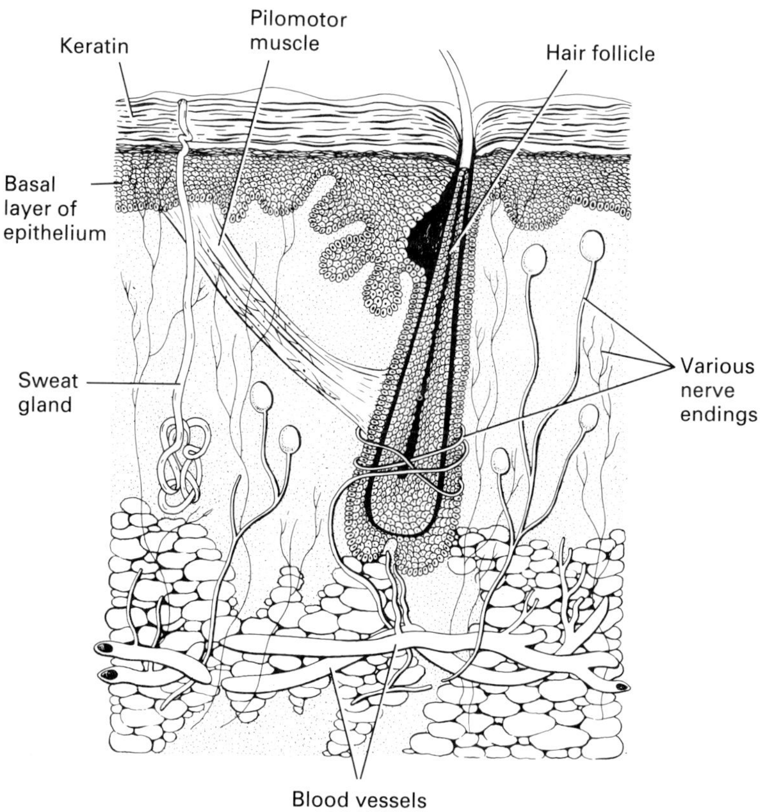

Fig. 19.1 Skin and immediately underlying subcutaenous tissues.

and on the back of the trunk, the thickness at any one side is kept constant by an exact balance between the rate of cell loss through normal desquamation and replacement by the basal germinal layer.

The sebaceous glands, sweat glands and hair follicles are all downgrowths of specialized epidermal cells into the dermal layers, and the nails arise from a further specialized area of epidermal tissue.

CYSTS

Sebaceous epidermoid cyst

This is the commonest type of skin cyst encountered in clinical practice. The name suggests that they arise from the sebaceous glands, but this is probably not so, and more likely they originate in hair follicles. They have a thin-walled capsule of stretched epidermal cells and the creamy-white cheesy content is a mixture of keratin and sebum. The name epidermoid cyst is therefore more appropriate, but the term sebaceous cyst has been used for so long that it is likely to continue in common clinical usage.

The cyst can occur anywhere on the skin surface except the palms and soles, and the commonest sites are in the scalp, behind the ears (Fig. 19.2), the back of the trunk and the scrotum. They may be multiple, and some patients may present with a succession of them over a period of years.

Unless infection is present the patient simply presents on account of the noticeable or palpable round soft swelling. The main diagnostic features are that clearly it is cystic, arises from the skin itself, since the skin cannot be moved over it, and close inspection usually, though not always, reveals a small dark spot or punctum somewhere over the summit of the swelling.

Excision of the cyst under local anaesthesia is usually a straightforward matter, but it is important to ensure that the entire capsule is removed, otherwise a recurrent cyst is almost certain to develop from even a tiny remnant. It is easier to ensure complete removal if the capsule remains intact during the procedure.

The only complication which may arise with a sebaceous cyst is infection, and if this supervenes there will be enlargement, pain, tenderness and often local throbbing. The cyst will have been converted into an abscess, and should be treated as such. This implies that incision and drainage of the pus is performed, and no attempt is made to excise the wall. Occasionally the infection will destroy the cyst wall and no further treatment will be needed. More often, however, once the infection has completely subsided the cyst will recur and it can be later excised under local anaesthesia, as already outlined.

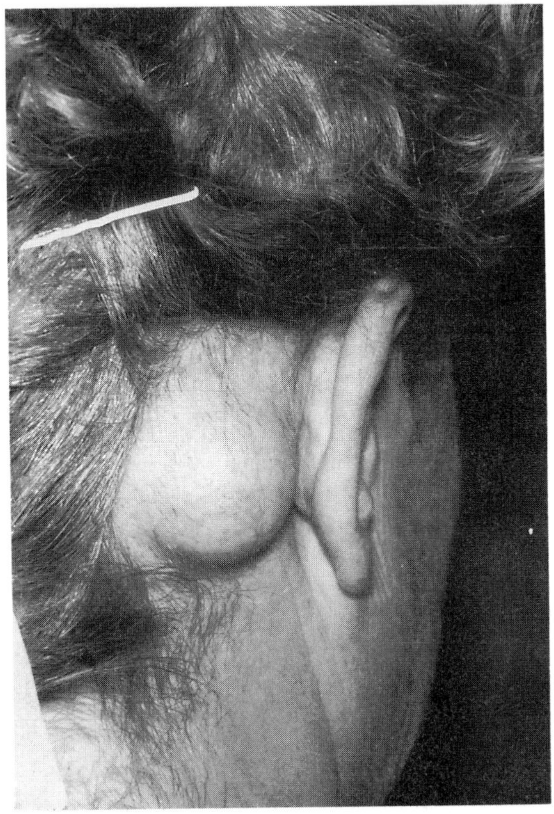

Fig. 19.2 Sebaceous cyst behind the right ear. This area and the scalp are the common sites for this common benign cyst.

Dermoid cyst

This type of cyst results from the deposition of one or two epidermal cells in the subcutaneous tissue. Such a downward displacement can occur either during embryonic development at sites where two embryonic folds fuse (Fig. 19.3), e.g. frontal and maxillary facial processes, the midline of trunk anteriorly etc., or as a result of puncture wounds, e.g. needle or pinpricks in the hands.

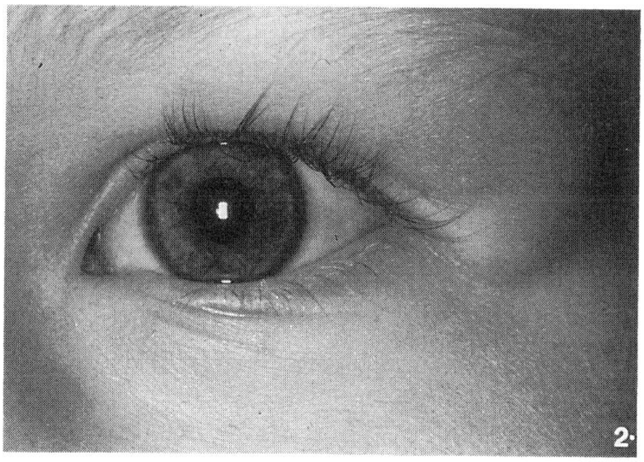

Fig. 19.3 Angular dermoid cyst in a child. This arises at the level of fusion between the frontal and maxillary embryological folds.

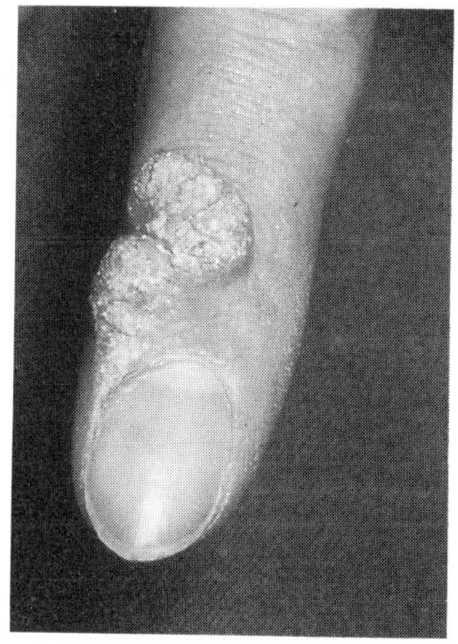

Fig. 19.4 Simple papillomas arising from the skin of a finger, probably of viral origin.

The wall of the cyst is squamous epithelium from the epidermis and the fluid content includes sebum, desquamated cell debris and occasionally hair. Clinically there is an obvious cystic swelling over which the skin does move to a limited extent. Sometimes, especially on the face, there is a degree of attachment deeply. Rarely do these cysts become infected, and it is usually a simple matter to excise them under local anaesthesia. A word of caution is required concerning those which arise at the outer angle of the orbit—the external angular dermoid. This is the most frequently encountered congenital dermoid coming from the fusion of the frontal and maxillary processes. On occasions the defect passes through the bony fusion line, with an 'hourglass' extension inside the skull, and it is therefore wise to X-ray the skull and if there is suspicion or confirmation of a defect in the bone, to follow this with brain computerized tomography scan. If there is an intracranial extension a formal neurosurgical approach will be required.

BENIGN LESIONS OF THE SKIN

Papillomas

These are exceedingly common innocent little growths. Practically everyone will find one or more on some part of the body. Favoured sites are around the head and neck, on the trunk, in the axilla or on the limbs. Most are tiny pedunculated or sessile projections from the skin surface (Fig. 19.4) and many are referred to by the old-fashioned name warts. Some are the same colour as the surrounding skin; others are pink on account of their liberal blood supply, and others are brown, pigmented with melolin, especially in the elderly. The surface generally has a finely wrinkled appearance, or if more than a few millimetres in size may have a cauliflower-like surface.

On histological examination a papilloma shows considerable proliferation of fairly organized squamous epithelial cells in leaf-like folds around a core of small blood vessels, lymphatics and connective tissue.

Advice is usually sought for cosmetic reasons or because the lesion causes minor irritation, or keeps getting caught in the clothes or knocked against objects, or on account of anxiety that it might be something more dangerous. Repeated minor friction or other trauma is undesirable as this might lead to local infection and if prolonged, malignant transformation.

It is generally a simple matter to excise the papilloma under local anaesthesia. A small ellipse, including all the base and a few millimetres of surrounding healthy skin, is removed and the small wound is closed by sutures, clips or tapes. When there is a narrow, stalk-like pedicle it is tempting to tie a tight ligature round this stalk. This leads to ischaemic necrosis and the papilloma becomes infarcted and drops off within a day or two. However, the base cells in the pedicle may not be destroyed and the papilloma may recur.

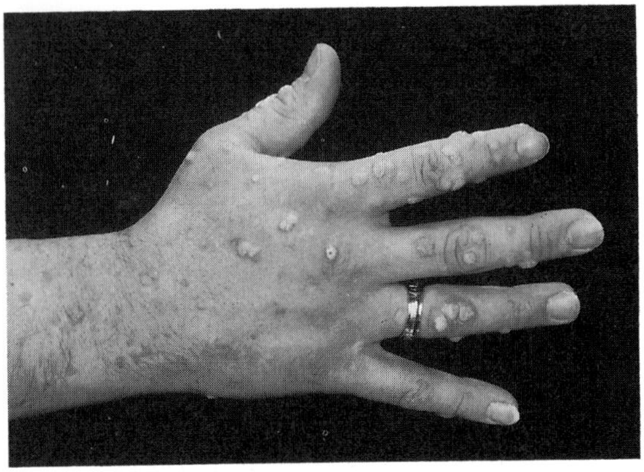

Fig. 19.5 Multiple viral papillomata.

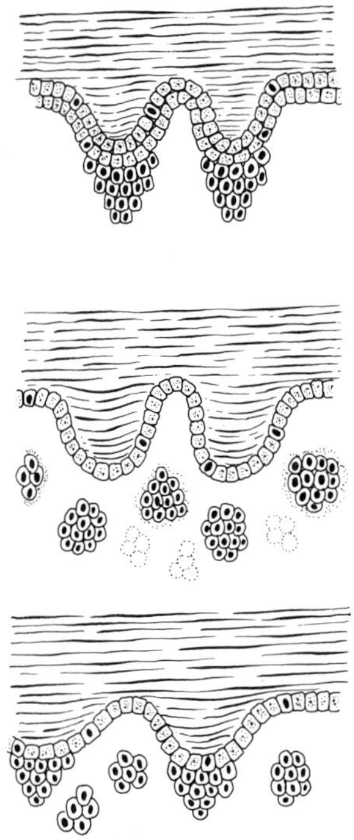

Fig. 19.6 Three types of pigmented naevi: (**A**) junctional; (**B**) dermal; (**C**) compound—see text.

Verruca is the name given to papillomas or warts which have a viral, infective origin. These are often multiple, occurring on the hands or feet, and have finger-like fronds (Fig. 19.5). There may be patches of pigmentation and the colour ranges from grey to brown. Spontaneous regression can occur, but the patient may be prone to recurrences, or even recurrent crops from time to time. Persistent ones can be treated by local applications of caustics or freezing.

A particularly troublesome variety occurs on the sole of the foot—plantar verruca—and since these have a tendency to arise in weight-bearing areas, e.g. the heel or under the metatarsal heads, they can make walking painful. Appropriate methods to remove these are either curettage with a Volkman's spoon, or the local application of liquid nitrogen.

Crops of infective warts occurring in the perineum are often of verrucal origin, and non-venereal ones of viral origin sometimes appear in patients on immunosuppression. When presented with large perineal warts the two specific possibilities of syphilis and lymphogranuloma should be kept in mind.

Pigmented moles or naevi

These are exceedingly common, and there must be few people who do not carry at least one or two such small pigmented lesions. Normally melanocytes are distributed at intervals along the basal layer of epidermal cells. In benign melanotic spots and nodules clumps of melanocytes accumulate either at localized sites in the epidermis or migrate into the dermis. This allows a pathological classification into three basic types (Fig. 19.6):

1. Junctional naevus, in which the clumps of melanocytes arise at the base of extensions of epidermal downgrowths into the dermis, but remain still within the true epidermis.
2. Dermal naevus, in which the clumps lie in the dermis proper, with no continuity with the overlying epidermis.
3. Compound naevus, in which there are elements of both the above.

Clinically there are several different patterns of presentation.

Junctional naevus

These are small, dark brown, flat, well circumscribed spots occurring most often in the distal parts of the limbs and in the perineum. All such spots in the palms and soles of the feet are of this type. They may become apparent and slightly enlarge during childhood, and remain static thereafter, or even occasionally diminish.

Giant hairy mole

These are usually solitary, projecting, fleshy lesions with varying amounts of hair growing from the surface (Fig. 19.7). The face and the buttocks seem preferred sites of origin, and these moles are present at birth. The pathological pattern is either compound or dermal.

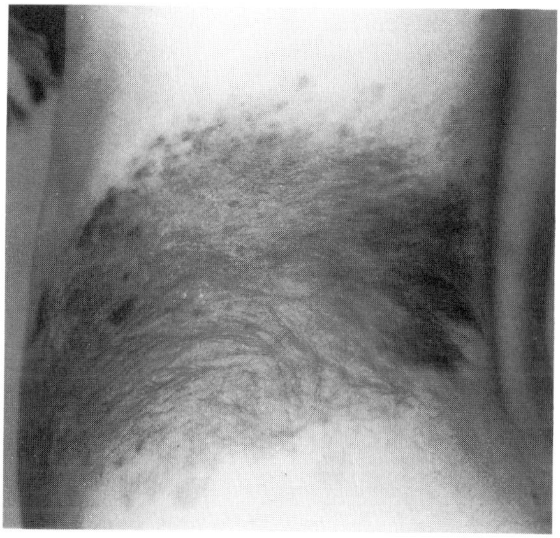

Fig. 19.7 Typical pigmented hairy naevus on side of trunk.

Blue naevus

These are flattened patches, varying in size from a spot to a large map-like area of skin, and the bluish appearance is due to the optical effect of the overlying unpigmented layers of epidermis over the melanocytes which are located deep in the epidermis or dermis (Fig. 19.8).

Halo naevus

In this lesion the brown pigmented spot or nodule is surrounded by a circular area of depigmented skin, which is lighter in colour than the normal skin of the individual. The ring of depigmentation is

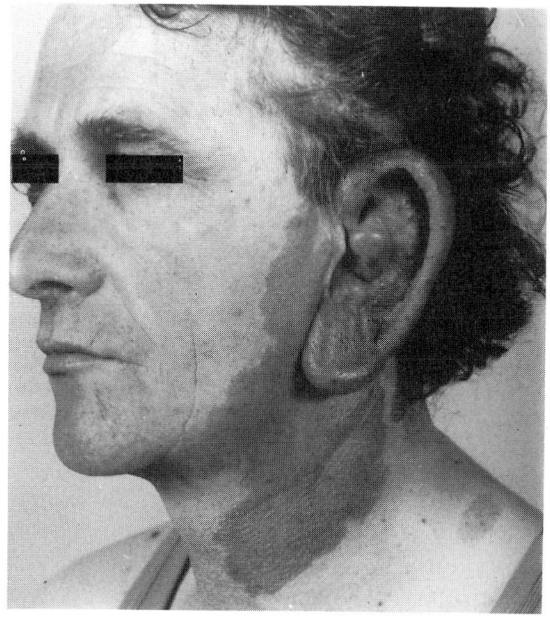

Fig. 19.8 Blue haemangiomatous naevus affecting side of face, neck and ear.

thought to be in some way a manifestation of a local immune reaction. The majority are seen in adolescents and after a period of weeks or months they may gradually and completely regress.

Clearly the main concern on making a clinical diagnosis in any case of a pigmented spot or nodule is that the lesion may in fact be malignant, or undergoing malignant change. A reasonably confident diagnosis can be made when the classical features of the above pigmented moles are present, and no active intervention is advised. However, suspicion of malignant change is raised by any recent increase in size, bleeding, itching, scaliness, or apparent deepening or extension of the pigmentation and wide local excision is then recommended. If removal of a typically benign mole is requested the excision should be complete, and include a margin of normal skin of 0.5–1 cm. Removal of a giant hairy mole will usually require a grafting procedure by a plastic surgeon.

Keratoacanthoma

The main clinical importance of this rare skin lesion is that it may be mistakenly diagnosed as a malignant epithelioma or squamous carcinoma. It

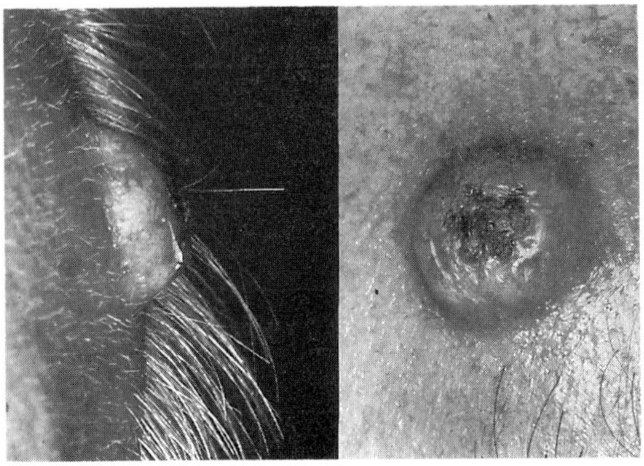

Fig. 19.9 Keratoacanthoma, showing characteristic raised, rounded dome-shaped protruberance, with central ulceration and necrosis. The uniform, regular, rounded outline generally distinguishes it from malignant skin tumours.

is encountered only in adults, generally older than 50 years, and almost always on the face. It starts as a small pimple-like nodule which grows very rapidly to become a raised, dome-shaped firm mass (Fig. 19.9). The skin over the summit ulcerates to reveal a mass of necrotic matter. There is often a mild, inflammatory reaction in the skin immediately surrounding the base, and as superadded infection arises in the ulcer, the local draining lymph nodes may become palpably enlarged and tender. If left alone the mass will become necrosed and disappear, leaving a shallow rounded scar, which may or may not remain visible. Even when the diagnosis is fairly confident on clinical grounds it is wise to take a small biopsy for pathological confirmation, and healing is often both hastened and improved by excising the bulk of the mass and curetting the basal layers.

The histological pattern strongly suggests that this curious lesion arises from the epithelium of the hair follicles.

Vascular neoplasms—angiomas

Most of these are due to abnormal development in areas of blood vessels, and the main component can be arterial, venous or capillary. From the gross pathology point of view they can be classed into either capillary or cavernous types, the former being made up of a network of fine endothelial-lined channels and the latter comprising large, blood-filled sinuses, again lined by endothelium.

Strawberry naevus

One type of capillary haemangioma—the so-called strawberry naevus—can undergo spontaneous involution. This presents as a bright red raised mass, with a lobulated surface (Fig. 19.10), which empties on gentle manual compression and very rapidly refills on removing the pressure. Occasionally the lesion may be more deeply situated, and then it may appear bluer, on account of the visual distortion of the overlying skin.

The usual sequence is that it appears shortly after birth, grows for about 6 months, lasts for 1–2 years and thereafter becomes smaller and paler and eventually disappears over the following years. This lesion is clearly best left alone and any attempt at surgical removal will almost certainly cause unnecessary deformity.

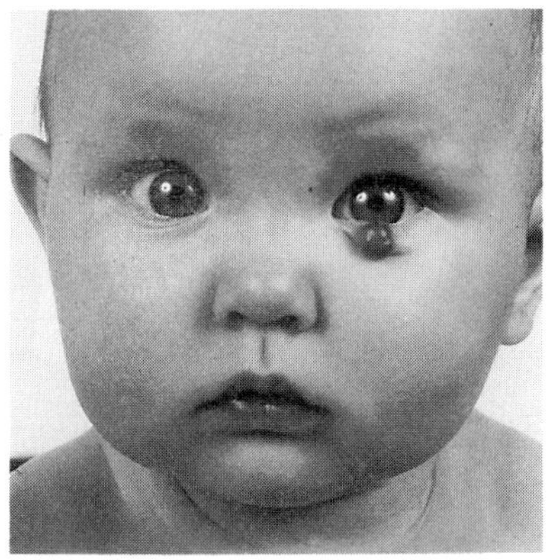

Fig. 19.10 Benign haemangioma of lower eyelid.

Port-wine stain

The other, commoner pattern of capillary haemangioma is the port-wine stain (Fig. 19.11). Some variation in size is encountered, but often they cover quite a large area, and unfortunately they are not uncommon on the face, head and neck. They thus may give rise to considerable and embarrassing cosmetic effects. The patches of red-to-purple discoloration are usually irregular, and sometimes appear to lie along the distribution of one or more cutaneous nerves. If undisturbed the lesions usually remain unchanged throughout life. While small ones may be amenable to cosmetically acceptable

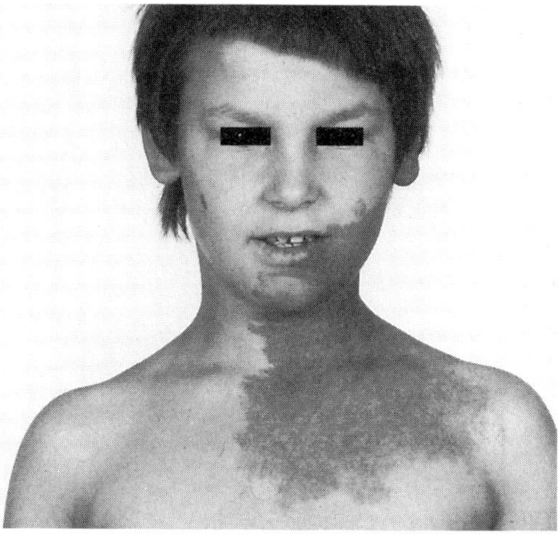

Fig. 19.11 Port-wine stain—capillary haemangioma.

local excision, attempts to remove larger ones are fraught with the risk of causing even greater disfigurement. Most sufferers choose to accept the condition and may use masking cosmetic substances or other means of disguising the blemish. When removal of any but the smallest lesion is urged by the patient, skin grafting, preferably by an experienced plastic surgeon, will be required.

Cavernous haemangiomas

Cavernous haemangiomas present as localized, blue or purple raised soft masses, which again empty on finger pressure, but rapidly refill on releasing the pressure. They usually start to appear during childhood and persist throughout adult life. If exposed to recurrent minor trauma there is, of course, the risk that they will bleed or become infected. Uncomplicated ones may be left alone, or if removal is demanded, may be locally excised.

Cirsoid aneurysm

Cirsoid aneurysm could be regarded as basically similar to a cavernous haemangioma, but with one or more arteries feeding directly into the mass of enlarged blood spaces. The whole mass therefore pulsates and in time the tortuous spaces may enlarge appreciably and may erode neighbouring bone. The scalp is a common location for this lesion and the presence of several vascular commmunications through the skull vault may lead to a similar collection of distended tortuous vessels and blood spaces arising on the inner aspects of the cranium, pressing in turn on the brain surface. Operative correction may be a tricky procedure, and unless all feeding vessels are isolated and divided the lesion will remain. There is, of course, the risk of severe bleeding during the procedure, and this may prove difficult to control.

Campbell de Morgan spots

These very common bright red, rounded, slightly raised spots, generally 2–3 mm in diameter, are of more historical than practical interest. Most often seen in patients aged 50 or over, on the abdomen, chest and less on the limbs, these are of no clinical significance and being so small do not cause symptoms or cosmetic complaints. Their true vascular nature is easily demonstrated and they are best left alone.

Glomus tumour

Glomus tumour is a rare, small, difficult to locate, painful and tender mass, generally occurring in the fingerpulp near the nail, and since there are prominent blood vessels as well as muscle, epithelium and nerve elements, on histological examination they tend to be classified along with other tumours primarily of vascular origin. Simple excision rids the patient of the annoying symptoms.

Benign tumours of nerve origin

Neurofibroma

Neurofibroma arises from nerve tissue which has developed abnormally. Solitary ones may be encountered or they may be multiple; the latter finding is characteristic in von Recklinghausen's disease. This is an inherited disorder, with a dominant genetic pattern, and presents at birth, in childhood or early adult life (Fig. 19.12). The neurofibromas vary; some project obviously above the skin surface, while others lie in the dermal layer and may only be apparent on running the fingers over them. They are distributed along the course of peripheral nerves. There are also quite often pigmented patches in the skin—the so-called cafe-au-lait spots.

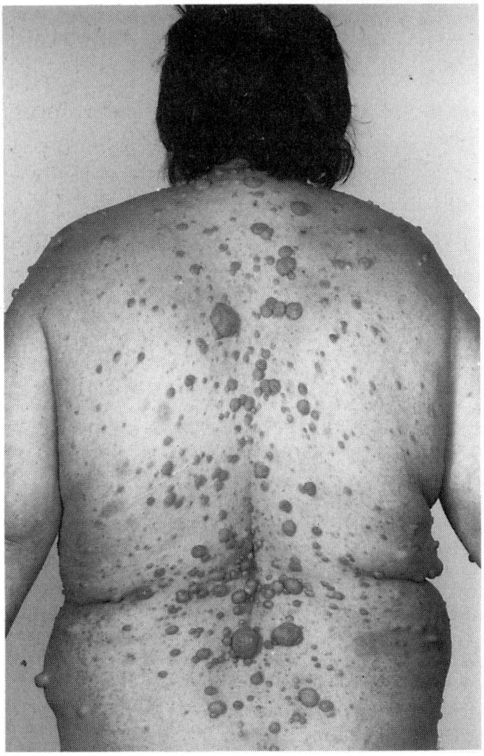

Fig. 19.12 Neurofibromatosis (von Recklinghausen's disease). Very numerous soft-to-firm nodules are scattered all over both trunk and limbs. They vary from tiny subcutaneous nodules to larger pedunculated masses. Occasionally one or more may undergo sarcomatous change, and this is usually suspected if the nodule rapidly enlarges, becomes firmer or starts to itch or cause discomfort.

Solitary neurofibromas are unlikely to change with the passage of time, but those associated with von Recklinghausen syndrome have a tendency to undergo malignant transformation into sarcomas, and therefore if any change in size, appearance or other local symptom is reported excision of that particular lesion is strongly recommended. Clearly it is impractical and unnecessary to remove all multiple neurofibromas, and apart from the above indications, the only reason for local excision would be concern of the patient about the appearance or repeated local minor trauma.

Nerve sheath tumours (schwannomas, neurilemmomas)

These are solitary, arising generally in either the neck, arms or legs, and as their name indicates, they are derived from the Schwann cells enveloping a superficial peripheral nerve. Because of the close application to the nerve this lesion is usually painful and tender and the pain may be referred distally along the course of the nerve. Simple excision is curative.

Other connective tissue benign tumours

Fibromas

Fibromas are occasionally found lying superficially in the subcutaneous layers. They are usually small rounded firm mobile lesions, the skin moving freely over them. They are usually symptomless and removal is sought on account of their appearance or nuisance value.

Lipoma

Although arising from subcutaneous fat, this common benign, lobulated soft mass is usually superficial and therefore often presents as a swelling raising the skin over it (Fig. 19.13). There is rarely real diagnostic doubt because of its characteristic soft, flabby feel, and often the lobulation can be felt easily, or brought into prominence by gently pushing the mass to one side. This slightly tenses the thin fibrous capsule and places the lobules under increased pressure. Whether the lipoma is solely in the subdermal layer or is arising from fat lying between muscle bundles can be determined by

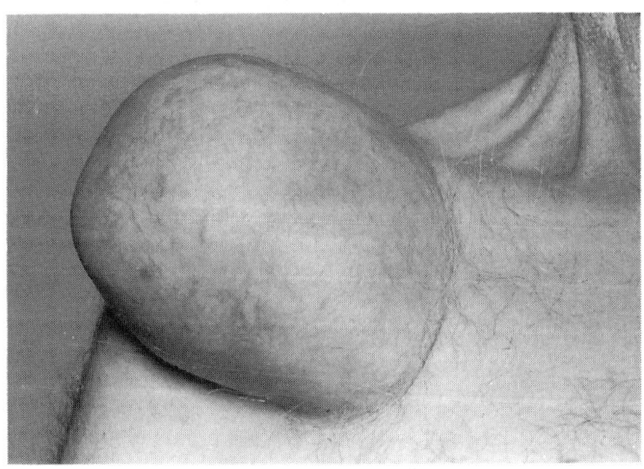

Fig. 19.13 Large lipoma on the right shoulder. This had been present and slowly enlarging over many years before the patient sought advice with regard to removal.

asking the patient to perform an action which will contract the muscle and feeling whether this restricts the mobility of it or not. Sometimes the portion of a lipoma just below the skin represents only the tip of the iceberg, with the greater part lying within or below muscle.

Lipomas are entirely benign and removal is recommended for cosmetic reasons, or because of gradually increasing local size and nuisance value. Superficial ones may be easily excised under local anaesthesia, but those lying more deeply may be more adequately explored and removed under general anaesthesia. It is very important to dissect carefully around the entire capsule of all component lobules to ensure removal is complete, otherwise recurrence is certain.

Sweat gland tumours

These are very rare adenomas showing a well organized acinar pattern of the epidermoid cells. They can be single or multiple, and appear just below the skin as rounded nodules. Local excision is required.

MALIGNANT TUMOURS

Basal cell carcinoma (rodent ulcer)

This locally invasive tumour occurs mostly in fair-skinned people who have been exposed for long periods to the sun, and like other skin tumours is relatively common in Australia. The vast majority arise on the skin of the face, in an area from the forehead, side of the nose, inner canthus of the eye and the cheek (Fig. 19.14). Rarely do they present at other sites.

As the name indicates, these tumours start in the basal layer of the epidermis, forming clumps of proliferating cells which extend down into the dermis, and ultimately into other deeper tissues, and also ulcerate through the more superficial epidermal layers. Although when left untreated, the lesion displays the locally invasive properties of a malignant tumour, it very rarely metastasizes by either lymphatic or blood routes, with the result that effective local removal is curative.

Clinically the usual presentation is of a very slowly growing pale nodule, which gradually ulcerates and

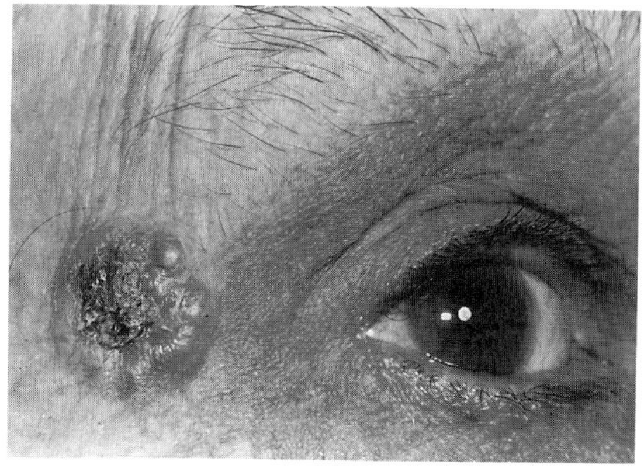

Fig. 19.14 Basal cell carcinoma or rodent ulcer in a common site, i.e. near to the eye. The edge is slightly raised in a rolled, nodular pattern and the centre is ulcerated.

may bleed slightly from time to time. A scab usually forms over the central ulcerated area and the slowly progressive edge is slightly raised up from the skin surface, giving a pearly appearance. The edge is usually well defined. Rarely there is cystic degeneration within the tumour which presents as a cystic, blister-like lesion (Fig. 19.15).

Although it should be rare to meet long-neglected examples of this tumour, occasionally these are still encountered, and widespread erosion and destruction of the underlying structures, e.g. facial bone, nasal cavity and orbit, may have taken place.

Two satisfactory methods of treatment are available. First, since they are of squamous epithelial origin they are as a rule very sensitive to

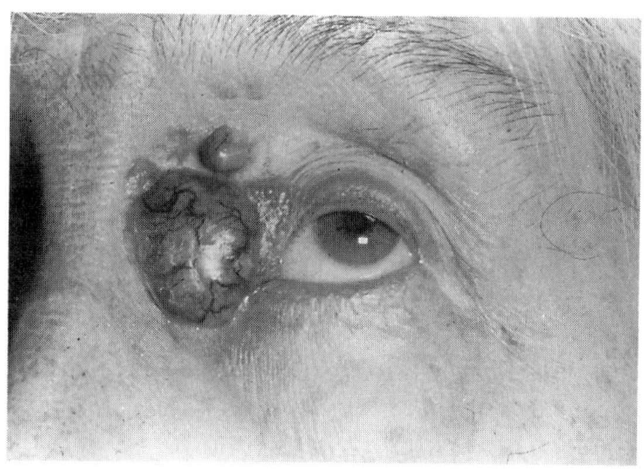

Fig. 19.15 Basal cell carcinoma of the rarer encysted type. The surface is covered by a layer of stretched skin; this one also shows prominent blood vessels. A second smaller one lies immediately above the main lesion.

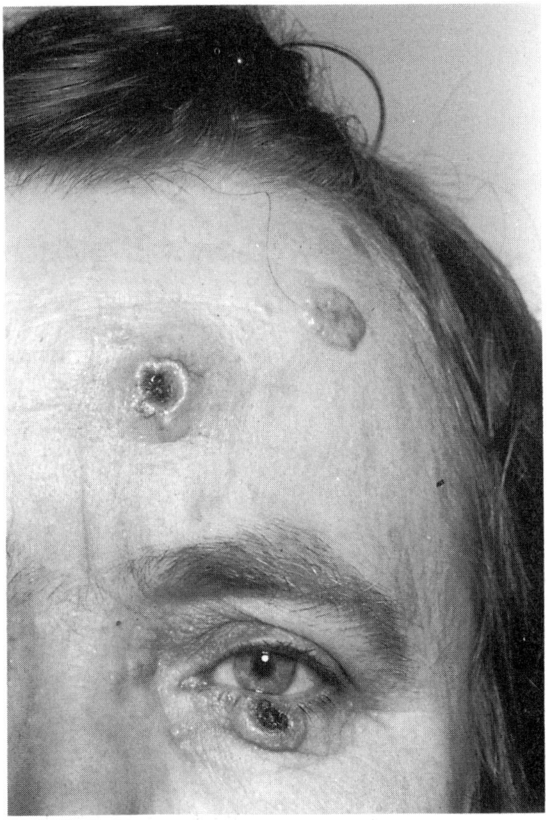

Fig. 19.16 Multiple simultaneous basal cell carcinomata: two with ulceration and a third with the skin still unbroken.

radiotherapy, and this is the preferred method when available. Second, local excision, including an all-round removal of a small margin of uninvolved skin and deeper tissue and closure of the wound by suture or if the defect is too large for this, by skin grafting, gives a good result.

Radiotherapy can be damaging to the eye, and to any closely underlying cartilage or bone, and therefore surgical excision is the treatment of choice whenever the lesion is close to those structures (Fig. 19.16). The removal of large neglected lesions may involve complicated plastic surgery procedures to give satisfactory functional and cosmetic reconstruction.

Squamous cell carcinoma (squamous epithelioma)

This skin tumour also tends to appear on areas exposed to the sun, but in addition to a variety of other forms of chronic mechanical and chemical irritation, and irradiation. Although a squamous cell carcinoma may arise anywhere where stratified squamous epithelium exists, the commonest sites are the ear, the lips, cheek, and the back of the hand. Areas in which hyperkeratosis has previously arisen, e.g. leukoplakia, are more prone to develop this pattern of malignant change, as are chronic ulcers, discharging sinuses or burn scars. In the past among city dwellers the specific occupational hazards to cotton spinners and chimney sweeps of local accumulation and irritation by hydrocarbons in the perineal region led to the development of scrotal epithelioma, and a present-day analogy is perhaps the Khangri cancers occurring in Kashmir, where the practice of applying charcoal burners to the lower abdomen in order to keep warm continues.

Whether or not there is a pre-existing predisposing change in the epithelium, the histological changes which characterize squamous cell carcinoma are irregular cells or groups of cells which penetrate into the dermis and other neighbouring tissues. Increased cellular activity is reflected in abundant mitosis, columns of dark-staining cells, and here and there in the microscopic field cell-nests. Metastatic spread to the regional lymph nodes is often an early occurrence, but since the primary tumour ulcerates at an early stage, leading to super-added infection, this may also be responsible for enlargement of the draining lymph nodes. Metastatic spread by the blood stream is unusual and if it occurs tends to be late.

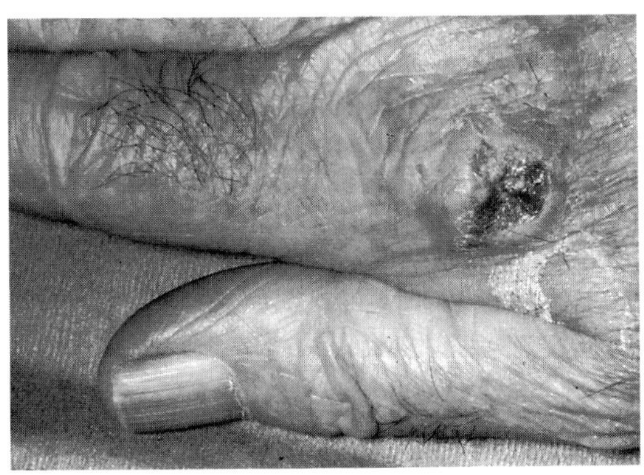

Fig. 19.17 Squamous carcinoma of skin over the first metacarpophalangeal joint: a raised, irregular ulcerated hard mass.

Clinically the lesion may start either as a raised papillary growth, which then breaks down on its summit to produce a raised, firm, ulcerated mass, or as a hard, indurated ulcer, with a slightly raised and everted edge (Fig. 19.17). This latter presentation is more likely if it develops on a predisposing condition, e.g. chronic infected ulcer or a burn scar. The regional lymph nodes should be examined and may be found to be palpably enlarged. The ulcerated area contains slough, is often mildly infected so that there is a continuous discharge of purulent material, and there are usually small areas of haemorrhage (Fig. 19.18).

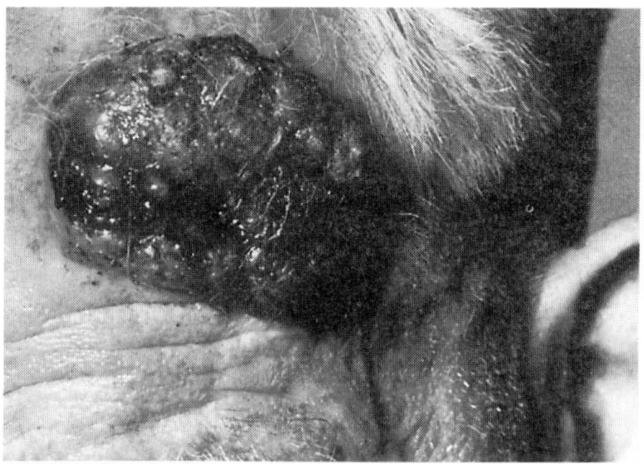

Fig. 19.18 A large neglected squamous carcinoma which has proliferated to produce a fungating mass which bleeds spontaneously or on the lightest contact and has superadded infection. Lymph node metastases were present in the preauricular area and jugular chain.

To confirm the diagnosis wedge biopsy of the edge of the ulcerated lesion is desirable, and it is wise also to X-ray the chest to determine whether any metastatic deposits are present.

When it comes to treatment there are again the two options of radiotherapy or surgical excision. The same contraindications to radiotherapy listed under basal cell carcinoma also apply, but where there are no such restrictions a good cosmetic cure can be obtained. As an alternative, wide local surgical removal and primary suture or graft closure may be equally successful (Fig. 19.19).

As far as the regional lymph nodes are concerned, these may rapidly return to normal after eradication of the primary lesion if the enlargement has been due only to infection, but if enlargement remains or there is strong clinical suspicion that they are enlarged due to metastases, biopsy should be performed, and if positive for malignant involvement, a block dissection of the nodes of that side of the neck carried out.

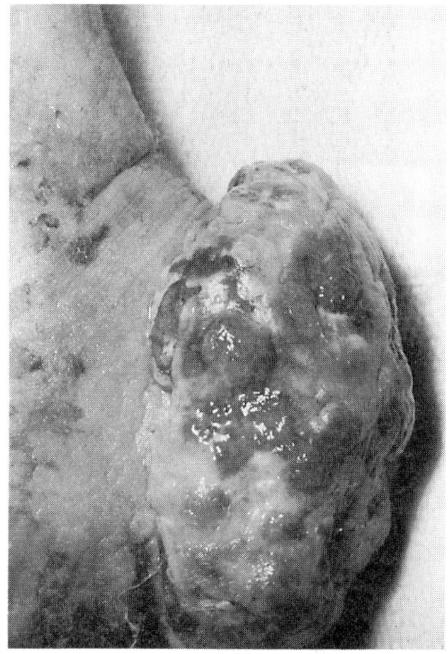

Fig. 19.19 Another large fungating squamous carcinoma on the heel.

Extensive involvement or recurrence may be palliated by either local irradiation, or chemotherapy with agents such as bleomycin.

Malignant melanoma

This is a highly aggressive tumour with a bad reputation. It may arise anywhere where melanocytes are located, namely the skin, the linings of the mouth, nose, vagina and in the choroid plexus of the eye, or the meninges (Fig. 19.20). White-skinned people are much more at risk than dark-skinned, and once again excess exposure to sunlight may be one of the aetiological factors. Most patients presenting with a melanoma have previously existing cutaneous benign melanotic spots or naevi. However, since virtually everyone has several of these it is difficult to be certain whether the malignant lesion has truly developed as a transformation of the pre-existing one or started de novo alongside other innocent ones. In any event it is clear that the vast majority of benign pigmented

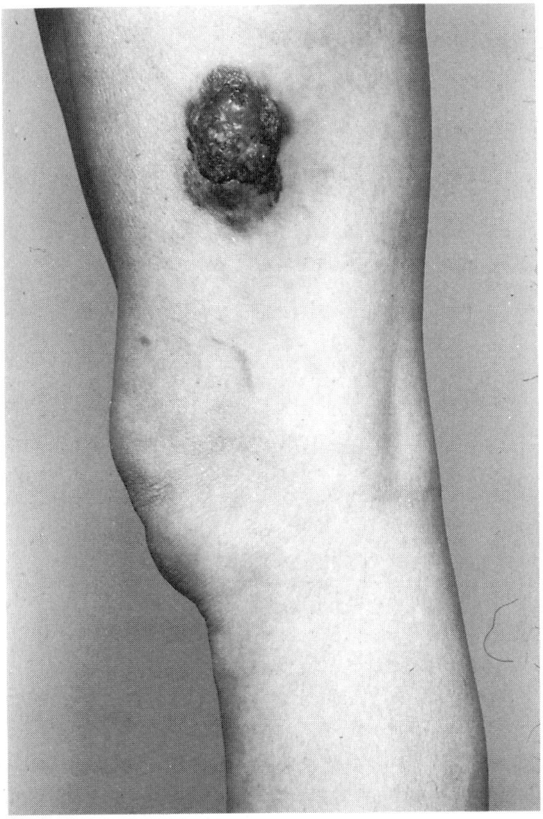

Fig. 19.20 Malignant melanoma: a deeply pigmented raised mass which has only been present for several weeks. Spreading distally from the main tumour mass is a halo of minute satellite nodules of the melanoma. This will require wide local excision and possibly block dissection of the groin nodes, if there is evidence of spread to them.

naevi remain entirely innocent throughout life, and removal of all such spots is unnecessary and impracticable.

Symptoms and signs which are suspicious of malignant change are distinct increase in size, local itch, bleeding on minimal or no trauma, deepening of the pigmentation, or the extension of it out from its original limits.

The histological features of malignant melanoma include clear penetration of masses of cells from the junctional layer between epidermis and dermis, down into the latter and perhaps also into deeper structures. Pigment granules may be seen in both the highly active, rapidly dividing cells and in the intercellular spaces. Some alveolar formation of the cells with large dark nuclei is often seen. Spread of metastases to the regional lymph nodes is a prominent and often early feature and widespread dissemination by the blood is an all too frequent later development. Although a rapid progression without interruption is common, sometimes there may appear to be a halt in the clinical course for months or even years after initial diagnosis and treatment during which no further evidence of tumour is apparent. However, after this prolonged lull there may appear a quickfire succession of more deposits at one or more sites, and these are usually resistant to all attempts at control, and prove rapidly fatal.

When blood spread does occur the liver seems to be a favoured site for metastatic deposits to lodge, but virtually any tissue may become the target.

From the clinical point of view there are several different main patterns of presentation.

Lentigo maligna (melanotic freckle)

This starts as a long-standing, but slowly extending dark brown patch of the skin, generally on the cheek, and nearly always in elderly females. A history of 10 years' presence of this lesion is not uncommon. When the malignant melanoma change develops it does so as a firm nodule to one or other side of the patch. The nodule increases in size, penetrates below the epidermis, ulcerates and then behaves as a fully malignant tumour.

Superficial spreading melanoma

This commoner pattern of melanoma arises most often on the trunk or legs, and has a peak incidence in middle age. It has a premalignant phase of about 1–2 years during which it appears as a slightly raised flat-topped pigmented area extending irregularly outward in several directions. Again frankly malignant development is indicated by the appearance of an induruated area which ulcerates or bleeds. At this point the proliferating melanocytes invade the dermis and perhaps also other deeper structures.

Nodular melanoma

This, unlike the other two varieties, starts de novo as an invasive collection of malignant melanoma in an area of skin with no previous pigmented spot

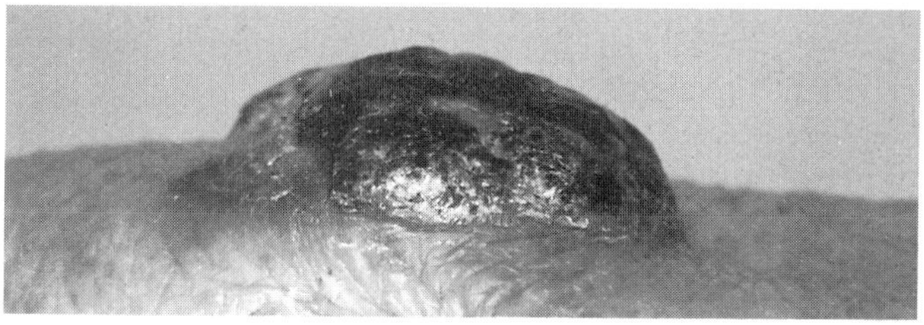

Fig. 19.21 Lateral view of a malignant melanoma showing the pigmented mass well raised up from the surrounding skin.

or area (Fig. 19.21). A common site is on the leg, particularly the lower leg in women. Characteristically it presents as a nodule, steadily deepening in colour from brown to almost black, stretching the skin over it so that it becomes shiny, ulcerating, bleeding to slight touch, scabbing over and often being the seat of itching. If allowed to progress without treatment further satellite nodules may later appear in the neighbouring skin.

Subungual melanoma (melanotic whitlow)

When a melanoma arises beneath or just lateral to a toenail or fingernail it is often first diagnosed as an inflammatory lesion (Fig. 19.22). This is because infection and abscess formation is common at these sites, and also because the initial symptoms may be of a painful and tender swelling in relation to the nail. It may soon become apparent, however, that treatment appropriate for a pyogenic infection is not leading to improvement and the real diagnosis is entertained. Most commonly the melanoma affects the thumb or great toe, but other digits may be affected. Usually the patient is middle-aged or elderly. One of the difficulties with regard to early diagnosis is that at first pigmentation may be slight or apparently absent, and is only obvious when the lesion enlarges.

It is important to note that although the majority of malignant melanomas are pigmented there is a minority in which no brown discoloration can be seen on naked-eye examination—the amelanotic melanomas which generally have a slightly pink hue.

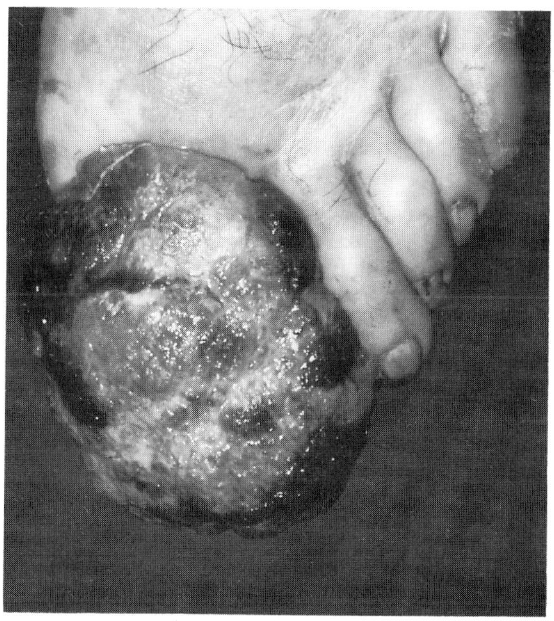

Fig. 19.22 Large malignant melanoma—which started as a swelling beneath the toenail—the classical subungual melanoma. This one, which had been ignored by the patient at first, grew to this size within 2–3 months.

Clinical features

The diagnosis of malignant melanoma is made or strongly suspected on the basis of history of development of the lesion and a combination of inspection and gentle palpation. The areas where the draining lymph nodes are located should always be palpated for detectable enlargement, and if this is present it virtually always signifies metastatic spread. When the primary lesion is on the leg, the abdomen should also be palpated to detect any grossly enlarged para-aortic nodes, and regardless of the site of original tumour the liver should be examined for enlargement due to metastatic deposits.

Treatment

At present the main hope of cure lies with surgical excision, but the successful eradication of the disease depends on how far the tumour has extended by the time operation is performed. If the diagnosis is uncertain, excision biopsy, preferably with frozen section reporting, is the first step. Taking any form of other biopsy, e.g. wedge excision, needling, or any other form of directly invasive procedure is to be avoided, since this will increase the risk of disseminating the malignant cells.

When the diagnosis is confirmed wide local excision including a margin of normal surrounding skin is performed, and the extent of this margin depends on several factors. About 1–2 cm will suffice when removing a lentigo malignum, whereas it is wise to excise at least 5 cm for more invasive tumours. The block of tissue removed should include skin and the whole thickness of subcutaneous tissue down to the deep fascial layer. Closure of the resulting defect will usually require skin grafting—generally a straightforward split-skin graft taken from another limb or area of the body. The only satisfactory way of removing a subungual melanoma is amputation of the digit.

If the regional lymph nodes are involved, or are close to the primary lesion, block dissection is advised. An alternative approach is the endolymphatic administration of radioactive isotope—but this has so far not proved too promising.

Prognosis

In keeping with the surgical management of several malignant tumours, the earlier the diagnosis and the less the invasion of the lesion, the better the chance of cure. Of particular importance is the depth of the tumour, and of the various ways of assessing this, the simple measurement by means of a micrometer gauge—the Breslow scale—is perhaps the most useful guide (Fig. 19.23). When the total depth is < 0.7 mm all should expect cure from local excision. When, however the depth is 0.7–1.5 mm 5-year survival rates are about 70%, and when >1.5 mm only 30%.

Other factors, e.g. the indices of cellular activity on microscopic examination, also influence the ultimate outcome, but the simple Breslow classification is easy to apply and is a good clinically applicable guide.

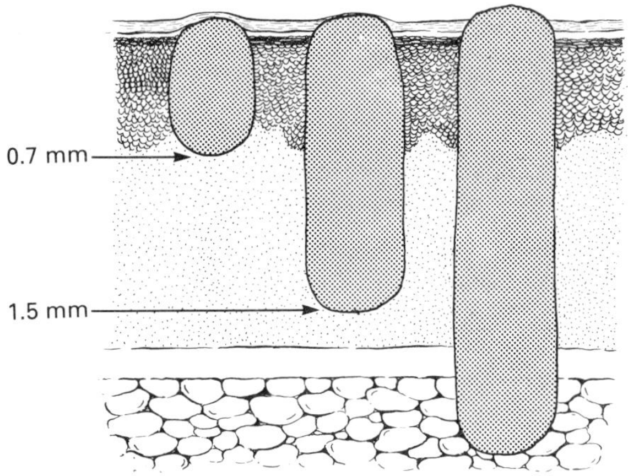

Fig. 19.23 Breslow scale for assessing depth of invasion by malignant melanoma—see text.

Treatment for those with advanced metastatic disease is generally unsatisfactory. The main hope is of one or more of the cytotoxic drugs given either systemically or by local intraarterial infusion, or BCG immunization or other attempts to provoke an immune response. At best temporary reduction in the spread of the disease may be hoped for.

Carcinoma-in-situ (Bowen's disease)

This can be regarded as an intradermal inactive form of cancer which, however, may become the seat of a frank squamous carcinoma with the passage of time. The condition presents with one or more flat but slightly raised plaques, often fissured on the surface, and of a red-to-brown colour. Local excision is advised.

Sweat gland tumours

These rare tumours, arising subdermally and having the characteristic histological appearance of sweat gland acinar tissue, are mostly benign, with no tendency to metastasize, but a very occasional adenocarcinoma of sweat gland origin has been reported.

OTHER DISORDERS OF SWEAT GLANDS

Hyperhidrosis

Excessive sweating can cause not only embarrassment, but also real disability. If it is mainly from the hands this can spoil paper, fabrics, cloth being handled at work and make dealing with food or fine objects more or less impossible.

If the problem with hands or feet is sufficiently troublesome it can be abolished permanently by sympathetic denervation, at the lumbar level for the feet and the upper thoracic level for the hands.

For profuse sweating from the axilla it is possible to offer relief either by excising a diamond-shaped area of the axillary skin, or by scraping the undersurface of the skin by means of a sharp curette introduced through a small incision. In either procedure it is helpful to mark out the usually limited area from which the excess sweating arises, e.g. by mopping the axilla dry, dusting with powdered starch and iodine and marking out the area which turns blue with the sweating.

Hidradenitis suppurativa

In this condition there is chronic pyogenic infection of the apocrine glands, and the three areas most commonly affected are the axilla, groin and perineum. It is more likely to arise in obese people and when the hygienic care is inadequate. Multiple small abscesses, sinus tracks, and discharging openings may appear over a wide area of the skin and continued sweating and irritation worsen the situation. Usually all attempts at treatment with local antiseptics, local or systemic antibiotics and other measures fail to clear the problem, and often local excision of the involved skin and subcutaneous tissues is required. It is important to ensure that all tracks are included in the excised material, otherwise recurrence is likely. If the wound cannot be closed without tension, skin grafting will be required.

SUBCUTANEOUS INFECTIONS IN HANDS AND FEET

Since both the hands and feet are more liable to minor injury, pyogenic infections are most commonly encountered there than at other sites in the body. The following are some of the most common clinical presentations.

Paronychia

The infection develops in the nailfold, and if it extends it may pass around or underneath the nailbed, and if unrelieved even into the pulp space. There is pain, swelling, redness, throbbing and tenderness most obvious to the side of the nail. Pus usually forms and may spontaneously point and discharge, with relief to the patient. However, if the patient presents with an undrained pocket of pus it is advisable to drain this through a longitudinal incision on the lateral aspect of the swollen nailfold (Fig. 19.24).

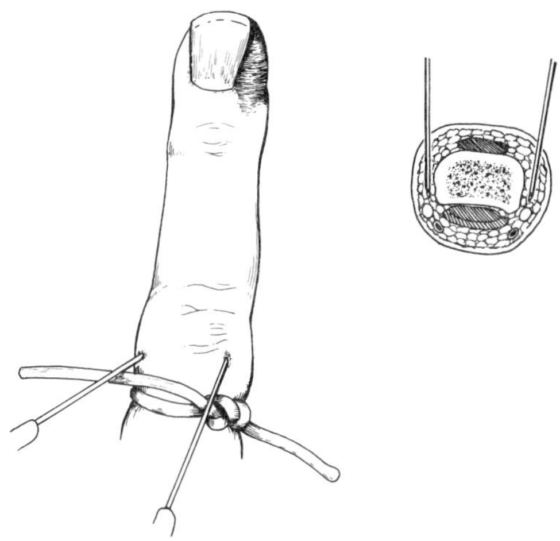

Fig. 19.24 Paronychia about to be surgically incised and drained under ring block local anaesthesia. The cross-section shows that after injecting local anaesthetic superficially the points are introduced to near the palmar aspect of the finger, to anaesthetize the digital nerves.

Ingrowing toenail

This is a form of paronychia caused by the erosive pressure of the edge of a grossly curved nail, nearly always on the great toe. If pus is present this may need surgical drainage, but often the patient presents with an already discharging, chronically thickened, raised red nailfold and the nail edge partly cut away. If the condition is mild and early the condition may be allowed to settle by taking care to open out the nailfold gently, clearing any obvious collection of dirt, applying an antiseptic and allowing the nail to grow longer and avoiding tight footwear. On the other hand, where the infection is well established it is better to avulse the nail under a brief general anaesthetic. As the new nail grows, hopefully it will be less curved than the former one, and it should be cut straight across after reaching its full length, avoiding any paring round the corner. If in spite of this the trouble recurs then permanent ablation of the nail and the nailbed is required (Fig. 19.25).

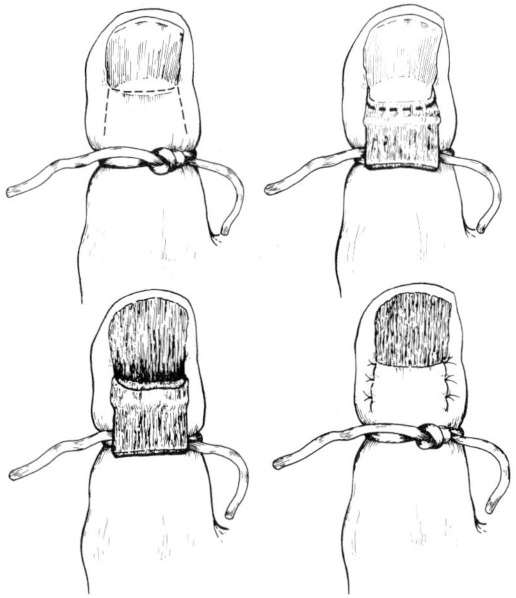

Fig. 19.25 Permanent ablation of toenail bed (Zadek's operation). Under general or ring block local anaesthesia, and after applying a simple rubber tourniquet, a skin flap is raised up to expose the entire nailbed, which is then excised with a small proximal margin around it. The flap is then replaced and secured with sutures along its edges.

Onychogryphosis

Although not primarily an infective disorder, this other fairly common toenail abnormality is appropriate to consider here. It is considerable overgrowth of the nail, leading to a projecting horn-like hooked mass arising from the nail bed (Fig. 19.26). It looks unsightly, but in addition may cause trauma and infection of the great toe from which it arises, or neighbouring ones. Treatment is by complete excision of the nail and nailbed.

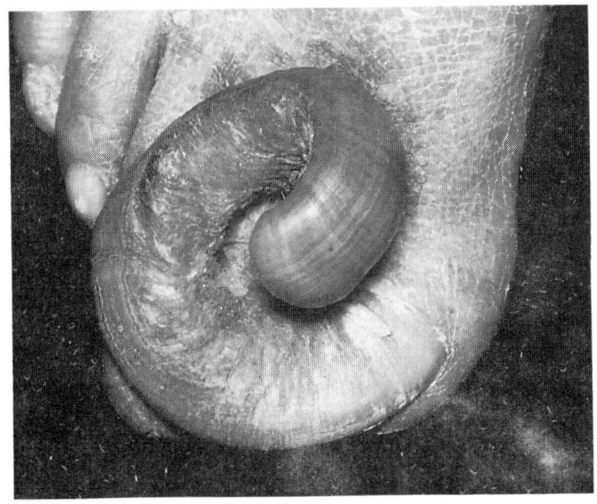

Fig. 19.26 An extreme example of onychogryphosis.

Hand infections

Pulp space infection

Since the distal pulp space is crossed from phalanx to skin by several fibrous septa, it is divided up into numerous loculi. Thus when pus forms considerable pressure builds up within these loculi. As a result, not only are pulp space infections very painful but also the pressure may compromise the blood supply to the phalanx. It is therefore important to achieve good surgical drainage as soon as an abscess is suspected. This is done through a longitudinal incision over the point of maximal swelling or the midline. The incision should not cross the flexor crease.

Web space infection

A puncture wound in the interdigital space or extension from an infected focus in nearby tissues can cause a collection of pus in the web space, and this is best dealt with by evacuation through a short incision in the dorsal aspect of the web.

Palmar space infections

These more serious deeper infections involve the mid palmar and thenar spaces and/or the flexor tendon sheaths, and are best treated by surgeons with a special expertise in the management of hand injuries. Correctly placed and timed incisions

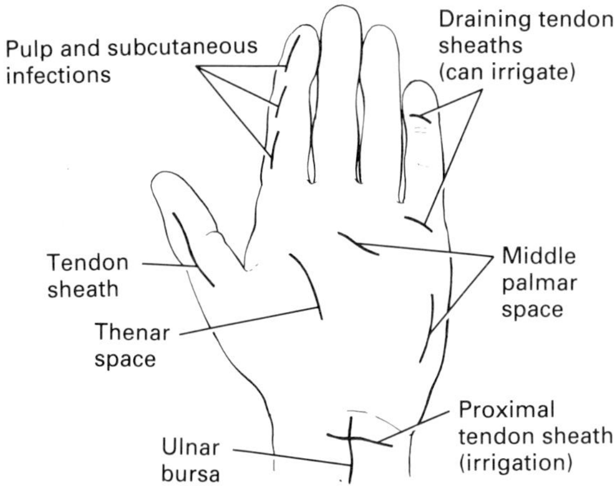

Fig. 19.27 Various sites for incisions to drain infections in different layers and structures of the hand.

(Fig. 19.27), exploration and drainage are required, otherwise there is a risk of damage to important structures and limited hand movements on resolution of the infection.

FIBROUS CONTRACTURES

Dupuytren's contracture

This is a relatively common affliction, particularly in middle-aged and elderly men, comprising a progressive thickening and contracture of the palmar aponeurosis (Fig. 19.28). In a proportion of cases there are predisposing factors, e.g. alcoholism, Epanutin treatment for epilepsy, repeated exposure of the hand to gripping actions at work and others, but many arise with no obvious pre-existing factors. In some families there may be a hereditary tendency to develop the condition.

The first sign is usually a hard nodule under the skin on the palmar aspect at the level of the metacarpophalangeal joint of the ring finger. As it extends it may in turn involve the little finger, and less often the other ones. The area of hard thickening becomes larger and the skin over it becomes adherent to it and in time the ring or little finger is drawn gradually more and more into a flexed position. Both the metacarpophalangeal and the proximal interphalangeal joints are bent, but the distal interphalangeal joint generally remains straight, with some range of extension and flexion. The other

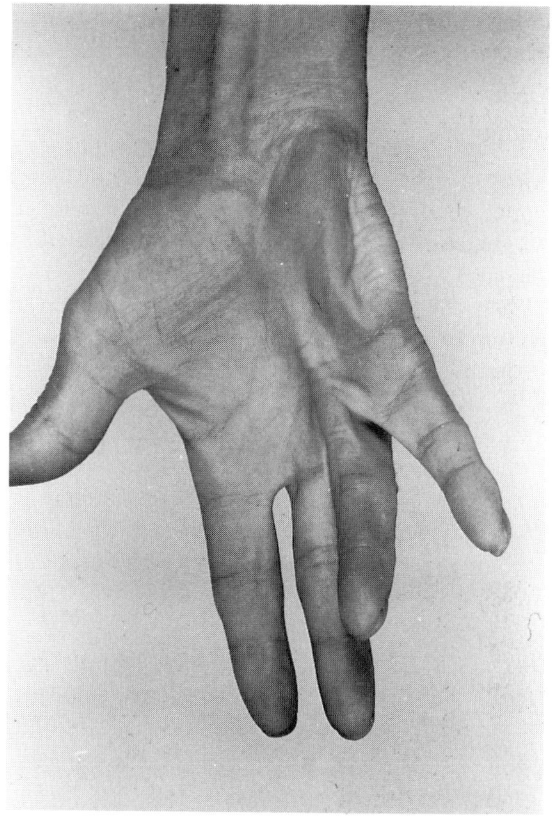

Fig. 19.28 Dupuytren's contracture. Palmar view showing the dense band of tight aponeurotic tissue affecting mainly the ring finger and to a lesser extent the little finger. The patient cannot straighten the ring finger any further than shown.

structures in the hand do not become involved in the fibrotic process.

The main clinical problems presented are difficulty in grasping objects properly, repeated accidental knocking of the bent finger or fingers on using the hand, and of course difficulty with fine movements of the hand and fingers.

Surgical relief can be obtained in mild examples of the deformity by the procedure of subcutaneous fasciotomy, in which a narrow tenotome is introduced laterally, passed to the region of the tight fascial bands, which are then divided; or when the condition is more advanced, by excision of the entire palmar aponeurosis. This involves raising skin flaps proximally and distally, under tourniquet control, and then dissecting out the entire triangular fascial layer with its extensions along the bases of the involved fingers. Occasionally amputation of a grossly bent, fixed finger is required.

Ganglion

Although this is not strictly of subcutaneous tissue origin, it presents as a rounded swelling occupying space predominantly in the subcutaneous space.

Ganglia are frequently encountered either on the dorsum of the wrist or the dorsum of the foot, less commonly on the palmar aspect of the wrist or other sites, e.g. distal interphalangeal joints and the knee. They arise from either joint capsule or tendon sheath, the former becoming more tense on flexing the relevant joint, the latter moving on contracting the appropriate muscle. The wall is thin and the content clear or slightly opalescent mucoid material. Although ganglia appear like herniations of the joint capsule or tendon sheath, they are more probably areas of degeneration of the fibrous tissue.

The patient usually seeks advice solely on account of the appearance of the swelling, but there may also be minor discomfort, particularly if he or she has to use the hand a lot.

The diagnosis is generally easy. The most satisfactory way of treating ganglia is complete surgical excision, preferably under general anaesthesia so that the root can be found, ligated and divided. If excision is incomplete recurrence is likely. Alternative but often temporary ways of dealing with them are dispersing them by applying strong digital pressure directly over the ganglion, or emptying through a large-bore needle. Recurrence will be almost inevitable.

20. The lymphatic system

STRUCTURE AND FUNCTION

The fine network of thin-walled channels directs the flow along via a series of nodes, and beyond these into slightly wider vessels emptying eventually into the systemic venous side of the blood circulation, mainly via the thoracic duct. The finest capillary-sized vessels resemble blood capillaries, but their walls are particularly permeable to macromolecules, e.g. proteins, micro-organisms and tissue debris. Lymph fluid brought to the nodes by afferent lymphatic vessels is filtered through the nodal tissue, with the opportunity for removing potentially harmful substances and organisms and mounting immune responses to foreign proteins (Fig. 20.1). The nodes therefore exert a basically defensive role. The filtered lymph then leaves by efferent vessels and travels to join that from other parts of the body, to reach the subclavian veins via the thoracic or other small ducts. In all but the finest lymphatic vessels there are numerous valves which direct the flow towards the veins, and the main force acting on the vessels is the mechanical pressure exerted by contracting muscles. The total volume of protein-rich fluid carried to the venous system by the lymphatics is between 2 and 4 l/day.

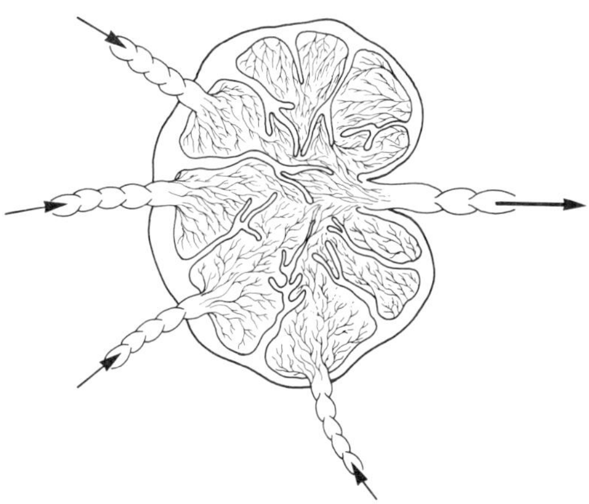

Fig. 20.1 Schematic diagram of flow through a lymph node. Several afferent vessels lead the fluid into a meshwork of nodal tissue, where organisms and other potentially harmful substances are removed, and immune responses are initiated or mounted. Once filtered, the lymph fluid leaves the node by a single efferent vessel.

DEFICIENT LYMPH FLOW

Since a main function of the lymphatic system is to remove protein-rich material from the tissue spaces, impairment due to an inadequate number and distribution of lymph vessels, varicosity in them, or blockage will lead to the accumulation of fluid and protein at the periphery—this is lymphoedema (Fig. 20.2). This may be due to congenital maldevelopment or secondary to damage by certain diseases or surgical intervention.

LYMPHOEDEMA

Regardless of the underlying cause the characteristics of lymphoedematous swelling will be the same. It arises most often in the lower limb, and at first there may only be a slight increase in girth of the foot and ankle towards the end of the day, and a return towards normal after a night lying flat in bed. As it progresses in extent and size of swelling it becomes more permanent, with little or no decrease after overnight elevation. The swollen area is not painful or tender unless episodes of cellulitis or lymphangitis occur—both of these are not uncommon complications. The feel of the part affected is firm and brawny, and on withdrawing the finger after a minute or so of sustained firm

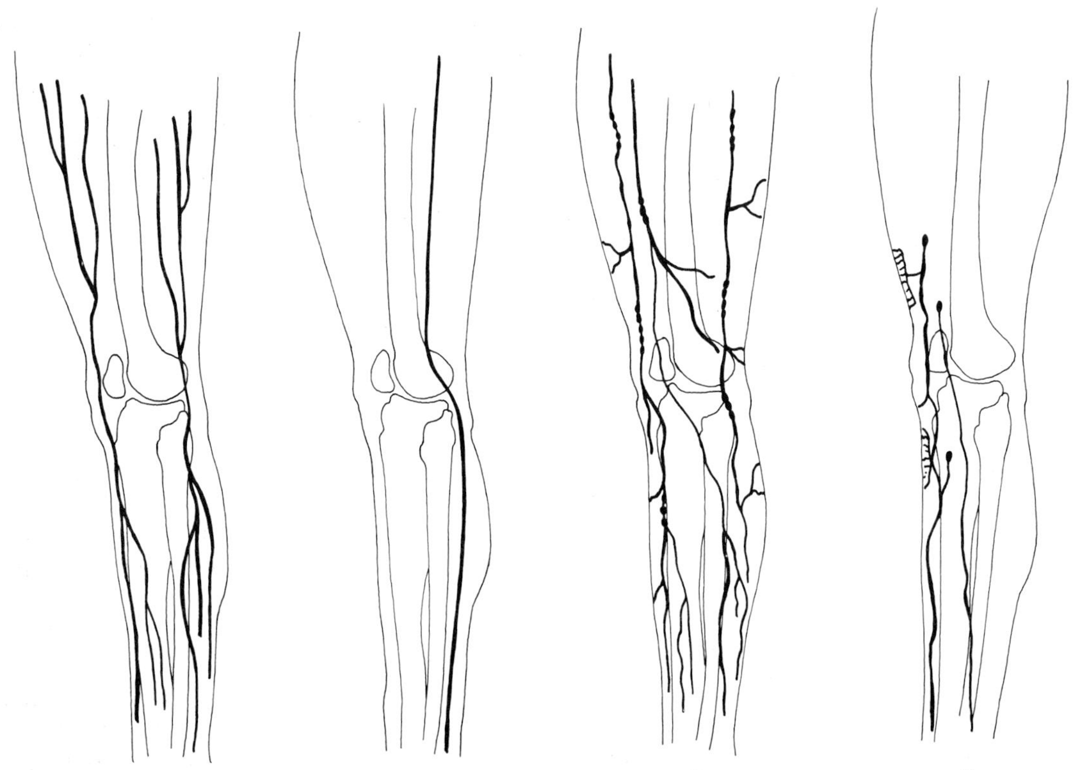

Fig. 20.2 Patterns of limb lymphatics, which can be demonstrated by lymphangiography. (**A**) Normal distribution; (**B**) gross congenital underdevelopment; (**C**) varicosity of some of the channels; (**D**) blockage of several main vessels, e.g. by surgery or malignant deposits.

pressure, there is either no pitting or at most only slight indentation, in marked contrast to the deep pitting oedema due to either venous impairment or congestive cardiac failure.

PRIMARY LYMPHOEDEMA

In this disorder the congenital defect is hypoplasia, aplasia, or variceal dilatation of the lymphatic vessels. The symptoms may first appear at or soon after birth, or may not become apparent until later childhood, adolescence or the early 20s. A variety of different names have been applied depending on the time of onset, e.g. truly congenital lymphoedema, lymphoedema praecox (Milroy's disease), lymphoedema tarda. It is probably not helpful to make these distinctions since the clinical problems and management are basically the same in any event.

Usually the obvious swelling is confined at first to the distal part of the limb, but extends gradually over months to a year to the entire leg. Although to begin with rest and elevation will allow partial diminution in the oedema, soon this makes little or no difference and the leg becomes permanently and often grossly enlarged. The subcutaneous tissue thickens, becoming hypertrophied as well as containing deposits of fluid and protein in the intercellular spaces.

The state of the lymphatics, both vessels and nodes, may be outlined radiologically by lymphangiography. In this investigation the superficial lymphatics are first visualized by injecting subcutaneously into one or more webspaces about 0.5 ml of 2.5% patent blue, a dye which is selectively taken up by the lymph stream. Under local anaesthesia a short transverse skin incision is then made over one of the outlined vessels, and a fine cannula is gently introduced into the delicate little vessel and held in place by a temporary ligature. After a test injection, under minimal pressure, with about 1 ml of water-soluble contrast medium, a larger infusion of up to 10 ml of an oil-based contrast liquid is then given very slowly, preferably by a slow constant-infusion pump. With good filling it should be possible to outline clearly the majority of the fine network of lymph vessels, and the collections of rounded or kidney-shaped nodes. The contrast medium will be slow to clear, and may remain visible on X-ray for weeks or months. The patient should be warned that the urine will be discoloured blue as the patent blue is cleared over the next 1 or 2 days.

In primary lymphoedema lymphangiography is most likely to demonstrate a dearth or even complete lack of identifiable lymph vessels.

Treatment

The conservative management includes advice to elevate the leg as much as possible; the wearing of a good-quality elastic support stocking, preferable of the graduated compression type, i.e. designed so that the compressing force is greatest in the foot, less in the calf, and least in the thigh; a trial of diuretics, and antibiotic, usually one of the penicillins, for any attacks of cellulitis or other infections.

Many young people with the disorder manage to remain remarkably active and indeed engage in vigorous sports in spite of the gross bulk of the affected leg, and accept the disfigurement, adapting their clothing and footwear accordingly.

The only contributions surgery has to offer are either wide excision of the subcutaneous tissues and re-grafting of the skin or the burying of dermal flaps to stimulate the drainage of lymph through the vessels situated more deeply within the muscle compartment (Fig. 20.3). Unfortunately the cosmetic result of either approach is often quite disappointing and there is reluctance to advocate their wide usage.

SECONDARY LYMPHOEDEMA

This occurs when disease, e.g. metastatic deposits, or infection blocks the nodes or vessels, or when the lymphatics have been surgically removed or obliterated by radiotherapy. While often, particularly when the ablation has been fairly complete, the limb swelling appears quite rapidly, sometimes it takes months or years for the gross oedema to become obvious.

In the upper limb the condition most often arises from invasion of the axillary lymph nodes with metastatic carcinoma, especially of the breast, and operations for this disease include excision of the axillary contents, e.g. the classical and modified radical mastectomies. The lower limb drainage may become blocked by metastases in the groin nodes from melanoma or other soft-tissue tumour, or in the pelvic nodes from malignancy in the female reproductive organs or bowel. Radical excision of the lymphatics in the pelvic wall may also lead to the disorder.

While damage from recurrent pyogenic and other infections in the area draining towards a particular group of lymph nodes may eventually lead to an

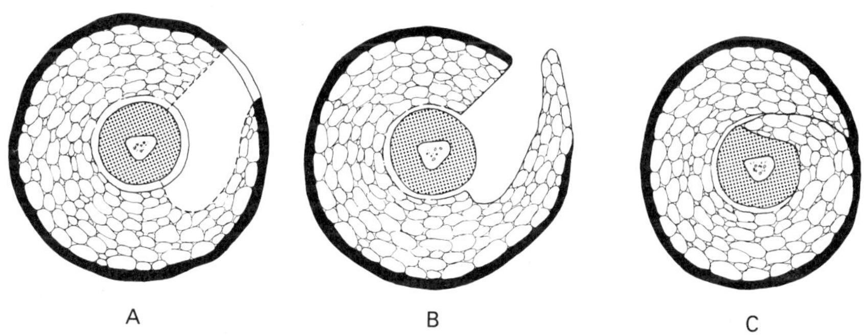

Fig. 20.3 The Thompson flap operation for chronic lymph-oedema. (**A**) After excision of a substantial segment of subcutaneous tissue, a flap is created; (**B**) the skin is shaved off from the leading edge of the flap; (**C**) the flap is then turned into the depths of the incision, fixed in place, and the skin edges are sutured together. This exposes a fresh raw surface for the development of new lymphatic channels.

overall deficiency in the lymphatic drainage, this is somewhat unusual. However, gross lymphoedema is a noted feature of infestation by filariasis—hence the term 'elephantiasis', often used for this disorder.

The management of secondary lymphoedema is along similar lines to that of the primary condition, discussed above. Generally there is little hope of significant improvement since the vessels and nodes are permanently destroyed or removed, and indeed a steady progression of the swelling and other symptoms is usual. However, as much elevation of the limb as possible plus the wearing of a suitable elastic compression garment are worthwhile measures to try to minimize size and discomfort.

INFECTED LYMPH NODES

Acute lymphadenitis

Some enlargement of one or more regional nodes draining an area infected by staphylococci, streptococci or other pyogenic organisms occurs in most people at some time in their lives. A common example is enlargement of the cervical nodes resulting from tonsillitis or other throat infections. The nodes become palpable and tender for a few days and then usually resolve as the infection dies off. Rarely pus will form in the node, forming a local abscess and this in turn may 'point' and require incision and drainage or, if medical advice is not sought, may discharge spontaneously.

Superficial pyogenic infections are common— almost universal—in the hands, feet and legs as a result of minor trauma during a normal active childhood and adult life, and since lymph nodes which have been enlarged as a result of these recurrent episodes may not always return to normal size, many people have a few palpable nodes, especially in the groins. This makes assessing the significance of palpably enlarged lymph nodes at times difficult, and often excision biopsy is required to be certain.

Clearly treatment for acute lymphadenitis is primarily at the site of infection from which the lymph drainage arises, and this will usually be an appropriate antibiotic, often one of the penicillins.

Chronic tuberculous lymphadenitis

Although very rarely other causes of chronic inflammatory enlargement of lymph nodes are met, tuberculosis of the nodes is by far the commonest cause clinically, and the commonest site is in the cervical nodes.

The nodes enlarge as part of a primary infection with the organisms, and when these enter by the mouth or pharynx the nodes affected are in the deep cervical chain; whereas when organisms enter via the lung, the supraclavicular nodes are involved. Similarly, when the bacilli are swallowed they may invade the Peyer's patches in the ileum and thereby travel to the nodes in the mesentery of that part of the small intestine.

When the nodes become directly invaded by the tubercle bacilli the typical sequence of histological changes leading to tubercle formation occurs, and this often includes caseation. A cold abscess therefore may form and track superficially, penetrating the deep fascia and resulting in the creation of a 'collar-stud' abscess (Fig. 20.4). The overlying skin may then break down so that a discharging sinus is formed. Not all tuberculous glands caseate and they may simply remain chronically enlarged over many months. The progress is of course influenced by the patient's own resistance to the organisms, and also by any treatment.

Clinically the presentation is usually simply the discovery of one or a group of painless lumps in the side of the neck. On palpation the nodes are firm, rounded and, if multiple, matted together. If a cold abscess has formed fluctuation may be demonstrable, but this sign requires the presence of at least several millilitres of liquefied material. There is rarely any symptom or sign to indicate the primary site of invasion of the organisms. General

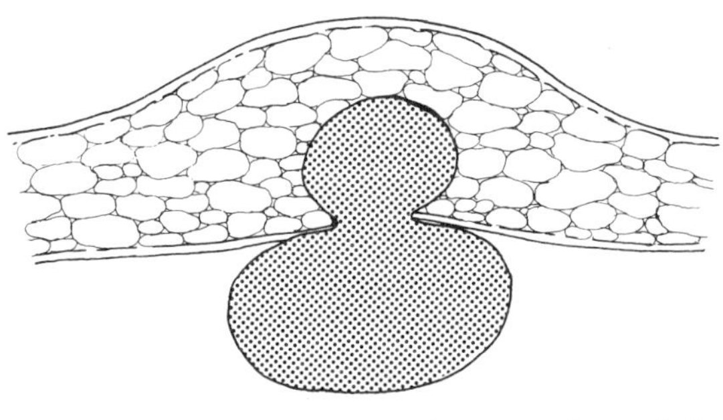

Fig. 20.4 'Collar-stud' abscess, such as may arise particularly with tuberculous infection in a lymph node. The abscess has simply extended through a gap in the deep fascia layer, so that a part of it lies in the subcutaneous tissue.

health is usually otherwise good, although there may be some weight loss and debility. The latter suggests that there may be concomitant active tuberculosis elsewhere in the body.

If there is a discharging sinus the diagnosis may be confirmed by culture of the pus, and needle aspiration of a cold abscess may also permit bacteriological identification. When liquefaction has not occurred a positive diagnosis may be made only after excision biopsy. As soon as the diagnosis is established a course of antitubercular antibiotics, including streptomycin, rifampicin and ethambutol, is given, and as long as abscess or sinus formation has not yet developed, slow but continuous resolution of the node enlargement can be expected. However, when this does not follow, or an abscess or sinus is present, local surgical excision of the mass of involved nodes is indicated. Lesser procedures, e.g. simple drainage, will not lead to healing, and only complete removal of the affected nodes is adequate. Since the disease process often spreads along a series of neighbouring nodes and through the deep fascia, quite an extensive exploration and mobilization of the deep cervical chain may be required.

LYMPHOGRANULOMA INGUINALE

This viral venereal infection is encountered most often in negro races. About 3-4 weeks after the eruption of a crop of small blister-like lesions on the genitalia multiple lymph node enlargement appears, usually in both groins. The masses have an indurated feel to palpation, and in due course the skin overlying them may break down, leading to sinus formation. In the female a rectal stricture may develop as a result of spread directly from the vulva.

The diagnosis can be confirmed by a positive skin response to a specific antigen—the Frei test. Treatment by systemic tetracycline is usually curative.

TUMOURS

Hodgkin's lymphoma

This neoplastic disorder of the reticuloendothelial system is characterized by progressive painless enlargement of lymph nodes, most commonly at first in the neck, and perhaps later involving the spleen, liver, kidneys and bones. A classical feature on histological section of an affected node is the presence of multi-nucleated giant cells of a particular pattern—the Reed–Sternberg cells. Most of the microscopic field, however, is filled with tightly packed lymphocytes and the relative proportion of these lymphocytes to other cell types can give a crude index of prognosis. Broadly speaking, the less the lymphocyte density, the worse the outlook.

Clinical features

There appear to be two peaks of incidence, at around 20 and again about 65 years and over. Men are more frequently affected than women. The commonest presentation is that of enlargement of a group of palpable nodes in the neck, and although these are nearly always painless, some patients note that drinking even small amounts of alcohol may cause the nodes to be temporarily painful and tender (Fig. 20.5). If the disease is localized to only one group of glands, the patient is usually otherwise well. However, if more generalized, there is often weight loss, malaise, recurrent sweating, local discomfort or itching, and anaemia.

On examination the enlarged nodes are well defined, rubbery in consistency, and often feel matted together. A full examination should be made of all the other main sites of lymph nodes, i.e. the opposite side of the neck, both axillae, both groins and the abdomen for palpable para-aortic nodes and for possible splenomegaly or hepatomegaly. Additional information regarding the state of deeply situated nodes can be obtained by lymphangiography or computerized tomography scanning, but an even more precise and direct method is surgical laparotomy to stage the extent of the disease.

Although this appears to be a somewhat drastic way to get basically diagnostic information, it can be justified because, with accurate assessment and thereafter the selection of the correct radical treatment, excellent results can be obtained in those with the disease confined to one region of the body. At the staging operation the spleen is removed, a biopsy is taken from the liver, and para-aortic nodes are explored from the level of the coeliac artery distally. At each level one or more nodes are excised

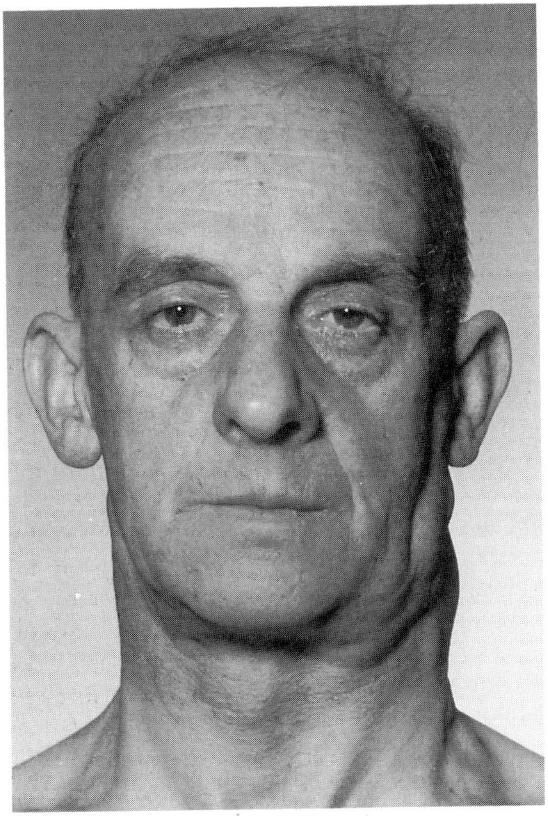

Fig. 20.5 Hodgkin's lymphoma, presenting as a mass of several prominently enlarged lymph nodes confined to one side of the neck. The mass of nodes in the left side of this patient's neck was the only presenting symptom in this instance.

and the points of removal are marked by a metal clip. This will enable exact positioning to be made of any nodes found on histological examination to be involved with the disease.

As a result of this detailed pathological assessment the patient can be defined as belonging to one of the following four stages:

Stage I: Involvement of only one node group or one extralymphatic site.

Stage II: Involvement of more than one lymph node group—or the combination of one extra lymphatic site plus lymph node area—on the same side of the diaphragm.

Stage III: Involvement of lymph node areas on both sides of the diaphragm, with or without additional involvement of the spleen.

Stage IV: Diffuse involvement of extralymphatic sites ± lymph node involvement.

Treatment

The mainstays of treatment are radiotherapy and chemotherapy and surgical procedures have nothing to offer apart from the assistance in accurate staging and the removal of the spleen, which reduces the field for irradiation.

For disease above the diaphragm the irradiation is applied to the neck, axillae and mediastinum, and for below the diaphragm, to the para-aortic, iliac and inguinal regions. For widespread disease chemotherapy is more appropriate, using a combination of agents, e.g. procarbazine, vinca alkaloids and nitrogen mustards, and possibly adrenocorticosteroids.

With this approach patients with stage I and II disease should have a 5-year survival expectancy of >80%, and a high proportion of stage I patients could be regarded as cured. The outlook is less good but steadily improving for stage III and IV patients.

Non-Hodgkin's lymphoma

This term embraces several types of lymphomatous disease, with differing gross and microscopic features. Basically the predominant cell is either lymphocytic or reticulocytic, although sometimes mixed types are present. The distribution of the disorder can be either nodular or diffuse, and this latter pattern tends to follow a relatively more benign course.

Clinical manifestations frequently arise in the gastrointestinal tract, the skin and the bones, and there is an increased incidence of the disease in patients with reduced immune defence mechanisms, e.g. transplant patients on immunosuppressive drugs. The surgeon may become involved either to perform lymph node biopsy for histological examination or, in the case of gastrointestinal lesions, to deal with perforation or obstruction. In either case excision of the diseased segment may be required and this, of course, gives ample material for pathological examination.

Again the main methods of treatment are radiotherapy and chemotherapy, often in combination.

A fairly standard regime is nitrogen mustard, vincristine, procarbazine and prednisolone. More often than not, only palliation is achieved, but sometimes for lengthy periods.

Burkitt's lymphoma (Fig. 20.6)

A specific type of lymphoma affecting African children in the tropical zones was identified in the 1960s. Indirect evidence points to it being the result of a viral infection, probably transmitted by an insect. Gross swelling over the jaw is most frequently the first manifestation, but it also spreads to involve many other structures, e.g. bones, central nervous system, kidney, and retroperitoneal tissues. An excellent and often dramatic shrinkage of the tumour masses is often seen after a short course of high dosage of an alkylating agent, but sometimes more prolonged or repeated courses of chemotherapy may be needed to bring about satisfactory suppression of the disease.

Metastatic lymph node deposit

Since so many of the commonest malignant tumours spread readily by the lymphatics, secondary spread to regional lymph nodes is far more frequent than any of the above primary tumours. Typically a node invaded by carcinoma is enlarged, rounded and extremely hard. At first still mobile in relation to neighbouring structures, it soon becomes fixed by direct invasion. Ulceration of the overlying skin may also follow.

The presence of metastatic tumour in lymph nodes indicates that the disease will almost certainly have spread even further, with microscopic deposits having passed through or bypassed the glands into either the next more proximal group of nodes, or on into the systemic blood stream.

Surgical removal of one or more invaded nodes may be indicated either to obtain definite histological confirmation of the diagnosis or to prevent or remove an unpleasant or painful ulcerating mass, and thereby make the patient more comfortable. In most instances there is little or no merit in trying to excise a whole mass of nodes if these are not causing symptoms, for this will not improve the outlook, and indeed may even encourage further dissemination of the tumour by spilling cells during the operation or removing what limited defences against the malignant cells may still reside in the nodes. Depending on the tissue of origin of the tumour, palliation may be sought from local irradiation or from chemotherapy.

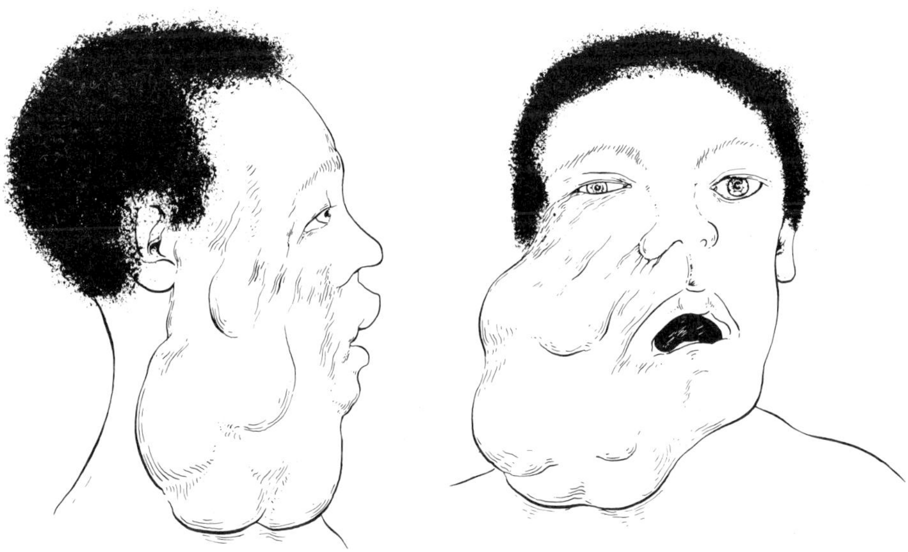

Fig. 20.6 Burkitt's lymphoma: the localized mass of enlarged lymph nodes may on occasions reach enormous proportions, as illustrated in this drawing.

Fields in which block dissection of regional nodes may still have a place, e.g. malignant melanoma or carcinoma of the lip or tongue, are discussed in the relevant chapters.

Leukaemia

In both acute and chronic varieties of this malignant disorder of the blood-forming elements there may be significant enlargement of the lymph nodes, and in the chronic forms this may be fairly generalized. Other features of the disorder, e.g. anaemia, bleeding, abdominal pain or discomfort, pyrexia and skin nodules, will usually dominate the clinical picture. Lymph node biopsy should rarely if ever be required, the diagnosis being established on blood and marrow examination.

21. The breast

DEVELOPMENT

In the human embryo, the breast develops as an ingrowth of ectoderm into the underlying mesodermal tissue at the end of the fourth week. In mammals with multiple breasts the ectodermal thickening extends as a continuous ridge from the site of the forelimb to the inguinal region, and this probably accounts for the site and types of occasional congenital anomalies, e.g. multiple breasts (polymasia) or ectopic nipples (polythelia). The mass of ectoderm grows in a flask-shaped fashion within the surrounding mesoderm and gives off a number of solid processes which represent the future ducts of the gland. These processes by further branching and division will form the future lobes, lobules and alveoli. The solid processes become canalized only at birth.

Postnatal growth and physiology of breast

The further development of the breast is delayed until puberty when it expands rapidly, with branching of the duct system and extension in the subcutaneous tissue. The main secretory activity happens only during pregnancy. In the first trimester duct growth occurs, followed in the subsequent months by the development of lobules and alveoli. At the time of delivery the breast is full of lobules, each of which is full of alveoli containing secretory cells.

The growth of the breast during adolescence, adulthood and pregnancy is influenced by hormones of the pituitary, ovaries, and adrenal glands, and also during pregnancy by the hormones of placenta (Fig. 21.1). Oestrogens from the ovary are responsible for the development of the ductal system, and

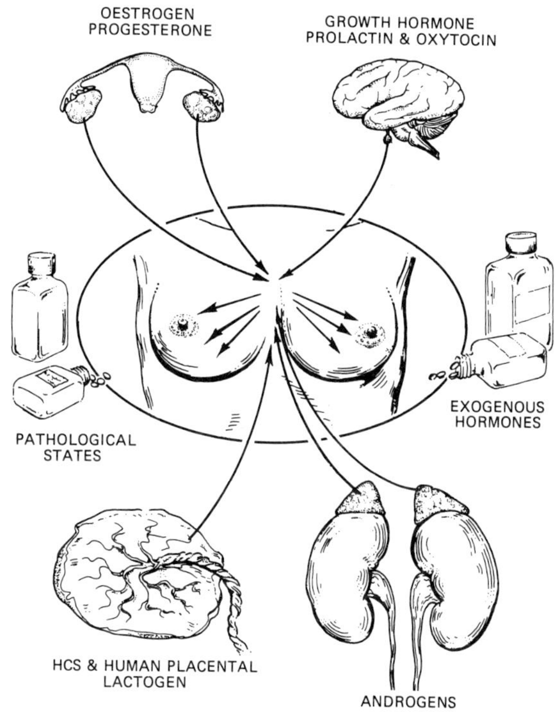

Fig. 21.1 Each of these hormones may influence the breast gland, or duct, or interstitial tissue growth, and of course more than one influence may be exerted simultaneously. HCS = Human chorionic somatomammotrophins.

for increasing the vascularization, fat deposition, elasticity and the volume of periductal connective tissue in the breast, while progesterone is mainly concerned with the development of the alveolar system. Growth hormone and prolactin from the pituitary gland also have effects on the development of the breast. During pregnancy human placental lactogen and human chorionic somatommotrophins have a metabolic and lactogenic effect on the breast, helping in the extensive growth of lobules and alveoli needed for lactation.

Production of milk starts after delivery. First, the act of suckling produces a transient increase in prolactin release from the pituitary gland, and oxytocin of the posterior pituitary gland causes milk ejection. For maintenance of established lactation there should be regular emptying of the breast, adequate diet and fluid intake by the mother, and an intact hypothalamopituitary axis. Cessation of lactation is produced by withdrawal of the stimulus of suckling, fluid restriction and firm support of the breast. Administered oestrogens, progesterone, androgen and various combinations also stop lactation.

Anatomy

The size of the mature female breast varies from one female to another, and in the same female asymmetry between two breasts is not uncommon. The base extends from the second to the sixth rib in the midclavicular line, and horizontally lies from the lateral border of the sternum to the mid axillary line. It overlies the pectoralis major muscle medially and extends beyond it on to serratus anterior and the external oblique muscles. A prolongation of the breast, the axillary tail, often extends towards the third rib in the axilla. The nipple lies normally in the fourth intercostal space, about 10 cm from the midline. The breast owes its shape and size to the amount of fat which surrounds the parenchyma, the stage of activity of the gland and the fibrous bands which run between skin and deep fascia (ligaments of Cooper) suspending it and anchoring it to that fascia.

The structure of the breast depends upon its activity. In the non-lactating state the breast consists of fat plus fibrous tissue with very scanty glandular ducts and alveoli. Before lactation starts new alveoli bud off from the ducts into the fibrous tissue and the organ enlarges considerably. In a normal adult female breast the number of ducts varies from 15 to 20, each one opening separately on to the summit of the nipple and showing a dilatation called the ampulla beneath the areola. The breast is divided into lobes by septa of fibrous tissue that radiate out from the centre of the breast. Each lobe is drained by one main lactiferous duct. The whole breast is embedded in the subcutaneous fat, which normally makes the lobules unable to be felt, and gives it its final shape. The skin on the nipple and areola is wrinkled and shows many small rounded projections due to modified sebaceous glands (of Montgomery). The nipple contains a number of plain muscle fibres and nerves which make it more prominent and firm on mechanical stimulation. The colour of the areola and nipple varies with the complexion of the patient and stage of development—it is usually pink in the young white female. The colour usually darkens during pregnancy and the areolar glands become more prominent and firm.

Nerve supply

The skin of the breast is supplied by the anterior and lateral branches of the fourth, fifth and sixth intercostal nerves. Sympathetic supply passes with the second to sixth intercostal arteries, taking fibres from the thoracic segment of sympathetic trunk.

Arterial supply

The arterial supply is derived from:

1. the lateral thoracic artery by the branches that curl around the lateral border of pectoralis major muscle and by branches which pierce through it;
2. the perforating branches of the internal mammary artery through the second, third and fourth intercostal spaces;
3. the intercostal arteries through the lateral branches of second, third and fourth intercostal arteries;
4. the pectoral branches of the acromiothoracic artery, supplying the upper part of the breast.

Venous drainage

The veins follow the above-mentioned arteries. The superficial veins radiate from the breast skin and, accompanied by the lymphatics, empty into neighbouring veins. The deep veins drain into the axillary, internal mammary and intercostal veins.

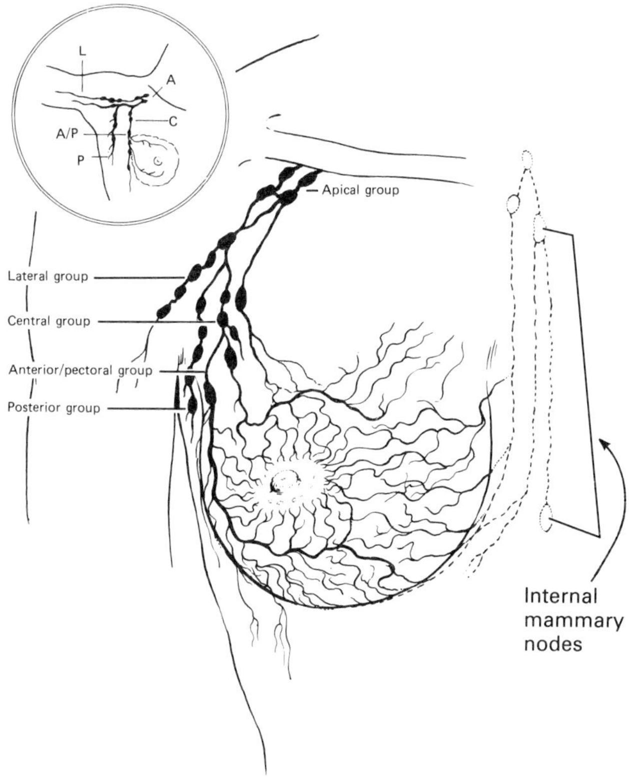

Fig. 21.2 Schematic diagram of the distribution of the main lymphatics of the breast and (inset) the groups of nodes into which they drain in the axilla, and internal mammary chain. L = Lateral; A = apical; C = central; A/P = anterior/pectoral; P = posterior.

Lymphatic drainage and lymph nodes in the axilla

The lymphatics of the breast drain mainly into the axillary and internal mammary lymph nodes (Fig. 21.2).

The axillary lymph nodes comprise five groups:

1. The anterior or pectoral group lies deep to pectoralis major, under the anterior axillary fold, mainly on the third rib. The axillary tail of breast is in contact with this group of lymph nodes, which are the main lymph glands of the breast receiving lymph drainage from the major part of the breast substance.
2. The posterior (subscapular) group lies close to the subscapular artery, along the medial wall of axilla in its posterior part. They receive some lymph from the axillary tail of the breast.
3. The lateral group lies on the medial side of axillary vein along the upper part of the humerus. They may receive lymphatics from the breast, but most of their drainage comes from the upper limb.
4. The central group lies within the axillary fat. The intercostobrachial nerve passes into the thorax close to this group. They drain mainly the floor of the axilla.
5. The apical group lies in the apex of the axilla, behind the clavicle. They receive from all the other groups and drain by the subclavian lymph trunk into the thoracic duct on the left, and the right lymphatic duct on the right. These ducts in turn open into the internal jugular vein of the respective side.

Lymph drainage of the breast

The overlying skin of the breast except that of the nipple and areola drains in a radiating fashion to the surrounding lymph glands. The parenchyma drains directly into either the axillary lymph nodes or the internal mammary chain, depending upon the quadrant of the breast.

The axillary lymph nodes receive directly about 75% of the lymph drainage from the breast tissue, mostly going to the anterior group and less to the posterior group. From here they drain into the central and apical glands. Some drainage from the deep surface of the breast may pass through the pectoralis major muscle and then travel to the axillary or internal mammary group, reaching the latter by lymph vessels passing either alongside the anterior perforating internal mammary veins or the lateral perforating intercostal veins.

Some lymphatics from the inner and lower quadrant of the breast pass downwards and communicate with the subperitoneal lymph plexus through the upper part of the linea alba. This communication may explain spread of carcinoma of the breast to the pelvic organs or to the surface of the liver.

That there are communicating lymphatic channels between the two breasts is suggested by the occasional metastasis spreading from one breast to the other.

Congenital anomalies of the breast

Aplasia

Amazia (absence of the breast) may be unilateral or bilateral. Athelia (absence of the nipple) may be unilateral or bilateral.

Hypoplasia

Hypoplasia, or underdevelopment of the breast, may occur with other anomalies like maldevelopment of the pectoral muscles or ribs.

Supernumerary

An additional nipple, with or without some underlying breast tissue, may be explained by the existence of a mammary ridge during the development of the breast. It is located along the line extending from the anterior axillary fold to the inguinal region.

Hyperplasia

Gross enlargement of the female breast may occur at puberty due to an excessive deposition of fat. The hypertrophy may be unilateral or bilateral, symmetrical or asymmetrical.

Congenital retraction or inversion of the nipple

This may become evident when puberty is reached. The cause is shortening of the ducts and retraction by the accompanying connective tissue. It is usually bilateral, and its importance lies in the fact that it may cause problems during lactation, and it may be confused with the recent occurrence of retraction of one nipple, which points to malignancy of the breast. It is liable to cause cracks of the nipple during breastfeeding, and the cracks in turn permit the entry of bacteria causing infection and abscess formation in the underlying breast tissue. The nipple should in such cases be prepared for lactation during pregnancy by repeated gentle manual eversion.

Disorders of growth

Premature breast development in girls, say at the age of 8 or 9 years, is usually due simply to the early onset of puberty, but rarely granulosa cell tumour of the ovary may be the cause. Failure of development of the female breast at puberty may be due to agenesis of the ovaries associated with Turner's syndrome; other features include infantilism, short stature, webbed neck and cubitus valgus.

Trauma to the breast

Although bruising and localized haematomas may arise from direct blows, or as the result of sudden compression, e.g. by car seat-belts, these usually resolve in the usual manner. One specific type of sequel of injury which may cause considerable diagnostic difficulty and confusion is traumatic fat necrosis.

Fat necrosis

This occurs more commonly in obese patients with pendulous breasts. There may be a clear history of localized trauma, followed weeks or months later by the finding of a firm, hard lump in the breast which may simulate carcinoma of the breast. The lump is formed by aseptic fat necrosis followed by saponification by lipase, and deposition of calcium in the mass, giving its firm consistency. Fibrous tissue reaction surrounding the fat necrosis adds to the size and firmness of the lump.

On examination of the breast there is usually a firm or hard, painless lump with well defined margins and an irregular surface. It may be attached to the skin but rarely to the deep structures. The nipple and the axillary contents are usually normal.

In rare cases fat necrosis of the subcutaneous tissues of the breast may be a local manifestation of Weber–Christian disease. The main clinical importance of fat necrosis lies in its differential diagnosis from carcinoma of the breast.

Treatment is excision of the lump and its histopathological examination.

BREAST INFECTIONS

Acute infections

Acute bacterial infection of the breast is commonest in women of child-bearing age. The infection is usually by staphylococci but other organisms may be involved. The vast majority of such infections occur during lactation, but a few are encountered in non-lactating women. The factors during lactation which greatly increase the risks are the engorgement of the breast with milk, and perhaps insufficient suckling by the baby. In turn the ducts become dilated and this milk is a good medium for infection by bacteria. The bacteria will usually gain access through a crack in the nipple or more rarely by blood spread from another focus in the body.

Clinical features

The patient usually complains that an area of the breast has become painful, tender, swollen and perhaps throbbing, and there may be generalized constitutional symptoms of infection like fever, chills and sweating. On examination there will be swelling which is either localized or diffuse, and the overlying skin is red, feels hot and is tender and firm in consistency. Fluctuation may be present if a definite abscess has formed, but it may be difficult to elicit on account of the tenderness and thick wall of the abscess. If the abscess remains untreated it may penetrate through the skin, discharging its content of pus. Rarely some pus may discharge from the nipple. It may be possible to locate the site of pointing pus by noting the most indurated and most tender part of the breast, with perhaps local oedema overlying it. Aspiration may confirm the diagnosis in doubtful cases.

The differentiation from the fulminating inflammatory variety of carcinoma should be borne in mind, especially if the history is longer, signs of inflammation are less pronounced, the breast is less tender and the induration is more pronounced. This particular, though fortunately rare, type of carcinoma is one which may occur in young women and during pregnancy or lactation.

Treatment

In the early stage of infection before a definite abscess has formed, an antibiotic effective against staphylococcus given for a few days may cause the inflammatory signs to subside. It is wise also to try and achieve proper evacuation of the breast by feeding, manually or by means of a pump. If the child can be weaned or bottle-fed, lactation may be stopped by the oral administration of stilboestrol. If the child has to be continued on breastfeeding for any reason, the milk should be expressed by evacuation manually or by breast pump, boiled, and then given to the child. If, in spite of the above management, pain continues and the local signs, such as increased induration, redness and oedema strongly suggest the presence of pus, the pus should be drained surgically. Persistence with antibiotics may lead to the formation of a chronic abscess which contains sterile pus or serous fluid and will present as a hard, indurated fixed mass.

To achieve adequate drainage of pus a suitable incision is usually made overlying the most tender part of the breast, all the pus and slough in the cavity are evacuated, and a sample of this pus is

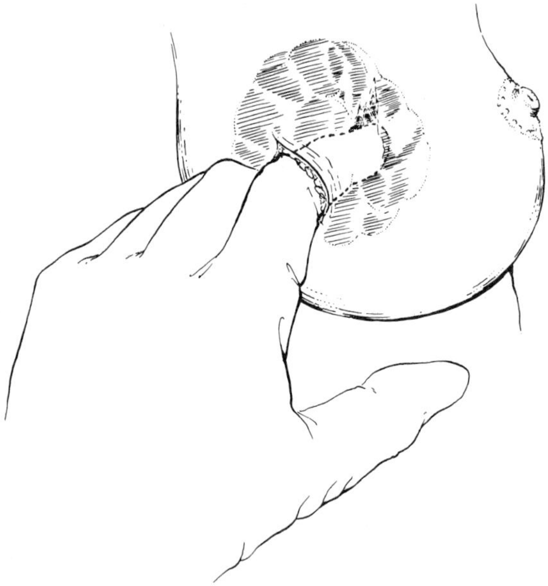

Fig. 21.3 Drainage of breast abscess: the septa between loculi of pus are being broken down by a finger inserted through the incision, to ensure complete emptying of all the pockets of pus.

sent for culture and antibiotic-sensitivity testing. It is important to break down all the septa in the cavity so that all the loculi containing pus and necrotic material drain freely (Fig. 21.3). If the incision is not at the most dependent part of the cavity it may be necessary to make a counter-incision at such a level. Suitable rubber or plastic drains are inserted and if the cavity is particularly large, light packing may also be used. Drains are usually removed in 2–4 days, depending on the rate of healing. Resolution is often rapid and complete after the operation, and as long as the patient is in good health otherwise, many surgeons would not prescribe antibiotics. If complete drainage is not properly achieved the lesion may go on to form an indolent chronic abscess which may require further exploration and excision.

Mumps mastitis

The breast may be a seat of inflammation during the course of mumps infection. One or both breasts may be affected and either sex may be involved. This inflammation subsides with the decline of the primary condition, i.e. mumps.

Subareolar mastitis

This is due to infection of the sebaceous glands of Montgomery in the areola. A retention cyst may first form due to obstruction of the duct, appearing as a small rounded swelling in the region of the areola. This cyst may then become infected and form an abscess. The cyst should be excised in toto, otherwise if incised a chronic sinus may result.

Chronic infections

Chronic pyogenic abscess

As mentioned, this may be due to improper management of acute infection either by the prolonged use of antibiotics (antibioma) or improper drainage at the first place. The chronic abscess will present as an indurated mass, firm or hard in consistency, painless or slightly tender. If a thick fibrous capsule forms round it, there may even be slight retraction of the nipple, and suggestion of tethering to the skin, making its confident differentiation from carcinoma difficult. Excision biopsy may be the only means of establishing the final diagnosis.

Treatment is excision of the mass and its histopathological examination.

Mammary fistula

This complication may occur as a result of recurrent abscesses that create openings into one of the lactiferous ducts and on to the skin. There may also be blockage of the main duct in the nipple by epithelial debris.

The only effective treatment is to lay open and excise the affected duct.

Plasma mastitis

This is a very rare condition arising from a foreign body reaction to the extravasation of milk from dilated ducts.

Tuberculosis of the breast

This rare condition of the breast is usually seen in areas where tuberculosis is common. Infection may be either due to blood-stream dissemination or by direct spread from an adjacent tuberculous focus. It is usually associated with either active pulmonary tuberculosis or cervical tuberculous lymphadenitis; multiparous, ill-nourished women with poor hygiene and social conditions are usually affected.

In advanced tuberculosis of the breast, there may be multiple suppurating sinuses and areas of necrosis and caseation and the regional lymph nodes are often involved. The clinical picture may be mistaken for advanced fungating carcinoma of the breast.

The diagnosis is to be made from the history, the presence of stigmata of tuberculosis either in lung or lymph nodes, by examination of the discharge from the sinus, by direct staining to show acid-fast bacilli, and culture for tubercle bacilli. Histopathological examination will reveal the classical features of tuberculous tissue reaction.

If the diagnosis of tuberculosis is confirmed, specific antitubercular therapy, usually by a combination of three drugs, is begun and continued for several months. If resolution does not occur or is incomplete mastectomy may be considered.

Very rarely indeed the breast may be affected by actinomycosis, or by syphilitic organisms.

Retromammary abscess

Pus may collect in the retromammary space between the superficial and deep fascia. This infection has no connection with the breast tissue proper. The pus may originate from an infected haematoma, a tuberculous rib or an empyema necessitans. The pus is deeply located, and thus will be very difficult to locate by physical examination.

Treatment involves dealing with the primary cause; the abscess may be drained through a submammary incision.

Mondor's disease

This is thrombophlebitis involving some of the veins of the breast. It appears suddenly and is a self-limiting condition, presenting as an indurated cord in the subcutaneous tissue of the breast. As the segment of vein involved is often close to the skin, when the arm is raised the cord may stretch the skin and a shallow groove alongside the cord may become visible. Its importance is the possible confusion with malignancy of the breast.

Once a confident diagnosis is made all that is required is reassurance that complete resolution will occur, usually in a few weeks.

Mammary duct ectasia (comedomastitis)

In this condition dilatation and fibrous thickening of the ducts occur. If fatty material accumulating in these ducts escapes from them into the breast, this will cause an inflammatory reaction and fat necrosis, followed by fibrosis. Due to the shortening of the ducts some retraction of the skin and nipple may occur, thus raising a suspicion of carcinoma.

Differentiation is by histological examination, a particular finding in duct ectasia being a large number of plasma cells.

Fibrocystic disease or fibroadenosis of the breast

This is a proliferative disorder of the stromal and glandular tissue, the latter undergoing degrees of papillomatosis, epitheliosis, cyst formation, fibrosis and adenosis. It is found most commonly in women between 25 and 45 years of age and 15% of all women are affected by it. It is rare after the menopause. It may be either unilateral or bilateral, affecting the whole breast or only one lobe. No definite initiating cause of the structural changes is known, but the various hormones known to influence the breast clearly have some role in promoting and continuing the disorder.

It is commoner in unmarried women, childless women or in those multipara who did not suckle their children. This may suggest its predominance in breasts denied their normal lactational function.

The patient generally presents with either a lump or an area of lumpiness in one or both breasts, and she may have noticed that the lump or area concerned is slightly painful and tender especially in the day or two before a menstrual period. There may also be a history of slight fullness, swelling or tightness in the breasts at this particular time of the monthly cycle. Usually the discomfort and tenderness rapidly decrease after the period starts, and indeed the patient may also note that the lump or lumpy area becomes a bit smaller at the same time.

On examination there is often a feeling of granularity to the substance of either one or more segments of either or both breasts; when the disorder is most widespread this consistency to palpation may be present throughout the two breasts. Even when the complaint is of a single localized lump it is very often possible to detect several areas elsewhere in the breast which have this characteristic finding. A single lump within such a breast will usually comprise either a mass of thickened fibroadenosis tissue or a cyst, and will form a discrete, well defined, mobile, smooth mass with no sign of any skin or deep tissue attachment, and is often slightly tender to direct compression by the examining fingers. This may be especially evident if she is examined just prior to a period, and much less obvious after it has ended.

Examination of unaffected portions of the breasts, the axillae and other lymph node areas should reveal completely normal findings.

If a solitary lump is thought to be a cyst it is reasonable to guide the tip of an aspirating needle into it, after temporarily holding the cyst firmly in position between thumb and fingers. If it is a cyst the fluid—nearly always green and opalescent—will be drawn into the syringe and the cyst will collapse completely (Fig. 21.4) It is customary to send the aspirated fluid for cytological examination in case there are malignant cells present, but it is highly exceptional if the cyst totally collapses, for there to be any malignancy.

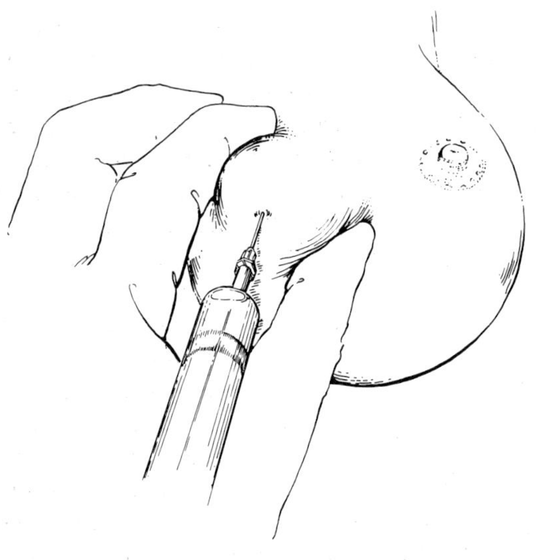

Fig. 21.4 Aspiration of a breast cyst: with the cyst held firmly and steadily between the thumb and index finger of one hand, the sterile needle, attached to a sterile syringe, is introduced directly over the summit of the cyst. Gentle aspiration confirms when the cyst is entered.

If no fluid is obtained on exploring with the needle, it may be possible to aspirate a small amount of the solid tissue by applying suction as the needle is passed down into and drawn out again several times through the mass, and submitting slides from the smears of the aspirated tissue to an expert cytologist.

Although some debate continues, the general consensus is that the presence of fibroadenosis does not increase (or decrease) the risk of frank carcinoma subsequently developing.

As far as treatment is concerned, where the symptoms are mild all that is often required is strong reassurance that the disorder is not cancer or a related disease, and advice to wear a bra which gives good support to the breasts and therefore usually improves comfort.

If, however, there is genuine diagnostic doubt, or the amount of local pain and discomfort is severe, or the patient remains unhappy or worried about the continuing presence of any lump, then it is wise to perform local excision, with a small surrounding area of apparently normal breast, through an appropriately sited incision.

Cystic lesions in the breast

Most commonly these are either solitary or multiple manifestations of fibrocystic disease. Occasionally a haematoma becomes cystic as it resolves, and also some carcinomas can develop areas of cystic degeneration. This may also be a feature of the uncommon cystosarcoma phylloides. A galactocele is a rare complication occurring almost always in the lactating breast. It is the accumulation of retained milk behind a blocked duct. A false capsule of fibrous tissue is laid down around the collection which extravasates through the dilated damaged duct. The treatment is local surgical excision of the cyst, including its fibrous wall.

TUMOURS OF THE BREAST

Fibroadenoma

This is one of the commonest benign tumours of the breast and should not be confused with the more general condition discussed above—fibroadenosis or fibrocystic disease. A fibroadenoma is a single, discrete, well localized benign tumour usually in a breast which is otherwise essentially normal. Clinically it may be either hard or soft, depending on the amount of fibrous tissue, which is more abundant in the hard type and less in the soft ones. The hard variety tends to be small, to occur in younger age groups and is very freely mobile—the so-called 'breast mouse'.

Histologically, there is a combination of fibrous tissue and epithelial tissue components which differ in amount from one fibroadenoma to another. Two histological types are described—pericanalicular and intracanalicular. However, usually both variants are often found in the same tumour.

In the pericanalicular picture fibrous tissue surrounds the alveoli and glandular tissue, which maintains its regular configuration. In the intracanalicular pattern the growth of the fibrous tissue is rapid and invaginates the ducts, making them appear as slit-like spaces.

Clinical features

The small hard type usually appears in an earlier age group (between 15 and 30 years), and the soft type in a slightly older age group (30–45 years). The patient usually complains of a painless lump in the breast discovered accidentally. In about 10% there may be more than one lump, and it may increase in size during pregnancy. It can occur in any part of the breast but the lower part is affected more frequently than the upper. Growth rate is slow, and if unattended some may increase to a huge size, especially when of the soft variety; these are then called giant fibroadenomata. A fibroadenoma may also become calcified and therefore very hard.

On examination, the skin of the breast, nipple and areola is normal. On palpation one or more lumps may be felt; they are well demarcated, firm in consistency, very mobile within the breast tissue, and not fixed to either skin or deeper structures. The surface is smooth and often bosselated and no lymph nodes are enlarged. Fibroadenomata are well encapsulated, and there is no known relation between them and carcinoma, although rarely a sarcomatous change has been recorded.

The fibroadenoma should be excised. For small hard ones this is usually a simple matter of enucleation through a small overlying radical or circumferential wound. Larger, deeper ones, often of the soft variety, may require a submammary approach and wider excision. Rarely simple mastectomy is the only way effectively to remove a giant fibroadenomatous mass.

Intraduct papilloma

This arises from one of the ducts of the breast, and usually presents with discharge of red blood from the nipple. It arises most commonly in females between 30 and 40 years of age. The patient may complain of frank blood discharge or of noticing staining of the underclothes with blood.

The discharge may be continuous or more often intermittent, and sometimes only precipitated by compression on self-examination. A few patients also complain of a lump just lateral to the areola, and pressure directly on this swelling may produce the discharge of blood from the nipple.

On examination, the breast may look completely normal or a small swelling to one side of the areola may be observed and pressure on this may cause blood discharge from the nipple. In the absence of any swelling, by careful palpation and pressure at points passing stage by stage all the way around the nipple, localization of the affected lobe may be determined. There should be no axillary lymphadenopathy.

The duct papilloma is usually small, and the only satisfactory way of ensuring its removal is to identify the duct from which the blood is escaping and excise a wedge of tissue to include the duct. If manual and other pressure on the breast is avoided for several days before the operation the duct opening can be located by radial pressure and then a fine lacrimal probe or other suitable fine instrument can be introduced into the duct. A wedge of areolar and surrounding skin, breast tissue and the duct can then be dissected around the probe, and the excised material sent for histological confirmation. The small wound is closed by primary suture after securing good haemostasis.

Cystosarcoma phylloides

This is a giant form of fibroadenoma which may remain benign, change to a frankly malignant sarcoma, or may start as a sarcoma right from the beginning (Fig. 21.5). It occurs in the same age group as carcinoma of the breast, the median age being about 45 years of age; it is rare before the age of 20 years. The patient usually presents with a large mass in the breast or apparent enlargement of the whole breast, as the mass may involve many parts of the breast. The skin overlying the tumour is often red and shiny, or even bluish to black due to necrotic patches. Dilated veins may be obvious around the area. Eventually the skin may ulcerate and a serosanguineous discharge exude from it.

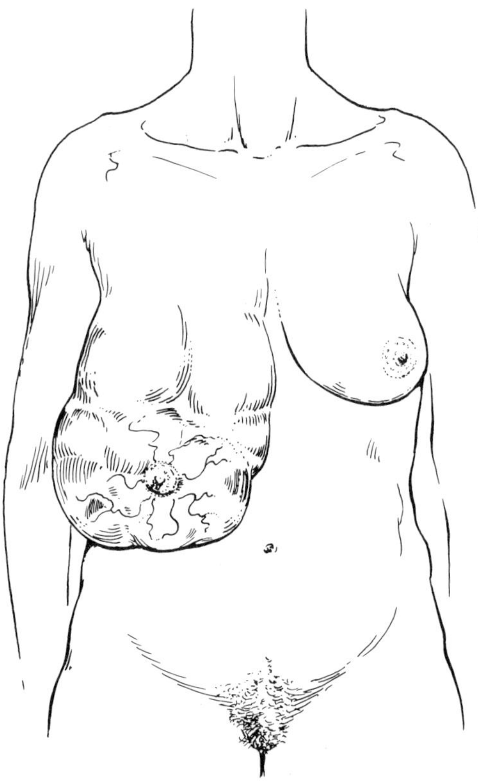

Fig. 21.5 Cystosarcoma phylloides may present with an enormous, lobular enlargement of the breast; the overlying skin is thin, stretched, and contains prominent blood vessels.

Pain is not common but the edge of any ulcer may be tender. On palpation the surface feels smooth and bosselated, and the consistency is firm to hard, but in places there may be soft cystic areas where cystic degeneration has occurred. If the tumour is still benign it is neither adherent to the skin nor to deep structures and the axillary lymph nodes are not enlarged. If, however, it becomes sarcomatous it may infiltrate both skin and deeper structures and there may be axillary lymphadenopathy.

Macroscopically cystosarcomata are usually well circumscribed, grey-white and firm. Areas of necrosis, cystic degeneration and haemorrhage are seen in larger tumours. In the benign form, the stromal component has almost always a fibrous appearance with the occasional interposition of mature adipose foci. In the malignant variant, the stroma may have the appearance of fibrosarcoma, liposarcoma, chondrosarcoma or osteosarcoma. The epithelial element is almost always not directly involved in the malignant process. The histological distinction between benign and malignant cystosarcoma can be difficult. Spread by the blood stream to the lungs or other sites is seen in about 15% of cases.

For small or moderate-sized benign lesions simple enucleation (local excision) is all that is necessary. Large ones involving the major part of or the entire breast or malignant ones will require simple mastectomy.

Malignant carcinoma of the breast

Carcinoma of the breast is one of the commonest malignant tumours affecting women. In the west it is estimated that one in 25 women will develop breast cancer. It appears to be more common in those who have never been pregnant or had few pregnancies, or in those who have not lactated or lactated little. It is comparatively less common in communities where early marriage and frequent pregnancies and prolonged lactation are the usual habits. Although until now no specific aetiological agent has been found, in a proportion of families there is a significant hereditary tendency for successive generations of females to be at higher risk of the disease than the rest of the population.

The commonest age of those affected is above 30 years; the incidence peaks in the 40s and 50s, but may arise at any later age. It is commonly unilateral but a second primary in the other breast may arise concurrently or consecutively in about 1%.

Breast cancer arises from the epithelium of the ducts and lobules of the breast. Histological features are variable depending upon the type of the carcinomatous epithelial cells and the amount of fibrous tissue which surrounds them.

Carcinoma of the breast spreads by direct local infiltration, the lymphatics, the blood stream and by transcoelomic spread.

The local spread is due to direct invasion by the malignant process of the neighbouring tissues such as the skin which may then become tethered or fixed, or the pectoral fascia or muscle or even the underlying chest wall.

As far as the lymphatics are concerned, the tumour cells spread either by lymphatic embolism or by permeation. In embolic spread the malignant cells are swept along the lymph flow to be deposited in the lymph nodes. With the permeation pattern of spread the cancer cells grow along the lymph vessels in the form of a continuous column of malignant cells. By these two methods lymph nodes in the axilla and the internal mammary chain become involved, and later those in the supraclavicular fossa, in the opposite breast, the mediastinum and even more distant ones are invaded. Lymphatics in the subperitoneal space from a cancer in the lower inner quadrant of the breast may be involved and this may lead to metastases by seedling in the peritoneal cavity or on the surface of the liver.

Carcinoma of the breast may metastasize by the blood stream to various organs, but mainly first to bones, e.g. the ribs, spine (particularly the lumbar vertebrae), femur, skull, humerus and pelvis. These metastases may result in pathological fractures. Soft-tissue organs like the liver, brain and lungs are next most likely to be affected.

Prognosis

Breast cancer becomes widely disseminated by both the blood stream and the lymphatics often at an early stage. The secondary deposits grow synchronously at a rate determined by the balance between the tumour and the host. Histological evidence of axillary node involvement remains one of the most important practical predicting factors in breast cancer. Outlook deteriorates as the number of involved axillary nodes increases. Tumour size, histological grade and oestrogen receptor status can also affect prognosis. Very early detection of the carcinoma is the main hope of improving the chances of completely successful treatment. For this reason it has been advocated that women should periodically examine their own breasts, and report for medical examination should they have any doubt about the presence of a lump in the breast. Various methods of screening women for the presence of early tumours have been proposed, e.g. thermography and mammography, but the problems of practicability, organization, and accurate interpretation of results are all matters of continuing debate.

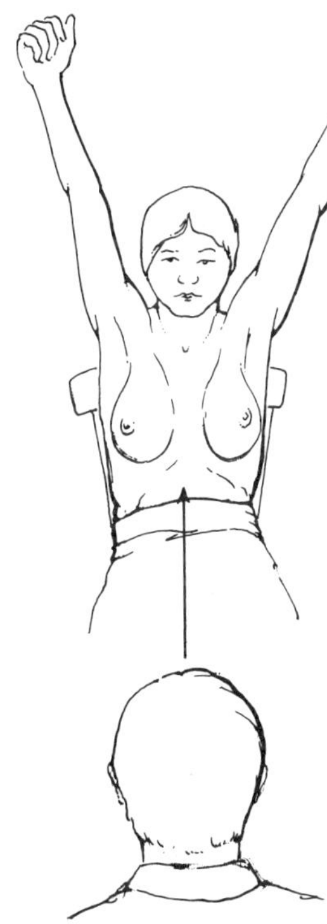

Fig. 21.6 After both breasts have been inspected with the patient's arms comfortably by her sides, she is asked to raise both arms up above her head. This action will often make obvious a lump which was not visible with the arms by the sides, or make an indefinite one more obvious. A further important clinical sign which may only be apparent with the arms elevated is dimpling, or tethering of an area of skin over a tumour.

The primary complaint of the majority of patients with carcinoma of the breast is the presence of a lump, which is usually painless and which has simply been felt accidentally by the patient herself, but rarely may cause mild aches or a pricking sensation in the breast. Less frequently the presentation may be on account of nipple disorders, e.g. erosion or eczematous changes, retraction, displacement or discharge of serous fluid or blood; alteration to the size or shape of the breast, or evidence of metastatic disease, e.g. an axillary mass, or pathological fracture due to a bone deposit.

The clinical examination should start by unhurried inspection, with the patient exposed from the waist up, sitting comfortably against a back support at an angle of about 60°, and in a good light. Any obvious abnormality of contour is looked for, and the position and appearance of the nipple are checked. The patient is then asked to raise gradually both arms above her head (Fig. 21.6) and this action may bring into prominence swelling or dimpling of skin overlying a tumour, or reveal indrawing or undue elevation of the nipple on the side of a carcinoma. Once thorough inspection has been completed, it is appropriate to begin palpation, at first with the flat of the hand systematically around all quadrants, and then more detailed palpation of any mass which is found.

Characteristic features of an early carcinoma are that it:

1. is painless and not tender;
2. is stony hard in consistency;
3. has ill defined margins due to local infiltration;
4. may cause dimpling or actual fixation of the overlying skin;
5. may cause retraction of the nipple—aggravated by direct pressure on the tumour.

With a larger, more advanced tumour there may be:

1. dusky red colour changes in the skin overlying the lesion (Fig. 21.7);
2. ulceration where the tumour has eroded through the skin (Figs. 21.8 and 21.9);
3. skin nodules;
4. oedema of the breast (peau d'orange);
5. fixation to the chest wall;

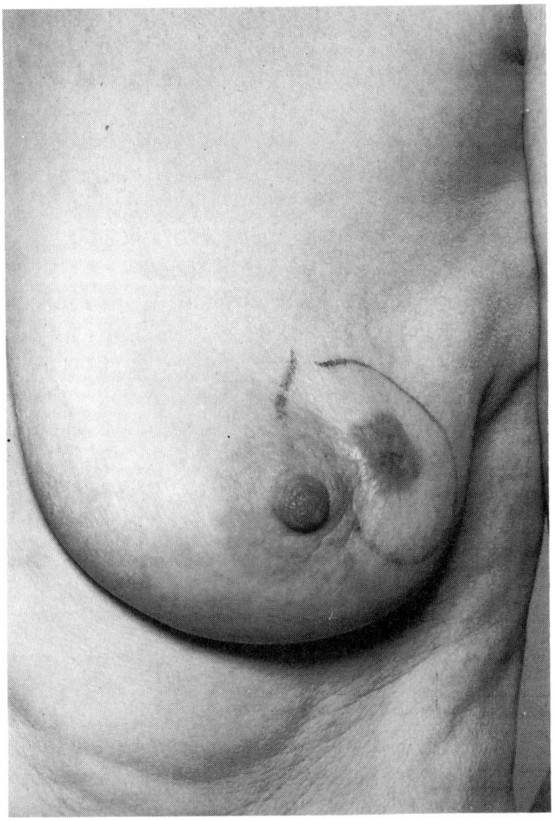

Fig. 21.7 Close-up view of the surface of a carcinoma. There is some direct involvement of the overlying skin, which has become dusky red, and deformity of the edge of the areola.

6. enlarged fixed lymph nodes in the axilla and supraclavicular lymph nodes;
7. distant metastases in the bones, liver, brain or lung.

Although all carcinomas are basically the same pathological process there are several well known patterns of clinical presentation and progress, which are characteristic enough to merit separate description for clinical purposes.

Intraduct carcinoma

In this rare variety of carcinoma the growth starts and may remain for some time within the ducts. The tumour contains thick-walled ducts with areas of normal-looking breast parenchyma in between and when pressure is exerted on the ducts wormlike masses of necrotic tissue may be extruded from

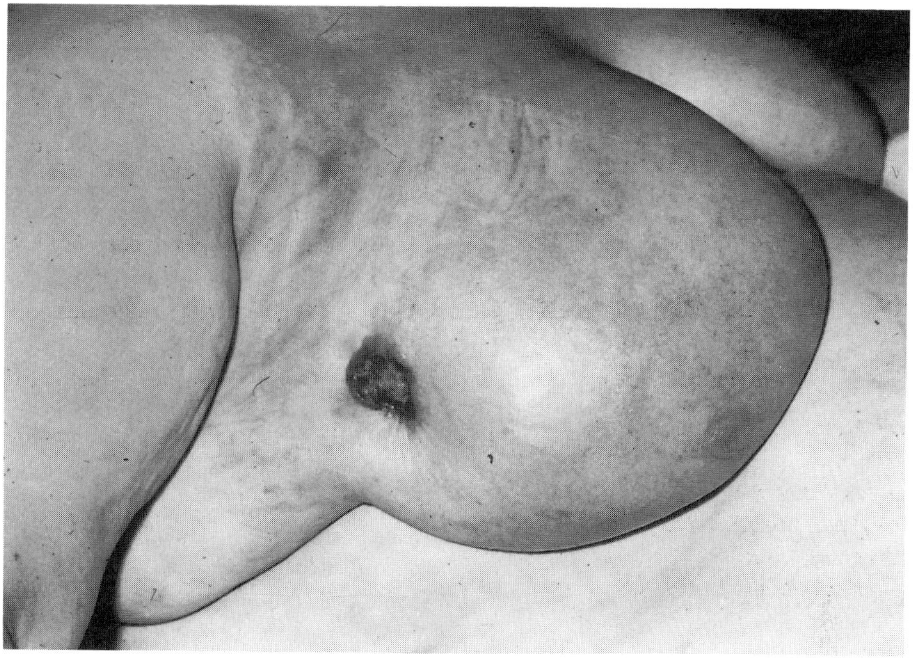

Fig. 21.8 More advanced carcinoma, which has ulcerated and destroyed most of the breast tissue.

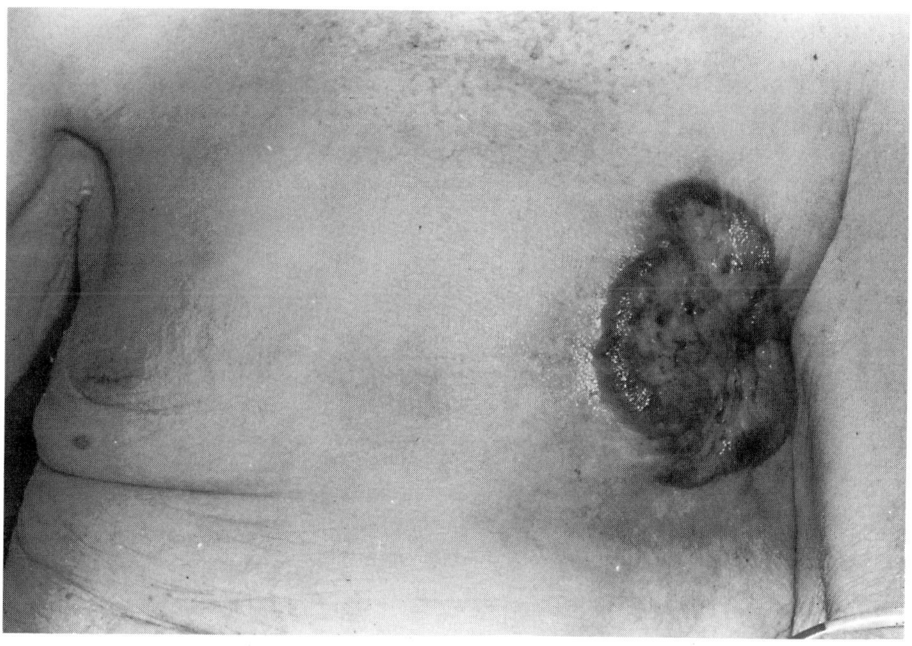

Fig. 21.9 This carcinoma has ulcerated through the skin and there is considerable indrawing of the surrounding skin and subcutaneous tissue.

them, hence the name comedocarcinoma which is sometimes given to this type. Intraduct carcinoma can be either invasive or non-invasive and metastases to the lymph nodes occur.

Atrophic scirrhous carcinoma

This type of carcinoma is seen in elderly females with small atrophic breasts. Here the fibrous element is much in abundance, and a slow rate of progression is usual, with a chronic course before ultimate ulceration. Retraction of the nipple, skin fixation and adherence to the deeper structures all occur, but sometimes cause little disability for long periods of time.

Inflammatory carcinoma

This pattern of carcinoma is also fortunately uncommon for it tends to run an unpleasant, aggressive and fatal course. Younger women, particularly during pregnancy or lactation, are quite often the victims of this particular variety. It is called inflammatory carcinoma because of its clinical presentation with pain in the majority of cases, which is not a usual symptom in carcinoma of the breast, and the appearance of redness, increased warmth and oedema of the overlying skin. The oedema is due to blockage of the subcutaneous lymphatics by malignant cells. This clinical picture may be confused with that of an inflammatory condition, but the absence of fever, leukocytosis and the extensive oedema and failure to respond to antibiotics if these have been given are all pointers to the correct diagnosis. The axillary lymph nodes will usually be enlarged, and may also be tender.

The prognosis is generally worse with this type of presentation than with most others and the patient may be dead within a few months. If detected reasonably early, management with mastectomy and radiotherapy may be life-saving. If the patient is pregnant, the possibility of termination of pregnancy may have to be considered. In advanced cases palliation by radiotherapy, chemotherapy or hormone may be the only possibilities.

Paget's disease of the nipple (Fig. 21.10)

The presentation is as a crusted lesion or eczema-like condition affecting the nipple, usually in patients over 50 years of age. It is the superficial manifestation of an underlying slowly growing in-

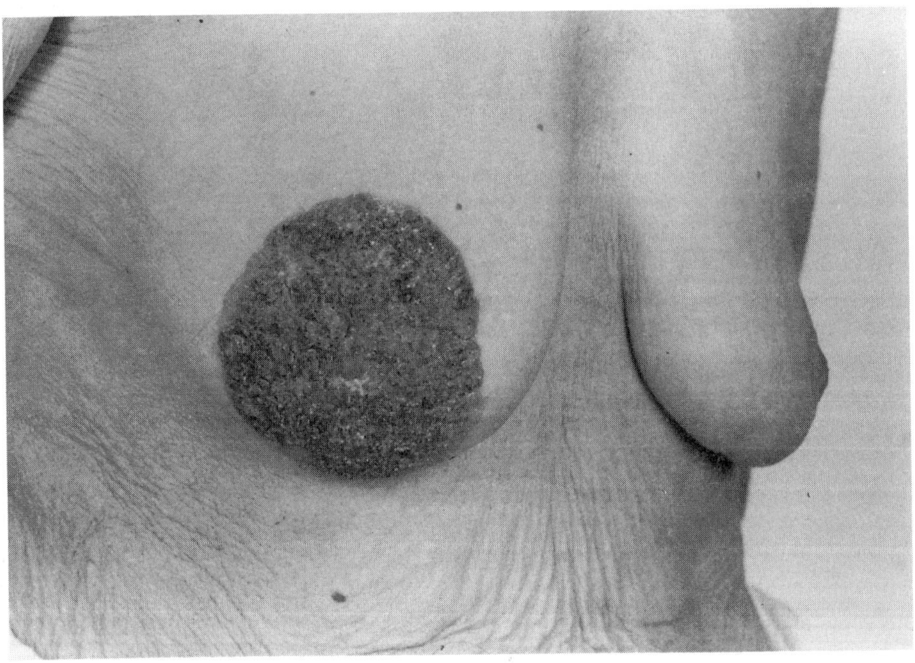

Fig. 21.10 Paget's disease of the nipple. This is a particularly extensive example; more frequently, a small area of scaliness and redness would be seen to one side of the nipple or areola.

traduct carcinoma of the breast and is almost always unilateral. The weeping eczema-like lesion appears on the nipple but later the areola and the surrounding skin will be involved. True eczema by contrast generally affects younger females during lactation, is usually bilateral and shows typical vesicles of eczema and responds to the standard treatment of eczema.

Microscopically, large tumour cells lie within the epithelium of the nipple and areola and these are identical to the tumour cells within the underlying ducts.

If a definite mass can be palpated beneath the affected nipple, the tumour is already of an invasive character whereas absence of a palpable mass in the breast indicates that it is more likely still confined to purely intraductal, non-invasive tumour, with a better prognosis.

The management of Paget's disease of the breast (nipple) is that of the underlying carcinoma.

Pathological classification of breast cancer

Many detailed classifications of the different histological patterns of carcinoma of the breast have been made over the years, and one holding the general acceptance and agreement of many pathologists was produced by the World Health Organization in 1982. The first main subdivision is into two broad categories of invasive and non-invasive, but the more detailed breakdown into numerous further categories dependent on different characteristics of the carcinoma and stroma cells is primarily of interest to the pathologist and of much less relevance to the surgeon.

However, some relatively straightforward histological grading of the aggressiveness and extent of the tumour can be of assistance in determining the prognosis in an individual patient.

Factors such as lymphocytic infiltration, "pushing" peripheral margins of the tumour, and well differentiated malignant cells have a better prognosis, regardless of the gross tumour type. By applying such general criteria to the classification of tumour types, Ackerman et al divided breast cancer into four well defined categories in 1970:

Type I: not invasive.
Type II: invasive, well circumscribed.
Type III: invasive, moderately metastasizing.
Type IV: invasive, highly metastasizing.

Another readily applied method of classification is Broder's grading, in which the grading of the tumour is done according to the percentage of cells which are undifferentiated, as follows:

Grade I: up to 25%.
Grade II: from 25 to 50%.
Grade III: from 50 to 75%.
Grade IV: more than 75%.

Clinical staging

It is important after the establishment of the diagnosis of carcinoma of the breast to complete as far as possible the clinical and pathological assessment of the extent the disease has reached and the local and distant spread of the malignant process. On this assessment shall largely depend the management of the individual case. The assessment also helps surgeons to compare the results of different modes of therapy in respective stages and degrees of malignancy, and gives an idea of prognosis in each case.

For clinical use, the Manchester and TNM classifications are most commonly used. These classifications are based on the size of the tumours, the relation to skin and deeper and neighbouring structures, lymph node involvement and the presence or absence of distant metastases, as found either clinically or as the result of appropriate investigations.

The Manchester classification

This defines four stages, the first being the earliest one with the best prognosis and the fourth the most advanced with the worst prognosis (Fig. 21.11).

Stage I. The growth is confined to the breast and is mobile; any skin adherent to the tumour is smaller in area than the periphery of the tumour; there are no palpable axillary lymph nodes. Ulceration of the skin does not affect the stage.

Stage II. This is similar to stage I with the addition that axillary lymph nodes are palpable, but mobile.

Stage III. The tumour in the breast has skin involvement greater in area than the tumour, and

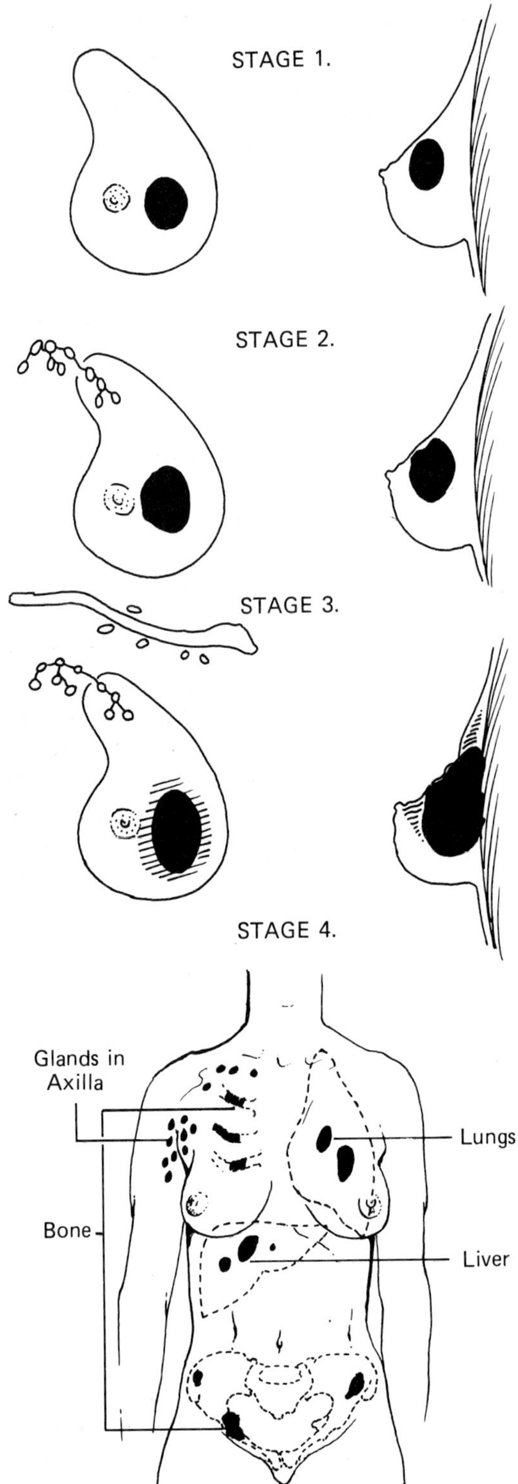

Fig. 21.11 Carcinoma of the breast: Manchester classification—see text for details.

the lymph nodes in the axilla are fixed. In addition there may be fixation to the pectoralis muscle, and/ or involvement of the supraclavicular lymph nodes.

Stage IV. This is the same as stage III with the addition that distant metastases, either via the blood stream or lymphatics, are found. In addition metastases may have spread to the opposite breast, opposite axilla, the supraclavicular lymph nodes or as satellite nodules to the skin.

The TNM classification

This system of clinical classification was recommended by the international union against cancer. Here T stands for tumour, N for lymph nodes and M for metastases (Fig. 21.12).

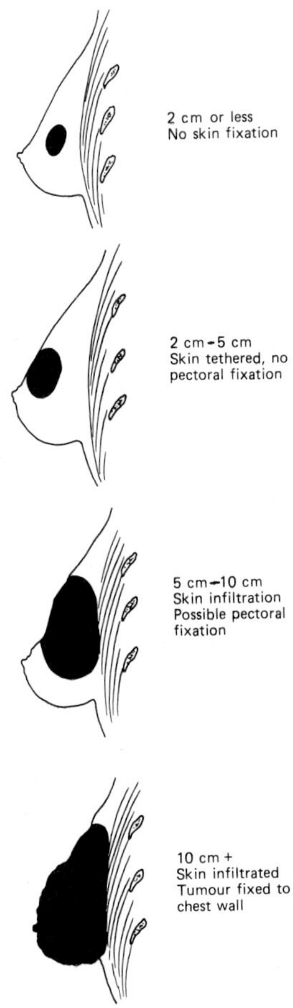

Fig. 21.12 Carcinoma of the breast: TNM classification—see text for details.

Tumour (T)

T_1 Tumour size 2 cm or less; no skin fixation.
T_2 Tumour size from 2 to 5 cm; skin tethered, no pectoral fixation.
T_3 Tumour size more than 5 cm up to 10 cm; skin infiltration or ulceration is present and there may be pectoral muscle fixation.
T_4 Tumour size more than 10 cm in diameter; skin is infiltrated but not beyond the breast and the tumour is fixed to the chest wall.

Lymph nodes (N)

N_0 No lymph nodes involved.
N_1 Axillary lymph nodes are palpable but mobile.
N_2 Axillary lymph nodes are palpable and fixed.
N_3 Axillary lymph nodes are involved, and also supraclavicular lymph nodes.

Metastases (M)

M_0 No metastases.
M_1 Metastases are present.

Confirmation of diagnosis

Where some or all of the classical features described above are present there will be little or no real doubt about the correct diagnosis. However, with very small lumps, or when uncertain whether a discrete nodule which might be carcinoma is present, several other investigative procedures, if available, may be helpful in confirming a suspicion. Mammography and thermography, mentioned already as possible screening methods, can sometimes clarify whether a nodule is benign or malignant, and ultrasound and various scintiscanning techniques may also be useful in the future.

However, regardless of how a lesion, or suspect lesion is detected, it is always important to have definite cytological or histological confirmation before embarking on treatment. This may be achieved by fine needle aspiration of the mass or area, passing the needle several times into the area concerned and applying firm suction during insertion and withdrawal, or by one of the special coring needles, e.g. Trucut. Special skills are required of the cytologist and pathologist in the interpretation of the material obtained by these methods.

Failing these, the most obvious way to secure the pathological diagnosis is to perform open surgical biopsy—either total excision biopsy if the lesion is small, or wedge biopsy if it is large. If frozen-section facilities are available this permits a rapid answer and planning of further treatment. More conventional paraffin section and staining usually takes 2–3 days to provide a full report.

Staging and prognostic indices

Carcinoma of the breast tends to spread early to the regional lymph nodes, lungs, bones, liver and pleura, and this may be occult at the time of clinical presentation. This makes truly accurate staging very difficult. An extensive surgical procedure in an advanced case with metastases is unwarranted. The presence of disseminated disease indicates the need for adjuvant chemotherapy, radiotherapy or endocrine treatment. Five year survival and prognosis are poor in those with lymph node involvement, and the more nodes involved, the worse they become. Oestrogen receptor-positive tumours have a better prognosis than negative ones, and there is a good correlation between oestrogen receptor content of breast cancers and their response to endocrine therapy. Preoperative staging should include chest X-ray, full blood count, liver function tests, fasting serum calcium and isotope bone scintigraphy (which has replaced standard skeletal X-ray survey).

Treatment

This may involve one or more of the following:

1. Surgery.
2. Radiotherapy.
3. Chemotherapy.
4. Hormone therapy.
5. Immunotherapy.
6. Combination therapy.

Surgery

Stages I and II. Opinions vary widely as far as the management of early breast carcinoma is concerned. Many trials have been conducted in many centres and the operations have ranged from simple removal of the lump (lumpectomy) to supraradical mastectomy with removal of the internal mammary chain and supraclavicular lymph nodes. In between these two extremes we have simple mastectomy, mastectomy with clearance of the axillary nodes, and various modifications of radical mastectomy. There is now good evidence that overall survival is not affected by the method of local treatment and there seems therefore no indication for the extensive radical or supraradical ablative operations. Current opinion favours a relatively conservative surgical approach: the following three methods of local treatment are perhaps the most frequently performed:

1. Modified radical mastectomy (Patey's procedure).
2. Simple mastectomy with either axillary node sampling or clearance, perhaps followed by local radiotherapy.
3. Local excision (lumpectomy) axillary node sampling plus postoperative radiotherapy.

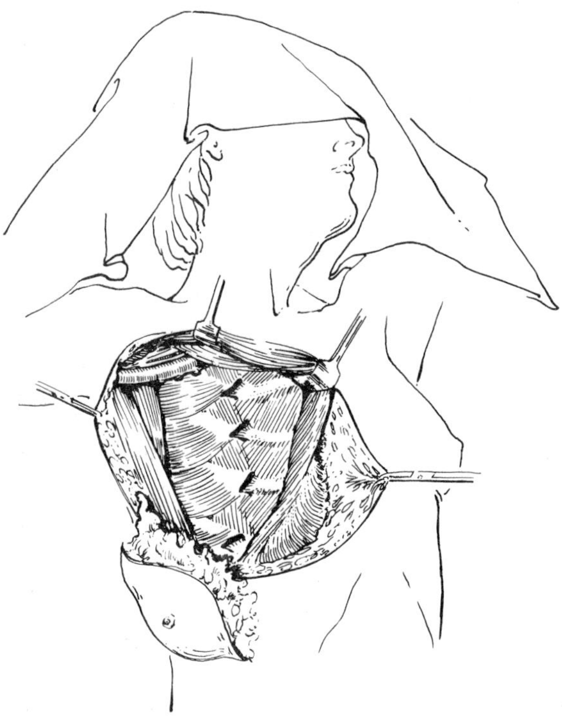

Fig. 21.13 Modified Patey's mastectomy. In this procedure, in addition to removal of all the breast through a transverse elliptical incision, the pectoralis minor muscle is removed and the axillary fat containing all the lymph nodes is dissected free from the axillary blood vessels, and removed en bloc with the breast.

Modified radical mastectomy. In Patey's procedure, the pectoralis major muscle is not removed but simply retracted during the approach to the axilla; the pectoralis minor muscle is excised in toto along with all lymph nodes from the axilla (Fig. 21.13). It gives a good cosmetic result compared to conventional radical mastectomy and is probably as effective an axillary clearance.

Modified radical mastectomy is practised by those surgeons who believe in a radical approach to the breast carcinomas.

Simple mastectomy. Here the breast is removed in toto but both the pectoral muscles are left intact (Fig. 21.14). The axilla is explored and either the axillary fat and nodes are stripped as far as possible from the space, or a few nodes are removed from the medial wall and any other part of the area where they are obvious. Postoperatively radiotherapy is usually given when tumour is identified in the nodes, but may be withheld if all are clear. The results of this procedure compare very favourably with those of radical mastectomy.

Lumpectomy. This involves wide local excision, followed by radiotherapy to the rest of the breast

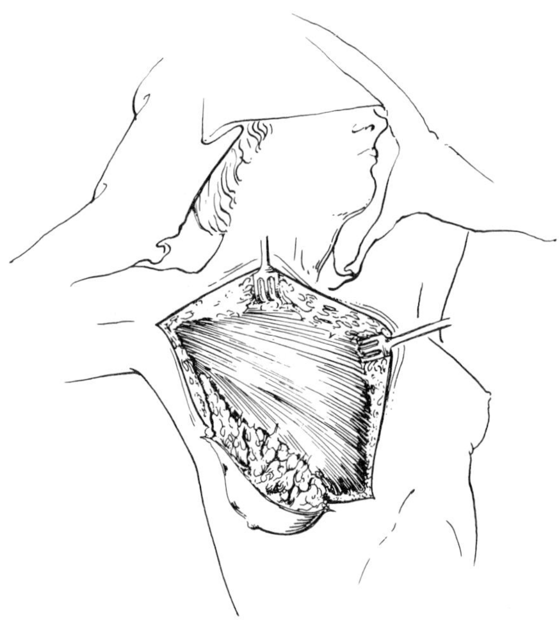

Fig. 21.14 Simple mastectomy involves excision of all the breast, including the axillary tail, but leaving intact both pectoralis major and minor. Any obviously enlarged axillary lymph nodes may be dissected free and removed, or sampling of non-enlarged nodes may be done.

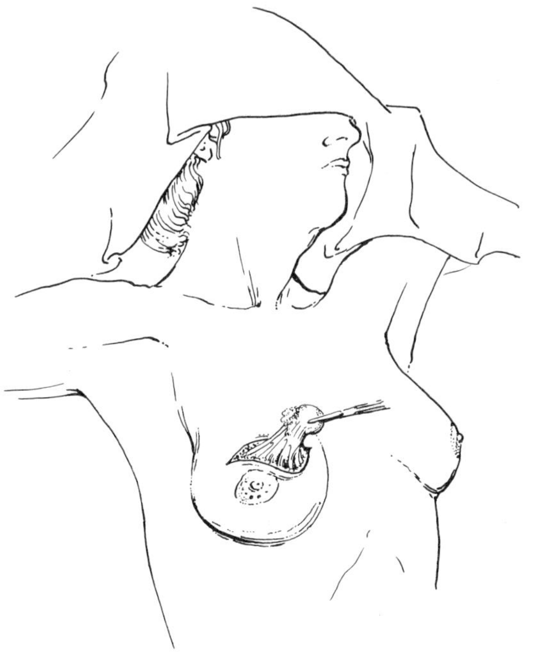

Fig. 21.15 Where local excision of the tumour with a clear margin of normal surrounding breast tissue is performed, radiotherapy is customarily administered to the remainder of the breast to minimize the chances of local recurrence from residual microscopic deposits.

and nodal areas (Fig. 21.15). This approach, as expected, has the advantage of an excellent cosmetic result. Some long-term studies have shown no difference in the survival and local recurrence rates comparing mastectomy with local excision plus radiotherapy.

Most surgeons perform either simple mastectomy with sampling or clearance of the axilla, or local removal of tumour (lumpectomy) with radiotherapy.

Stages III and IV (advanced disease). Curative surgical clearance of the disease at this stage is impossible, and the management can be considered under three headings:

1. The primary breast lump and the regional lymph nodes.
2. Local recurrence.
3. Metastases.

Management of the primary breast lump. If the primary tumour is resectable with a good chance of the wound edges meeting without tension and healing by primary intention, it is usually desirable to proceed with local excision or simple mastectomy. This is particularly so where the tumour is about to ulcerate or has already broken through the skin, as it will avoid the unpleasantness to the patient of a discharging, smelling, bleeding, fungating mass which is difficult to conceal or ignore.

If the mass is too large or accompanied by involvement extensively along the chest wall (cancer en cuirasse) the overall mass may be reduced in size by local radiotherapy, and if the shrinkage is sufficient local excision or mastectomy may then become feasible and helpful. However, if neither local surgery nor radiotherapy is practicable or beneficial, reliance has to be placed on other modes of treatment such as chemotherapy or hormone therapy.

Management of recurrent or metastatic disease. The main approach is usually a combination of local or field radiotherapy and either hormone or chemotherapy. There has been a general move away from surgical clearance of the axilla when nodes are involved in this area, and rather to rely on the effects of systemic therapy or to use radiotherapy to diminish their size if causing symptoms. Surgical excision is now more often limited to biopsy for histological confirmation or removal of a symptomatic local recurrent deposit.

Distant metastases in bone, if causing pain, may be treated by local radiotherapy, often with substantial relief, and pathological fractures may heal surprisingly well with a combination of internal fixation and radiotherapy. Secondary deposits in the thorax and abdomen may cause pleural effusion or ascites, either of which may be helped by aspiration and the instillation of cytotoxic drugs.

For detailed consideration of the various chemotherapeutic and hormone agents consult Chapter 10. The following general comments, however, may be made: the vast majority of oestrogen receptor-negative tumours are unresponsive to hormone therapy and of the receptor-positive ones only 60% respond to endocrine therapy. The effect of hormones on breast cancer is not permanent. The tumour may undergo a fresh surge of proliferation on withdrawal of the drug, or may be unresponsive to the same hormone repeated at a later date. If the tumour stops responding to one hormone, a change to a second hormone may sometimes be beneficial.

In general, for premenopausal patients or early postmenopausal patients, i.e. up to 5 years, ovarian ablation either by irradiation or surgery is usually first recommended. For postmenopausal patients either stilboestrol or an antioestrogen agent, e.g. tamoxifen, is used. It binds to the oestrogen receptor within the tumour cell. Stilboestrol (oestrogen) has side-effects, e.g. water retention with headache, nausea, hypertension and even congestive cardiac failure. Since tamoxifen has minimal side-effects it is used most commonly as the first line of endocrine treatment.

Summary of treatment for advanced carcinoma of the breast

1. *Surgery*: Localized lesions should be excised if they are solitary or producing symptoms.
2. *Radiotherapy*: This is especially useful for secondary deposits in bones, e.g. secondaries in spine causing backache.
3. *Hormones*: Depending upon menstruation.
   a. Premenopausal—ovarian ablation: surgical or by irradiation.
   b. Up to 5 years after the menopause—ovar ian ablation followed by tamoxifen or androgen therapy.
   c. More than 5 years after the menopause—tamoxifen or oestrogen therapy.
4. *Cytotoxic therapy*: Combination chemotherapy, especially in premenopausal patients, may be of use where hormone therapy has failed. Three or four drugs may be given together in well spaced courses.
5. *Hypophysectomy/adrenalectomy*: This is now not much in favour because of the morbidity and postoperative sequelae.
6. *Immunotherapy*: At present this is experimental.

Carcinoma of the breast during pregnancy

Carcinoma of the breast usually shows an accelerated rate of growth and acute inflammatory signs when occurring in a pregnant woman. This is probably due to the increased levels of hormones during pregnancy and lactation. The prognosis is generally poor and most surgeons advise termination of the pregnancy.

Sarcoma of the breast

Fibrosarcomas of the breast stroma are usually large, firm and well circumscribed. They account for 0.5% of all malignant tumours of the breast. Some of them arise in pre-existing intracanalicular fibroadenomas.

They look like medullary carcinoma but are distinguished by their large size and the fact that, unlike carcinoma, they do not get attached to the skin. On cutting the tumour, pale colour and friable consistency are characteristic. The peak age incidence is between 30 and 40 years.

The prognosis is bad. Treatment consists of simple mastectomy followed by radiotherapy. Other types of sarcoma may very rarely arise in the breast.

THE MALE BREAST

Gynaecomastia (or gynaecomazia) means enlargement of the male breast, and can be either primary (idiopathic) or secondary.

Idiopathic gynaecomastia

There is enlargement of the male breast occurring before the age of 25 years; this is usually attributed to pubertal hormonal changes. If the condition presents after 25 years of age, it is usually secondary to an underlying disease (Fig. 21.16). It may be unilateral or bilateral and may attain the size of a fully developed female breast. It does not, however, affect virility.

Secondary gynaecomastia

This may result from hormonal disturbances, drugs or different diseases.

Hormonal disturbances

Patients on oestrogen therapy, e.g. for carcinoma of the prostate, often develop a degree of gynaecomastia. Oestrogen-producing tumours like teratoma, chorion epithelioma of the testis, adrenocortical tumours, bronchial carcinoma and pitui-

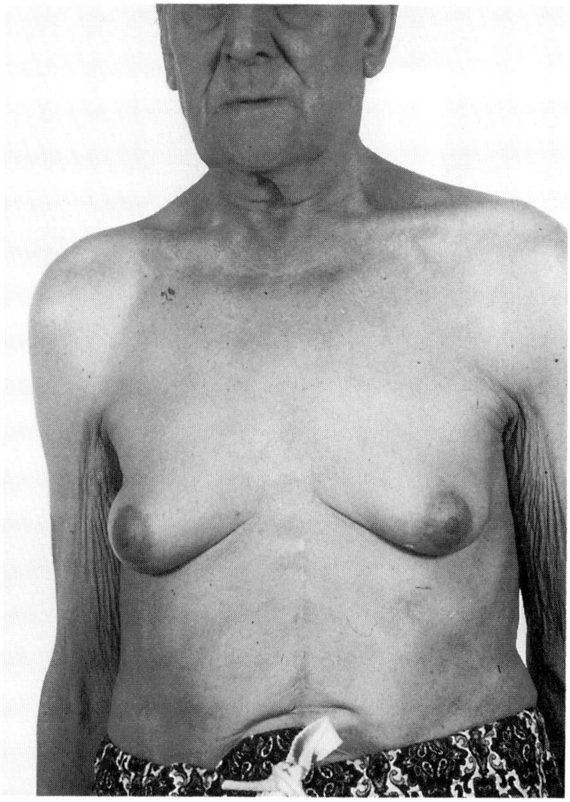

Fig. 21.16 Gynaecomastia. Whereas in young men this may occur as an idiopathic disorder, in older men it is more likely to be due to abnormal hormonal influence. In this patient it was caused by the administration of stilboestrol for carcinoma of the prostate.

tary tumours can also produce gynaecomastia. Patients after castration and those workers who work in oestrogen-producing factories may also develop gynaecomastia.

Drugs

Certain drugs like digitalis, isoniazid, spironolactone, dilantin, methyldopa and cimetidine have gynaecomastia as one of the reported side-effects.

Diseases

1. Leprosy: male patients with leprosy suffer from gynaecomastia. This is probably due to testicular atrophy which usually accompanies leprosy.
2. Cirrhosis of the liver: oestrogens are metabolized in the liver and in cases of liver failure these oestrogens may not be fully metabolized and may produce gynaecomastia.
3. Gynaecomastia may be a feature of Klinefelter's syndrome.
4. In carcinoma of the bronchus, especially the oat-cell pathological variety, there is sometimes ectopic production of feminizing hormones leading to the breast changes.
5. Addison's disease may produce gynaecomastia.

Treatment

If the factors responsible for secondary gynaecomastia can be removed or treated there may be resolution of the secondary condition. In the idiopathic type, mastectomy with preservation of the nipple and areola is recommended.

Carcinoma in the male breast

The incidence of male breast cancer in the USA is about 1% of all breast carcinomas, and may be a little higher in certain tropical countries. There is no documented evidence to suggest any relation between pubertal gynaecomastia and carcinoma. However, there is a suggestion of an increase in the risk of carcinoma arising in the gynaecomastia induced by oestrogen administered to patients with cancer of the prostate, and in patients suffering from Klinefelter's syndrome.

Clinical presentation:

It usually appears in elderly males as a painless lump or nodule. There may be nipple discharge or bleeding. The axillary lymph nodes are likely to be involved and skin involvement is frequent (Fig. 21.17). The naked-eye appearance and microscopic picture of male breast carcinoma are identical to that of the female breast.

Involvement of the skin and surrounding chest wall occurs early due to the small size of the breast, and since the malignant process infiltrates surrounding structures earlier, prognosis is generally worse than for carcinoma of the female breast.

Treatment

Stages I and II are treated surgically as in the fe-

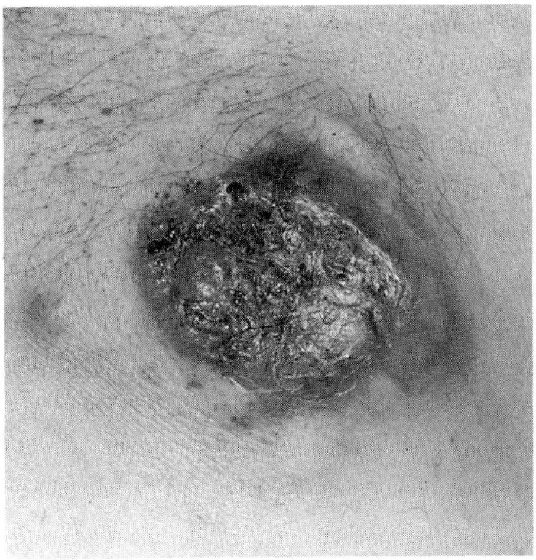

Fig. 21.17 Carcinoma of the male breast. The nipple and immediately surrounding area have been eroded and replaced by an ulcerating raised nodular malignant mass.

male. In inoperable cases bilateral orchidectomy is usually much more beneficial in controlling the disease than oophorectomy is in females. In those cases showing recurrence, or where the effect of orchidectomy has disappeared, oestrogen therapy can be of help. Radiotherapy and chemotherapy, either alone or with surgery, can be used—depending upon the stage and condition of the patient—in advanced cases with metastases or inoperable cases.

Fibroadenoma and fibroadenosis are exceedingly rare in male breasts.

22. Hernia, umbilicus and abdominal wall

A hernia may be defined as a protrusion through a defect in the wall of a body cavity or tissue compartment, containing a viscus or tissue not normally present in this situation. The defect may be primarily a normal anatomical area of weakness or one resulting from mechanical or pathological abnormality.

From the clinical point of view the hernias most frequently presenting for surgical attention are those arising from the abdominal cavity—inguinal, femoral, paraumbilical, epigastric and incisional hernias. Much rarer are ones such as obturator, lumbar, spigelian and the various internal hernias in congenital pockets within the peritoneal cavity. Diaphragmatic hiatal hernias are considered separately in Chapter 27. Portions of muscle and other tissue can occasionally also herniate out through gaps in the overlying fascia, but rarely do these merit operative repair.

As far as abdominal wall hernias are concerned these characteristically comprise a protruding peritoneal sac covered by subcutaneous tissues and skin, and they may contain either omentum or a loop of intestine, rarely portions of other viscera, or a mixture of both gut and omentum. If the neck of the sac is narrow there is a risk of the hernia becoming irreducible or incarcerated by which is implied that the contained gut or omentum is physically prevented from being returned into the main abdominal cavity, but the tissue is still viable and healthy. If in addition to the hernial content not being able to return into the abdomen a contained loop of bowel is occluded by the pressure, this is referred to as an obstructed hernia. When the blood supply to an obstructed, incarcerated loop of gut is compromised by still further increase in local pressure the hernia is then a strangulated one, and there is considerable risk of gangrene of the bowel segment, and dire consequences if urgent surgical relief is not obtained.

Obstruction and strangulation may occur with most types of hernia, but perhaps most threat of such complications arises with femoral hernias, slightly less with indirect inguinal and paraumbilical and less still with other varieties.

An uncommon pattern, but a dangerous one, which may lead to strangulation without complete obstruction, is the Richter hernia (Fig. 22.1) in which only a part of the circumference of a segment of small intestine is trapped in the hernial sac. The blood supply to this segment can still be compromised sufficiently to cause local infarction and rupture. If the damaged portion is reduced either spontaneously or by manual pressure, the infarcted area may subsequently leak and cause dangerous peritonitis.

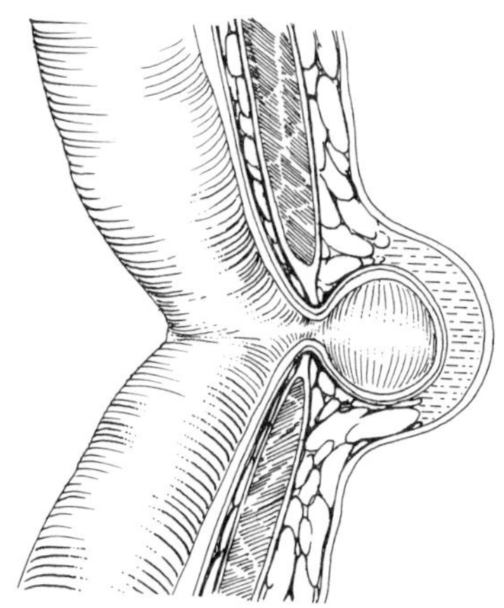

Fig. 22.1 Richter's hernia: only a part of the circumference of the bowel wall is trapped in the hernial sac, and forward passage of the bowel content is not completely impeded.

INGUINAL HERNIA

This is the commonest hernia and operations for its repair are perhaps the commonest abdominal operations performed by surgeons throughout the world. The inguinal canal forms a relatively weak part of the anterior abdominal wall, particularly in males. In fetal life, during the descent of the testis from the posterior abdominal wall where it is formed towards the scrotum, a small part of the peritoneum is brought through the internal inguinal ring. This is the processus vaginalis. Normally the lumen of the greater part of the processus vaginalis is obliterated by birth, and it degenerates into a fibrous cord. The lower end of the processus remains patent to form the tunica vaginalis of the testis. Sometimes the lumen of the proximal part of the processus persists so that a communication exists between the peritoneal cavity and the lumen of the processus. Through this communication abdominal contents may come through the internal inguinal ring and the patent processus vaginalis becomes the sac of a hernia. Abdominal contents do not always descend into the sac before birth and this descent may occur later in childhood or in adult life. Many inguinal hernias develop in this way and are therefore basically congenital in origin. In others, a part of parietal peritoneum may prolapse through the internal ring or the posterior wall of the inguinal canal as a result of recurrent increases in the intra-abdominal pressure due to coughing in chronic bronchitis, obstruction to bladder outflow, or constipation. Sometimes a single sudden violent effort, as in lifting a heavy weight, may be the precipitating cause of the herniation. Frequently, however, herniation may appear in the absence of a history of any such factors. These may be attributed simply to a gradually acquired weakness of the abdominal muscles. However, many surgeons believe that these are really examples of hernia in which there is a delayed descent of abdominal content into a preformed congenital sac.

The sac may be empty or occupied and, as mentioned, the most common contents are either a part of the small intestine or of greater omentum. More rarely a portion of large intestine or the appendix, and in the female the ovary or part of the fallopian tube can be included in the sac.

Occasionally the peritoneal surface of the caecum on the right side or of the pelvic colon on the left side, or a segment of the bladder on either side, may become incorporated as a part of the wall of the sac, and the hernia is referred to as a sliding one (Fig. 22.2).

There are two types of inguinal hernia — direct

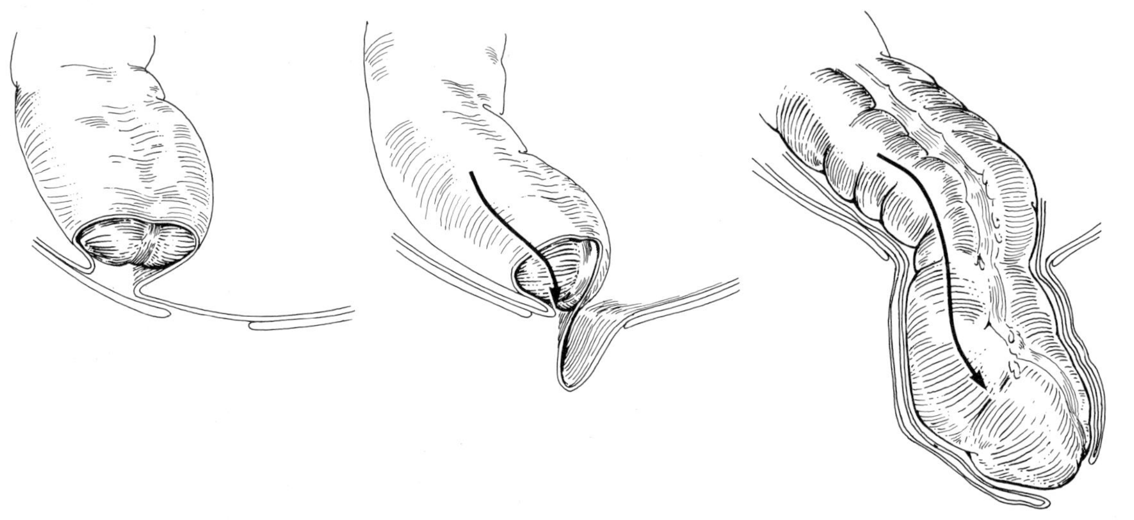

Fig. 22.2 Right-sided sliding hernia: the lower pole of the caecum progressively protrudes down posteriorly along with the developing peritoneal sac. As the hernia enlarges the prolapsed portion of the caecum comes to be incorporated in the wall and may be at risk of damage during operative repair, unless steps are taken to free it and return it to the peritoneal cavity.

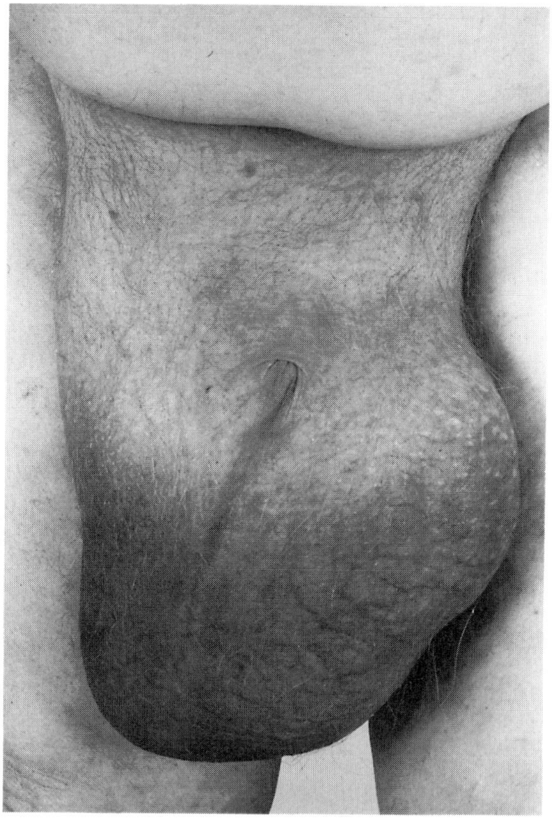

Fig. 22.3 Bilateral huge indirect inguinal hernias, both extending well down into the scrotum, and distorting the appearances by stretching and taking up space within the penile skin.

and indirect. Indirect hernias are by far the most common in both sexes and at all ages. In this variety the sac begins to protrude through the internal inguinal ring, passes along the inguinal canal, and if large enough emerges through the external inguinal ring, and may even extend down into the scrotum (Fig. 22.3). The direct hernia starts through an area of weakness in the medial end of the posterior wall of the inguinal canal and as it enlarges pushes, above the spermatic cord, straight forward to emerge through the external inguinal ring. The neck of the direct type is generally wide and lax in contrast to the often quite narrow one of the indirect hernia.

Clinical features

The most common complaint is simply that of a swelling in the groin. Many patients (or the parents of an infant sufferer) notice that the swelling either disappears or is reduced in size on lying down, and increases on coughing, crying or otherwise straining.

A proportion of patients also complain of a dull dragging pain in the abdomen and sometimes the complaint of occasional pain in the groin during heavy work or straining precedes the appearance of the definite hernial swelling.

The patient is best examined first in the standing position, being completely uncovered from the umbilical level down. A swelling may be clearly visible in the inguinoscrotal region. Whether or not a swelling is seen, the patient is next asked to cough while turning the face away from the examiner. The cough impulse may either make the temporarily reduced hernia appear, or make an already visible one enlarge, in both cases confirming the presence of a definite hernia.

On palpation, the upper limit of the swelling appears to merge imperceptibly with the abdominal wall, and when the patient coughs again while the examiner's fingers are pressed gently over the swelling, a good cough impulse should be felt.

At this stage of the examination, the patient is asked to lie down and in some cases, particularly of a smaller hernia, it may become reduced spontaneously. If this does not happen, an attempt is made to reduce it by applying gentle pressure on the lower part of the swelling in alternately a directly inwards, and inwards, upwards and lateral direction. During reduction of larger hernias, a gurgling sound may be heard as coils of intestine return to within the abdominal cavity from the hernial sac. If the contents of the hernia cannot be reduced by this manoeuvre a diagnosis of irreducible hernia should be made.

After reducing the hernia, the index finger or preferably the index and middle fingers apposed of the clinician are pressed over the internal inguinal ring, which is situated about 1 cm above a point on the inguinal ligament midway between the anterior superior iliac spine and the pubic tubercle and the patient is asked once again to cough, while steady pressure is maintained with the fingers. In an indirect hernia, no swelling appears in the groin and the thrust of the cough impulse is felt beneath the occluding fingers, whereas a direct hernia will protrude and can be clearly seen and felt emerging medial to the fingers.

Usually the examination procedures just described are all that is needed to reach a confident diagnosis of inguinal hernia and its type, but if doubt still persists another method of digital examination may give additional helpful information. This is the gentle invagination of a loose portion of the scrotal skin by the index or little finger of the examiner, with the aim of introducing it through the external inguinal ring along the course of the canal itself so that the fingertip lies at the level of the internal inguinal ring (Fig. 22.4). The patient

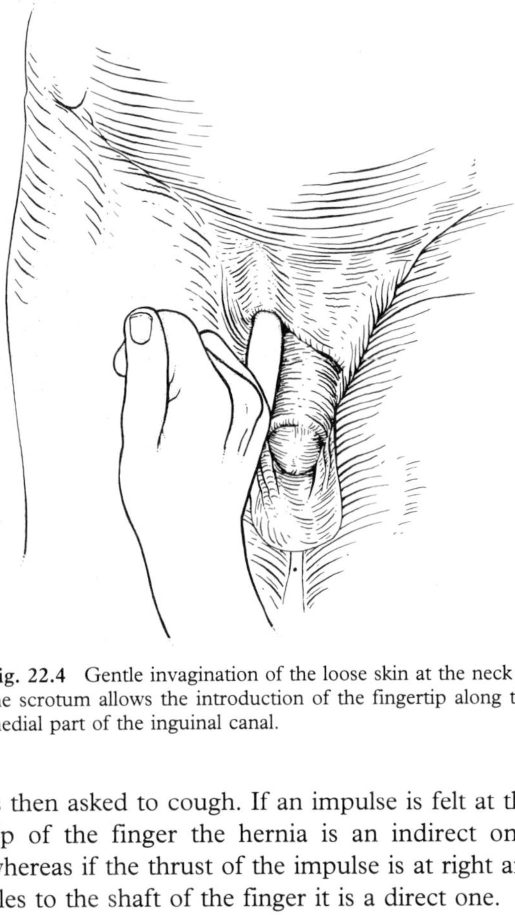

Fig. 22.4 Gentle invagination of the loose skin at the neck of the scrotum allows the introduction of the fingertip along the medial part of the inguinal canal.

is then asked to cough. If an impulse is felt at the tip of the finger the hernia is an indirect one, whereas if the thrust of the impulse is at right angles to the shaft of the finger it is a direct one.

Several other groin swellings may come into the differential diagnosis of inguinal hernia, but these are usually recognized confidently by simple differences in the clinical signs as follows.

First, femoral hernia should be distinguished by the neck of the sac being identified below and lateral

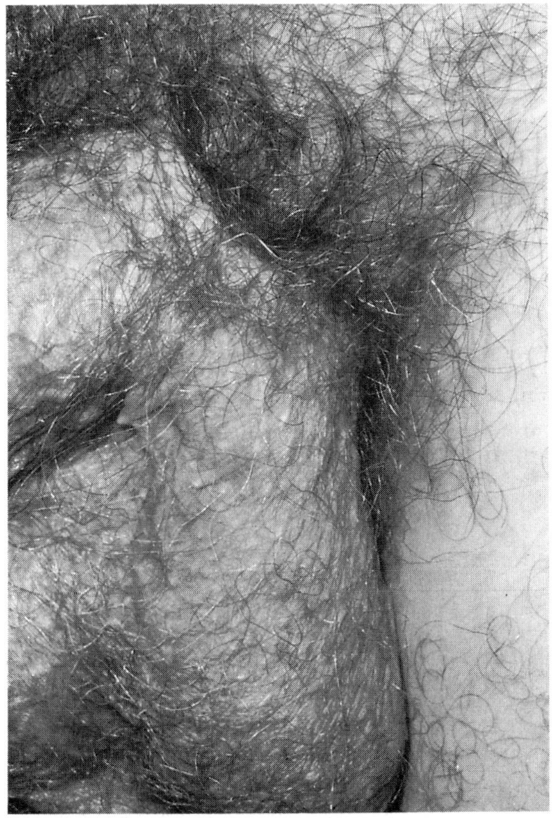

Fig. 22.5 Varicocele presenting as a bulge—a soft swelling at the neck of the scrotum. On palpation it is said to feel like a bag of worms.

to the pubic tubercle, as distinct from above the tubercle and inguinal ligament in inguinal hernia. A varicocele has a characteristic feel to the examining fingers, described graphically as like a bag of worms, and the venous nature of the swelling can be confirmed by gentle manual emptying and rapid spontaneous refill (Fig. 22.5). When a very large indirect inguinal hernia passes down into the scrotum it can be differentiated from a hydrocele by the inability of the examiner's fingers and thumb to grasp a normal-sized spermatic cord above the swelling, whereas this will be readily accomplished with a hydrocele. Furthermore most idiopathic hydroceles will transilluminate quite vividly. Rarely a small cyst of the cord, an isolated cystic remnant of the tunica vaginalis lying at some point along the spermatic cord, may mimic an inguinal hernia, but it will not reveal a true cough impulse and its edges can be clearly defined on palpation.

Treatment

Indirect inguinal hernias should be surgically repaired, the only exceptions being in infancy, and in the elderly patient with concomitant incurable life-threatening disease. Most surgeons prefer to use general anaesthesia, but the operations may be performed adequately under local anaesthesia and this or spinal anaesthesia can make repair in the elderly high-risk case feasible and safe.

Most direct inguinal hernias are also suitable for surgical repair, but very small bulges and large wide-necked ones which present virtually no risk of becoming obstructed or strangulated may be left alone, particularly if there is present some chronic disorder such as emphysema, myocardial ischaemia or prostatic obstruction.

In babies born with an inguinal hernia the question of operation can safely be postponed till the age of about 2 years, although the parents should be advised to seek medical advice at any time should the hernia become irreducible. By the age of 2 the hernia may have disappeared spontaneously as the inguinal canal develops and the internal and external inguinal rings move apart and no longer overlap. In this case operation will not be required. If, however, the hernia persists an operation should be recommended—the procedure being simple excision of the peritoneal sac, i.e. herniotomy.

In older children and adults it is necessary not only to remove the sac, but also to carry out a repair of the internal ring and strengthening of the weakened posterior wall of the canal. Many different techniques for achieving these objectives have been described over the years. It is unlikely that one is distinctly superior to all the others, and probably it is more important that the surgeon should be familiar with and competent at the method. The first step in all approaches is to divide the external oblique aponeurosis in the line of its fibres, starting from the edge of the external inguinal ring and continuing laterally to open up the anterior wall of the entire canal. After dissection of the sac from the cord structures, right up to the neck, opening it, ensuring it is empty, transfixing the neck and ligating it with an absorbable suture and excising the sac distal to this stitch, the edges of the enlarged internal ring are defined and drawn together snugly around the emerging cord structures by one or two sutures. Next is the choice of method to strengthen the posterior wall of the canal and for this there are three popular techniques.

The Bassini technique

The Bassini pattern involves suturing the lower edge of the conjoint tendon down to the reflected part of the inguinal ligament behind the spermatic cord (Fig. 22.6). Non-absorbable suture material is used, but individual surgeons prefer a series of interrupted sutures, or a continuous approximating one, or a darn, using several layers of continuous sutures introduced across the gap between these two structures in different directions to form a loose but even scaffolding of material among which fibrous tissue will develop. Whatever technique is employed the suturing starts precisely at the pubic tubercle and is continued laterally until there is just enough room to accommodate the passage of the spermatic cord and no more. This is a matter of good judgement, making the closure on the one hand tight enough not to allow the escape of any further hernial sac, but on the other hand not so tight that it will compromise the blood supply to the testis. Should undue tension arise on approximating the conjoint tendon to the inguinal ligament, some decrease of this tension may be achieved by making a release incision in the anterior rectus sheath a few centimetres above the groin, to allow the lower fascial layer to slide downwards—the so-called Tanner slide manoeuvre. Once the posterior repair is completed, the incision in the external oblique tendon is closed anterior to the cord by a continuous absorbable suture and the skin approximated by sutures or clips, with or without the addition of subcutaneous stitches.

The Shouldice repair

In the Shouldice repair stress is laid on careful dissection of the transversalis fascia in the posterior wall of the canal after mobilization of the cord structures and reinforcement of the internal ring. Once the edges of the weakened area in the fascia are identified and defined these edges are sutured together by the surgeon's preferred method, but again using non-absorbable material. Further strengthening of the posterior wall is next achieved

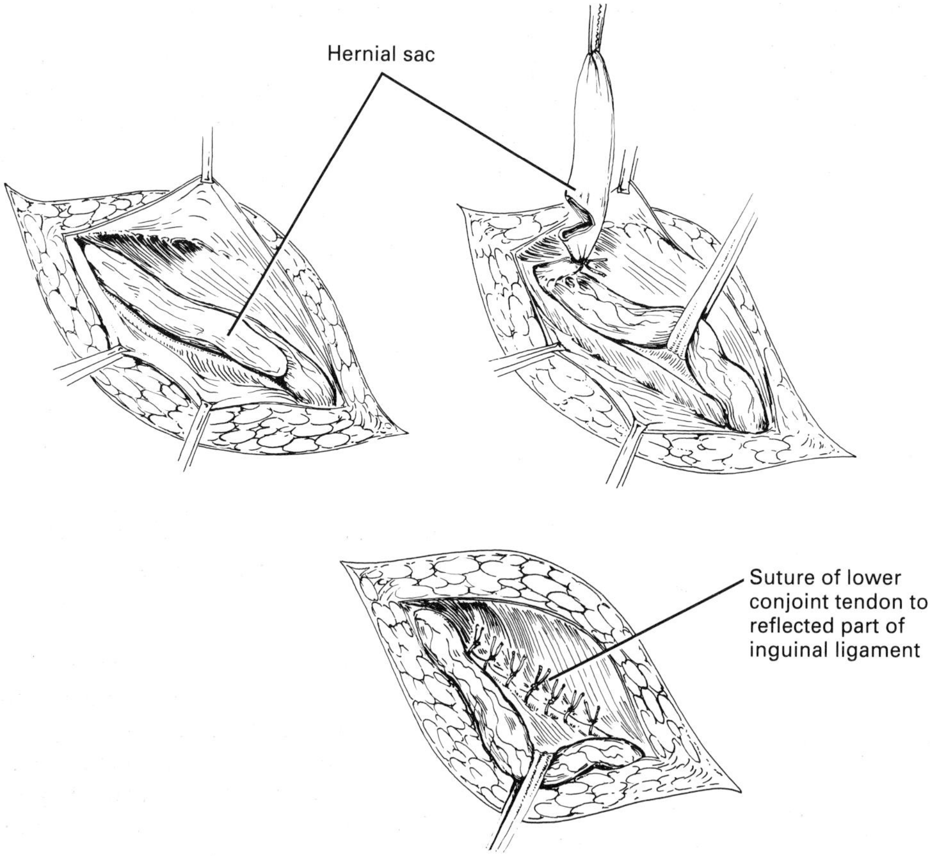

Fig. 22.6 Bassini type of hernia repair. The peritoneal hernia sac is gently dissected from the anterior layers of the spermatic cord, emptied, opened and ligated at its neck. The posterior wall of the inguinal canal is then strengthened by suturing the lower end of the fibrous conjoint tendon to the tough reflected part of the inguinal ligament.

by suturing the conjoint tendon to the inguinal ligament behind the cord, much as in the Bassini type of repair. Once more, if there is a risk of undue tension a relaxing incision may be made in the anterior rectus sheath. The external oblique aponeurosis is resutured and the wound closed.

The Halsted technique

The Halsted operation differs from the above two procedures in that the lower end of the divided external oblique aponeurosis is brought down behind the spermatic cord in addition to the conjoint tendon, and sutured as a separate layer to the inguinal ligament. The cord is thus placed in a more anterior position at completion of this procedure and the tougher fibres of the external oblique aponeurosis give additional strong support to the posterior wall.

Whatever technique is used it is important to achieve good haemostasis, to define layers accurately, and to appose without tension. Precision, care and thoroughness in the performance of the operation are as important as the type of procedure selected.

Sliding hernia presents additional problems in the repair operation. Usually the exact diagnosis is made only during the dissection of the sac from the cord structures, but there may have been a preoperative suspicion in the case of a large indirect hernia with obvious bowel content, or when there have been associated bladder symptoms.

On discovering the true nature of a sliding hernia at operation great care should be taken on completing the clearance of the sac not to damage bowel or bladder. In some cases, once the neck of the sac has been reached it may be possible to insert a series of inverting sutures through the peritoneum on either side of the bowel or bladder and step by step reduce the viscus back into the abdominal cavity proper. If this is not feasible, however, it will then be necessary to open the sac away from the area in which the bowel or other organ is incorporated, and cut a fringe of peritoneal attachment, as shown in Figure 22.7.

The organ can then be returned, and perhaps fixed by suture within the abdomen, and closure of the remaining neck and excision of surplus sac may be performed. One of the repair procedures already discussed is now possible, and since this particular type of hernia is usually large and associated with weak stretched muscle and fascial layers, a particularly thorough repair is advised.

For the very small number of hernia patients in whom there is no realistic possibility of surgical repair under any form of anaesthesia the only alternative is to recommend a truss. The most commonly prescribed comprises a spring steel band passing around the waist to the groin, where it keeps in place a pressure pad. It is vital to ensure that the hernia is fully reduced before the appliance is put on, and that the pad is placed precisely over the site of the hernial weakness, otherwise not only will it fail to control the hernia during normal activity, but the wrongly applied pressure may aggravate matters and even precipitate obstruction. The truss is kept in place by simple retaining straps.

Direct inguinal hernia

As mentioned, this variety protrudes through an acquired area of weakness in the posterior wall of the inguinal canal and is often associated with disorders causing increased intra-abdominal pressure. If there is a means of dealing with such an underlying factor, e.g. prostatic hypertrophy, this should be corrected first since obviously it will reduce the chance of further hernial recurrence. As far as the operative repair of the hernia itself is concerned a small sac may simply be inverted, but a larger one is best dissected cleanly and excised. The neck is generally too wide to deal with by transfixation/ligation, and requires formal suturing with a continuous absorbable peritoneal stitch. The direct sac usually occurs just medial to the inferior epigastric blood vessels, and care should be taken not to damage these structures. Repair of the posterior wall can then be carried out using one of the techniques described for indirect hernias.

A minority of patients present with simultaneously a direct and an indirect hernial sac and it is wise when performing operations to repair one variety to check that a second or double-barrelled sac is not present. If so this second component should also be removed and a conventional repair of the posterior wall effected.

Complicated inguinal hernia

If an inguinal hernia becomes irreducible, but there is no evidence of obstruction, i.e. no colicky abdom-

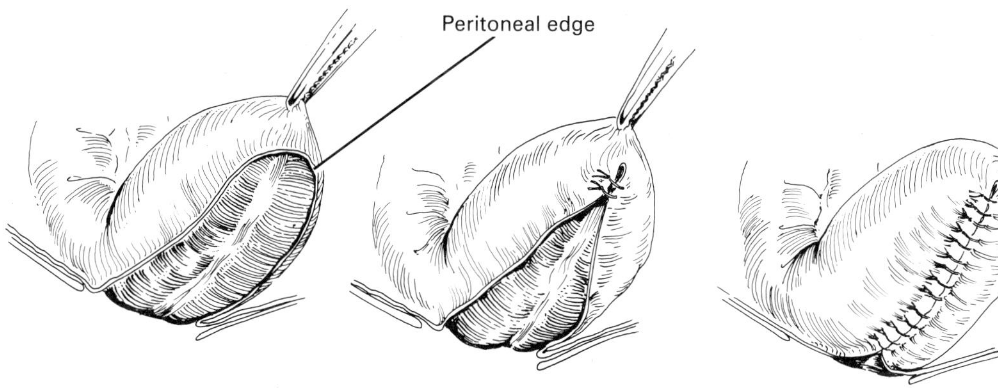

Fig. 22.7 Repair of a sliding hernia, involving caecum. A fringe of peritoneum is cut around the pole of the caecum, from the hernial sac. This allows the reperitonealized caecum to be returned into the peritoneal cavity, and the resulting opening of the hernial sac is sutured at the level of the internal inguinal ring.

inal pain, abdominal distension or vomiting, then an initial gentle attempt to reduce it is permissible. The patient should be admitted to hospital, confined to bed with the foot of the bed elevated and sedation and analgesia may reduce muscle tone sufficiently for reduction to occur either spontaneously or on gentle pressure over the swelling. It is then wise to advise surgical repair in the next few days. Clearly if reduction is not achieved operation should be performed on the next available theatre session.

When there is an obstruction in the hernia urgent exploration is required since it is difficult on clinical grounds alone to determine whether strangulation has occurred in the segment of bowel. The signs which raise the suspicion of this degree of damage are severe pain and tenderness locally in the hernial swelling itself; any signs of peritoneal irritation, e.g. guarding and rebound tenderness, and toxicity as manifest by rapid tachycardia, pyrexia, restlessness and sweating. As with other forms of intestinal obstruction it is important to aspirate the gastric contents by means of a nasogastric tube and to set up a good intravenous line for the administration of fluids.

Most obstructed and strangulated hernias can be dealt with by direct exposure of the inguinal canal as for an elective repair of an uncomplicated hernia. The sac can be opened, the trapped segment of bowel examined and if clearly viable returned to the abdomen after, if necessary, widening or releasing the neck of the sac. If a portion of bowel is infarcted it is best to open the abdomen formally to resect the piece of bowel and perform end-to-end anastomosis. The abdomen should also be explored if there have been clear signs of peritoneal irritation, or a markedly raised white blood cell count, or if the sac is found to be empty but to contain dark or blood-stained liquid. These latter signs suggest that although the previously trapped piece of bowel has returned into the abdomen, it is very likely to be non-viable and will perforate and cause dangerous peritonitis.

Recurrent hernia

Recurrence after an operative repair of a hernia is always a great disappointment to the patient and to the surgeon. Even in spite of careful technique and attention to detail, recurrences after primary repair of inguinal hernias vary from 1–2% to 7–10%. Higher rates may be expected with large defects in elderly and debilitated patients and those with sliding hernias. In some cases the recurrence may be due to an overlooked second sac at the primary repair, others to incomplete excision of the sac or to the weakening effects of postoperative haematoma or infection. Repeated coughing or other forms of straining may also be important factors leading to the second hernia.

In most cases a second repair should be carried out, with the same basic principles of complete excision of the sac and some procedure to strengthen further the posterior wall of the canal. A range of manoeuvres may be necessary to achieve the soundest repair, e.g. use of fascial strips, sheets of collagen or synthetic material to close the defect, removal of the spermatic cord and testis etc. Repeated recurrences after several competent repair operations suggest some basic defect in formation of collagen tissue and a stage may be reached when further attempts at repair are futile.

FEMORAL HERNIA

A femoral hernia descends from the abdomen into the thigh through the femoral ring, which is a potential gap between the medial end of the inguinal ligament and the upper border of the pubic bone, just lateral to the pubic tubercle. It is bounded anteriorly by the inguinal ligament, posteriorly by the fascia covering the pectineus muscle, laterally by the fascial sheath of the femoral vein and medially by the sharp edge of the lacunar ligament. Normally a lymph node and some extraperitoneal tissue occupy the ring. The ring is bounded on three sides by unyielding structures. A hernia passing through it is, therefore, more liable to become obstructed and strangulated than is an inguinal hernia.

Femoral hernia is comparatively more common among European and American people and constitutes about 5% of all hernias. It is far less common among the Indian population. In women this hernia accounts for about 20–30% of all hernias, whereas in men it represents only about 2–3% of the total. Nothing is known about its aetiology. Its relative frequency in women has been ascribed to their comparatively wider pelvis and to the changes which occur in the soft tissues of the pelvis during pregnancy. As the peritoneal sac descends through the femoral ring, it usually pushes ahead of it a lymph node (Cloquet's), and some of the extraperitoneal fat and fascia. Further enlargement will pass in a forward direction, through the cribriform fascia, and as this is attached to the fascia lata at this level, any further extension of the hernia can pass only superiorly. The fundus can, therefore, move above the medial end of the inguinal ligament (Fig. 22.8).

The Richter's type of hernia, in which only a part of the circumference of the intestine enters the sac, may occur in this region.

The content of the hernial sac is most likely to be either omentum or small intestine, and less commonly a portion of colon, bladder, appendix or adenexae of the uterus. Rarely, the sac contains only fluid.

Clinical features

The patient may present either with a rounded swelling in the groin, or with the picture of small bowel obstruction (Fig. 22.9). In the latter case there may or may not have been an awareness of a pre-existing swelling. Where obstruction is present the main symptoms will, of course, be colicky abdominal pain, localized pain in the region of the

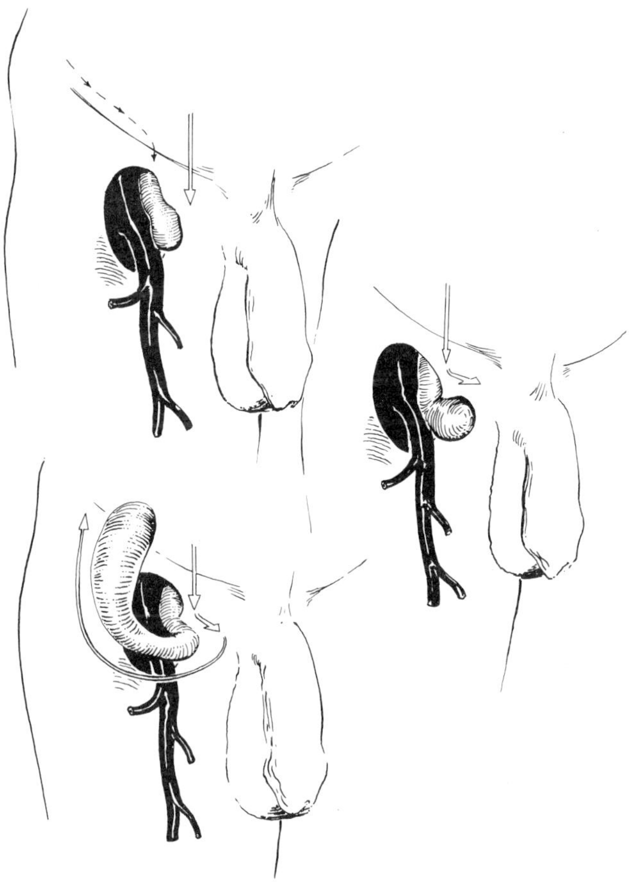

Fig. 22.8 Most femoral hernias are small and simply project downwards directly through the femoral canal. If, however, the sac further enlarges, its fundus projects anteriorly through the saphenous opening in the deep fascia, and still further extension may turn proximally towards or even over the inguinal ligament.

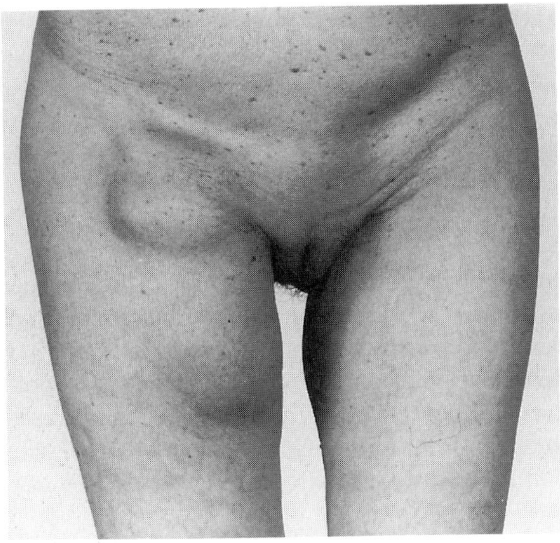

Fig. 22.9 Large femoral hernia, located clearly below the inguinal ligament. The lower swelling in the thigh is a coincidental lipoma. More commonly, this hernia presents as a small swelling or cough impulse precisely through the femoral canal, and it can be very much less obvious.

hernia, nausea, vomiting, constipation, and abdominal distension. If the hernia is of the Richter's pattern there may not be constipation.

On examination with the patient standing the femoral hernia may be easily seen in a thin patient. There is a reducible swelling below and lateral to the pubic tubercle, and an impulse on coughing is present. The swelling either disappears or becomes smaller when the patient lies down and can be reduced by pushing the contents upwards and backwards, and this may be facilitated by flexing the patient's thigh. In an obese patient, no swelling may be visible and the presence of a hernia may be difficult to ascertain by palpation. A useful landmark is the femoral artery just below the inguinal ligament, the swelling being sought medial to the artery.

A femoral hernia may have to be distinguished from a saphenous varix, a dilatation of the terminal part of the long saphenous vein. This will also exhibit a cough impulse, but usually in a direction more obviously continued along the anatomical course of the vein. It will also either disappear or become very much smaller on lying down. Saphenous varix is nearly always associated with varicosities of the superficial veins of the lower limbs and on tapping one of the varicose veins, with the patient standing up, a thrill can be felt transmitted to the saphenous varix.

Some confusion may also arise in differentiating a femoral from an inguinal hernia, but careful attention to the relationship with the inguinal ligament, the pubic tubercle and the direction of the cough impulse should allow a confident diagnostic decision.

Confusion is most likely to arise when the femoral hernia has enlarged sufficiently to bring the fundus up anteriorly over the medial end of the inguinal ligament. In this situation, however, it should be possible to follow the course of reduction first downwards, then directly backwards and finally upwards behind the inguinal ligament, whereas the direction of an inguinal hernia is upwards and backwards above the inguinal ligament from the start.

If the femoral hernia is irreducible it has sometimes to be distinguished from an enlarged lymph node in the inguinal region. In the absence of abdominal pain or of any focus of infection in the drainage area of the inguinal lymph nodes, the question can be difficult to settle prior to exploration.

An obstructed femoral hernia in an obese person is sometimes extremely difficult to diagnose and tragedies can be averted if this possibility is kept in mind whenever a patient presents with symptoms and signs indicating small-bowel obstruction.

Treatment

Surgical reduction of the hernia and closure of the femoral ring is the only treatment of the condition and although a general anaesthetic is usually preferred, it is possible to effect a repair satisfactorily and comfortably for the patient under local anaesthetic, if fitness for general anaesthesia is doubtful. In unobstructed cases, this operation can be performed through an incision either below or above the inguinal ligament. In obstructed cases, a suprainguinal approach is safer, in case resection of a piece of damaged bowel or further exploration of the abdomen is required. Femoral hernia cannot be controlled by any truss. Recurrence of femoral hernia after surgical repair is uncommon.

INCISIONAL HERNIA

An incisional hernia may occur through any abdominal incision but is commoner with vertical as opposed to oblique or transverse incisions. The most important predisposing factor is wound infection. Some are examples of incomplete burst abdomen, where only the skin has been left intact. Other factors are wound haematomas, obesity, persistent postoperative cough, paralytic ileus, muscular weakness, anaemia, diabetes and the presence of malignant disease. The use of absorbable sutures in wound closure is also likely to favour the development of incisional hernia.

Pathology

The size of the hernia is variable (Figs. 22.10 and 22.11). Rather than there being a distinct well defined sac there is more often a diffuse bulge under the line of the scar and as the neck of the hernia is usually wide, the chances of complete obstruction are small. Irreducibility and intermittent partial obstruction may, however, occur because the contents tend to become adherent to the innermost layer of the hernial covering and to each other.

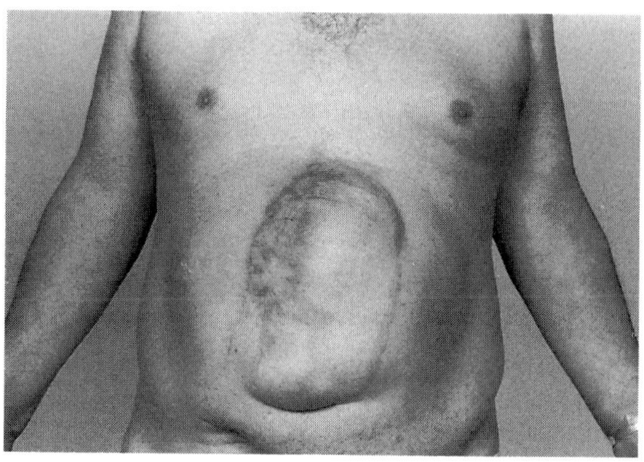

Fig. 22.10 Large incisional hernia following an upper abdominal operation. These are more common when vertical wounds have been made, as opposed to transverse or oblique wounds.

Clinical features

A bulge in the operation scar is the presenting complaint. If it is large there may be considerable local discomfort, and if the wall of the hernia is thin and stretched the writhing movements of contained loops of intestine may be obvious. On examination the majority of hernias are unmistakable, except where a small hernia occurs in a fat person. An impulse on coughing is present but the best way of making it most prominent is to ask the patient to raise the head and shoulders or straighten the legs from the bed to tense the abdominal muscles (Fig. 22.12). In reducible hernias, the circumference of the opening in the abdominal wall can usually be clearly defined, again by asking the patient to tense the abdominal muscles, when the separated medial edges of the rectus abdominis muscles can be felt.

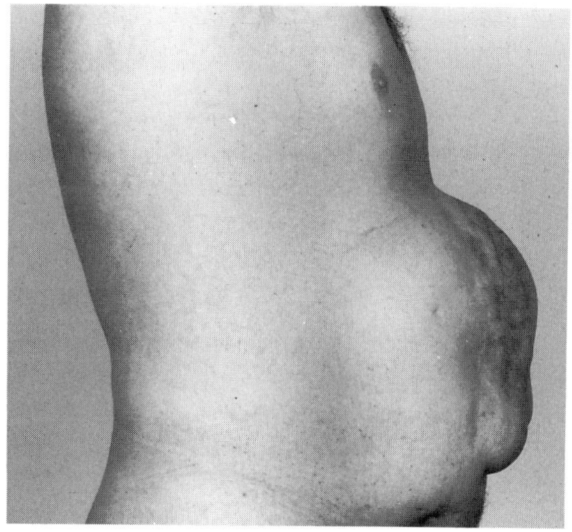

Fig. 22.11 Lateral view of the same incisional hernia as in Figure 22.10, showing marked protruberance of the sac and its thin coverings of skin and small amounts of subcutaneous tissue.

Treatment

It is reasonable to offer surgical repair of the hernia unless there are severe uncorrectable health problems which would make operation risky, or the defect is so wide and the muscles and fascial layers so weak and attenuated that the repair is very unlikely to succeed. Under either of these latter circumstances the patient is usually fitted with an abdominal support corset or even a binder.

When operation is feasible the edges of the defect

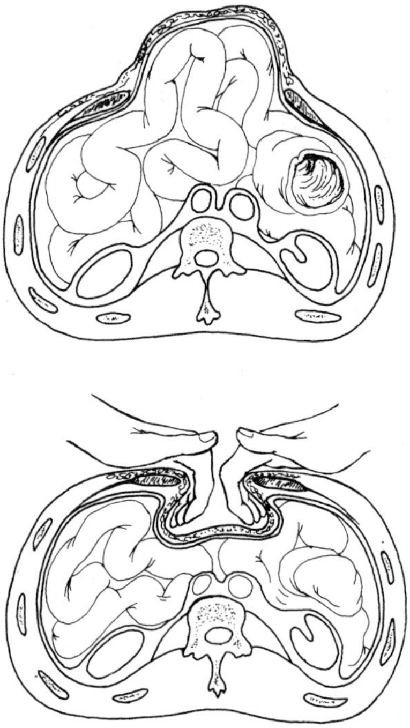

Fig. 22.12 Palpation of the edges of the incisional hernia. With the patient prone and relaxed, normally the abdominal viscera will protrude into the thin covering of peritoneum and skin. The fingers of each hand can be gently insinuated as shown and when the patient tenses the abdominal muscles the edges are usually clearly felt.

are dissected out, preferably without opening the peritoneal cavity, and the edges are approximated by one or more rows of non-absorbable sutures with little or no tension. A popular technique is progressively to invaginate the thin fibrous wall with layers of sutures, to create a 'keel', each layer bringing the muscular edges slightly closer together, for final approximation by sutures. Occasionally it is not possible to achieve a satisfactory repair with the patient's own tissues, and the insertion of a sheet of synthetic material such as Marlex mesh or Goretex over the defect may be used. In all repairs it is important to secure complete haemostasis.

UMBILICAL HERNIA

There are three patterns of umbilical hernia we have to consider: two arising in infants— exomphalos and true umbilical hernia—and one in adults—the paraumbilical hernia.

Exomphalos is a developmental defect in which a part of the anterior abdominal wall has failed to develop and the abdominal viscera are covered with a thin, transparent membrane. The membrane consists of three layers—amniotic membrane, Wharton's jelly and peritoneum, in that order from the outside inwards. In the majority of cases other congenital defects like club foot, hare lip and hydrocephalus are also present.

Urgent surgical intervention is called for. It is not usually possible to carry out a formal reduction of the hernia and repair of the abdominal wall at a single sitting, as the abdominal cavity is too small to contain all the viscera, which have not so far been inside it. A two-stage operation is therefore usually undertaken. In the first stage, skin is mobilized by undermining it in the surrounding area, and covering the defect with the mobilized skin flaps alone. The second operation is performed when the baby is 1 year old and at this operation a formal repair of the abdominal wall is carried out in layers.

A true infantile umbilical hernia is always acquired in the sense that it develops after the baby is born and the cord is cut. The only complaint is that there is a reducible umbilical swelling which increases in size when the baby cries. Obstruction and strangulation almost never occur in this hernia. Moreover, most of the hernias disappear as the child grows. Operative repair is only required if the hernia persists after 2–3 years of age.

A paraumbilical hernia is a hernia through the anterior abdominal wall near the umbilicus. Middle-aged, multiparous and corpulent women are the usual victims, though it occurs in men also. The hernia is usually small, but may grow to a large size. Greater omentum is the commonest content, but a loop of small intestine or even colon may enter the sac. The neck of the sac is often small, well defined and tight in relation to the size of the hernia, and there may be loculations due to adhesion of the contents to the sac wall. Irreducibility, obstruction and strangulation may arise in this type of hernia.

Advice is usually sought either simply on account of a lump near the umbilicus or for abdominal pain, if the hernia becomes incarcerated or obstructed.

Surgical repair should be recommended to remove

the risk of obstruction or strangulation. The usual approach is through a transverse elliptical incision embracing the umbilicus, but if there is a strong desire to preserve the umbilical pit, careful dissection of the thin umbilical skin with the upper flap of a linear transverse incision below the umbilicus may be possible. The neck of the sac is generally dissected out easily, the sac emptied, opened and excised at its neck and then repair is effected by overlapping upper and lower flaps of the dense rectus sheath and linea alba layers (Fig. 22.13). The skin is then closed over the repair. Sound repair is expected and recurrence should be rare.

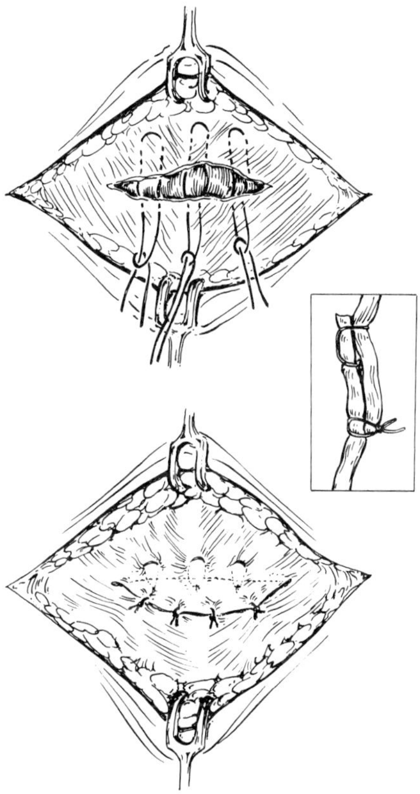

Fig. 22.13 Mayo repair of a paraumbilical hernia. After freeing and excising the peritoneal sac, the defect in the linea alba is extended slightly laterally and two rows of sutures are inserted to overlap the upper flap over the lower one.

EPIGASTRIC HERNIA

An epigastric hernia occurs in the midline through a defect in the linea alba, usually 2–3 cm above the umbilicus. Nothing is known about its aetiology, but probably it occurs through a congenitally weak spot in the linea alba. Sometimes only extraperitoneal fat herniates through the defect. In other cases, a true hernia develops. Usually it is small and empty, but in a few cases omentum or a part of stomach or intestine may occupy the sac.

The majority of these hernias are symptomless, but they may be associated with vague abdominal pain which may become aggravated on straining or worse after meals. If the hernia is irreducible the swelling may be quite obvious to inspection and palpation and may also be slightly tender on even gentle compression. When a patient does present with upper abdominal pain or other upper gastrointestinal symptoms and has an epigastric hernia it is important to be sure that these symptoms are arising from the hernia and not from some other cause, e.g. peptic ulcer, gallbladder disease or hiatal hernia. If these are clearly excluded operative repair of the hernia should be advised. This is usually a simple straightforward procedure, using non-absorbable sutures to close the defect in the linea alba.

RARER HERNIAS

Obturator hernia

This rare hernia is more likely to be encountered in women than in men, and unlikely to be diagnosed unless a loop of small bowel becomes trapped in it. The peritoneal sac passes directly through the obturator foramen, which accommodates the obturator nerve and blood vessels. The classical description of the hernia pressing on the obturator nerve and thereby causing pain referred along the distribution of this nerve, down the inner aspect of the thigh and knee is very rarely encountered.

The clinical presentation, as mentioned, is most likely to be that of a small-bowel obstruction and the nature of the hernia is discovered only at exploratory laparotomy. Repair should be straightforward.

Lumbar hernia

In the majority of cases, a lumbar hernia emerges through the lower lumbar triangle, (triangle of Petit)

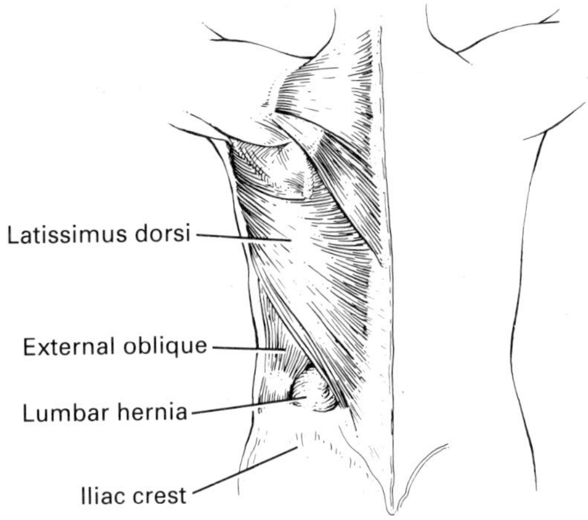

Fig. 22.14 Anatomical relations of lumbar hernia.

which is bounded by the iliac crest inferiorly, latissimus dorsi posteriorly, and the external oblique muscle anteriorly (Fig. 22.14). In a minority of cases, the hernia emerges at a higher level through a space bounded in front by the internal oblique muscle, behind by the erector spinae muscles and above by the 12th rib.

Hernias through these triangles have to be distinguished from cold abscess, lipoma, renal tumour, haematoma and muscle strain. An impulse on coughing is diagnostic. Many of these hernias cause pain and discomfort and they should be repaired surgically. This may require considerable dissection to mobilize flaps of neighbouring fascial layers.

Spigelian hernia

Spigelian hernia is the name given to a rare hernia in the aponeurosis of the lateral abdominal wall muscles as they meet the lateral edge of the rectus abdominis sheath. This hernia may be difficult to feel in an obese patient. Its usual level is below and lateral to the umbilicus at the level of the arcuate line (of Douglas). Obstruction is likely to develop as the neck of the hernial sac is surrounded by rigid fascia. Surgery should, therefore, be advised unless there are definite contraindications.

Internal hernia

A variety of congenital or postoperative pockets in the peritoneal cavity may, from time to time, entrap a segment of bowel and present as intestinal obstruction. Examples are the foramen of Winslow, the intersigmoid fossa, various paraduodenal fossae, and any gaps left by the surgeon after dividing peritoneal coverings, mesentery, etc. The nature of the hernial sac comes to light at the exploratory operation.

THE UMBILICUS

Apart from umbilical and paraumbilical hernia the following disorders affecting the umbilicus may be encountered.

Umbilical sepsis

Infection in the newborn may arise on account of non-sterile applications to the region after severance of the umbilical cord, and various organisms may be introduced in this way. The most serious threats to the infant are tetanus neonatorum, or fatal extension of the sepsis along the umbilical vein to cause portal thrombophlebitis, jaundice and portal hypertension. Any sign of infection in the neonate should be promptly treated by local cleansing with an effective antiseptic solution or antibacterial powder.

In the adult local sepsis is nearly always due to inadequate cleanliness and the accumulation of inspissated sebum and other material in the umbilicus. A local inflammatory response with perhaps the discharge of obvious pus is the usual presentation. Once the acute episode is under control with local removal of foreign material and cleansing, local excision of the umbilicus is advised to eradicate the infected area.

Tumours

Rarely primary tumours, such as squamous carcinoma of the skin or melanoma, can arise in the umbilicus, and it is also a possible site of metastatic tumour, either from widespread blood dissemination or from retrograde passage along the ligamentum teres from the liver or porta hepatis.

Congenital abnormalities

First, remnants of the urachus, which runs from

the apex of the urinary bladder to the umbilicus, may persist, either as a cyst or fistula. In either case local excision is required.

Second, likewise, portions of the vitellointestinal duct may persist after birth, leading to a variety of abnormalities. It will be recalled that in fetal life this duct connects the yolk sac to the intestine at the level of the distal ileum and within the abdomen incomplete obliteration of the duct may lead to a Meckel's diverticulum, an enclosed antimesenteric cyst, or a fibrous band running right forward to the umbilicus. If, on the other hand, it is the more anterior part of the duct which fails to disappear, a raspberry-like tumour, an enteroteratoma, may present at the umbilicus. Again patency along the duct may persist, causing a fistula. In both cases surgical excision is indicated.

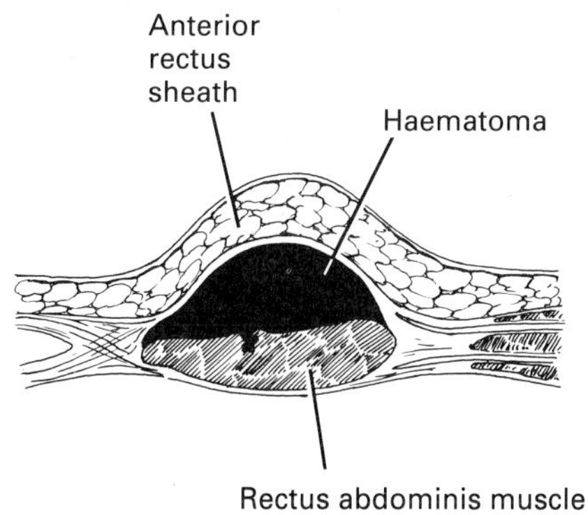

Fig. 22.15 Haematoma of rectus sheath. The bleeding arises from a torn vessel, e.g. inferior epigastric artery or vein, leading to a collection of blood confined beneath the dense anterior rectus sheath.

OTHER DISORDERS AFFECTING THE ABDOMINAL WALL

Haematoma of the rectus sheath

A tear in the inferior epigastric vessels may occur either as the result of direct trauma, during pregnancy, or on occasions apparently spontaneously. The result is a painful and tender rounded mass behind the rectus sheath (Fig. 22.15). The pain is aggravated by actions which tense the rectus muscle and there is generally guarding in this muscle. The finding that both pain and tenderness are more marked when the patient tenses the abdominal muscles than when they are relaxed is an important way of differentiating the lesion from a truly intra-abdominal one. If diagnosed within a few hours it is often worthwhile exploring the area, ligating the torn vessel and evacuating the clot. If, however, it is some days since the onset of symptoms the haematoma will often resolve and mild to moderate analgesics may suffice during these few days.

Tumours

Benign tumours, e.g. lipoma, fibroma, neurofibroma and angioma, are fairly common and require removal only if causing local discomfort or if the patient wishes to be free of them.

Most malignant tumours are metastatic deposits from blood spread or direct invasion from within the abdomen.

A particular type of tumour which can cause considerable problems is the desmoid tumour. This, fortunately rare, lesion arises, more often in women, in the fibroaponeurotic layers of the abdominal wall. Commonly its appearance starts in operation scars, or after parturition. The fibrous intersections in the rectus abdominis muscle seem particularly prone sites for the neoplastic change. Very wide local excision is required to reduce the chances of local recurrence, and there is also the risk of these recurrences becoming frank fibrosarcoma, with fatal results.

23. The mouth, jaw and salivary glands

MOUTH

Cleft lip and cleft palate

No definite cause has been found to account for these congenital defects, though it is probable that a number of factors may influence their occurrence. However, in view of the complexity of the development of the face and oropharynx it is not surprising that abnormalities of fusion of the various embryological processes may occasionally arise. Sometimes the deformities are associated with other congenital anomalies such as congenital blindness, hydrocephalus and mental retardation. Rubella infection in the first trimester of pregnancy has been found to be a factor in some cases, and maternal hypovitaminosis, exposure to X-radiation, excessive use of cortisone and drug sensitivity have also been implicated.

In the simplest form, the upper lip alone is involved. There is a gap between the lateral and central parts of the lip. This is due to failure of the mesoderm of the maxillary process to fuse completely with the frontonasal process. In second-degree cleft, the lip and the corresponding alveolus are affected. In third-degree, in addition to the cleft of the lip and alveolus, the palate is also involved. There may also arise a cleft of the palate alone, which may be partial or complete. In many cases the deformity is bilateral. The various defects may be classified as follows (Fig. 23.1):

1. Partial cleft lip alone.
2. Complete cleft lip and cleft alveolus.
3. Double cleft lip and alveolus.
4. Cleft soft palate.
5. Cleft soft and hard palate.
6. Partial cleft of palate and lip.
7. Complete cleft of palate, alveolus and lip.
8. Double complete cleft lip, alveolus and palate.

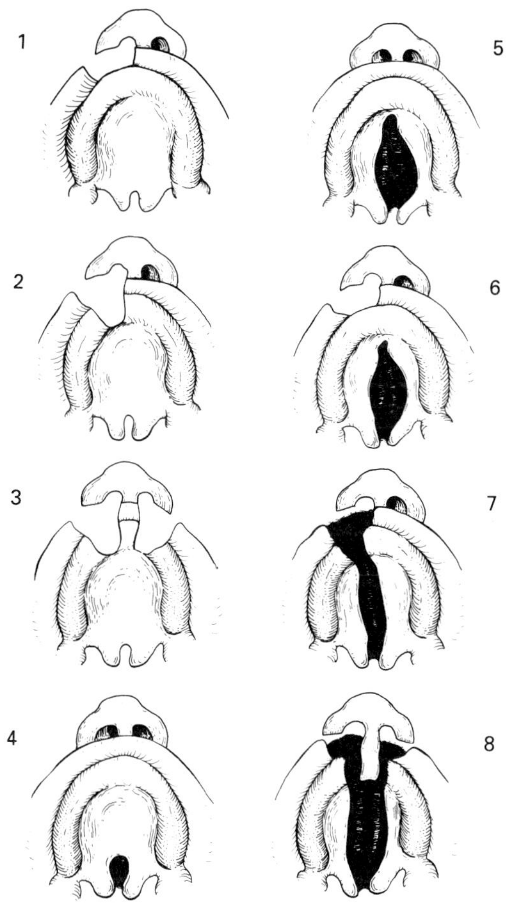

Fig. 23.1 Various degrees of cleft lip and palate: see text for details.

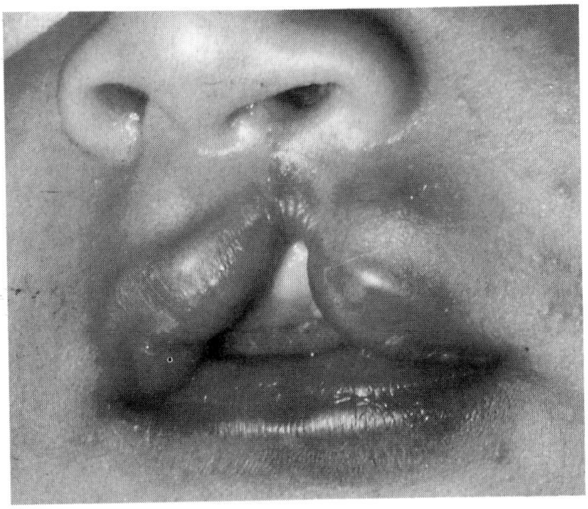

Fig. 23.2 Cleft lip – affecting only one side, the gum and palate being fully developed and intact.

The presenting problem with cleft lip (Fig. 23.2) is the obvious deformity, and cosmetic improvement is the main consideration. Cleft palate is a more serious disability (Fig. 23.3). In infancy, the baby cannot suck properly as the milk regurgitates through the nose and the negative pressure necessary for sucking is defective. If the defect remains unrepaired, speech is grossly affected and in particular consonants cannot be pronounced properly. Because of the defective oropharyngeal mechanism the child becomes prone to develop inflammation of the nasopharynx as a result of regurgitation of food. This may in turn lead to oedema of the eustachian tubes, otitis media, and defective hearing.

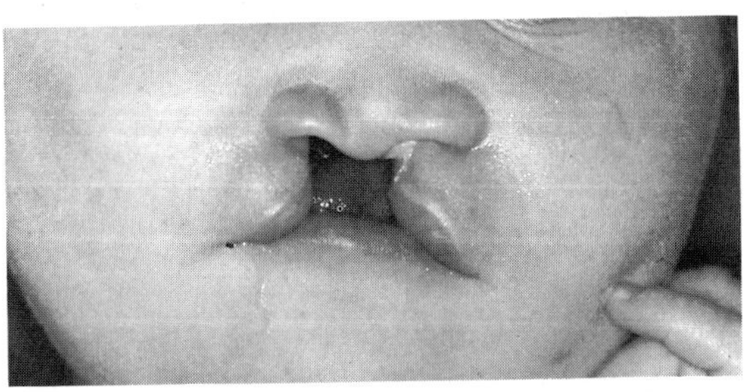

Fig. 23.3 Combined cleft lip and cleft palate deformity, with the tongue being visible between the incomplete lip and alveolar edges. A large gap is also present in the hard and soft palate, allowing the tongue to become displaced upwards.

Treatment is usually planned jointly between the plastic surgeon, the paediatrician and the orthodontist. In simple cleft lip, no emergency measures are needed. In cleft palate, the baby has to be fed by means of a dropper. Since there is no abnormality in the swallowing mechanism it should be possible to feed the baby adequately as long as the milk is delivered to the back of the mouth. Breast-feeding is usually out of the question, but enlargement of the holes in the teat of a feeding-bottle to allow easier escape of the milk can make feeding easier. Use of a compressible plastic bottle is also preferred.

It is also a wise precaution to hold the baby at about 45° posture to encourage the milk to flow over the back of the tongue into the pharynx and discourage regurgitation into the nasal passages. Definitive treatment of the cleft lip may be undertaken 3 months after the birth or when the baby weighs about 5–6 kg. Cleft palate is repaired before the baby starts to speak, i.e. between 12 and 18 months of age. Pending repair, a dental prosthesis may be used to prevent regurgitation of food.

The aim of surgery in lip deformity alone is to improve the appearance of the child. This generally involves transposition of the displaced lip edges, freeing of attachments to underlying tissues, and some form of Z-plasty to achieve a proper length to the upper lip. Good careful, precise apposition of the full layers of the lip is required, without any tension, and the operation should preferably be undertaken by a specialist plastic surgeon. In cleft palate, the most important aims are the correction of speech and normalization of the feeding process. For these purposes the mobility of the soft palate is an important factor as well as the closure of a gap in the hard palate. Mainly by mobilizing and advancing mucoperiosteal flaps from each side it is aimed to bring these together without tension and at the same time give the soft palate posteriorly enough mobility to be able to close off the nasopharynx from the oropharynx during phonation. If good closure does not occur there will continue to be a speech defect. Hopefully the repair can be completed in a single stage, but on occasions the advancement of the palatal flaps may need to be staged over several procedures.

Results of treatment depend upon the degree of the deformity and the skill of the surgical repair.

Leukoplakia

This is a condition in which there are one or more patches of thickening of the mucosa with whitish discoloration. It is due to the formation of a thick keratin layer on the surface of the epithelium, and there is often overgrowth of the underlying prickle cell layer. At a later stage abnormal cells with large nuclei, some showing mitosis, may appear in the deeper layers, and sometimes frank malignant changes may develop.

In many cases leukoplakia develops as a result of chronic irritation from sharp edges of teeth or ill fitting dentures, or from spices, spirits or tobacco. In India, the habit of keeping lime and tobacco between the cheek and the gum is an important irritating factor. Syphilis, particularly in its tertiary stage, appears to be a precipitating factor in communities in which this disease is still fairly frequently encountered. In quite a proportion of patients presenting with the condition, however, there appears to be no obvious underlying cause (Figs. 23.4 and 23.5).

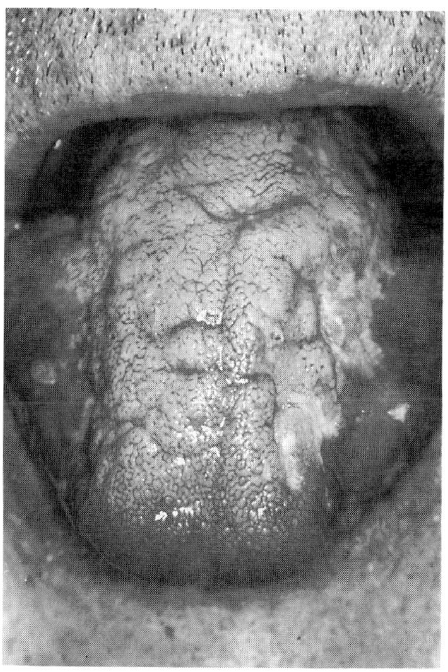

Fig. 23.4 Leukoplakia: multiple white, thickened patches over the dorsum and lateral edges of the tongue. The smoother areas, where the roughened papillary prominences have been flattened and the edge diffuses gradually into the surrounding normal appearing parts of the tongue, are the areas with greater premalignant potential.

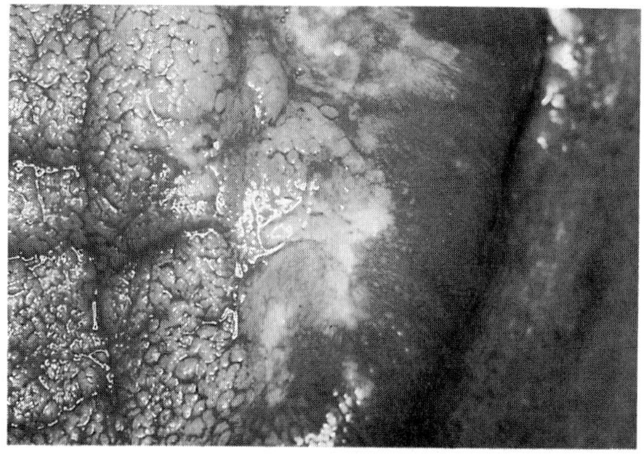

Fig. 23.5 Close-up view of an area of transition from roughened papillae to smooth white to normal appearance tongue surface.

Clinically the condition presents usually as simply the observation that there is a white patch on the tongue or cheek, or the complaint of some local irritation or pain, often at the edge of a patch. On inspection the area may be uniformly white and slightly indurated, or there may be some papilliferous portions or some fissuring. This latter occurrence raises the question as to whether malignant conversion may be taking place.

A commoner cause of white patches appearing on the tongue or other parts of the mouth is *Candida* infection (thrush). In this condition, however, the white patches are only loosely adherent and can be scraped off gently by means of a spatula, leaving reddened raw areas of mucosa. Confirmation of the infection can be made from microscopic examination of the scrapings.

As far as the management of patients with leukoplakia is concerned the first step is obviously to remove any precipitating factors. The majority will not develop malignant change and it is reasonable simply to keep the condition under periodic review. Excision biopsy is indicated if there is any suspicious change, e.g. warty projection, fissuring, local pain, bleeding, etc. If suspicion is increased or frank local malignant change detected local excision with a clear margin of healthy tissue is required.

Ulcers of the mouth

The lips, cheeks and tongue are quite common sites of superficial ulceration (Fig. 23.6). This may be due to local trauma, or a manifestation of vitamin

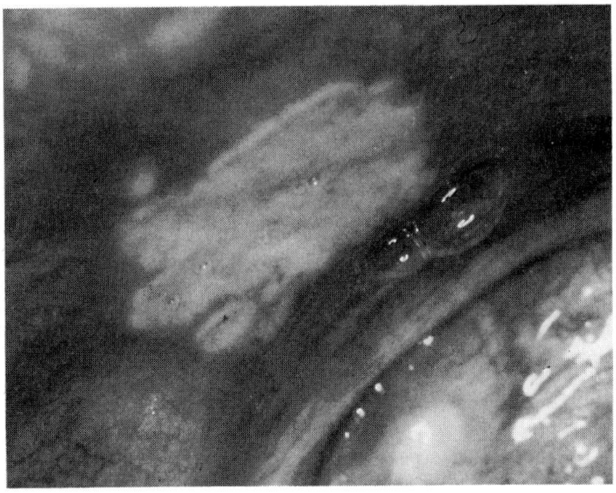

Fig. 23.6 Solitary shallow ulcer on posterior inner aspect of cheek.

deficiency or a specific infection such as tuberculosis, syphilis, or Vincent's angina. Apart from these conditions, there are some small recurrent mouth ulcers which are quite non-specific and tend to be referred to as aphthous ulcers (Fig. 23.7).

Ragged teeth and ill fitting dentures commonly produce ulceration of the cheek and the side of the tongue. It is often painful, and the cause is usually apparent on oral examination. Treatment consists of removal of the cause, but if this does not produce healing in a week or two, the diagnosis should be reviewed and biopsy considered.

Ulcers developing as a result of external trauma usually do not present any special problem and are treated with mouthwashes and analgesics. Antibiotics are only exhibited if there is gross infection.

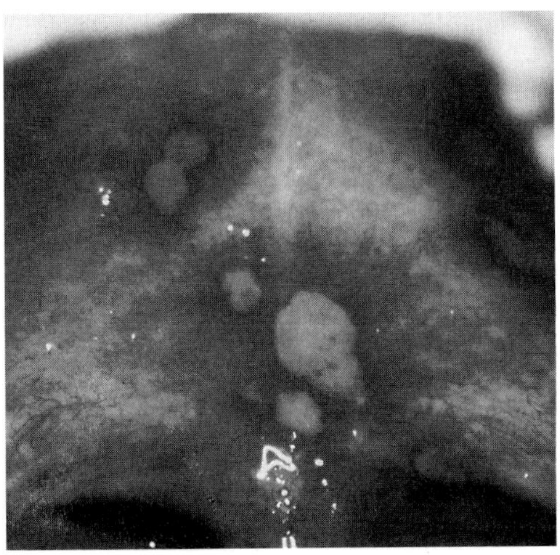

Fig. 23.7 Multiple discrete shallow aphthous ulcers on the palate.

Nicotinic acid deficiency gives rise to pellagra. As a part of the clinical picture, ulcers may develop on the tongue. Nicotinic acid in adequate doses is curative.

Tuberculous ulcers are uncommon in the mouth, but may develop as a complication of pulmonary or laryngeal tuberculosis, and may be multiple. A typical ulcer is oval in shape and greyish in colour, with reddish margins, and painful. Antituberculous drugs are given and are usually effective in allowing the ulcers to heal without surgical intervention. For pain, local amethocaine lozenges are often helpful.

Syphilis may involve the lips, tongue or tonsils in the primary, secondary and tertiary stages. In the primary stage, a painless indurated papule develops, which undergoes ulceration. Regional lymph nodes enlarge but are painless. *Treponema pallidum* can usually be demonstrated in a slide prepared from a swab taken from the ulcer. Serological tests are usually negative in the first few days. Penicillin-G is curative, and a course of 14 days' duration is recommended. Untreated, the ulcer heals in a few days and the patient passes into the second stage of the disease.

Multiple shallow ulcers, mucous patches and warts (Hutchinson's) are the manifestations of secondary syphilis. Ulcers appear on the sides of or on the under-surface of the tongue. Mucous patches may involve the tonsils also. Hutchinson's warts are papillomatous structures which develop on the dorsal aspect of the tongue generally in the midline. This is a very infective stage of the disease. Diagnosis is confirmed by serological tests and the demonstration of spirochaetes. History of contact 2–12 months previously may be available, and treatment is on general antisyphilitic lines.

In the tertiary stage, a gumma may develop on the dorsum of the tongue or on the palate. On the tongue a typical ulcer with punched out edges and wash-leather slough appears. On the palate, perforation may occur. Serological tests are positive in most cases, and again full antisyphilitic treatment is carried out.

Aphthous ulcers are small, multiple and painful and present as shallow rounded defects 1–5 mm in diameter with a white floor and slightly yellow edge. They may develop on the lips, the mucosa of the cheeks, the tip or the sides of the tongue. The aetiology is unknown. There appears to be an occasional association with chronic inflammatory bowel disease, iron deficiency anaemia, various forms of allergy and mental stress, but most often there is just no associated factor. Treatment is therefore largely empirical, and the local application of pellets containing hydrocortisone, or triamcinolone or simple chlorhexidine mouthwash may be helpful.

BENIGN TUMOURS AND CYSTS OF THE MOUTH AND JAWS

Angiomas

Among the benign tumours, haemangiomas and lymphangiomas are not uncommon. It is now agreed that angiomas are not true tumours but rather manifestations of congenital malformations (Fig. 23.8).

Angiomas have a soft consistency and are of variable size. The colour is predominantly that of the overlying mucosa, although underlying collection of blood may be obvious. Microscopically two types of haemangiomas are encountered, a capillary variety in which endothelial-lined channels are very narrow and may appear to be packed with red blood cells, and a cavernous variety, in which there are large spaces which intercommunicate and are filled with blood.

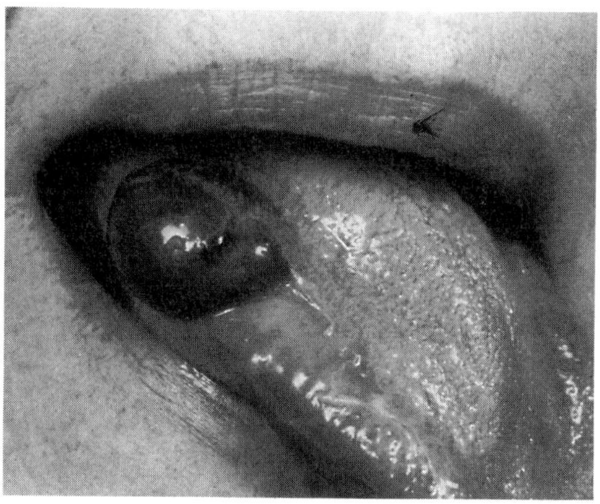

Fig. 23.8 Benign angioma on the lateral aspect of the tongue.

Lymphangioma of the mouth presents similar changes, with the exception that the endothelial-lined spaces are filled with lymph instead of blood. A diffuse form may give rise to one type of macroglossia, if it occurs on the tongue.

Advice is sought because of deformity if the tumour is situated on the lip or because of difficulty in speaking when it arises on the tongue. They are slow-growing and painless. The size of the tumour decreases on compression.

Since there is no fear of malignant change, treatment is on conservative lines. A considerable reduction in size may be obtained by inducing sclerosing injections under anaesthesia. Surgical excision is indicated for cosmetic purposes in small lesions.

Cysts

Two types of cyst develop most commonly in the floor of the mouth: retention cysts and dermoid cysts.

Retention cysts develop as a result of obstruction of the outlet of mucous glands of the lips or cheeks or the glands of the undersurface of the tongue. These cysts are usually translucent. One particular form is referred to as a ranula because of an alleged resemblance in appearance to the belly of a frog (*rana*—a frog). Sometimes the swelling is so large that a part of it protrudes below the chin through the floor of the mouth. The duct of the submandibular salivary gland may be seen traversing it through the mucosa of the mouth.

Small retention cysts can be removed under local anaesthesia. When the cyst is large it may be easier to remove it after aspirating some or all of its contents. If it is very large indeed it is adequate to remove as much of the wall as is accessible, empty the contents and suture the edge of the residual wall to the surrounding mucosa, thereby making it a part of the floor of the mouth—so-called marsupialization.

A dermoid cyst occurs either in the midline or slightly to one side of it in the floor of the mouth and a part of it may protrude below the chin. It usually does not transilluminate. Treatment consists of complete excision through an external incision.

Benign solid tumours

Tumours may arise in the small salivary glands of the mouth, most commonly on the palate. Although these are usually benign, malignant change can occur and the tumour may attain considerable size. Their true nature is only established after excision, on histological examination. The benign lesion is generally a pleomorphic adenoma, the so-called mixed tumour, and when malignant the tumour is most often a cylindroma. This latter grows slowly and may metastasize to the regional lymph nodes. Complete excision is the treatment of both the varieties.

Papilloma, fibroepithelioma and lipoma are other tumours occasionally encountered in the mouth. Excisional biopsy is carried out for diagnostic and therapeutic purposes.

Epulis

A swelling arising from the gum is called an epulis. Three types of epulis are described— fibrous, giant cell and granulomatous. The first two are true neoplasms while the third is of inflammatory origin.

The fibrous epulis is a small, firm swelling covered with normal coloured mucosa of the gum, usually in the incisor or premolar region (Fig. 23.9). Sometimes it is pedunculated. A rare form is the fibrosarcomatous epulis which grows very rapidly. The majority of epulis are slow-growing and should be excised and examined histologically. Rapidly growing tumours should be subjected to biopsy, and if the report reveals sarcoma the growth together with a wedge of bone containing the tumour should be excised, and the adjoining tooth or teeth extracted.

The giant cell epulis is a soft, sessile swelling with a lobulated surface covered by dark red or purple mucous membrane. It usually begins in the interior of the alveolus and may project into the bone, expanding it and giving rise to a cystic swelling. The neighbouring teeth may become loose and ulceration and haemorrhage may occur. Microscopically the epulis is characterized by the presence of foreign body-type of giant cells and a vascular stroma. The tumour should be excised and the bone, if involved, curetted.

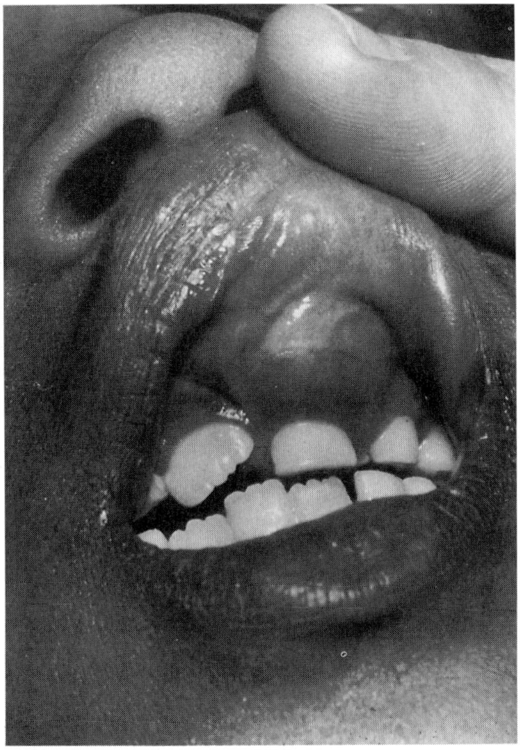

Fig. 23.9 Fibrous epulis at the base of an upper canine tooth in a child.

The granulomatous epulis develops near a carious tooth or in relation to an ill-fitting denture and this coexistence may be obvious on simple inspection of the mouth (Fig. 23.10). Excision biopsy is curative provided that the offending tooth is extracted or the ill-fitting denture is changed.

Odontome

This is the term used to describe a cyst or tumour in relation to a tooth. Dental cyst, dentigerous cyst and adamantinoma are the common varieties.

A dental cyst arises in relation to a normally erupted tooth which is usually infected and may be pulpless. The common site is the incisor or the canine region of the upper jaw. The swelling develops in an adult and appears as an expansion of the alveolus. It may protrude into the maxillary antrum or the floor of the nose, but usually does not open into these cavities. The cyst contains a clear fluid and is lined with squamous epithelium. It does not cause any pain and advice is usually

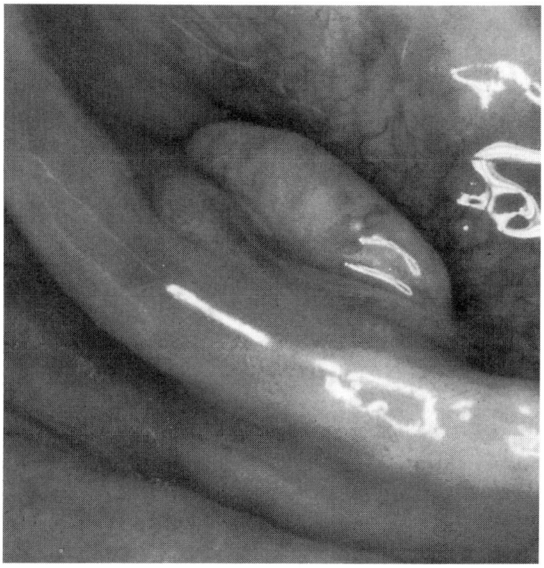

Fig. 23.10 Benign chronic granuloma caused by long-standing irritation by ill-fitting denture.

sought because of the presence of the swelling. Radiography reveals a cystic space in relation to the neck of a tooth. Treatment consists of the removal of the cyst through an incision over the alveolar mucosa.

A dentigerous cyst arises in the place of an unerupted tooth, usually in the molar region, and causes expansion of the gum. The unerupted tooth or a part of it is found inside the cyst, and it is lined with squamous or rarely cuboidal epithelium. Sometimes bony ridges may form subjacent to the mucous lining. X-ray shows a cyst containing a tooth or a part of it and if bone ridges are formed, there may be a soap-bubble like appearance. Treatment is complete excision of the cyst. The gap in the bone, if big, can be filled with bone chips obtained from the iliac crest.

MALIGNANT TUMOURS

The commonest malignant tumour is carcinoma, and at the present time it is more common in the Indian subcontinent than in western countries. It may arise in the lip, cheek, gums, tongue, floor of the mouth or palate. Both sexes are equally affected, and it is the disease predominantly of middle and old age.

Tobacco and betel nut chewing have been found to be important aetiological factors in the Indian subcontinent. Leukoplakia is also a predisposing factor in all countries. All the elements which favour the development of leukoplakia therefore favour the development of cancer, e.g. chronic irritation due to ill-fitting dentures, sharp edges of teeth and chronic dental sepsis.

Carcinoma of the lip (Fig. 23.11) usually presents as either a superficial flat chronic ulcer with no eversion of the margins and very little induration, on the vermilion border, or as a deep ulcer with everted margins and considerable surrounding induration. More rarely it is a cauliflower-like type of growth. Elsewhere in the mouth, cancer manifests itself as a wart, a cauliflower growth, a nodule, a fissure or as an ulcer, the last being the commonest. Microscopically, the tumours are squamous cell carcinoma in the majority of cases.

The first important mode of spread is by local infiltration. Thus, a tumour of the cheek may involve alveolus and the underlying bone—the mandible or the maxilla. Cancer of the gum may involve the floor of the mouth, the tongue and, in the posterior part, the tonsillar region. Carcinoma of the tongue may spread to the surrounding tissues in such a way as to make it immobile.

The next important mode of spread is by way of lymphatics to the regional nodes in the neck. Spread is also possible to the contralateral side as well as to the ipsilateral. Blood-borne metastases are less common. The patient usually dies before its

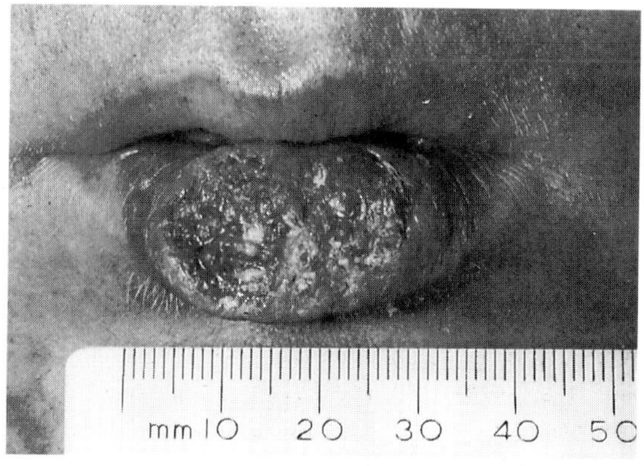

Fig. 23.11 Squamous carcinoma affecting the central portion of the lower lip. The lesion is ulcerated and its floor is irregular and nodular.

occurrence, due to sepsis, haemorrhage or malnutrition.

Advice is sought because of an ulcer or a lump in the mouth. Sometimes swelling in the neck due to secondary lymph node involvement is the only complaint, especially in carcinomas of the posterior third of the tongue. Pain is also complained of in advanced disease and particularly when there is ulceration and there may be referral to the ear. Profuse salivation, foetor and bleeding are other symptoms of advanced disease.

The management of oral cancer can be discussed under three headings—prophylactic, curative and palliative measures.

Education warning against the dangers of chewing betel nut and tobacco should be promulgated. Irritating factors such as dental sepsis, ill-fitting dentures and sharp-edged teeth should be promptly and effectively corrected and patients with leukoplakia managed as described above.

In suspected cases biopsy should always be taken (Fig. 23.12). In lesions less than 1 cm in diameter, excisional biopsy with surrounding healthy tissue is all that is required by way of curative treatment.

For larger lesions there is a choice between surgical removal or radiotherapy, each having approximately the same chance of success in treating the primary lesion. Operation involves wide excision, including a good margin of apparently uninvolved tissue, and may therefore include removal of a portion of the mandible, palate and other structures. Complicated grafting and other reconstruction procedures may be required. Since squamous-type carcinoma is generally sensitive to irradiation, a good response should be expected. The dose is usually delivered from an external megavoltage beam source of X-rays or gamma rays,.

As far as treatment of metastatic lymph nodes is concerned, irradiation is not so effective and therefore any direct attack on them is likely to be surgical.

A good policy is to treat the primary growth and administer antibiotics in full doses in the post-radiotherapy or post-operative period since the node enlargement may be due to secondary infection of an ulcerated lesion. If the glands persist after 2–3 weeks of treatment, a block dissection of the cervical lymph nodes of the affected side is recommended. If there are involved nodes on both sides, bilateral block dissection can also be carried out, provided that the internal jugular vein is spared on one side.

Tumours considered initially to be inoperable may become smaller and more amenable to a surgical approach as a result of radiotherapy or regional cytotoxic drug therapy, e.g. with amethopterin.

OTHER TUMOURS

Ameloblastoma, formerly called adamantinoma, is a solid tumour arising from ectodermal elements, but cystic degeneration may give a honeycomb or multilocular appearance (Fig. 23.13). Clinically, painless swelling of the jaw is present and the diag-

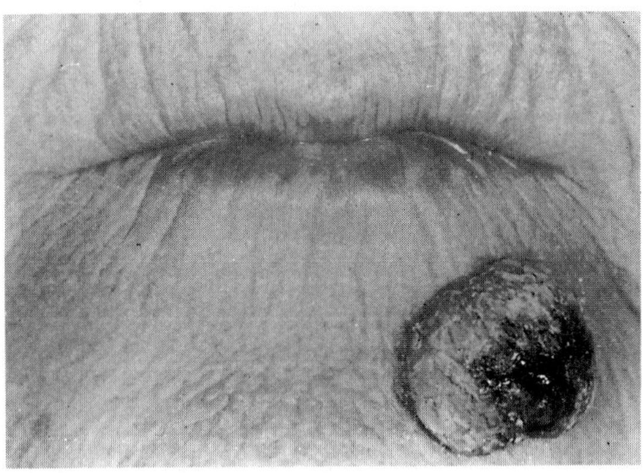

Fig. 23.12 Keratoacanthoma arising below the lower lip in an elderly patient. This raised, rounded, well circumscribed, and ulcerated lesion can cause diagnostic confusion as it may be mistaken for a squamous carcinoma. Biopsy may be required to confirm the diagnosis.

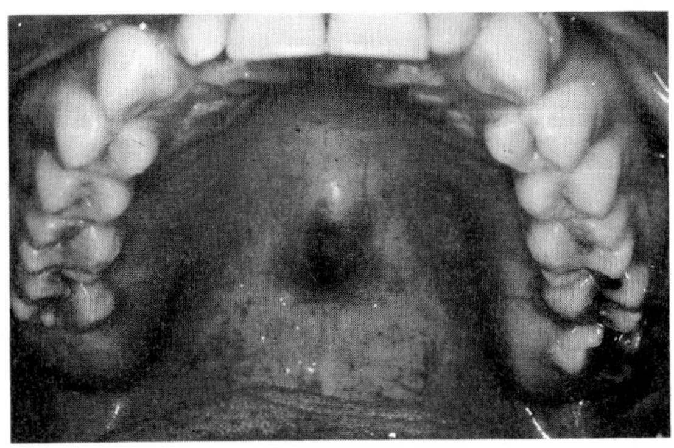

Fig. 23.13 Salivary gland tumour in ectopic site in palate.

nosis is made by the radiologically characteristic honeycomb appearance on X-ray. It is treated by excision of the tumour-bearing part of the jaw, together with a margin of adjoining healthy bone. Inadequate removal or local curettage is followed by recurrence of the ameloblastoma, although it does not show any tendency to metastasize.

The maxilla and mandible may occasionally become the seat of any bone tumour, e.g. osteoclastoma. Fibro-osseous dysplasia may also occur. The main complaint is of swelling in the involved part of jaw or face. The diagnosis can usually be clearly established by X-ray and rarely, biopsy and local excision may be performed if necessary. Any residual bony gap, if large, can be filled with bone chips while smaller defects are left to granulate.

The maxilla may become the seat of a cancer arising from the mucosa of the maxillary antrum, which may present itself in several ways, depending upon the site of origin. A tumour arising in the roof of the antrum may present with proptosis, while one in the floor as a swelling of the hard palate, and one in the anterolateral part as a deformity of the face. Those extending medially may block the tear duct or the nasal passages. An X-ray shows distortion and opacity of the antrum. Treatment is usually by interstitial or megavoltage irradiation followed by surgical removal of the antrum. If the growth is large the entire maxilla may be removed after a full course of radiotherapy.

SALIVARY GLANDS

Parotid gland

The common diseases of the parotid gland are either inflammatory or neoplastic.

Acute parotitis can be due either to a viral or bacterial infection. Of the former the commonest is mumps, which usually involves both the parotids. It is a self-limiting disease and its only surgical importance is that it is occasionally complicated by an acute viral orchitis, which has to be differentiated from other painful disorders in the scrotum, especially torsion. It is, of course, important not to miss the latter and to explore it urgently, whereas the mumps orchitis should be allowed to settle spontaneously.

Acute pyogenic parotitis, which is much rarer than in former years, usually occurs as a complication of a systemic disease or in the postoperative period, whenever there is a marked decrease in the flow of saliva due to dehydration. Patients suffering from typhoid fever or cholera and uraemic or septicaemic subjects are more liable to develop the condition. Obstruction to the flow of saliva by a stone in the parotid duct is rare, but when it does occur it may be another precipitating cause of acute parotitis. The offending organism is most commonly *Staphylococcus aureus*. The inflammation is usually multicentric in origin but later on the whole gland becomes swollen, and if the inflammation does not subside, an abscess develops. Clinically the patient complains of a painful swelling on the side of the face. Other symptoms of toxaemia such as fever and anorexia tend to be overshadowed by the symptoms of the general disease from which the patient is suffering prior to the development of the parotitis. The only prominent physical sign is a tender swelling in the parotid region, though inspection of the orifice of the parotid duct may show this to appear congested and sometimes a spot of pus may be seen to exude from it.

Correction of dehydration is the most important part of management, and frequent mouthwashes are advised both to remove any pus or debris and stimulate salivary flow. Antibiotics and analgesics are usually exhibited. Should an abscess form this should be drained surgically, and this may be done under local anaesthesia if necessary. An incision is made over the most prominent part of the swelling, and on deepening the wound to the level of the fascia this is incised transversely, parallel to the branches of the facial nerve. A safe way of making this opening is to use blunt-ended forceps to separate the blades in the longitudinal direction of the nerve branches (Hilton's method). A small drain is left in the cavity for a day or two.

A few patients become troubled by recurrent episodes of painful swelling of the parotid glands and even between attacks there may be continuing residual enlargement of the glands. In some there is stenosis of the orifice of the main duct, and sialography should be attempted to outline the duct system. Occasionally the X-ray examination itself will lead to marked improvement or disappearance of the symptoms and signs, probably on account of gentle dilatation of the duct orifice to introduce the contrast medium. If not, simple surgical enlargement of the opening in the mouth may relieve the condition.

Tumours of the parotid gland

These are relatively common. They may be benign, benign with a tendency to recur locally, or rarely undergo malignant change, or frankly malignant.

Pleomorphic adenoma. This is the commonest parotid tumour. It is also known as a mixed parotid tumour, because microscopic examination reveals areas of varying histological appearance, some of which even look like cartilage. However, these latter are simply areas which contain mucoid material, and although the histological pattern may vary, all the cells are basically of the same epithelial origin. The tumour is not, therefore, truly a mixed one. Very occasionally malignant changes may occur. The pleomorphic adenoma has a capsule formed by the condensation of the surrounding parotid tissue, and although this appears on gross inspection to be a well defined wall, microscopic cellular extensions beyond this capsule are relatively common, and excision immediately outside this layer is very prone to be followed by local recurrence on account of leaving tiny pockets of these cellular protrusions behind.

The tumour may appear first in early adult life or later, and both sexes are affected equally. It usually arises in the superficial part of the gland, i.e. that part which lies superficial to the facial nerve, but can, of course, also arise in the deeper part. The first complaint is simply the awareness of a small lump or nodule which grows slowly and may eventually attain a large size (Fig. 23.14). It may appear to remain stationary for years. On examination the lump is rounded, of firm consistency, free of attachment to the overlying skin, and often has a degree of mobility in relation to fixed deeper structures since, unless large, the portion of gland from which it arises will move along with the tumour. There is no tenderness and examination of the facial nerve function shows no defect (Fig. 23.15). The complete absence of any facial nerve involvement is one of the main clinical features differentiating it from malignant tumour of the parotid, in which some nerve damage is common.

It is unwise to biopsy parotid gland tumours in

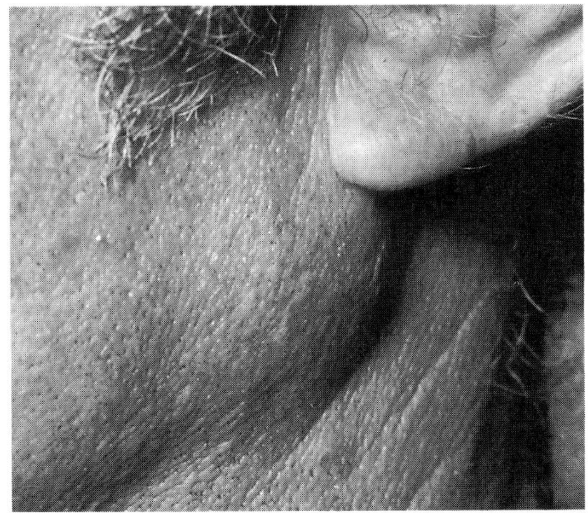

Fig. 23.14 Typical presentation of parotid tumour—most likely pleomorphic adenoma—with small, rounded, firm painless nodule behind the angle of the mandible.

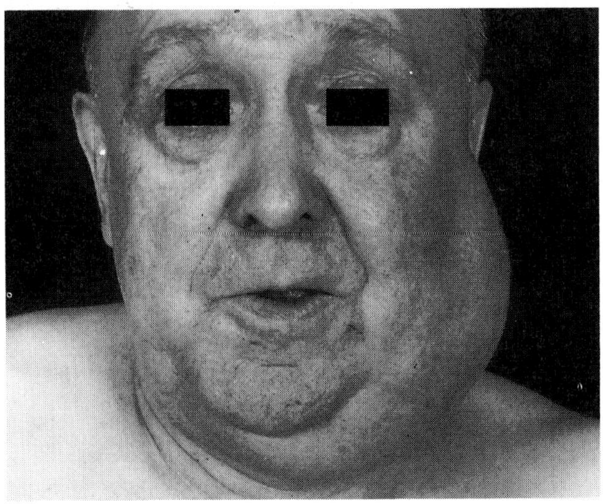

Fig. 23.15 Much larger pleomorphic adenoma of the parotid—a steadily enlarging mass which has been present for several years. However, no other symptoms or signs were present, hence the delay in seeking medical advice.

case of causing local implantation of cells, and therefore treatment is most often planned on the basis of a fairly confident clinical diagnosis. The primary approach to a tumour thought to be a pleomorphic adenoma is formal superficial parotidectomy. This involves excision of all the gland substance, enclosing the tumour, external to the several branches of the facial nerve. An S-shaped incision passing in front of the ear, back to the mastoid process and curving forwards behind the angle of the mandible is usually made. The main trunk of the facial nerve is exposed and the various branches are traced forwards into the gland. Carefully all the superficial parts of the gland are then dissected off these branches, the anterior end of the duct is divided, and all the excised material is examined microscopically. It is hoped that the line of section will prove to be well beyond the limits of the capsule.

Carcinoma of the parotid. This is fortunately less common. It affects both sexes and the patients are usually elderly. The majority arise in previously healthy glands, but occasionally a mixed tumour which has been stationary for years undergoes malignancy and starts to grow rapidly. The consistency is hard and it may become fixed to the surrounding structures, involving among other tissues the facial nerve. The surface may be smooth or irregular.

Microscopically, the pattern may show tubular formations lined by epithelial cells—the so-called cylindroma. In other cases, the picture is that of adenocarcinoma, anaplastic or squamous cell carcinoma. The tumour spreads by local infiltration, and soon metastasizes by lymphatic channels to the regional nodes. Blood spread to distant sites may then follow.

Clinically, the patient usually complains of a fairly rapidly growing swelling in the parotid region, which may be painful. When the facial nerve becomes involved there is paresis or paralysis of some of the ipsilateral facial muscles, and such a finding makes the diagnosis fairly certain.

Carcinoma of the parotid gland is not as a rule amenable to cure by radiotherapy, although its use as an adjuvant or postoperative treatment may have some benefit to confer. The main approach to treatment is total parotidectomy. No attempt is made to save the facial nerve at the expense of complete removal of the tumour. Resulting facial deformity may be corrected by plastic procedures at a later date. Postoperative radiotherapy is usually recommended. In advanced cases, palliation may be obtained by radiotherapy, but the prognosis is generally poor.

Adenolymphoma. Adenolymphoma or Warthin's tumour is a relatively uncommon benign neoplasm occurring more commonly in men, and said to be confined to white people. It usually arises near the angle of the jaw, either superficial or deep to the parotid fascia. It is soft and occasionally even fluctuant. Microscopically, lymphoid tissue containing epithelial elements is seen.

The appropriate treatment is simple local excision.

Other causes of parotid enlargement

Mikulicz's disease. In this disorder there is bilateral enlargement of the parotid, submandibular salivary and lacrimal glands with narrowing of the palpebral fissures and dryness of the mouth. Sometimes only one or more of the glands mentioned above is involved. Aetiology of the disease remains obscure, but it is thought by some to be due to a low-grade infection, as on microscopic examination lymphocytic infiltration is found in the affected glands. In its fully fledged form there is usually no difficulty with the diagnosis. However, when only one gland is affected only biopsy can reveal the true nature of the disease.

The fully fledged disease is treated by radiotherapy or corticosteroids. If only one gland is affected it can be removed surgically. Surgery may also be undertaken for cosmetic reasons.

Boeck's sarcoidosis. This is also a disease of uncertain origin. It is thought by some to have an allergic basis. One or both glands may be enlarged and the enlargement is associated with inflammatory changes in the uveal tract and sometimes with cutaneous lesions.

If an allergen can be identified it should be removed, and treatment with corticosteroids is sometimes recommended. If only one gland is affected, excisional biopsy may establish the diagnosis.

Stone in the parotid duct

The parotid gland is rather an uncommon site for stone formation, whereas in the submandibular salivary gland this is quite common. The stones are mainly composed of calcium and/or magnesium phosphate and are radiopaque.

The chief symptom is repeated attacks of painful swelling appearing in the parotid region, especially on eating, or even thinking about food. If the stone lies in the anterior portion of the parotid duct, it can be felt on bimanual examination.

Sialography may also be helpful in locating the size, number and site of the stones. Incision over the anterior duct and widening the opening on the inner aspect of the cheek will usually suffice to allow the stones to escape.

Other parotid disorders

Congenital parotid sialectasis is a rare condition in which the ductal system is dilated and the gland becomes the seat of repeated inflammation. The secretion becomes viscid and contains epithelial debris. The aetiology of the disease is not known. The symptoms appear early in life and the chief complaint is of recurrent attacks of pain and swelling in the parotid region. The diagnosis is established by the sialographic findings, which show dilatation of the ducts. If an allergen can be identified, its avoidance sometimes cures the condition. In other cases, parotidectomy may be indicated.

A parotid fistula may develop as a result of injury to the parotid gland, whether accidental or surgical. Dribbling of saliva at meal times, or even at the sight or thought of food, is the main presenting feature. Sialography may identify the site of the fistula in the duct system. A number of operations have been described to cure the condition. One approach is to convert the external fistula into an internal one, draining into a freshly created opening on the inner aspect of the cheek.

Submandibular salivary gland

The submandibular salivary glands may become the seat of inflammatory and neoplastic lesions similar to those occurring in the parotid gland. The basic approach to treatment is comparable to that discussed above. As far as total excision of the gland for the tumours which rarely arise, there is of course less hazard to vitally important structures such as the facial nerve. However, care has to be taken during dissection of the deep part of the submandibular salivary gland not to damage the lingual nerve, unless it is already compromised by a malignant lesion. Sacrifice of this nerve will lead to deviation of the tongue to the same side, since the main muscles of the tongue will be paralysed.

Stones in the submandibular ducts

Salivary calculi are most commonly found in the submandibular gland ducts. They may be either in the distal main duct or in the smaller branches within the gland proper. In both situations, the stones present clinically by the typical symptoms of swelling and pain, aggravated by eating or anticipating tasty food. Examination of the floor of the mouth with the patient rolling the tongue upwards may reveal inflammation lateral to the frenulum, around the opening of the duct. Occasionally a

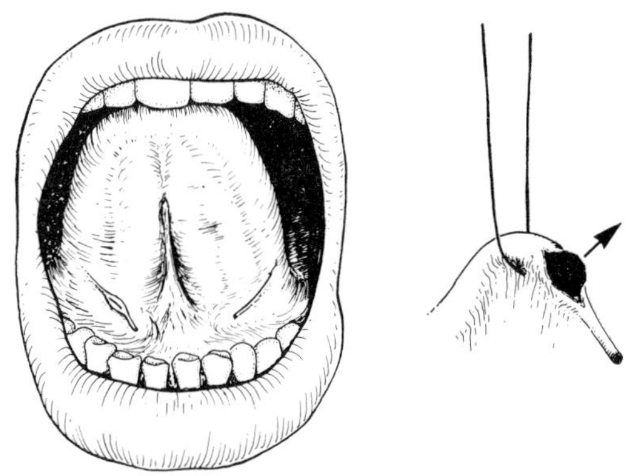

Fig. 23.16 Removal of stone from the anterior part of the right submandibular gland duct. A suture is first passed behind the stone, to prevent it slipping back out of reach. A longitudinal incision is made over the stone, and after removal the wound is left open to ease drainage from the duct.

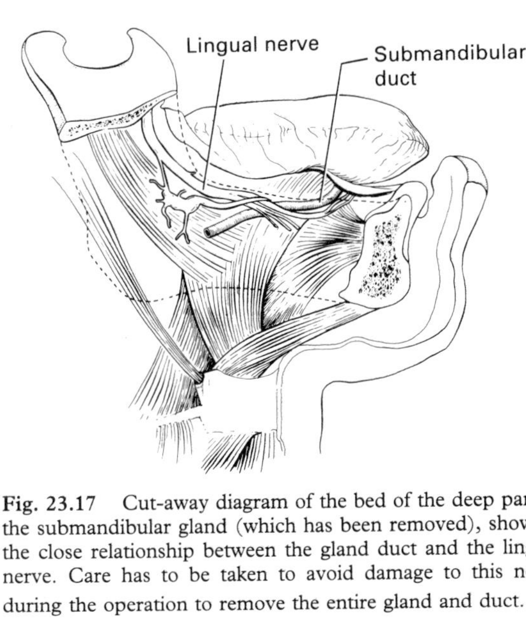

Fig. 23.17 Cut-away diagram of the bed of the deep part of the submandibular gland (which has been removed), showing the close relationship between the gland duct and the lingual nerve. Care has to be taken to avoid damage to this nerve during the operation to remove the entire gland and duct.

stone may be seen protruding through the orifice. The majority of the stones in the duct can be palpated by inserting the index finger of one hand into the floor of the mouth and placing the fingers of the other hand below the mandible in the suprahyoid region. The intraoral finger can palpate the duct from the frenulum to the medial side of the last lower molar tooth.

An X-ray examination of the floor of the mouth, including a vertical view through the floor of the mouth, is desirable, as many small stones may not be felt, and even bigger stones in the gland may otherwise escape detection.

Stones in the main duct can be removed under general or even local anaesthesia through a longitudinal incision along the duct in the floor of the mouth (Fig. 23.16). It is helpful to anchor a visible stone temporarily by a suture passed behind it, to prevent proximal dislocation during the procedure. Once the stone is removed through the opening in the duct, this is left open to drain freely, and no attempt should be made to suture it.

Stones in the gland and those in the duct which cannot be felt are best dealt with by the formal removal of the entire gland, through a submandibular incision (Fig. 23.17).

24. The neck

The main clinical exercise in dealing with this part of the body is the differential diagnosis of lumps or swellings in the neck. Many of these have been described in other chapters, e.g. swellings in the thyroid (Ch. 25), the parotid (Ch. 23) the submandibular salivary glands (Ch. 23), and in lymph nodes (Ch. 20).

Also to be considered in this chapter are wounds involving important structures in the neck, and infections in the various compartments.

SWELLINGS OF THE NECK

Branchial cyst

This benign, soft, fluid-filled cyst arises from some congenital abnormality in the formation and fusion of the embryonic branchial arches and clefts. Although the precise mechanism is uncertain, it is likely that the main defect lies in the second cleft since the rare persistence of a track from the depth of the cyst passes between the internal and external carotid arteries. These are the vessels supplying the first and second branchial arches respectively. The cyst wall is smooth, lined usually by stratified squamous epithelium, but occasionally by other types, and the liquid content is either clear or slightly opalescent, containing appreciable amounts of cholesterol.

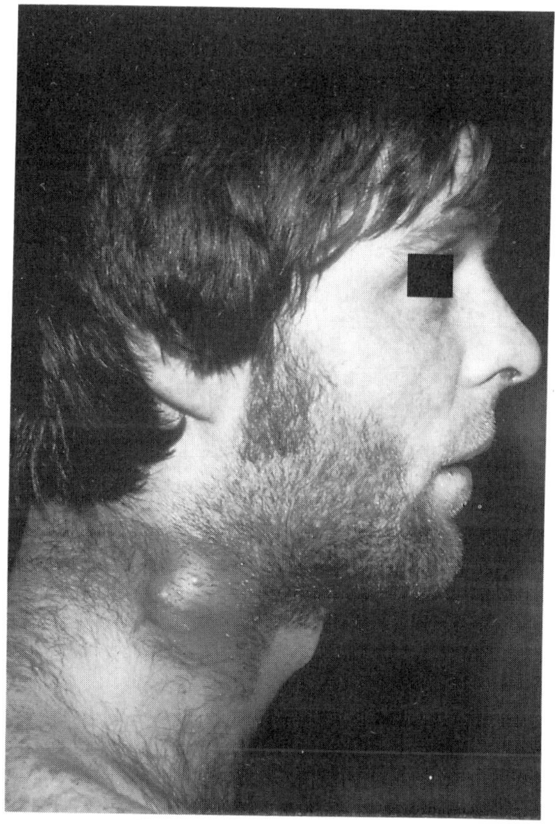

Fig. 24.1 Branchial cyst: usual site and age group. Signs of infection are present in this case.

Although the cyst is congenital in origin, it rarely presents clinically until the late teens or early 20s, and the patient seeks medical advice solely on account of the presence of the swelling. It is exceptional for there to be any other local symptoms. Rarely it may become infected, and present as an abscess (Fig. 24.1).

On inspection the rounded swelling is seen classically anterior to the sternomastoid muscle at the level of the hyoid bone, 1 or 2 cm below the angle of the mandible. Tensing the sternomastoid against resistance often makes the cyst more prominent and confirms that it is projecting forwards from underneath the muscle. On palpation the cyst feels soft and uniform and fluctuation is nearly always easy to elicit (Fig. 24.2).

A confident diagnosis can usually be made without recourse to any further investigations, and surgical removal is advised. The operation, under general anaesthesia, is generally straightforward. Through a transverse curved incision over the cyst, the dissection is gently deepened, the wall preserved intact and freed from all surrounding structures. This usually presents no great problem since it strips easily away and complete enucleation is achieved. It is, in fact, highly exceptional for there to be any obvious deep extension between the carotids, so that these vessels should not be put at serious risk. It is important to remove all of the cyst wall, otherwise recurrence is very likely.

Branchial fistula

Although this does not present as a neck swelling it is appropriate to consider it here since it has a similar origin to branchial cyst. However, in this case the track often does pass quite deeply in the neck between the internal and external carotid arteries. If the track is complete it will extend right up into the pharynx at the level of the tonsils (Fig. 24.2). More often there is a blind ending to the track when it is traced from the external opening in the neck, so that it is more correct to refer to the lesion as a sinus. The lining comprises squamous or cuboidal epithelium and there are usually patches of lymphatic tissue around or adjacent to it.

The characteristic site for the opening is along the anterior border of the lower part of the sternomastoid muscle, just 1–2 cm above the level of the suprasternal notch. The tiny hole may be noted from birth, but frequently it only becomes apparent in later childhood, when not only is the opening larger, but the upper edge takes on a crescentic appearance. There is usually an intermittent discharge of clear liquid or pus, but no other troublesome symptom.

The classical history and appearance make the diagnosis fairly certain, and the extent of the sinus or fistula may be determined by gentle probing, or more accurately by outlining by radiopaque material to give a sinogram.

Treatment is by surgical excision of the entire length of the track. This is approached by first mobilizing the lower part through a transverse elliptical incision which includes the lower orifice, and then dissecting out the higher reaches of it through one or more further transverse incisions at a higher level. Unless all of the track is removed there is a high chance of recurrence.

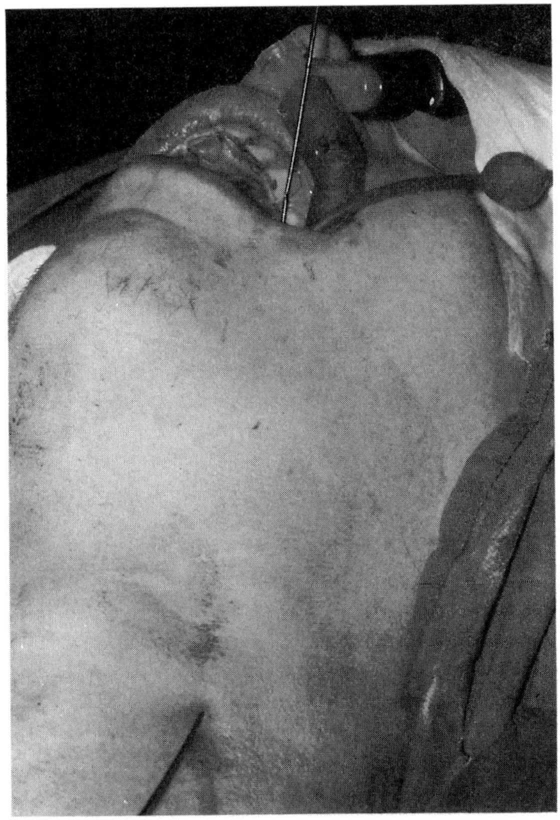

Fig. 24.2 Branchial fistula. With the patient under general anaesthesia and endotracheal intubation it has been possible to pass a probe right through from the external opening near the lower end of the anterior margin of the sternomastoid muscle to the internal opening in the pharynx. The track usually passes between the internal and external carotid arteries.

Cystic hygroma

This is a developmental abnormality of lymphatic origin present at birth or appearing within the first 1–2 years of life. A soft lymphomatous mass arises almost always in the lower part of the posterior triangle of the neck (Fig. 24.3). The size may vary from a small to a very large mass and in the latter case this may cause difficulty during delivery. Occasionally small ones may spontaneously resolve, but more often they persist and enlarge, mainly within

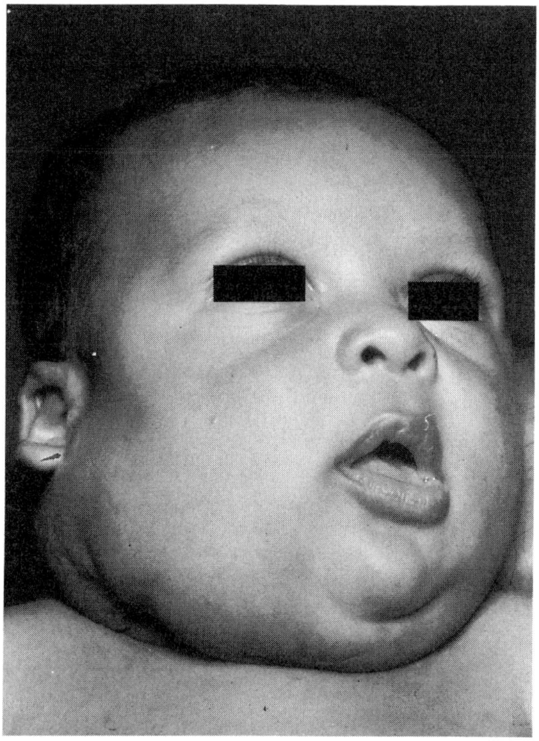

Fig. 24.3 Cystic hygroma: moderately large, typical site in an infant.

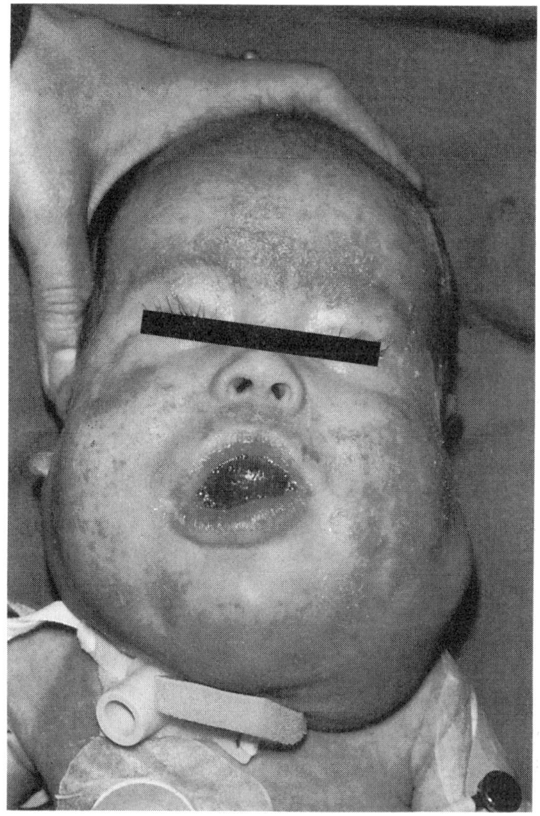

Fig. 24.4 Larger cystic hygroma involving the floor of the mouth and causing respiratory difficulty. A tracheostomy was required in this infant.

the subcutaneous layer, but sometimes extending down into the mediastinum, the axilla, or even up into the base of the skull (Fig. 24.4).

Clinically, the mass is very soft to palpation, and characteristically it transilluminates brilliantly. Sudden enlargement may arise from coughing or straining, or due to haemorrhage into the spaces. If haemorrhage occurs transillumination will be lost.

Whereas a short period of observation may be permissible in the case of small asymptomatic hygromas, to see whether spontaneous shrinkage will occur, it is better to recommend surgical excision for larger and persistent ones. This may require quite an extensive dissection where there is extension into other deeper planes. The aim is to remove all of the component multilocular cysts.

Cervical lymph node enlargement

Palpable lymph nodes are perhaps the commonest of all neck swellings, and reference to their presence is made in chapters dealing with infections and tumours of the mouth (Ch. 23), tumours of the thyroid (Ch. 25), tuberculous adenitis (Ch.12), the lymphomas (Ch. 20) and skin tumours of the face, head and neck (Chs 23 and 24). The following generalizations may be made.

If the node enlargement is due to acute infection in the drainage area the swellings are tense, fleshy and tender, whereas with chronic infection, e.g. tuberculosis, they are firmer, often matted together and there is little or no tenderness. Lymphomatous nodes are rubbery and discrete, and metastatic carcinoma in nodes makes them hard, and usually free of all pain and tenderness.

The distribution of lymph nodes in the neck comprises:

1. A horizontal ring of aggregates starting anteriorly near to the midline in the submental group, and passing to the submandibular region, the pre-

and postauricular areas, round to the mastoid and occipital regions.

2. A vertical chain of nodes descending along the main vascular compartment, and mainly related to the jugular veins down into the root of the neck.
3. A transverse series of nodes along the floor of the supraclavicular fossa (Fig. 24.5).

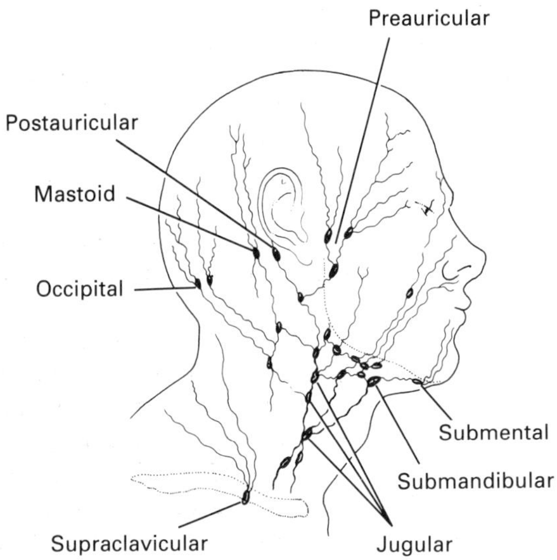

Fig. 24.5 Distribution of the main lymph nodes in the head and neck.

Short-lived enlargement and tenderness in one or more groups of the upper horizontal ring of nodes and the upper part of the vertical cervical chain are not uncommon as a result of staphylococcal or streptococcal infections of skin lesions in the scalp or face, teeth, tonsils or pharynx. While in most instances appropriate treatment of the primary infection leads to complete resolution of the lymph node enlargement, on occasions the node suppurates and presents as an abscess. Local incision and drainage may then be required.

Chronic inflammatory enlargement of nodes may rarely persist from drainage from non-specific infections, but steady slow enlargement suggests tubercular involvement. Rarely chronic swelling will be a manifestation of primary or secondary syphilis, but other indications of this disease should be apparent to lead to the correct diagnosis.

The clinical features and management of patients presenting with tuberculous adenitis are discussed in Chapter 12. The main characteristics are a tendency for several nodes to become matted together, for caseation to develop, and the possibility of a 'collar-stud' cold abscess. A full course of antituberculous drugs is usually effective in achieving healing with local calcification, and surgical excision may be required for removal of an abscess and the several nodes from which it arises. On occasions the observation of small calcified deposits along the course of the lymphatics on X-ray of the neck may be the only sign of an earlier tubercular infection which has healed up completely (Fig. 24.6).

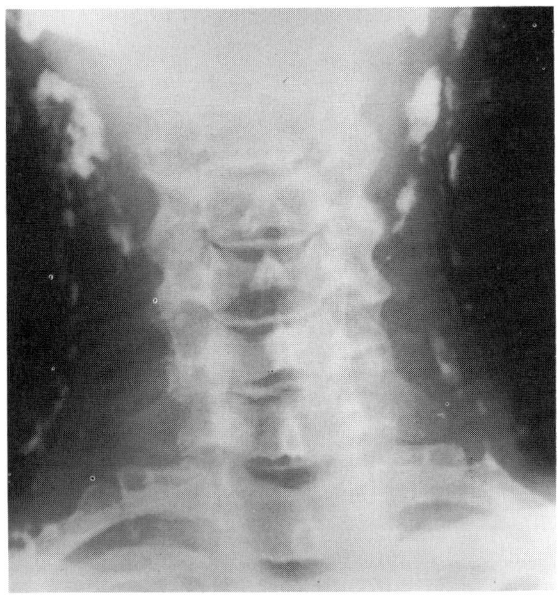

Fig. 24.6 Numerous lymph nodes mainly along the jugular chains on both sides of the neck, which are calcified as a result of previous tuberculous infection (see also Chapter 12).

In glandular fever several groups of nodes may be enlarged and tender, particularly those in the postauricular mastoid and occipital areas and there is of course general malaise and debility. A rare cause of inflammatory enlargement, and at times caseation and discharge, is cat-scratch fever due to infection with a mycobacterium by scratching or a bite by a cat. If the condition is recognized, treatment with an antibiotic such as rifampicin is often successful.

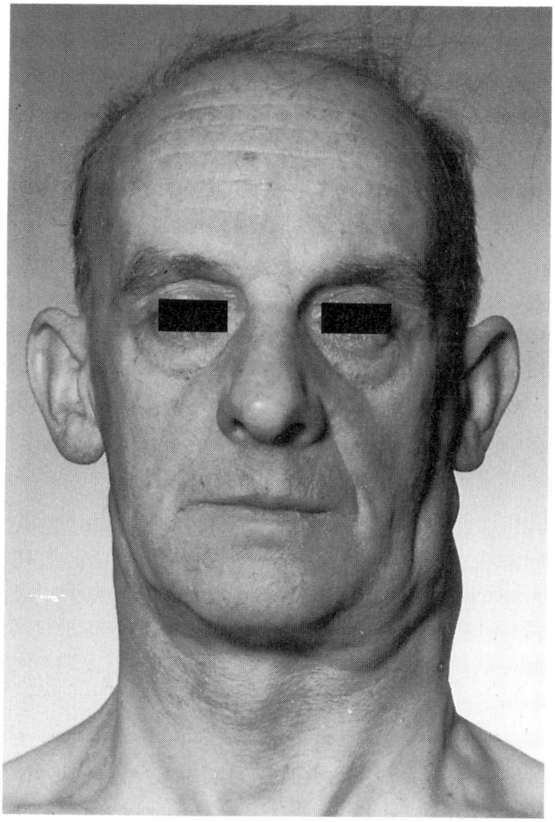

Fig. 24.7 Hodgkin's disease. The patient presented with a mass of several enlarged lymph nodes only on the left side of the neck.

Cervical lymph nodes which are enlarged in reticuloses, e.g. Hodgkin's disease (Fig. 24.7), are usually located in the middle of the vertical chain, and biopsy is the usual method of establishing a firm diagnosis. Further procedures to define the stage of the disease will then be required to decide on the best approach to treatment.

When the node enlargement is due to metastatic carcinoma the site of the primary tumour may or may not be obvious. Carcinoma of the lip and mouth tends to spread to the submandibular and upper cervical nodes, whereas primaries in the thyroid, larynx or pharynx are more likely to pass into the middle cervical chain. Metastases in the supraclavicular fossa point to primary tumour in the bronchus, breast or, if on the left side, stomach or other part of the gastrointestinal tract.

Carotid body tumour (chemodectoma)

This very rare, essentially benign tumour arises at the bifurcation of the common carotid artery into its internal and external carotid branches. It is similar to paraganglionoma, lies between the adventitia and the media, is very vascular, enlarges in a rather lobulated pattern slowly over several years, and it is not hormonely active. It presents clinically either simply as a slowly enlarging mass behind the upper part of the sternomastoid, or on account of local pressure symptoms. These latter may be on nearby nerves, producing pain up or down the neck, towards the ear, or voice changes, or there may be attacks of dizziness and faintness developing either spontaneously or when any local pressure is applied to the tumour. The commonest age group in which these are encountered is between 30 and 50 years.

Small asymptomatic chemodectomas in elderly patients may be left alone to avoid any risk of compromising the internal carotid supply to the brain. In younger patients and those with symptoms excision is recommended. Useful preoperative information is obtained from an arteriogram of the aortic arch and its main branches. This will show whether the main carotid arteries are displaced or narrowed by the tumour, and will demonstrate the degree of vascularity of the mass itself. If possible it is best to dissect the tumour from the vessels without opening into the arterial lumen, but this may not be feasible, and resection of the involved segment may prove necessary. This will need temporary arterial bypass to the internal carotid artery, and replacement of the excised segment by a graft from the long saphenous vein.

THYROID, SUBMANDIBULAR SALIVARY GLAND AND PAROTID GLAND

Swellings arising from these organs are discussed in Chapters 25 and 23 respectively.

CERVICAL RIB

An abnormal bony, or bone plus fibrous tissue development may articulate with the seventh cervical vertebra on one or both sides, and this can vary from a small vestigial stump to a full-length rib running above the normal first rib. In the latter circumstance the anterior end of the extra rib may end as a rounded prominent knob, and this may be clearly palpable low in the supraclavicular fossa. The bony hardness and fixity of the mass make the diagnosis obvious. The rib or any dense fibrous extension of it anteriorly may cause pressure on either the subclavian artery or the lower parts of the branchial plexus. The former may lead to aneurysmal dilatation of the artery, local thrombus deposition and subsequent small distal emboli in the fingers, or other more severe vascular problems in the hand (see Ch. 43). The latter may produce sensory disturbance in the ulnar side of the hand and arm.

An asymptomatic cervical rib should be left alone, unless there is any reason to suspect vascular changes such as aneurysm formation. The presence of either vascular or neurological symptoms merits surgical excision of the rib and any fibrous extension of it.

STERNOMASTOID 'TUMOUR' (CONGENITAL TORTICOLLIS)

This condition is not neoplastic, but because there is a palpable mass within the substance of the sternomastoid muscle, and the term has been used for many years in clinical practice, it is difficult to discontinue the name.

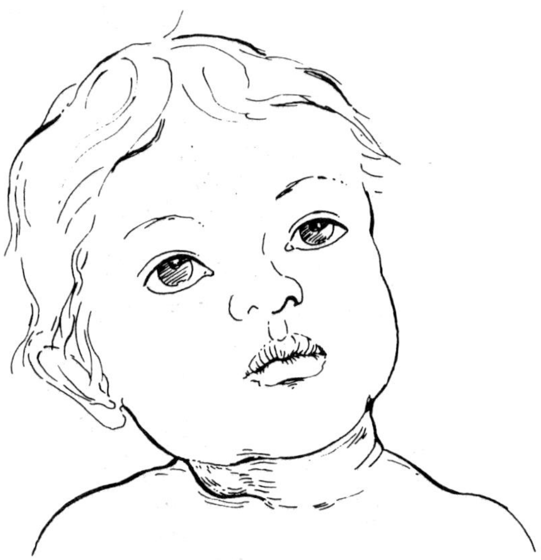

Fig. 24.8 Congenital torticollis. The fibrous nodule in the lower part of the sternomastoid muscle is generally visible and palpable. The contracture pulls the head over towards the same side, and deviates the chin to the opposite side.

The mass is a deposit of dense fibrous tissue in response to a tearing injury of the muscle fibres at birth (Fig. 24.8). It is more likely to occur if the birth has been a difficult one. It may be noticed immediately the baby is born, or sometimes not until a few weeks have passed. The 'tumour' is hard, oval and free of pain or tenderness, and it may resolve gradually and completely. However, when it persists the sternomastoid of the affected side will shorten, pulling that side of the head downwards towards the shoulder. If no steps are taken to correct the deformity a degree of facial asymmetry may develop as the child grows. For this reason, and on account of the obvious and embarrassing deformity, active treatment should be advised. A regular regime of putting the child's head through a full range of rotation, flexion, and extension movements several times each day may lead to a steady correction to normal. If this fails, operative division of the sternal and clavicular heads of origin of the muscle is recommended.

MIDLINE SWELLINGS

All the swellings so far described in this chapter lie to a greater or lesser extent lateral in the neck, but the following few are to be found in the midline.

Submental dermoid

As is discussed in Chapter 19, dermoid cysts arise at points of fusion of embryological folds, and as the jaw and chin are formed by the mandibular arches, which meet precisely in the midline, a dermoid cyst may thus develop. The cyst is usually small, no greater than 1–2 cm, lying superficial to or incorporated in the median raphe joining the two mylohyoid muscles. It does not move upwards on protrusion of the tongue: this differentiates it clinically from a thyroglossal cyst. Local excision should present no particular problem.

Subhyoid bursa

A small encysted collection of clear mucoid fluid, oval with its longer axis lying transversely, occasionally arises behind the body of the hyoid bone and the fibres of insertion of the sternohyoid strap muscle; these fibres are attached to the upper posterior border of the hyoid. If the bursa persists it can be excised.

Thyroglossal cyst

This is described fully in Chapter 25.

A solitary nodule arising in the isthmus of the thyroid gland may also appear truly in the midline, as may a central pretracheal lymph node.

ACUTE INFECTIONS OF SKIN AND SOFT TISSUES OF THE NECK

Skin

The back of the neck is a common site for infected hair follicles and boils of various sizes, particularly in young men. These sometimes occur as solitary lesions, and sometimes as part of acne vulgaris. Usually the small superficial abscess develops over a few days, discharges pus and then heals and only rarely local incision be required.

Carbuncle

This larger and much more troublesome condition starts as an infected hair follicle, but the infective process extends along both the skin and the subcutaneous tissues to produce a large raised, reddened, hot tender mass with multiple points of discharge of pus on to the surface. The vast majority of carbuncles develop on either the back of the neck, or a little lower down on the upper interscapular region. The central part of the mass becomes necrotic, blackened, and pieces of it may separate, leaving a mucky discharging crater. There is usually pyrexia, anorexia and a marked general systemic upset. Full dosage of an antibiotic to which the organism—usually staphylococcus—is sensitive is required, and in addition wide local excision of all the infected area may be necessary.

DEEP INFECTIONS

These are serious, dangerous infections if they reach one or more of the spaces enclosed deep to the deep cervical fascia. A knowledge of the anatomical arrangement of this fascial layer is important to an understanding of the progress of these deep-sited infections and how they may exert their harmful effects.

The deep cervical fascia

There is first of all a strong completely encircling sleeve of deep fascia starting posteriorly from the cervical spinous processes, enveloping the trapezius muscle, joining into a single sheet at the anterior border, passing over the posterior triangle, opening again into an inner and outer layer to enclose the sternomastoid muscle, coming together again at its anterior border and continuing across the anterior triangle to meet that of the other side in the midline. From the two lateral sides there are extensions around the carotid and jugular blood vessels and then passing across in front of the prevertebral muscles, behind the pharynx, the dense prevertebral layer of fascia.

These layers are strong dense fibrous sheets. In addition there are weaker fascial layers investing the thyroid gland, and fixing it to the trachea—the pretracheal fascia (Fig. 24.9).

This disposition of the fascia determines the direction in which collections of pus and other infected material may extend in the neck. For example, pus in the anterior triangle may travel down into the anterior mediastinum, and pus from

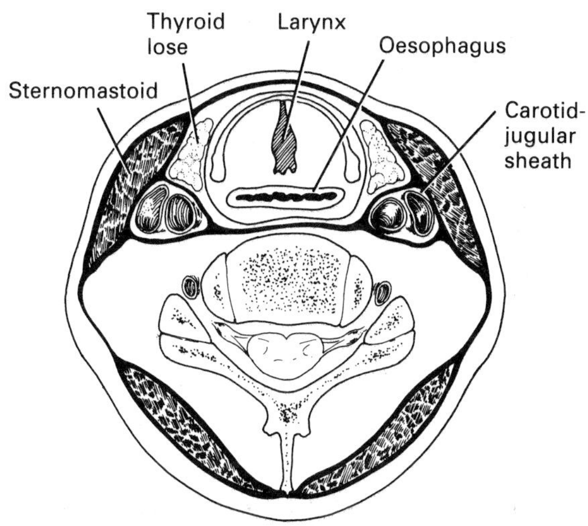

Fig. 24.9 Cross-section through the lower neck, showing the main layers of the deep cervical fascia.

the vertebrae may be forced either laterally into the posterior triangle of the neck, or may bulge forward into the posterior wall of the pharynx.

The commonest sources of infection going into the deep soft tissue spaces of the neck are from the mouth, fauces, teeth, salivary glands, larynx or pharynx. Although various organisms may be responsible, often the culprit is a streptococcus. Cellulitis and oedema can greatly increase local pressure, causing gross swelling across the floor of the mouth, difficulty and pain on swallowing, or if in lower compartments dyspnoea, dysphagia and speech difficulties. Pyrexia and severe toxic symptoms are to be expected.

A particular pattern of infection in the floor of the mouth, not seen so frequently as in past years, is Ludwig's angina (Fig. 24.10). This is a very gross cellulitis arising from an infected tooth socket or salivary gland, and spreading perhaps among all the muscles of the tongue and suprahyoid region.

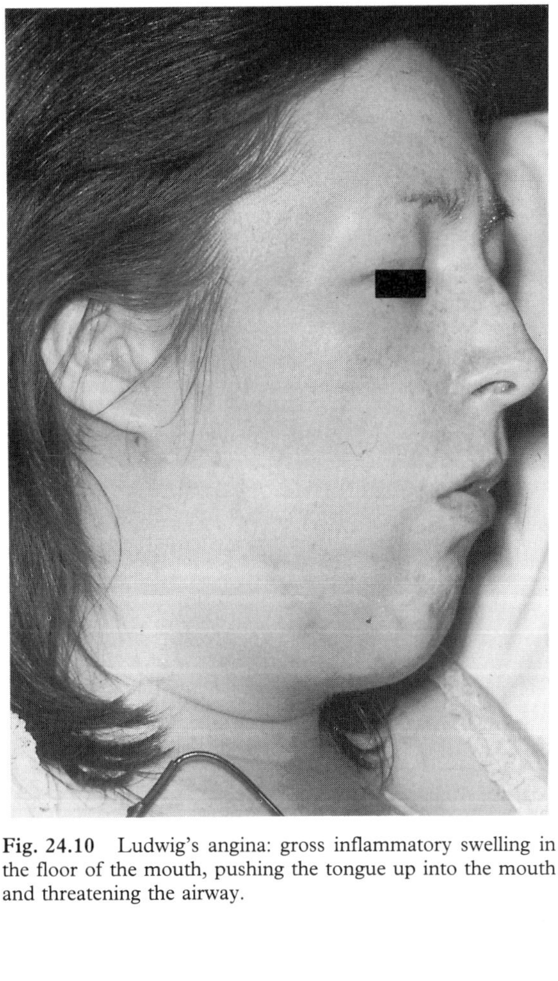

Fig. 24.10 Ludwig's angina: gross inflammatory swelling in the floor of the mouth, pushing the tongue up into the mouth and threatening the airway.

Large doses of one of the penicillins or broad-spectrum antibiotics are given and if there are any signs of mechanical compression on airway or blood vessels surgical decompression and drainage may be necessary. On rare occasions tracheostomy may even be required.

TRAUMATIC WOUNDS OF THE NECK

The two commonest varieties of wound are cut-throat, usually self-inflicted as a suicide attempt, and stab wound, by an assailant. Clearly in either type of wound there are risks of serious, indeed life-threatening injuries to major structures, e.g. carotid arteries, jugular veins, trachea, oesophagus, thyroid gland, brachial plexus, and particularly with stab wounds, pleura and apex of lung. On the left side the thoracic duct may suffer. Often the intending suicide will inflict the cut-throat wound with the neck extended, and this posture places the carotid and internal jugular vessels in a relatively posterior position. In this case these vessels may escape damage while other more anteriorly placed structures are divided.

The most immediate problems are control of haemorrhage, and maintenance of a satisfactory airway.

Haemorrhage

Where there is an open, incised wound the bleeding is of course external, and it may be very copious even from damage to the superficial neck veins, e.g. the external jugular. As a first-aid measure the patient should be transported with the head slightly elevated and efforts should be made to calm him or her and avoid straining, which can aggravate the bleeding. The patient should not, however, be sat totally upright or encouraged to stand up, in case air is aspirated into an open vein, thus giving rise to air embolism. A large accumulation of blood in the deeper cervical compartments may quickly arise after a stab wound, deep vessels being punctured by the point of a narrow blade. In this case pressure symptoms especially on the airway may need urgent relief, either by enlarging the small wound or making a rapid new relieving incision.

In either event, if the haemorrhage is severe, ultimate control will require surgical exploration and clear exposure of the damaged vessels. Minor ones may be ligated, and small tears in more major ones may be sutured. Severe damage or complete severance may need re-anastomosis or rarely the insertion of a graft. Once the bleeding has been dealt with the wound should be further explored to determine whether other structures are also damaged and repair made by an appropriate method. Blood transfusion may be required.

Airway

Immediate respiratory distress can arise from severance of the trachea or the inhalation of blood into opened air passages. It may, therefore, be necessary rapidly to aspirate secretions and blood from the back of the throat and upper trachea and either pass an endotracheal tube or establish a tracheostomy. A further potential cause of airway obstruction is falling back of the tongue, if the hyoglossus and mylohyoid muscles are divided, or if there is damage to the recurrent laryngeal nerves. In both instances intubation may be required.

Unlike surgical wounds in the neck, which carry a small risk of infection, there is a relatively high chance of organisms contaminating both types of traumatic wounds, and of course, collections of extravasated blood form an ideal medium for bacterial growth. It is wise, therefore, to give a broad-spectrum antibiotic to patients with these injuries and this is especially important when there is any reason to suspect damage to the pharynx or oesophagus.

Once good recovery and satisfactory wound healing are apparent the patient who has self-inflicted the injury should be assessed and further supervised by a psychiatrist.

25. The thyroid gland

DEVELOPMENT

The greater part of the thyroid gland develops as a diverticulum from the foramen caecum of the tongue (Fig. 25.1). The connection with the tongue, called the thyroglossal duct, becomes obliterated in the majority of cases, but may persist in some, to give rise to a thyroglossal cyst. A small part of the gland containing the parafollicular cells is thought to develop from ultimobranchial bodies which arise from the fourth branchial pouch.

ANATOMY

The thyroid is the largest of the endocrine glands, weighing about 20–25 g in an adult, and consisting of two lobes joined by an isthmus. The lobes lie on either side of the larynx and the upper part of the trachea and the isthmus crosses the second and third and sometimes also the fourth tracheal rings. The lobes extend vertically from the middle of the lateral side of the thyroid cartilage to the sixth tracheal ring. The gland is covered by the strap muscles on either side, namely sternothyroid lying deep to the sternohyoid. These muscles lie under cover of the deep cervical fascia, an encircling layer which divides to include the substance of the sternocleidomastoid muscles laterally. The whole of the thyroid gland is invested with a fibrous capsule connected with the pretracheal fascia, which explains the movement of the gland on swallowing. Each lobe consists of three surfaces—superficial, medial and posterior—and two poles—upper and lower. The superficial surface is related to the strap muscles while the medial surface lies in relation to the larynx, trachea and oesophagus. The parathyroid glands lie in relation to the medial

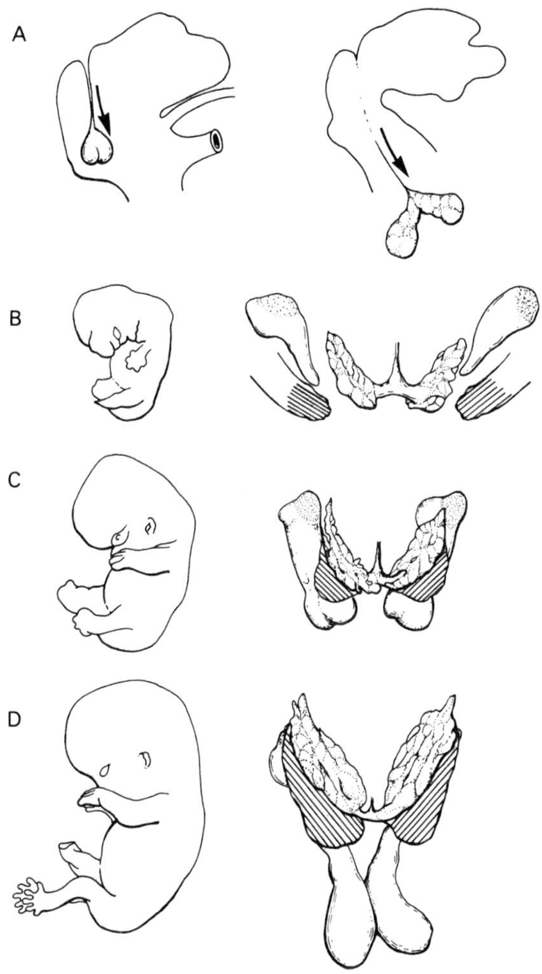

Fig. 25.1 Stages in embryological development of the thyroid gland. (**A**) Downgrowth of the main thyroid bud from the back of the tongue (foramen caecum region) on the left: it is more developed on the right, and beginning to be defined as a two lobe structure. (**B–D**). Left: the overall appearance of the embryo; right: the gradual migration of segments of the branchial arch (the cross-hatched area) to join up as part of the lateral lobes. The lower parts of this arch development fuse and descend as the thymus.

surface, the upper one near the upper pole and lower one near the lower pole of the thyroid.

The functioning unit is the lobule, supplied by a single arteriole and consisting of 20–40 follicles lined by cuboidal epithelium. The resting follicle contains colloid in which thyroglobulin is stored.

Blood supply

The thyroid gland receives its main arterial blood supply from two pairs of arteries, the superior thyroid artery which is the first branch of the external carotid artery and the inferior thyroid which is the terminal branch of the thyrocervical trunk arising from the first part of the subclavian artery (Fig. 25.2). The recurrent laryngeal nerve lies closely related to the inferior thyroid artery. The superior thyroid artery is intimately related to the external laryngeal nerve and enters the gland near the superior pole. Sometimes an additional artery, the thyroidea ima arising from the arch of the aorta, supplies the isthmus. In addition, numerous small branches from the arteries supplying the trachea and oesophagus may also supply the gland, anastomosing freely with the branches of the main arteries.

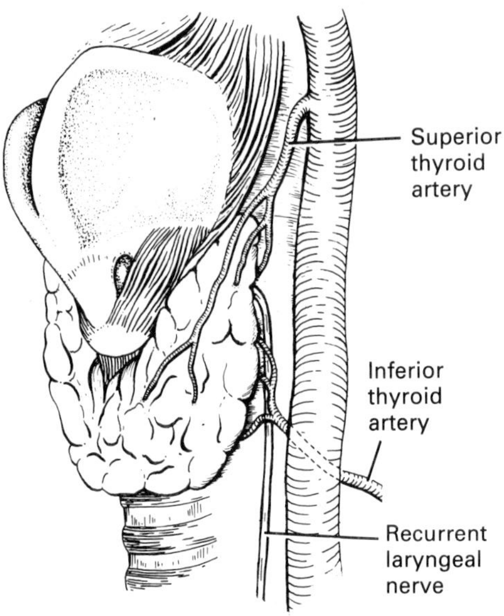

Fig. 25.2 The main arterial blood supply to the thyroid: the superior thyroid artery arising from the external carotid artery, and entering at the upper pole of the gland; the inferior thyroid artery, a branch of the thyrocervical artery, which in turn arises from the subclavian artery, emerges from behind the common carotid and travels to the posterior aspect of the lateral lobe. As it approaches the gland, it or its terminal branches are closely related to the recurrent laryngeal nerve.

Three pairs of veins—superior, middle and inferior thyroid veins—drain the gland; the superior and the middle ones drain into the internal jugular vein, and the inferior into the innominate vein.

Nerves

The thyroid gland is supplied by both sympathetic and parasympathetic nerves. Sympathetic fibres come from the middle cervical ganglion and travel alongside the blood vessels. The parasympathetic nerves are branches of the superior and recurrent laryngeal nerve (Fig. 25.3). The latter lies in the tracheo-oesophageal groove posterior to the inferior thyroid artery, and injury to it leads to hoarseness of the voice and respiratory difficulty.

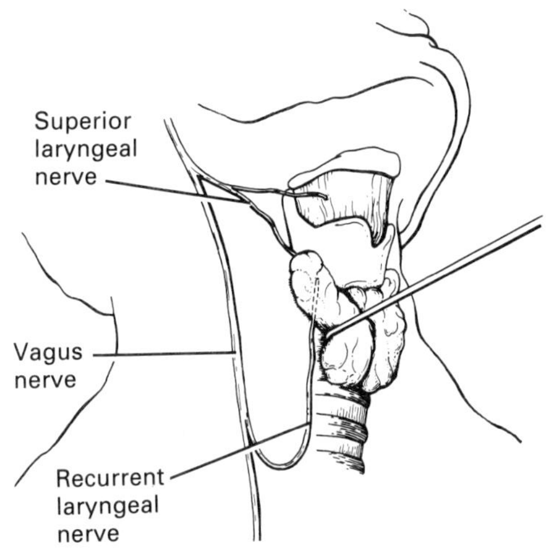

Fig. 25.3 Parasympathetic nerve supply to the thyroid gland: both the superior and recurrent laryngeal nerves are branches of the vagus nerve.

Lymphatics

Two sets of lymphatics drain the gland, an ascending and a descending system. In the ascending set the medial channel drains into the lymph nodes in front of the larynx, and the lateral lymphatics drain into the nodes along the upper part of the internal jugular vein. The descending lymphatics from the isthmus and the medial part of the lobes drain into pretracheal and retrosternal lymph nodes, while lymphatics from the lateral part of the lobes drain into nodes along the lower part of the internal jugular vein.

PHYSIOLOGY

Iodine is an essential constituent of the diet, the daily requirement being about 100–125 μg. After absorption from the gut, it circulates in the form of iodide in the blood and is extracted selectively by the thyroid gland where it is converted into iodine by the enzyme peroxidase. In the cells of the thyroid gland it combines with tyrosine to form mono-iodotyrosine (MIT) and di-iodotyrosine (DIT). Two di-iodotyrosine molecules combine to form tetraiodothyronine which is thyroxine (T^4), and mono- and di-iodotyrosine compounds combine to form tri-iodothyronine (T^3). These combinations occur under the influence of coupling enzymes.

T^3 and T^4 are stored in the acini of the gland in combination with a protein, globulin in the form of thyroglobulin, from which small quantities of the hormones are released in the blood according to metabolic requirements. Most of the thyroid hormones circulate in combination with a protein whereas a small quantity remains in the free state. T^3 and T^4 affect the general metabolism and growth of the body, and T^3 is four times more active metabolically than T^4. The exact mode of action of T^3 and T^4 at the cellular level is not properly understood but they are known to cause an increase in the consumption of oxygen and so stimulate cellular respiration and increased heat production.

The activities of the thyroid gland are regulated by the thyroid-stimulating hormone (TSH) secreted by the basophil cells of the anterior pituitary gland. This hormone is released partly under the influence of thyrotropin-releasing hormone (TRH) from the hypothalamus and partly under the direct influence of the level of circulating T^3 and T^4. TSH stimulates both the synthesis and the release of the thyroid hormones.

Thyroid hormones act on the nervous system, muscles and metabolism.

Nervous system

All three components of the nervous system are affected, i.e. the central, the peripheral and the autonomic nervous systems.

In the central nervous system the deficiency of thyroid hormone produces apathy, lethargy and somnolence whereas an excess produces excitation, irritability, nervousness, quickening of reaction times, emotional instability and insomnia.

In the peripheral nerves, T^3 and T^4 maintain the health of neuromuscular junctions. In deficiency states, the tendon jerks are sluggish with slow relaxation whereas in hyperthyroid states they may be brisk or exaggerated.

As far as the autonomic system is concerned thyroid hormones appear to enhance or make the tissues more susceptible to the action of catecholamines (adrenaline and noradrenaline).

In the cardiovascular system excess thyroid hormone causes tachycardia and the force of contraction of cardiac muscle is also enhanced, resulting in increase in the cardiac output. Blood pressure, especially systolic, may also be increased partly because of increase in the cardiac output and partly due to increase in the peripheral resistance. In extreme forms of thyrotoxicosis, this combination of enhanced cardiac output and increased peripheral resistance may lead to cardiac failure. Hyperexcitability of cardiac muscle may lead to extrasystole, paroxysmal tachycardia or atrial fibrillation.

The alimentary system is also affected, in that excess of thyroid hormones produces hypermotility of the intestines, resulting in diarrhoea. Constipation, on the other hand, is one of the cardinal features of thyroid deficiency state.

METABOLISM

As far as carbohydrate metabolism is concerned there is glycogenolysis, neoglucogenesis and a tendency towards hyperglycaemia in hyperthyroid states. There is also increased catabolism of both fat and protein, which partly explains the neoglucogenesis and excess production of creatinine. It also explains the loss of weight in spite of an increased appetite in this condition. In the hypothyroid state, on the other hand, there is abnormal deposition of fat.

Tests of thyroid function

The principal value of these tests is in assessing the thyroid status when the clinical picture is equivocal. However, even if the clinical diagnosis appears quite certain, it is valuable to have confirmatory evidence. In the absence of access to a biochemical laboratory, the measurement of sleeping pulse rate is useful, an elevation being indicative of thyrotoxicosis.

Assessment of thyroid function

Many tests have been proposed over the years, but as far as current practice is concerned, relatively few are needed to answer specific clinical questions.

The most useful tests are:

1. Serum T^4 by either radioimmunoassay or competitive protein binding. This is usually the most direct and reliable way of confirming either the euthyroid state (normal) or hyperthyroidism (elevated). Levels may also be elevated in acute thyroiditis, and during pregnancy or oestrogen administration. Although reduced T^4 levels are seen in hypothyroid states it is not the primary test for these disorders. Several drugs, e.g. androgens, salicylates, phenytoin and anabolic steroids may also depress T^4 concentration.
2. Serum T^3 is also measured by radioimmunoassay and in general levels mirror those of T^4. In severe debilitating illness and in old age there may be some depression of T^3 levels.
3. Serum thyrotropin or TSH, also by radioimmunoassay—this is the test of choice to confirm hypothyroidism, in which it is elevated.
4. T^3 resin uptake (T^3RU) gives an estimate of the amount of unsaturated thyroid-binding globulin available; it is increased in hyperthyroidism. However, many drugs can also increase the uptake, e.g. salicylates, large doses of penicillin, anabolic steroids, phenylbutazone. Pregnancy and contraceptive pills containing oestrogen, on the other hand, diminish resin uptake.
5. The radioactive iodine (RAI) uptake and scan give an overall measurement of the clearance of iodide from the plasma by the thyroid gland. The uptake will be increased when the gland is overactive or where there is iodine depletion, and decreased in all forms of hypothyroidism, when iodine is given in exogenous forms, including X-ray contrast media, and in some forms of thyroiditis.

All of these tests, apart from RAI, are unaffected by iodine administration, unlike previously used ones, e.g. the protein-bound iodine. As these tests are more reliable, they have now replaced these older ones.

One or two other physiological and biochemical measurements may be abnormal in specific disorders of the thyroid and these will be mentioned where relevant. They are not included in this preliminary list since they are not used as primary diagnostic tools.

CONGENITAL DISORDERS OF THE THYROID GLAND

Ectopic thyroid tissue

A collection, often rounded, of normally appearing thyroid gland tissue may rarely be found at any level from the junction of the middle and posterior one-third of the tongue, i.e. the foramen caecum, down through the floor of the mouth to the midline of the upper part of the neck. When it lies in the upper surface of the tongue it is referred to as a lingual thyroid. If large, it may give rise to impairment of speech, interference with swallowing, or even respiratory obstruction. Bleeding may occur into or from the mass.

Occasionally the ectopic thyroid is the only functioning thyroid tissue present, and so it is desirable to perform scanning to determine whether this is so, or if there is in fact normally sited functioning thyroid tissue present. If causing symptoms the ectopic mass is surgically excised. Clearly, if no other thyroid tissue is present, either autoimplants into a suitable site in the neck (e.g. sternomastoid muscle) or lifelong thyroid hormone supplements will be required.

Anomalies of the thyroglossal tract

A thyroglossal cyst is an uncommon developmental defect, in which the whole or part of the thyroglossal duct persists and appears as a cystic swelling in the midline of the neck, situated anywhere between the suprahyoid region and the thyroid gland. A strand of tissue usually connects it with the foramen caecum and that strand may make a loop or kink in front of or behind the hyoid bone. Due to the presence of lymphoid tissue in its wall, the cyst is liable to infection. If it discharges spontaneously or is incised, a thyroglossal fistula usually develops, lying to one or other side of the midline, usually the left. The treatment of the cyst or fistula is excision along with the removal of any remnant of the thyroglossal duct.

THYROID ENLARGEMENT AND THYROID MASSES

The term goitre usually refers to generalized increase in bulk of the gland—this may be uniform diffuse enlargement or a more irregular, nodular one.

Clinically there are four distinct types of simple, i.e. non-toxic, non-inflammatory and non-malignant, change in the gland:

1. Physiological goitre is a smooth, soft increase in prominence of the entire thyroid gland, seen mostly in girls at around puberty or during pregnancy. Usually the swelling subsides with the passage of time, and no specific treatment is required.
2. Endemic goitre was formerly commoner than today and arose classically in areas where iodine was relatively deficient in the diet, often in locations well inland from the sea. Examples of such sites are the Rocky Mountains, the Alps and the Himalayas; Derbyshire in the UK, and the mountainous areas of Jabal-Akdar in Libya. The thyroid enlargement results from increased production of TSH from the pituitary in response to the low circulating levels of thyroid hormones, which are in turn due to the iodine lack.

   The condition is largely prevented now by the simple addition of iodine to salt and could be eliminated by the worldwide extension of this practice, where appropriate. Where cases are still encountered surgical removal of the excess tissue, which on occasions may be very bulky indeed, may be required either for cosmetic reasons or because of mechanical compression on the trachea.
3. Sporadic goitre is uniform enlargement of the gland, occurring often for no apparent reason in areas where the supply of iodine is plentiful. Rarely the ingestion of goitrogens, e.g. thiocyanates in green vegetables, or drugs such as para-aminosalicylic acid will be responsible.

   Here again partial thyroidectomy will be indicated if the enlargement is cosmetically unacceptable or if pressure symptoms arise.
4. Non-toxic multinodular goitre: although the cause of this disorder is not really known, it may in part result from alternate stimulation and inhibition of growth by TSH or other factors, leading to an irregular pattern of histological change, some areas showing activity and cellular proliferation while others are relatively inactive, with collection of colloid, involution and formation of cysts of varying sizes. From time to time local haemorrhage may occur into cysts or other areas, causing sudden enlargement of that part of the gland and perhaps slight local tenderness.

   The patient usually presents simply on account of the obvious enlargement in the front of the neck and is euthyroid. Sometimes there are pressure symptoms such as dyspnoea or dysphagia, particularly if there is so much enlargement of a lower pole of one lobe that it extends down behind the sternum, where space is limited. The nodules are often visible and certainly palpable, being of firm consistency (Fig. 25.4). Retrosternal extension is suggested by the inability to get the examining fingers clearly below the relevant lower pole, even when the gland is elevated during a swallow by the patient. Other physical signs of retrosternal extension are dullness to percussion over the area, and increasing prominence of the neck veins (if there is pressure on the main venous return in the upper mediastinum).

Non-toxic multinodular goitre is a common condition in western communities and the main indications for partial thyroidectomy are once again unhappiness about the disfigurement or any pressure symptoms. However, since there may be uncertainty as to whether other diseases, e.g. thyroiditis or tumour, are present, it is

A
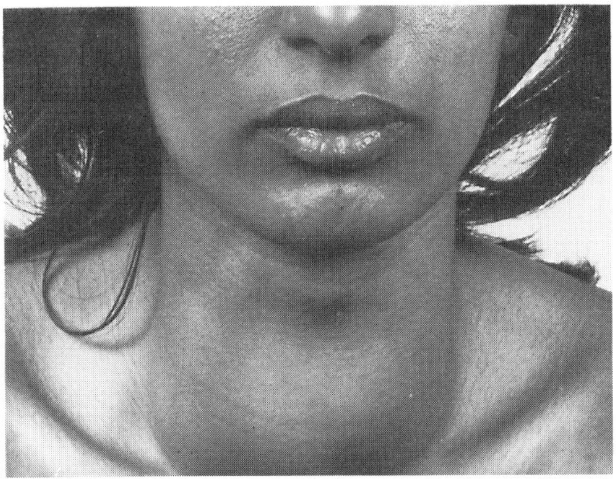

B
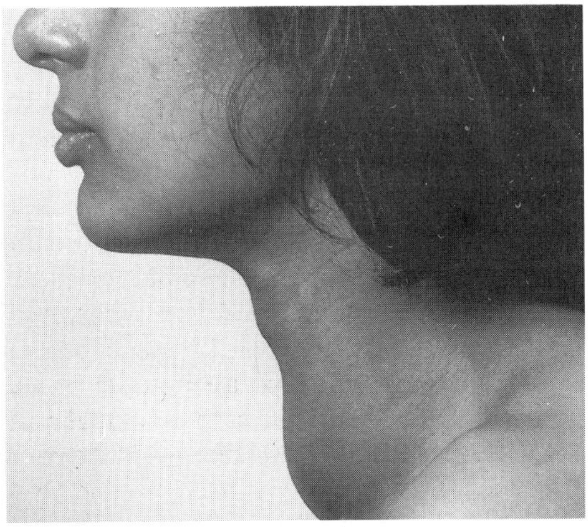

Fig. 25.4 (**A**) Anterior and (**B**) lateral view of a non-toxic multinodular goitre. The anterior view shows that there is more enlargement of the gland on the left lobe than on the right.

usually wise to proceed with a limited number of investigations. Thyroid hormones should be measured, as should thyroid antibodies to exclude thyroiditis, e.g. Hashimoto's disease. X-rays will look for any tracheal deviation or compression, and retrosternal extension. Ultrasound and radionuclide scanning will give further useful information about the presence of cysts and hot or cold nodules. Since there is nothing to prevent the coexistence of a tumour with non-toxic multinodular goitre, suspicious scan findings may lead to surgical exploration. In a proportion—perhaps as high as 20–30%—of patients with non-toxic multinodular goitre, thyrotoxicity will develop in the later follow-up period, and this is referred to as secondary thyrotoxicosis, distinguishing it from the primary form (Graves disease), discussed later. The onset of secondary thyrotoxicosis is usually an indication for surgical excision.

If operation—usually subtotal removal of the gland—is performed for multinodular goitre, either non-toxic or toxic, it is generally recommended that a small regular dose of thyroxine, e.g. 0.1 mg/day, is prescribed, in the belief that this will diminish TSH secretion and therefore further stimulation to proliferation of the remaining small portions of thyroid gland tissue.

Solitary nodule

This is defined as the clinical presentation with an apparently single nodule in an otherwise normal gland. Most of the patients with solitary nodule are females between the ages of 30 and 50 and are otherwise asymptomatic.

In a proportion of patients presenting in this way the apparently solitary nodule will be part of a multinodular goitre, the other nodules being so relatively small and normal in consistency that they are not identified on simple palpation. In these patients the prognosis is very good and the management is that of the non-toxic multinodular goitre.

Of those with truly a solitary nodule and no abnormality in the rest of the gland, the majority prove to be benign adenomas or cysts, but about 10% will be one or other form of thyroid malignancy, notably the papillary or follicular patterns.

Since clinically it is impossible often to be sure of the correct diagnosis, it is wise to perform some or all of the following investigations in someone presenting with an apparently solitary nodule: measurement of circulating thyroid hormone levels; ultrasound scanning, to determine whether solid or cystic; isotope scanning, to distinguish hot (i.e. active) from cold (i.e. inactive); X-ray of neck and chest, and serum thyroid antibody estimations.

Those nodules which are found to be cysts may be emptied by needle aspiration under local anaesthetic. These are usually retention cysts or cystic degeneration in an adenomatous area of thyroid tissue. If they refill after aspiration they may require local surgical excision. Very occasionally the cyst may arise in a tumour and for this reason it is wise to submit any aspirated fluid for cytological examination. A suspicious or definite report of malignant change would, of course, lead to formal surgical exploration of the gland.

Turning to solid nodules, a tissue diagnosis may be obtained by needle or aspiration biopsy under local anaesthesia. This is a simple procedure with minimal risk, but its usefulness primarily depends on the availability of a competent, experienced pathologist to interpret the findings on such limited samples.

Benign solitary solid nodules are either true adenomas or simply areas of hyperplastic tissue and can be removed along with an appropriate segment of the lobe from which they arise.

The treatment of malignant nodules is that recommended for the appropriate type of tumour.

TUMOURS OF THE THYROID GLAND

Benign tumours

Simple adenoma

A true thyroid adenoma has a complete fibrous capsule and is well delineated from the surrounding thyroid tissue. It consists of small thyroid follicles with or without colloid material in them. There may be central fibrosis and areas of haemorrhage may be detected within the substance of the adenoma. The cells may be of variable size and have a trabecular arrangement.

Depending upon the degree of thyroid function, the adenoma may be hot or cold on radioiodine scan.

Hürthle cell adenoma

This is a much rarer tumour than simple adenoma. Microscopically it has large cells with abundant granular pink cytoplasm, and well defined prominent nuclei. Cells are arranged in solid masses or columns. The cells are small, containing little amounts of colloid.

Clinical features

The patient, usually female, may be asymptomatic, and the lump may be found incidentally by either the patient or the clinician. Alternatively, the patient may have noticed a lump in the neck, which was small at the beginning, and has gradually increased in size, but without pressure effects. A sudden increase in size may have been due to haemorrhage into the adenoma. Symptoms of hyperthyroidism may develop if the adenoma is grossly hyperactive.

The clinical diagnosis of adenoma should be confirmed by histological examination of either a biopsy or the formally excised lesion. A wide excision, preferably a subtotal lobectomy, should be done.

Malignant tumours

Malignant tumours of the thyroid gland may be primary or secondary, but metastatic deposits in the thyroid from primary tumours in other organs are very rare.

There are three distinctive types of primary carcinoma of the thyroid—papillary, follicular and anaplastic. In general these are all less common than other malignancies of the human body. Irradiation of the neck region in childhood or the previous uptake of radioactive isotopes of iodine may increase the risk of a thyroid malignancy developing, and some, e.g. the papillary pattern, often show a degree of dependence on thyroid hormones. Carcinomas also appear to occur more often in areas where other thyroid disorders are more frequent.

Papillary carcinoma

Papillary carcinoma is the commonest of the cancers affecting the thyroid gland. In the USA 70% of thyroid cancers are of papillary type and 90% of the radiation-induced carcinomas are of papillary type.

It is commonest in children and young adults, and females are three to four times more commonly affected than males.

Papillary carcinoma is a non-encapsulated tumour of hard consistency arising usually as a solitary nodule in either one of the lobes or in the isthmus of the gland. Multiple foci may occur in the same lobe or rarely in both lobes because of spread by the lymphatics within the gland. The commonest spread is to the local lymph nodes.

Blood-borne metastases are most unusual. Occasionally the tumour may be too small to be noticed and the enlarged lymph nodes bring attention to the primary condition of papillary carcinoma.

Microscopically the pattern shows a papillary architecture or a mixture of a papillary and follicular pattern. Nevertheless if any papillary structure is present, it will behave as a papillary carcinoma.

Clinical features

A painless lump in the region of the thyroid gland is the most common presenting feature. The lump is hard and moves up and down on deglutition. Being a slowly growing tumour, it may be present for some years before it comes to notice. Less frequently it presents as one or more hard, discrete palpable lymph nodes in the jugular chain, usually level with the thyroid gland. Occasionally the nodes are bilateral. They may be mobile or fixed but are usually not attached to the skin.

A thyroid scan of a papillary carcinoma will reveal a 'cold' nodule.

Management

A hard nodule in the thyroid gland, with or without palpable lymph nodes in the neck, should be diagnosed and treated as carcinoma unless proved otherwise by histological examination.

In view of the possibility of either a truly multifocal origin or intraglandular lymphatic spread, many surgeons recommend total thyroidectomy with preservation of the parathyroids. An alternative surgical approach is to perform total lobectomy on the side of the obvious lesion, and subtotal removal of the other lobe. Any enlarged lymph nodes should be dissected out and removed, but block dissection is not recommended.

After operation the suppression of TSH is achieved by giving 0.3–0.4 mg thyroxine daily, and this should be continued for the rest of the patient's life. This is often quite effective in keeping known established secondary deposits under control for many years.

The prognosis generally in papillary carcinoma of the thyroid is good, with 10-year survival expected in at least 80% of cases, even when lymph node metastases are known to be present.

Follicular carcinoma

This is a well differentiated tumour where the cancer cells retain the normal follicular pattern to some degree. These follicles may contain small amounts of colloid. The tumour is usually solitary and invades the venous system, spreading to bones, the brain and the lungs.

A certain degree of anaplasia may be present, but in some instances the features are hardly different from a normal thyroid gland, the only difference being a clearcut invasion of the thyroid parenchyma. The secondaries may grow slowly, but they may be very vascular and even pulsatile, and they also avidly take up radioactive iodine.

Clinical features

Follicular carcinomas are commonest in adults between the ages of 30 and 50 years and again with an increased incidence in females. The patient may present with a swelling in the thyroid or a secondary deposit may be the first indication of the primary tumour. Cervical lymph nodes may be enlarged. The lump is painless and hard in consistency and the lymph nodes, if enlarged, are discrete and hard in consistency. Secondaries in the lung may cause haemoptysis and bone deposits may present with local bone pain or a pathological fracture.

Management

Total thyroidectomy should be performed, with every attempt to preserve the parathyroid glands. Any involved lymph nodes should also be excised, and on occasions this may involve block dissection.

Once the main thyroid tissue has been removed it should then be possible to detect metastases by giving radioiodine and scanning for uptake in lymph nodes, bones or other tissues. It is pointless doing such a scan before thyroidectomy as the normally situated gland will avidly take up the isotope and prevent uptake in any metastatic deposits.

Metastases which are identified by isotope scanning, and therefore are capable of taking up iodine, can be treated by therapeutic doses of radioiodine, and TSH suppression by the oral administration of T_4 or T_3 is advisable.

If no metastases are detected immediately after total thyroidectomy repeat scans should be undertaken at intervals in the follow-up of these patients, as deposits may appear later. The overall prognosis for this type of tumour is distinctly worse than for papillary carcinoma: 10-year survival rates are only around 50%.

Anaplastic carcinoma

This tumour has the worst prognosis of all thyroid tumours. Microscopically the majority of the tumours show spindle cells and giant cell formation, with a lack of any follicular pattern. It is a highly undifferentiated tumour and spreads locally by infiltrating neighbouring structures, e.g. the muscles, the trachea and the oesophagus.

Clinical features

The patients are generally old, between the ages of 60 and 80 years, and females are more commonly affected than males. The patient usually presents with a diffuse swelling of the neck rather than a localized lump. There may be a dull ache in the neck, hoarseness or a change of voice because of involvement of recurrent laryngeal nerve or dyspnoea due to tracheal obstruction. Pain in the bones or pathological fractures due to bony metastases may occur. On examination, only one lobe may be affected in the early stages but later the whole gland is enlarged, perhaps massively so, and the tumour mass feels solid. There may be skin changes due to infiltration, and the movement of the thyroid gland on swallowing may become restricted due to the infiltration of the neighbouring structures. Deep cervical lymph nodes may be palpable, hard and fixed. Examination of the vocal cords may show weakness or paralysis.

Anaplastic carcinomas are very lethal and death occurs within months rather than years. Curative resection is not usually possible. Surgical measures are usually limited to simple debulking and decompression of the trachea, if this is feasible. External irradiation may temporarily diminish the size of the mass, but as the tumours rarely take up iodine, giving radioiodine is generally quite ineffective.

These are the three main types of carcinoma arising from the glandular epithelium of the thyroid gland proper. There are in addition two other forms of malignancy which very rarely grow in the thyroid, although arising from other cells—medullary carcinoma and malignant lymphoma.

Medullary carcinoma

These very rare tumours arise from the parafollicular cells (C cells) of the thyroid gland which are derived from the ultimobranchial body. Macroscopically, the tumour is solid, with a uniform yellowish-grey surface, and is well delineated from the rest of the thyroid tissue. The cells are in solid nests, regular in size and shape, with granular cytoplasm. The stroma may contain amyloid, which is characteristic, and may calcify.

The incidence of the tumour is highest in the fourth decade but younger patients between 20 and 30 years may be affected. Females are more affected than males. Clinically the patient usually presents with a lump which is firm, smooth and discrete. Occasionally the condition appears as part of a multiple endocrine neoplasia (MEN) syndrome, with tumours of other glands, especially phaeochromocytoma also occurring in the same patient. There may be a family history of similar disorder.

Although several different hormones may be released by the tumour, the commonest is calcitonin, and indeed the finding of elevated levels of calcitonin in the serum can be a useful diagnostic aid.

Both lymph node and blood-borne metastases are common by the time of clinical presentation.

Management

The tumour is not hormone-dependent. The treatment is by total thyroidectomy and resection of the involved lymph nodes. Five-year survival figures of only 50% are usual.

Malignant lymphoma

Primary malignant lymphoma of the thyroid gland

is also very rare, and may be associated with Hashimoto's disease or may arise per se in a normal thyroid gland. The thyroid gland may be involved alone or along with the regional lymph nodes. The treatment is by irradiation with adjuvant chemotherapy, even if regional lymph nodes are involved. Surgical resection is not needed, except for the relief of any mechanical compression symptoms. The prognosis is good if the lymph nodes are not involved; it is worse if the thyroid disease is a part of widespread malignant lymphoma.

Secondary deposits in the thyroid gland are rare, but occasionally they may arise from malignant melanoma or from carcinoma of breast, lung, kidney or uterine cervix.

THYROID DYSFUNCTIONS

Hyperthyroidism

The state of overactivity of the gland is usually accompanied by obvious diffuse or nodular enlargement of the gland, in which case the disorder is often referred to as toxic goitre.

There are three recognizably different syndromes which account for the vast majority of all presentations of hyperthyroidism:

1. Primary thyrotoxicosis—Graves disease.
2. Secondary, arising with a multinodular goitre.
3. Toxic adenoma—the excess hormone production arises from a single functioning adenoma.

Primary thyrotoxicosis—Graves disease

The exact aetiology of the syndrome is not clear. However, there is no doubt that the normal relationship between the TSH of the anterior pituitary and the circulating thyroid hormones is disrupted in the disease, and in spite of large quantities of thyroid hormone in the circulation, TSH is either not suppressed or the control normally exercised by the anterior pituitary over the thyroid secretion is lost in some way and the secretion of the thyroid hormones continues unchecked.

Recently it has been shown that a specific globulin is produced in hyperthyroid states and this competes with TSH for combination with receptor sites on the membranes of thyroid cells. Having combined with it, it continues to stimulate the cell. Thyroid-stimulating antibody is thought to be a part of an autoimmune phenomenon. Whatever the primary mechanism may be, the net result is that the thyroid gland becomes endocrinologically autonomous and continues to secrete T_4 and T_3 independent of any control which is normally exercised in the production of these hormones by the anterior pituitary.

Pathology

The gland becomes more vascular and increases in size. The thyroid cells lining the acini multiply and, instead of one layer, many layers of cells are found. The acini appear to be devoid of colloid and the lining cells appear in the form of convoluted ribbons inside the acini.

Clinical features

The majority of patients are young women, and they present with a diffuse goitre and a varying number of the classical symptoms of hyperthyroidism listed in Table 25.1.—both the goitre and the functional symptoms appear about the same time. While nervousness, tremor, irritability, weight loss and eye changes are common in this disorder, cardiac manifestations are rare.

Palpation reveals generalized enlargement, often symmetrical but perhaps more apparent on one side than the other, and the pyramidal lobe may be quite prominent. The consistency is soft to firm and the increased vascularity may be reflected in a palpable systolic thrill and a bruit heard on auscultation over the lateral lobes.

Eye signs. Some amplification is perhaps needed regarding the definitions of the signs listed in Table 25.1. By exophthalmos is meant true forward displacement of the eyeball on account of an increase in the cellular and fluid content in the retrobulbar tissues (Fig. 25.5). Clinically, the examiner is able to see sclera between the lower eyelid and the iris, with the patient looking straight ahead. Rarely the degree of proptosis is so extreme that there is papilloedema, corneal ulceration and virtual inability to move the eyeball. This serious con-

Table 25.1 Symptoms and signs of hyperthyroidism

	Symptoms	Signs
Increased metabolic heat production	Feeling of warmth Heat intolerance Preference for cold weather Sweating	Warm, moist skin Maybe pyrexia
Gastrointestinal system	Weight loss in spite of increased appetite Increased frequency of bowel motions—frank diarrhoea Thirst	Loss of body fat
Cardiovascular system	Palpitations Shortness of breath Angina	Tachycardia Raised sleeping pulse rate Hypertension and increased pulse pressure Atrial fibrillation Cardiac failure
Neuromuscular system	Undue fatiguability Muscular weakness Tremor of hands General restlessness	Weakness of the proximal limb muscles Brisk tendon reflexes Tremors in the fingers Hyperkinetic movements
Genitourinary system	Polyuria Oligo- or amenorrhoea	
Psychiatric	Irritability Anxiety	Instability Insomnia Frank psychosis
Eyes	Prominence of eyes Increased lacrimation Double vision	Exophthalmos Lid retraction Lid lag Ophthalmoplegia

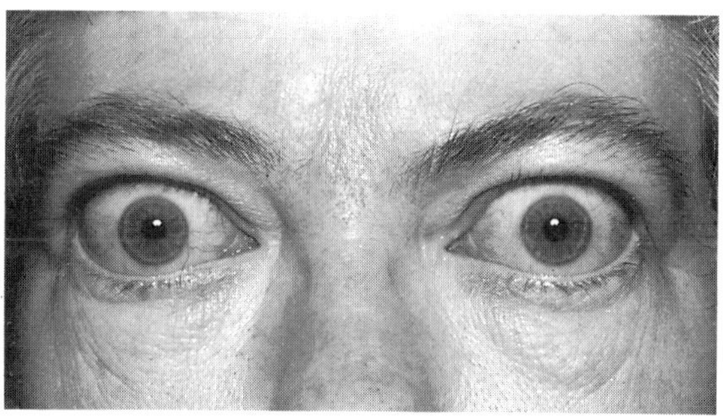

Fig. 25.5 Exophthalmos in Graves disease—thyrotoxic goitre. A clear margin of sclera is seen all around the iris, and the eyes appear to be staring. The prominence of the eyeball is best detected by looking either laterally at the patient or from above, looking down over the forehead.

dition, which carries a danger of loss of sight, is called ophthalmoplegia.

Lid retraction implies that a rim of sclera can be clearly seen between the upper eyelid and the iris, again with the patient looking directly ahead.

Lid lag is detected by the examiner when he or she sees sclera between the upper eyelid and the irises as the patient follows a finger brought steadily down from above within the patient's field of vision, while the patient's head remains fixed in position.

Diagnosis

Before direct measurement of thyroid hormones became available various clinical diagnostic indices, e.g. that of Wayne, were used in ascertaining the status of the thyroid gland. Numerical scorings were allotted to the different symptoms and signs, the most important symptoms being loss of weight with increased appetite, palpitations, preference for cold weather and excessive sweating, and the most important signs being the presence of a goitre and exophthalmos in a nervous and excitable patient, and a raised sleeping pulse. All clinical features are not present in every patient of thyrotoxicosis, nor are they of equal importance in establishing the diagnosis. Some, like tachycardia, tremor of the fingers and nervousness, may be present in other common disorders, e.g. anxiety neurosis. Loss of weight with increased appetite may also be a feature of diabetes mellitus.

Although the diagnosis of thyrotoxicosis can usually be fairly confidently established on clinical grounds it is desirable to confirm it by finding elevated serum levels of T_3 and T_4, with low or absent TSH. Other tests, e.g. the TSH response to TRH, may give added information regarding the TSH reserve supplies.

Secondary hyperthyroidism—toxic multinodular goitre

In this condition the toxic symptoms appear in a patient known to have had a nodular goitre for some time previously, and the patient is usually middle-aged or elderly. Generally there are fewer eye symptoms and signs, but cardiovascular manifestations are commoner. It may be either that the areas of glandular tissue between the nodules become overactive in the production of hormone, or occasionally that one or more nodules become autonomous and overactive. Isotopic iodine uptake scans will give helpful information on the distribution of overactive tissue within the whole gland.

Toxic adenoma

The presence of a pre-existing benign non-toxic adenoma may have been known for some time before the onset of thyrotoxic symptoms. Here again the eye changes tend to be minimal and the cardiovascular symptoms are more frequent than with Graves disease. The single overactive adenoma should be clearly identified on isotope scan.

Treatment of hyperthyroidism

There are three forms of treatment available: antithyroid drugs, surgery and radioactive iodine.

Antithyroid drugs

Antithyroid drugs act by depressing the production of thyroid hormones and their release from the gland. Although in the past other agents, such as potassium iodide, potassium perchlorate and the thiourea group of drugs, have been used, today the drug of choice is carbimazole, in a dose of 10 mg up to three or four times per day. There is usually a period of 7–14 days after starting the preparation before any clinical improvement is noticed. It is desirable to space the doses evenly throughout the day in an attempt to maintain adequate levels. When the patient becomes euthyroid the dose should be reduced to a maintenance level of 5 mg two to three times per day.

Carbimazole is generally the first line of treatment for primary hyperthyroidism and Graves disease and a proportion may go into spontaneous remission after treatment for 12–18 months and many physicians therefore recommend stopping the drug after this period of time, keeping the patient under follow-up surveillance in case there is a later relapse.

If prolonged carbimazole treatment is used the patient needs to be checked for side-effects which occur in a very small minority—such as vomiting, skin rashes or, most serious of all, agranulocytosis. Routine blood counts at intervals of 2–3 months are desirable and the patients should also be told to seek medical advice should they develop a sore throat or fever.

Although carbimazole and indeed other antithyroid drugs are effective in achieving a euthyroid state, they may lead to an increase in the size of a goitre, probably by promoting an increase in circulating TSH levels. For this reason these drugs are usually not the first choice where there is a large goitre, and particularly in both toxic multinodular goitre and toxic adenoma, surgical resection is generally preferred.

Surgery

Surgical removal of the greater part of each lobe plus the isthmus, i.e. subtotal thyroidectomy, is certainly the quickest and easiest way of correcting hyperthyroidism and removing the obvious goitre. As has already been stated, it is the treatment of choice in toxic multinodular goitre and toxic adenoma, although in the latter some surgeons advocate lobectomy alone if the adenoma is confidently located to one side and can be adequately removed by this procedure. In Graves disease subtotal thyroidectomy is also preferred when the goitre is large, when relapses have occurred after antithyroid drugs, or where there is any sensitivity to these drugs. Also some patients given the options of prolonged medication or operation will prefer the latter.

Of course there are risks to every operation, as there are to other forms of treatment. The mortality risk is extremely small in experienced hands. There is, however, about a 5% chance of recurrence of hyperthyroidism in later years, as the remnants of the lateral lobes left at the operation enlarge and hypertrophy, and there is also about a 20% chance of hypothyroidism subsequently. This is simply because it is difficult to judge with precision exactly how much gland to leave at operation. Any hypo-thyroidism is easy to correct by simple oral administration of T_4.

Rarely parathyroid deficiency will arise after the operation due to removal or damage to all functioning parathyroid tissue, and this may be quite difficult to control. Its management is further discussed on page 224.

Preparation for operation. Ideally the patient should be completely euthyroid by the time he or she comes to surgery, and the commonest way of achieving this is by carbimazole. In the past it was common practice to stop antithyroid drugs about 2 weeks before operation and administer an iodine preparation during this time in the belief that this decreased the vascularity of the gland. However, there is little evidence of its effectiveness in this regard, and many surgeons no longer use this approach.

Increasingly popular in preparation for operation, however, is beta-adrenergic blockade by propranolol. This, either alone or combined with antithyroid agents, will particularly control the cardiovascular manifestations of the hyperthyroid state, and as these are both the most distressing to the patient and the important features of the disorder, it is a highly effective method of preparation for operation.

Before thyroidectomy it is also important, in addition to other regular preoperative checks, to examine the vocal cords to detect any weakness or paralysis in case of doubt about any postoperative damage to the recurrent laryngeal nerves. It is also useful to know whether thyroid antibodies are present and the level of serum calcium, in case of postoperative hypoparathyroid problems.

Technique. General anaesthesia with endotracheal intubation is used. A collar incision in the crease of the neck is made and upper and lower flaps of skin are mobilized; pretracheal (strap) muscles are separated in the midline and retracted or divided. Middle thyroid veins are identified, ligated and divided, the lobes are mobilized and then the superior and inferior thyroid arteries are ligated. The inferior thyroid artery is ligated in continuity. The superior thyroid vessels are tied close to the gland while the inferior thyroid artery is tied as far away from the gland as possible to avoid injury to the superior and recurrent laryngeal nerves respectively. Special care is taken to avoid injury to the recurrent laryngeal nerves, preferably by exposing them at the lower pole and following the course of the nerves upwards. After devascularization of the thyroid lobes, subtotal resection of each lobe is done: seven-eighths to nine-tenths of the thyroid gland is removed, leaving behind 4–5 g of thyroid tissue on each side. The parathyroid glands, lying close to branches of the inferior thyroid arteries, should be identified and safeguarded. Absolute haemostasis is achieved. A drain (Redivac) or drains are left to prevent any haematoma following operation. The wound is then closed in layers, using fine clips to appose the skin, as these leave less noticeable scarring than stitches.

Postoperative complications. These are very rare, but the ones which are of particular relevance—and all are potentially very serious—are the following:

1. *Haemorrhage*: The danger here is that a collection of blood may accumulate in a closed space, behind the strap muscles and in front of and at each side of the trachea, causing asphyxia. Treatment is urgent. The wound should be immediately opened in the ward, strap muscles separated or divided and haematoma evacuated. It is important to realize that the haemato-

ma is behind the strap muscles, so simple skin and platysma opening will not relieve the obstruction. Once the haematoma has been evacuated, the patient can be taken to the operating theatre, and proper haemostasis secured.

2. *Thyrotoxic crisis*: This should very rarely occur if the patient is rendered euthyroid by proper preoperative preparation. It is thought to develop as a result of excess of thyroid hormones entering the circulation due to handling of the gland during the operation. The syndrome consists of hyperpyrexia, restlessness, air hunger, tachycardia, mental confusion and even delirium. In serious cases even death may occur in spite of treatment. The treatment consists of rapid beta-adrenergic blockade with propranolol, and intravenous hydrocortisone. Iodine has also been recommended but is of doubtful value. Sedation and sponging to reduce hyperpyrexia may also help.
3. *Tetany*: This may start immediately or shortly after operation. It is due to damage to parathyroid glands. The glands may have been excised, but commonly it is due to interference with their blood supply. The result is hypoparathyroidism with a resultant fall in serum calcium and a rise in the serum phosphorous level. Clinically it presents with carpopedal spasm, twitching and paraesthesia, especially around the mouth. The serum calcium should be immediately estimated. Treatment consists of giving intravenously 10–20 ml of 10% calcium gluconate immediately. In most cases the symptoms improve and parathyroid function returns to normal. In cases in which no improvement is achieved, oral calciferol (400 000–500 000 u) may be given, followed by 100 000 units every day. The dosage depends upon the level of the serum calcium. In some cases dihydrotachysterol may be tried to restore the serum calcium to normal.

Voice changes. Some degree of transient weakness or other changes in the voice is fairly frequent after thyroid operations. Most of these are understandably due to the trauma of both the surgery and the endotracheal intubation. If the vocal cords have been seen on direct laryngoscopy at the end of the operation to be moving normally, the patient can be clearly reassured that full recovery can be expected.

Rarely hoarseness will be due to damage to a recurrent laryngeal nerve. Again the majority are due to mechanical pressure or stretching of the nerve and recovery will gradually ensue. Minor changes in the voice may also result from damage to the external laryngeal nerve, which passes near to the upper pole of the lateral lobe.

If the very rare occurrence of bilateral damage to the recurrent laryngeal nerves occurs, the patient may choke or have severe stridor, and urgently require tracheostomy.

Radioactive iodine

Because of the theoretical risks with any radioactive material that carcinogenesis or mutation within germ cells may arise, there is great reservation about using this form of treatment in those under 40 years of age.

Although the idea of simply drinking a single dose of the isotope and thus suppressing the overactive glandular cells is indeed an attractive one, there are several problems, in addition to the potentially oncogenic ones, which have led to this mode of therapy being less popular than at first hoped when it was introduced.

One of the main difficulties is judging the correct dose which will suppress just the right amount of overactive thyroid to leave the patient euthyroid. Unfortunately up to 80% of patients treated by this method will become hypothyroid in the months or years after dosage and thus lifelong follow-up is required if it is employed. The initial effect may also be quite slow, taking several months to appear.

In those patients with other medical disorders which render them at high risk for general anaesthesia, and in those few developing recurrent hyperthyroidism following previous thyroidectomy, radioiodine administration is the treatment of choice. Some would also argue that it is a satisfactory way of managing toxic adenoma in those over 40.

THYROIDITIS

Autoimmune thyroiditis

Under this heading comes a range of degrees of damage to the thyroid gland by lymphocytic infiltration, accompanied by the presence of circulating antibodies to thyroid globulin and to subcellular fractions of the acinar cells. The lymphocytic infiltration damages the normal hormone-producing cells, and as it progresses leads to frank hypothyroidism. The antibodies are believed to result from the damaged thyroid rather than being the cause of the disorder. There may be a family history of other autoimmune diseases, e.g. pernicious anaemia or gastritis.

When the pathological changes are minimal there are only a few scattered foci of lymphocytic deposits, usually organized into follicles as in normal lymph nodes, and the intervening thyroid gland tissue appears normal. The most severe and widespread changes produce generalized enlargement, i.e. a goitre, with a characteristic firm consistency and the condition is referred to as Hashimoto's disease.

Hashimoto's disease

This is 10 times commoner in women than men and the majority of patients are in their 40s or 50s. The thyroid gland is diffusely enlarged, although one part may be much more obvious than the rest (Fig. 25.6). It may be large or small and of variable consistency from soft to firm, depending upon the degree of cellularity or fibrosis. Microscopically the gland shows diffuse lymphocytic infiltration of the gland with lymphoid follicles, many plasma cells and variable change from destruction to hyperplasia with eventual fibrosis. Some of the follicular cells are enlarged and eosinophilic in appearance, and are known as Askanazy cells.

Clinically, the onset of the disease may be slow and asymptomatic, or on the other hand so virulent that it may resemble an acute form of granulomatous thyroiditis. In the beginning there may be evidence of hyperthyroidism but sooner or later hypothyroidism is bound to occur due to increased loss of functioning glandular cells.

The diagnosis of autoimmune thyroiditis can be confirmed by the demonstration of autoimmune antibodies in the blood. Thyroid hormone levels should be measured in the blood. The condition may be difficult to differentiate from nodular goitre, carcinoma and malignant lymphoma. A needle or open biopsy may be necessary to reach a final diagnosis.

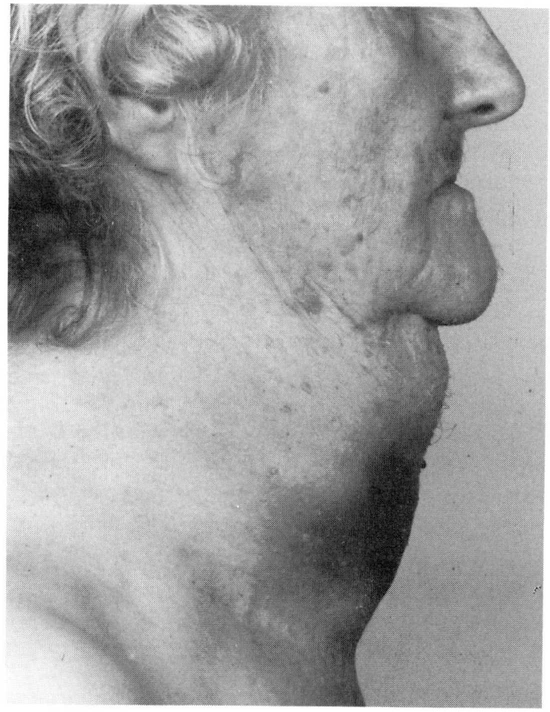

Fig. 25.6 Thyroiditis. This produces a massive thickened, often 'woody' swelling which, as it extends through the gland may come to occupy most of the front of the neck, as in this patient.

Treatment

When the diagnosis has been established the treatment is to give full replacement dosage of T_4, because eventual hypothyroidism is inevitable and undesirable. The dose should be sufficient to suppress TSH secretion, and this may lead to a decrease in size of the goitre. Surgery should not be recommended unless to remove a particularly large goitre or relieve any pressure symptoms. This is rarely required.

Riedel's thyroiditis

This is an extremely rare cause of thyroid enlargement. It is characterized by the occurrence of dense fibrosis in the thyroid which may extend beyond the confines of the gland to involve neighbouring structures. The aetiology is not known but there is no evidence of it having an autoimmune basis, and it is most probably a collagen disease. The goitre may be unilateral or bilateral and is stony hard on palpation. Pressure symptoms due to tra-

compression commonly arise. It may produce hypothyroidism when the thyroid tissue is extensively replaced by fibrous tissue. It may be difficult to differentiate this condition from anaplastic carcinoma of the thyroid except by biopsy.

The only treatment available is the removal of as much abnormal thyroid tissue as possible in order to relieve compression of the trachea and to make the patient as comfortable as possible.

Acute bacterial thyroiditis

The thyroid is very rarely invaded by pyogenic bacteria, but when this does occur, the patient complains of a painful swelling in the region of the thyroid, and usually has constitutional symptoms in the form of fever and malaise. The thyroid gland is tender and enlarged. An appropriate antibiotic may cause resolution of the inflammation. If pus has formed drainage is necessary.

De Quervain's thyroiditis (subacute thyroiditis)

This very rare clinical condition is probably due to a virus infection, as it frequently follows an upper respiratory tract infection. There are usually symptoms of muscle ache and fatigue and there is no leukocytosis. It varies in severity, and may start with an acute onset of pain and tenderness in the thyroid gland, and the pain may radiate to the mandible and the ears.

On examination the thyroid gland is usually uniformly enlarged and tender, and the skin over it may be red. The erythrocyte sedimentation rate is raised.

The condition pursues a variable course but usually subsides within a few weeks to a few months, although relapses may occur. Usually no treatment except analgesics is needed.

Hyperparathyroidism

The main disorder of the parathyroids for which surgical treatment may be required is primary hyperparathyroidism, usually arising from a single parathyroid adenoma. Less commonly there is functioning hyperplasia of more than one gland, or of all four glands. Even more rarely the disorder is due to a malignant parathyroid tumour.

When there is generalized diffuse hyperplasia of all the parathyroid tissue in response to lowered circulating levels of calcium, e.g. in renal failure, malabsorption or, rarely, vitamin D and calcium deficiency, this is referred to as secondary hyperparathyroidism. Management in this situation is directed at the primary disorder or appropriate supplements.

The clinical manifestations of hyperparathyroidism include urinary tract stones, peptic ulcer, bone pains, the detection of bone cysts, psychological disturbance and pancreatitis. The detection of an elevated serum calcium level points to the diagnosis, which should then be confirmed by the finding of elevated levels of parathormone in the serum.

The only satisfactory treatment for primary parathyroidism is surgical removal of either the solitary adenoma or the greater part of the total functioning glandular tissue in the case of hyperplasia. Although a number of methods of locating the glands preoperatively have been advocated, none has found easy universal applicability, and it is better to proceed to direct operative exposure of all four glands on mobilizing the thyroid before deciding on what excision is required in each individual case.

Where an adenoma is obvious in one of the glands this is excised, and some surgeons also recommend removal of one or two of the remaining ones. If there is uniform enlargement of all four glands, three should be removed and a segment of the remaining one may also be excised.

26. The adrenal glands

Surgical removal of one or both adrenal glands may be indicated for either endocrine tumours or for functioning hyperplasia of the cortical tissue. In the past bilateral adrenalectomy used to be used in some patients with widespread carcinoma of the breast, mainly where there was reason to believe that the tumour was hormone-influenced. However, this operation is now rarely performed in this clinical situation, and in any event adequate suppression of adrenal function, if desired, can be achieved by the drug aminoglutethamide.

It will be recalled that the right adrenal lies medial to the upper pole of the right kidney and is also tucked closely behind the lateral aspect of the inferior vena cava. The left gland is applied to the medial pole of the left kidney and to the aorta, though generally it is not so closely applied to it as the right one is to the vena cava. The arterial supply is from a variable number of branches arising directly from the aorta. The adrenal veins are more constant in pattern, the right one passing from the anterior aspect of the gland to the posterolateral part of the vena cava, whereas the left adrenal vein passes downwards from the lower pole to join the left renal vein. It is often joined by the left inferior phrenic vein before entering the renal vein.

The two distinctly different parts of each gland—cortex and medulla (Fig. 26.1)—have quite different physiological roles: the cortex produces various steroid hormones, while the medulla manufactures and secretes catecholamines, notably adrenaline and noradrenaline. Furthermore, the cortex can be subdivided into three separate functioning layers—the outer glomerulosa zone producing aldosterone, the middle fasciculata and inner reticularis zones producing cortisol and various sex-active hormones with both androgenic and oestrogenic properties.

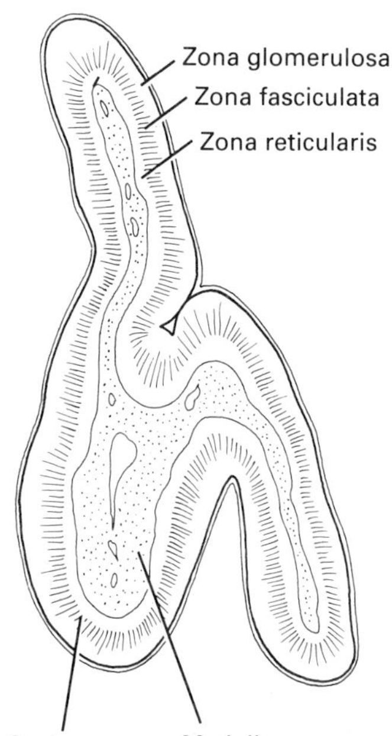

Fig. 26.1 Diagrammatic cross-section through the adrenal gland, showing the medulla and surrounding cortex. The cortex is in three layers—the inner zona reticularis, middle fasciculata, and outer glomerulosa.

PHAEOCHROMOCYTOMA

This tumour, arising from adrenal medullary tissue and secreting excessive quantities of adrenaline or noradrenaline or both, is nearly always benign. The majority are solitary tumours, so that there is a very good chance of complete cure of the condition after removal of the gland containing it. However,

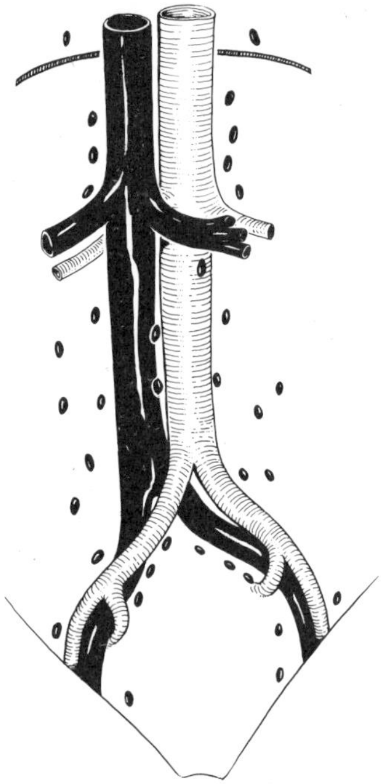

Fig. 26.2 Various possible sites of ectopic adrenal gland tissue, from above the diaphragm to deep in the pelvis.

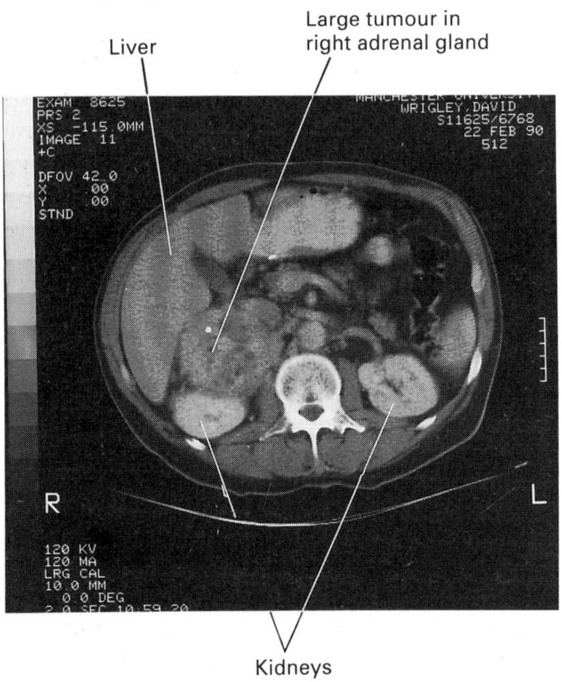

Fig. 26.3 Computerized tomography scan showing the clear outline of an adrenal tumour.

a small proportion arise in ectopic sites (Fig. 26.2), e.g. the retroperitoneal para-aortic region, or rarely the chest, neck or pelvis, and very rarely the tumour is frankly malignant.

The dominant clinical feature is hypertension, which may be either persistent or episodic. In the latter there are bouts of headache, tachycardia, sweating, possibly tightness in the chest and either pallor or flushing of the face. During the attack, blood pressure readings of greater than 200/100 mmHg may be recorded. Sometimes the paroxysms are brought on by exercise, local mechanical pressure in the abdomen or sudden changes in body position, but at other times there appears to be no obvious precipitating factor. Visual field disturbances and other eye symptoms may also occur and these are a feature of the more persistent hypertension presentation.

Glycosuria and thyrotoxicosis are two metabolic manifestations which may also arise from the excess quantities of the catecholamines. Most patients with hypertension will have either essential, otherwise unexplained hypertension, or one of the many other causes, but when it occurs in young persons or the pattern is paroxysmal the possibility of phaeochromocytoma should be borne in mind. The diagnosis can be readily confirmed by the finding of grossly elevated levels of the metabolite vanillylmandelic acid in the urine. If the laboratory facilities are available then even more detailed analysis of both adrenaline and noradrenaline levels in either blood or urine can be done.

The diagnosis having been made, the next problem is localization of the tumour, and this is probably best accomplished by computerized tomography (CT) scanning (Fig. 26.3) and possibly by magnetic resonance imaging (MRI) when this is more widely available. Alternative though less reliable techniques include X-ray tomography with or without intravenous contrast pyelography, and retropeitoneal gas insufflation radiography (Fig. 26.4)

Treatment

Assuming accurate localization has been obtained the relevant adrenal gland is approached via either a transabdominal route or through a lumbar, renal type of approach.

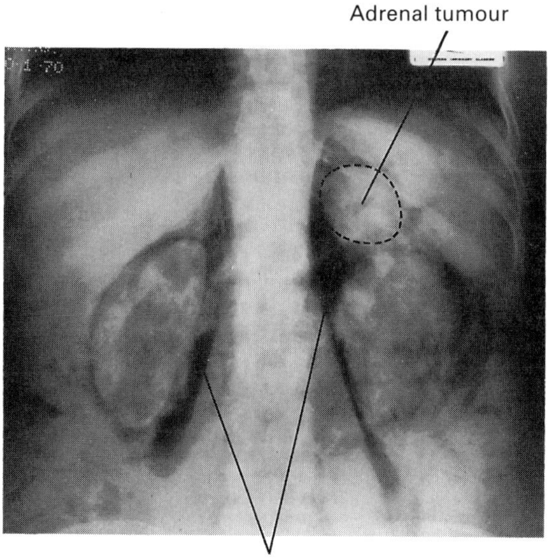

Fig. 26.4 An adrenal tumour outlined by the older and less reliable technique of retroperitoneal gas insufflation.

In view of the hazards of hypertension and the very real chance of sudden exacerbations occurring from even gentle pressure on the tumour during the operation it is extremely important to have good pre- and peroperative control of the blood pressure. It is usual practice to give an alpha-blocking agent, e.g. phenoxybenzamine, for about 10 days before the operation, with perhaps the addition of a beta-blocker, e.g. propanolol, to minimize tachycardia. Immediately before operation the anaesthetist should establish preferably two good intravenous lines, and have continuous monitoring of heart rate and blood pressure. Repeated doses of either alpha- or beta-blockers may be required and sodium nitroprusside, which has a rapid direct action on blood vessels, is often needed throughout the procedure, until all venous drainage of the tumour has been clamped and divided.

Indeed the successful reduction of blood pressure on removal of a tumour is a good guide that it is the only source of excessively functioning tissue. If the pressure does not fall, search should be made of the other adrenal gland, and of the other ectopic sites where glandular tissue may reside.

ALDOSTERONISM

One of the main actions of aldosterone, the most powerful mineralocorticoid produced by the adrenal gland, is on the distal renal tubule, where it promotes the exchange of sodium for potassium, causing retention of sodium and increased loss of potassium. Therefore, when excess levels of aldosterone are released into the circulation by tumour or hyperplasia of the aldosterone-producing cells of the adrenal cortex, there is hypokalaemia, loss of hydrogen and therefore alkalosis, sodium retention and consequent hypertension.

Primary hyperaldosteronism is that which results from a tumour , usually an adenoma, or essential hyperplasia. However, increased levels of aldosterone can also arise in response to primary renal disease, hypertension from other causes, and various disorders producing oedema, and under these circumstances it is referred to as secondary hyperaldosteronism.

The usual clinical presentation is that a patient found to have hypertension is also noted to have a low serum potassium concentration. It is as well to have one or two repeat estimations of the serum potassium, and if hypokalaemia is confirmed then it is possible to measure the aldosterone levels directly by radioimmunoassay. If there is doubt as to whether the condition is primary or secondary, plasma renin levels may help to discriminate. In the primary disorder they will be normal, while they are almost always elevated in secondary hyperaldosteronism. Localization of a tumour in the primary disorder is sought, as for other adrenal tumours, by CT scan or MRI.

Treatment

Spironolactone, the aldosterone antagonist, should keep the condition under control, and in particular maintain a normal blood pressure, and is useful in preparing patients with primary hyperaldosteronism for operation. It can also be used on a more long-term basis in those who are unfit for surgery, and is of course the mainstay of treatment for those with uncorrectable secondary hyperaldosteronism.

However, for the primary disorder, excision of the gland containing a single adenoma or bilateral adrenalectomy for hyperplasia are the relevant procedures. In the latter some surgeons choose to leave a small remnant of one of the glands—estimated at no more than 20–30% of that gland—in an effort to leave at least some functioning tissue. The patient may still need postoperative hormone replacement, and those having complete removal of both glands will certainly require lifelong maintenance therapy, with hydrocortisone and perhaps also fludrocortisone.

CUSHING'S SYNDROME

This well known syndrome, chiefly characterized by 'moon-face' truncal obesity, striae and hypertension (Fig. 26.5), is due to an excess production of cortisol and related hormones, and it may arise from a pituitary chromophobe or basophil adenoma (commonest cause), or inappropriate secretion from tumours in bronchus or other sites, or primary tumours of the adrenal cortex. Once again the adrenal tumours are most often benign, i.e. adenomas, and solitary true carcinoma is rare. There is a distinct female preponderance.

Clinical features in addition to those already mentioned include amenorrhoea, mild diabetes mellitus, acne, cyanosis especially on the face, hirsutism, weakness of muscles, osteoporosis and purpura. The onset and progression of the syndrome are usually gradual, and it is often possible to have a high diagnostic suspicion before the full-blown picture is developed. Occasionally when the source of the excess hormone is ectopic the history is much more rapid and dramatic.

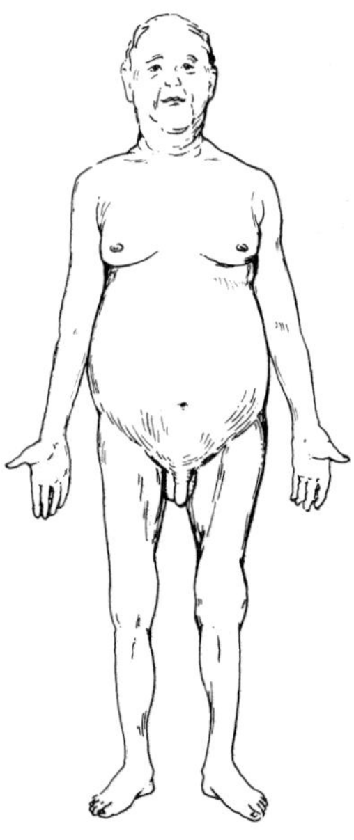

Fig. 26.5 Characteristic clinical features of Cushing's syndrome—'moon-face', truncal obesity, abdominal striae and gynaecomastia.

Cortisol levels can be measured in blood, and as there is normally a diurnal variation with higher values in the morning, it may be helpful to make several measurements at different times of the day. In Cushing's syndrome the levels remain constantly elevated throughout the day, since hormone secretion is autonomous. Once an elevated plasma cortisol level is established the next test to consider is the dexamethasone suppression test. An overnight dose of 1 mg will suppress cortisol output in normal individuals, but will have no such effect on Cushing's syndrome. Finally the measurement of circulating adrenocorticotrophic hormone (ACTH) should discriminate between an adrenal tumour, where the plasma ACTH is low; ectopic ACTH production, where plasma ACTH remains high, and Cushing's syndrome (or disease) of pituitary origin, where the plasma ACTH remains normal.

Where an adrenal tumour is suspected, again localization is pursued using either CT scanning or MRI. In the absence of these expensive techniques success may be achieved with X-ray tomography or perirenal gas insufflation.

Treatment

Suppression of cortisol synthesis can be achieved by the drugs metyrapone or aminoglutethamide, and these are used where surgery is contraindicated on account of other life-threatening disease, and also as preoperative preparation.

Where there is a pituitary tumour the aim should be either to enucleate it by microsurgical excision through a neurosurgical approach, or to ablate the pituitary by radiotherapy.

For a single adrenal adenoma removal of the single gland from which the tumour arises is adequate. When hyperplasia is present, total bilateral adrenalectomy should be performed, and any attempt to leave a small remnant of gland is unwise as postoperative hormone control is difficult, and recurrence is common. Of course, following bilateral adrenalectomy lifelong maintenance therapy is necessary. Initially high doses, e.g. 100 mg cortisol, are given intramuscularly and this is gradually reduced over the next few days under close clinical and biochemical supervision until a regular long-term dose of hydrocortisone of around 20–30 mg/day is reached. It may also be necessary to add a daily dose of 0.1 mg fludrocortisone.

It will be appreciated that patients with Cushing's syndrome are vulnerable to many complications, e.g. wound infection, excess bleeding, hyper- and hypotensive crises, and also gastric erosions and ulcers and pulmonary embolism. Their operative and nursing care is demanding, but once safely over the postoperative convalescent period there should be a steadily progressive diminution in all symptoms and signs over several weeks or months.

OTHER ADRENAL TUMOURS

These are all rare. Both virilizing and feminizing tumours may occur and in addition a genetically determined enzyme deficiency may induce hyperplasia of the adrenal cortex to release excess quantities of androgens. This disturbs growth in both sexes and causes virilizing signs in females. Conversely, feminizing signs in males may denote the presence of an oestrogen-producing adrenal tumour.

Non-functioning carcinoma is likely to present with the manifestations of either local or distant spread. Cysts, neuroblastoma and ganglioneuroma complete the list of rarities.

27. The oesophagus

EMBRYOLOGY

An understanding of the outline of the embryological development of this organ is helpful in appreciating some of the disorders encountered in clinical practice, particularly the congenital abnormalities.

In the early embryo the oesophagus is represented by a column of cells stretching from the developing pharynx to the dilated part of the upper gastrointestinal tract which in due course will form the stomach. The oesophageal column elongates, and then develops into a tube from which an outpouching occurs anteriorly to form the lungs and upper respiratory passages. Normally the separation of the latter from the developing oesophagus is complete, but it is easy to understand that on occasions when the process is incomplete various forms of fistula communication between the two systems may arise.

Imperfect cannulization of the developing oesophagus will also explain the occasional occurrence of congenital webs partly encircling the oesophagus.

It is believed that the stratified squamous epithelium, which normally lines the oesophagus from pharynx to oesophagogastric junction, begins somewhere in the middle of the oesophagus, and thereafter extends both proximally and distally. Incomplete migration of this stratified squamous epithelium may well account for occasional isolated pockets of columnar-type epithelium in the oesophageal lining.

ANATOMY

In adult life, the oesophagus, about 25 cm in length, passes through the posterior mediastinum behind the trachea and major air passages above, and the heart and pericardium below. The lower end passes through an opening in the right crus of the diaphragm to enter the proximal fundus of the stomach at a fairly precise line normally just below the diaphragm.

As already mentioned, the inner lining of the oesophagus is of stratified squamous epithelium, outside which there is a submucosal layer containing numerous small simple tubular glands secreting mainly mucus, and also containing numerous small blood vessels, lymphatics, and loose connective tissue. A double layer of muscular fibres surrounds these inner layers, the innermost layer being mainly circular in distribution, and the outer layer running longitudinally. At the upper end these smooth muscle coats merge with the skeletal muscles of the pharynx, and at the lower end they are continuous with the muscular layers of the stomach.

The oesophagus has both a parasympathetic nerve supply via the vagus nerve, and a sympathetic one from the regional sympathetic ganglionic chain.

PHYSIOLOGY

The main function of the oesophagus, of course, is simply to conduct the various materials which are swallowed from the mouth into the stomach, and furthermore a mechanism at the lower end of the organ normally ensures that there is minimal or no reflux of the material from the stomach back into the oesophagus. This is important, since the acid, digestive enzymes and any refluxed bile which may be present in the stomach are potentially harmful to the mucosa of the oesophagus.

A co-ordinated series of movements takes place

immediately after swallowing. First, there is relaxation of the musculature at the pharyngo-oesophageal junction, but as soon as the bolus enters the upper oesophagus the pharyngeal constrictor 'sphincter' contracts once more to ensure onward and downward passage of the material. Co-ordinated peristaltic contractions sweep the swallowed material down the oesophagus towards the stomach, and at the same time the area of high pressure in the lower oesophageal musculature, which normally prevents regurgitation, relaxes ahead of the propulsive wave to ensure complete transit into the stomach. As soon as the bolus has entered the stomach there is again a swift increase in pressure in the lower oesophageal musculature to prevent regurgitation. This finely co-ordinated sequence of propulsive movements is, of course, under the influence of several local reflex mechanisms involving both central nervous and autonomic reflex pathways, and it follows that damage or disease of any of the co-ordinated mechanisms may result in difficulty with swallowing.

In addition to the primary peristaltic wave which occurs normally on swallowing, there are two other types of contraction which may be seen in the oesophagus.

If there is abnormal distension of the oesophagus by either material sticking at any level on its passage through the organ, or as a result of reflux from the stomach, secondary muscular contractions may arise proximal to the distended area. These secondary contractions are an obvious local attempt to propel the obstructed or reflux material distally, and they again follow a co-ordinated pattern of downward sweeping waves.

Irregular ineffective contractions may occur in a localized segmental fashion, particularly in elderly patients. These tertiary contractions do not appear to be purposefully co-ordinated, and probably represent the effects of degenerative changes in the mechanisms regulating normal oesophageal motility. They are usually of no clinical significance.

SYMPTOMS OF OESOPHAGEAL DISEASE

Dysphagia

This is perhaps the commonest symptom of oesophageal disease, and it covers a wide range of symptoms from occasional difficulty in swallowing only relatively large fragments of solid food, to complete inability to get even liquids down. In some disorders, for example those associated with spasm or the early stages of achalasia of the cardia, the difficulty may be intermittent, whereas in diseases leading to gradual progressive obstruction of the lumen, for example carcinoma or fibrous stricture, the symptom of dysphagia will be continuous and indeed progressive.

The difficulty in swallowing may arise because of painful lesions in the mouth, pharynx or tonsils, or from inco-ordination of the swallowing mechanism as a result of damage to the supplying nerves, as in poliomyelitis. Occasionally pressure on the oesophagus from enlarged mediastinal lymph nodes, tumours such as bronchial carcinoma, or enlargement of the heart chambers or aorta can lead to some difficulty in swallowing.

However, more common than these various causes are those arising from physical narrowing of the oesophagus itself by tumours, principally carcinoma, by fibrous strictures, mostly the consequence of reflux from the stomach, and achalasia of the cardia, due to thickening and failure to relax of the musculature of the lower segment of the oesophagus.

Heartburn

This symptom, described as a sensation of burning or gnawing deep behind the sternum, is a reflection of inflammation or irritation of the delicate lining of the oesophagus, and is most often associated with reflux of irritating material from the stomach. It is often described as radiating upwards towards the neck or even into the mouth, when it may be accompanied by an acid-feeling at the back of the throat.

If it is associated with reflux from the stomach the symptom is most often troublesome when the patient lies flat or bends down, and is to some extent relieved by sitting up or standing.

Regurgitation

Where there is physical obstruction at some level in the oesophagus, or a pouch large enough to accommodate swallowed material, the patient may suddenly bring up some or all of the most recently ingested solids and/or liquids and, as is to be expected, this usually occurs very soon after an act of swallowing. The fact that the food is quite recognizable, with virtually no sign of digestion having taken place, and it is free from both acid juice and bile, usually distinguishes this regurgitation quite clearly from true vomiting.

Oesophageal pain

In addition to the recurrent and usually short-lasting symptom of heartburn described above, a more persistent, deep-seated pain deep within the chest and perhaps radiating up to the root of the neck or through to the back may arise from more continuous inflammatory changes and spasm of the musculature of the oesophagus. This pain is sometimes quite difficult to distinguish from that due to ischaemia of the heart. Furthermore, like the latter, pain arising from marked oesophageal spasm may be partially or completely relieved by glyceryl trinitrate. This type of oesophageal pain may occur spontaneously, or be triggered off by swallowing food or drink, and even after it is relieved it may be followed by a lesser feeling of discomfort in the same region, which gradually fades over a period of minutes or hours.

Respiratory symptoms

Because of the close proximity of the oesophagus to the air passages, it is not surprising that when there is obstruction to the oesophagus or other interference with the swallowing mechanisms, some aspiration of regurgitated material into the trachea and other respiratory passages may occur. This is most likely to happen when the patient lies down. Symptoms arising from the respiratory tract, e.g. cough, sputum, breathlessness and wheezing, may therefore be part of the medical history in someone with primary oesophageal problems, and indeed the respiratory symptoms may be the dominant ones.

Other symptoms

In various disorders of the oesophagus, particularly those associated with reflux, the mouth on occasions may rapidly fill with clear fluid, most of which is an increased flow of salivary juice, and this symptom is called 'water-brash'.

Although regurgitated material, particularly in carcinoma of the oesophagus, may on occasions contain a small streak of blood, frank haematemesis is rare as a result of any of the disorders already mentioned. Severe, profuse haematemesis can occur, however, from oesophageal varices which arise secondary to portal hypertension, and which will be discussed separately in Chapter 31.

EXAMINATION OF THE OESOPHAGUS

Since the organ is inaccessible to simple inspection and palpation, the principal physical signs to be looked for are in the neck for any sign of a mass which might be exerting pressure in the root of the neck, or evidence of enlarged lymph nodes in the supraclavicular fossa. The chest should also be examined for signs of respiratory infection. Finally, the liver may be enlarged from metastases from carcinoma situated at the lower end of the oesophagus.

The special investigations which are required to establish a clear diagnosis in oesophageal disorders include outlining of the organ by barium swallow, endoscopy and, where relevant indications arise, measurement of pressure and/or pH measurements within the lumen of the organ. In most cases the endoscopic examination is the one which will yield the most precise and clinically useful information, and even when the radiological appearances show the classical features of one or other disorder, it is usually wise to obtain the additional information from direct inspection and possibly biopsy through the endoscope. In addition, X-ray examination may detect one or two features which will warn the endoscopist of potential hazards during the subsequent introduction of the instrument.

X-ray

The examination should start with straight antero-posterior and lateral views of the neck and chest. These may reveal signs of respiratory infection, gross osteophyte formation on the cervical vertebrae which could increase the risk of damage to the oesophageal wall during endoscopy, or a soft-tissue shadow of a grossly dilated oesophagus characteristic of severe achalasia of the cardia.

Following these straight X-rays the entire oesophagus, stomach, and duodenum can be outlined by barium swallow and meal contrast radiography. This will give evidence of any structural abnormality such as diverticula, ulceration, or narrowing due to stricture, tumour or extrinsic pressure. The pattern of swallowing movements in the oesophagus can also be observed. The opportunity is also taken to examine both the stomach and duodenum for pathological lesions such as ulcers and tumours. It should be routine during this radiological investigation to test the competence of the oesophagogastric junction against regurgitation by applying increased pressure to the abdomen, or tilting the patient into the head-down position, or a combination of both manoeuvres. Finally, an assessment can usually be made of the state of the oesophageal mucosa, if a mixture of air and thin barium is used (double contrast).

Oesophagoscopy

Two types of instrument are available for this examination. The first is a rigid, slightly tapered metal tube approximately 45 cm in length, carrying a light source (Fig. 27.1); the second is the newer range of flexible fibreoptic instruments, the most modern of which have facilities for variable illumination, washing, suction, a channel for the passage of a special biopsy forceps, and fitments for taking either still or cine-photographic recordings (Fig. 27.2). It is also possible to introduce guide wires for special instruments to dilate strictures through these latter instruments.

Introduction of the rigid instrument usually requires complete general anaesthesia, and many surgeons prefer to use this type of instrument for the examination and biopsy of lesions high in the oesophagus or in the pharyngeal region, and to dilate benign strictures under direct vision. The flexible fibreoptic instruments can be passed without distress to the patient under a combination of local anaesthesia to the throat and sedation by an agent such as diazepam. In addition to the obvious advantage of avoiding a general anaesthetic, the very small risk of damage to the oesophagus during the procedure is even further diminished by performing the procedure with the patient still awake and co-operative, since the patient is able to assist the passage of the instrument by swallowing, and there is less likelihood of undue pressure on the oesophageal wall being exerted.

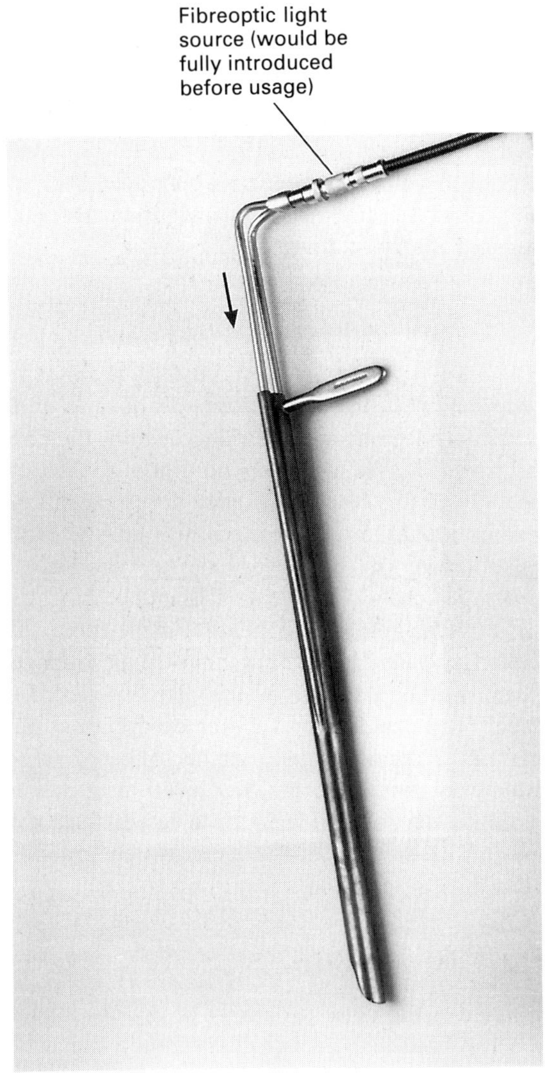

Fig. 27.1 Rigid oesophagoscope (Negus pattern).

In addition to direct inspection of the oesophageal lining the opportunity can be taken with either instrument to aspirate material for cytology, and to take small multiple biopsies from any area which appears to be the site of inflammatory, fibrous or malignant change. Thus a precise diagnosis based on histological evidence can usually be achieved.

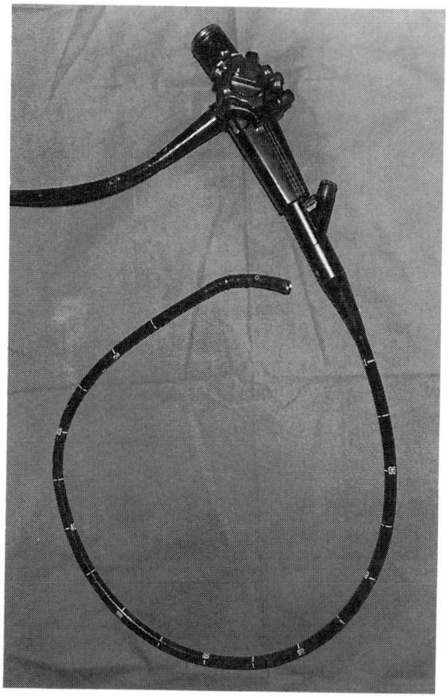

Fig. 27.2 Flexible fibreoptic oesophagoscope.

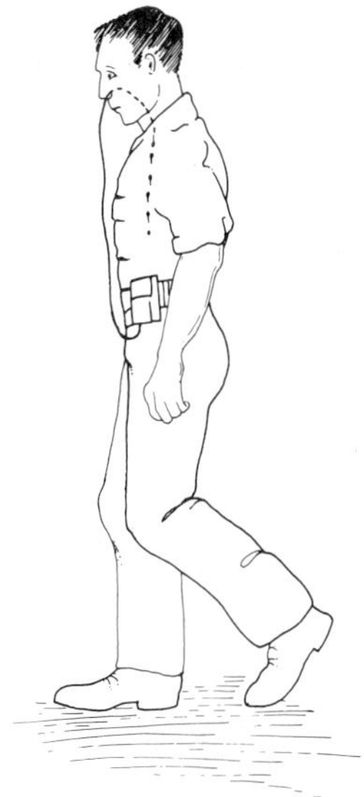

Fig. 27.3 Continuous recording of intraoesophageal pH by means of a pH-sensitive electrode fixed at the end of a nasogastric tube, and readings traced on a portable recorder. This allows normal ambulatory activities, and a more normal measurement of pH changes due to gastro-oesophageal reflux.

Acid measurements

As has been mentioned in the introductory parts of this chapter, the musculature at the lower end of the oesophagus normally acts in a manner to prevent or minimize reflux of gastric contents. The pH within the oesophageal lumen should therefore normally be alkaline. It is possible to make an estimate of the amount of reflux of the acidic gastric juice by passing a pH-sensitive electrode fixed to the end of a small–bore tube through the mouth or nasal passages, and locate the electrode at the desired level in the oesophagus (Fig. 27.3). This will permit the study of pH levels over a prolonged period of time, and as an additional test of competency at the oesophagogastric junction a known quantity of 0.1 normal hydrochloric acid can be directly introduced into the stomach by another tube. Other clinically useful tests involve measuring the rate at which small quantities of 0.1 normal acid introduced directly into the oesophagus can be emptied distally by repeated acts of swallowing by the patient, or by introducing into the oesophagus slow perfusions of either physiological saline or 0.1 normal hydrochloric acid, with the patient being kept unaware of the nature of the perfusing solution. In this latter (Bernstein) test, if the patient's complaints are reproduced only on perfusing the acid material this is further suggestive evidence that the symptoms are truly due to reflux.

Pressure measurements

It is possible to measure intraluminal pressure at various levels within the oesophagus by placing pressure-sensitive devices carried at the end of long fine tubes and these can be used to draw up a profile of pressure changes at rest, during acts of swallowing, and other physical manoeuvres. This can be useful not only in the investigation of gastro-oesophageal reflux, but also in disorders associated with abnormal motility in the organ, e.g. achalasia.

CONGENITAL DISEASES OF THE OESOPHAGUS

Although congenital conditions like web formation, stenosis, and duplication of the oesophagus may be encountered rarely, the commonest congenital abnormality, and indeed the one with most clinical

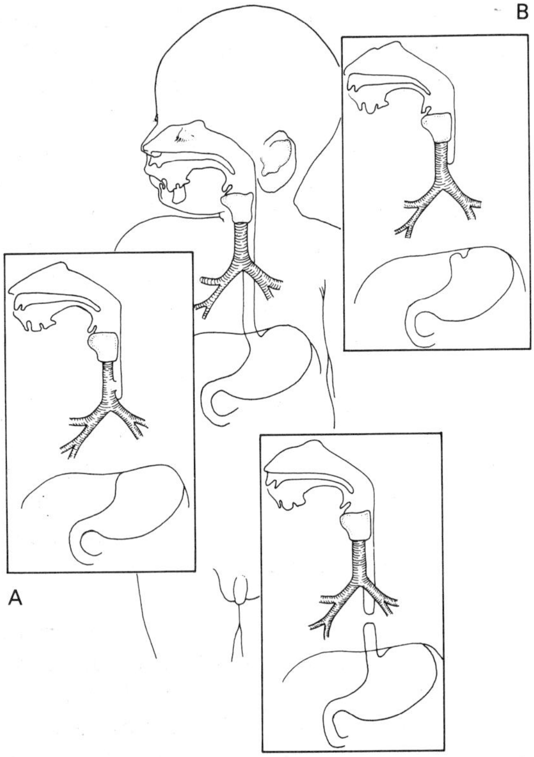

Fig. 27.4 Various patterns of congenital atresia of the oesophagus.
(**A**) Long gap between upper oesophagus and distal segment; (**B**) similar to (**A**), but with fistula between the upper oesophageal lumen and the trachea; (**C**) short segment undeveloped between patent upper and lower oesophagus.

relevance, is congenital atresia. As explained in the introductory section on the embryological development of the organ, the defect arises from some abnormality in the separation of the oesophagus from the developing air passages. Although a variety of anomalies may occur, as illustrated in Figure 27.4, in 90% of cases the upper end of the oesophagus ends as a blind pouch, and there is a fistula connection between the trachea and the distal end of the oesophagus.

The incidence of the defect is approximately 1 in every 2000–3000 live births. It should be remembered that a newborn baby presenting with atresia of the oesophagus has an approximately 1 in 3 chance of having some other congenital defect in addition, and therefore a careful examination should be made for such defects in other systems.

Clinical features

The presentation is usually quite dramatic. The first attempt to feed the newborn baby leads to distressing spluttering, coughing, regurgitation, and indeed if efforts are persisted with he or she may become cyanosed. Even before feeding is attempted, excessive dribbling of fine frothy mucus from the mouth may be observed. In the commonest variety, with a fistula between the trachea and the distal oesophageal segment, there may also be intermittent distension of the abdomen since, when the child cries, air passes from the trachea into the oesophagus, from where it passes readily into the stomach.

The diagnosis may be confirmed by passing a soft, preferably radiopaque catheter through the mouth into the upper oesophagus: inability to pass it much more than 8–10 cm from the alveolar margin is strongly suspicious of the lesion. Furthermore, radiography can be performed after gently introducing about 1 ml of a water-soluble X-ray contrast medium through this tube. The upper blind pouch of oesophagus may be thereby outlined and, in addition, if a distal fistula is present, the translucent shadow of air in the stomach and/or upper intestine may be seen.

Management

As soon as the diagnosis is suspected all attempts at feeding are stopped, and an intravenous line should be established. Aspiration of the proximal blind oesophageal pouch should be performed through the indwelling catheter, to minimize the chances of aspiration of any further material into the upper air passages. Urgent operation should then be performed as soon as fitness for general anaesthesia is obtained. Ideally, a single-stage procedure at which the two ends are freed, mobilized, and anastomosed, usually through a right thoracotomy, is the treatment of choice. However, if the gap between the two ends of the oesophagus is too great for such an approach, or if the child is generally unfit, it may be wiser as a first stage simply to establish a cervical oesophagostomy and a separate gastrostomy (Fig. 27.5), leaving the final reconstruction of the oesophagus to a later stage. The oesophagostomy allows satisfactory aspiration

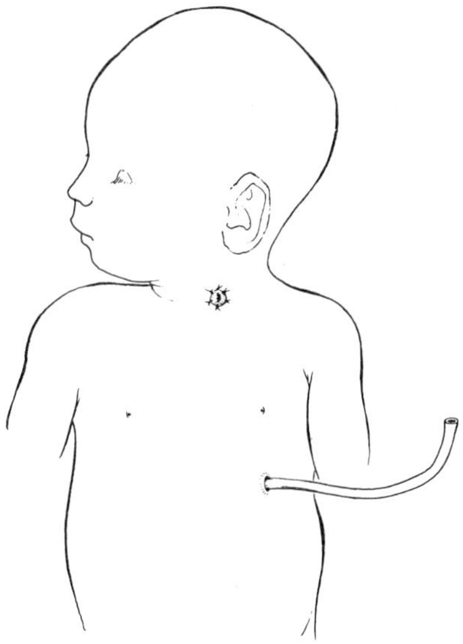

Fig. 27.5 Cervical oesophagostomy. The upper oesophagus is brought out to the skin surface, usually on the left side of the neck, and in addition a tube-feeding gastrostomy is formed.

of saliva and other secretions, thereby avoiding the risks of aspiration into the trachea, and the gastrostomy permits the maintenance of adequate nutrition. The subsequent reconstruction, which may be deferred until the child is between 1 and 2 years of age, may require the interposition of a segment of intestine in cases where the gap between the two ends of oesophagus is large.

It is preferable for the operative management of this condition to be conducted in centres with experienced surgical and nursing care, particularly where there is the possibility of this two-stage approach being required.

OESOPHAGITIS

The delicate lining of the oesophagus may be irritated by various factors including physical or chemical trauma, disease processes adjacent to the oesophagus, or by irradiation, but by far and away the commonest cause is the reflux of irritating material from the stomach or proximal small intestine. It follows, therefore, that the lower end of the oesophagus is most often affected. Two of the most irritant materials are first the acid gastric juice, and secondly duodenal and jejunal content containing bile, lysolecithin, and other irritant substances.

When such substances come in direct contact with the oesophageal epithelium, they cause first of all increased vascularity and therefore increased redness on direct inspection, oedematous swelling, and if the irritation persists interruption of the integrity, i.e. ulcer formation. Also as a result of continuing irritation there will be reflex increase in the muscular spasm, particularly within the longitudinal layers, which in turn produces spasm and some degree of contraction of the oesophagus proximally with a tendency to shortening of the oesophagus and consequent pulling of the gastric fundus towards the thoracic cavity. Long-standing continued irritation of the lower end of the oesophagus may also lead to the deposition of fibrous tissue in the wall of the oesophagus which may produce contraction and narrowing of the lumen of the organ so that a fibrous stricture may result.

Such a sequence of events is most commonly produced by incompetence at the oesophagogastric junction associated with hiatal hernia, but gastro-oesophageal reflux may also occur without there being such an anatomical abnormality, and the entire sequence of events described above may therefore be present without the demonstration of such an anatomical abnormality.

Small amounts of gastro-oesophageal reflux probably occur at some time in every person's life, for example, after unduly large meals, excesses of alcohol, after activities involving much stooping or bending, etc., and in women during the latter months of pregnancy but in these situations the symptoms are usually transient and regarded as no more than a temporary inconvenience. In the absence of such factors persistence of the symptoms requires further investigation.

Common to the foregoing situations is an imbalance between an increase in intragastric or intra-abdominal pressures, and the factors within the thorax and in the lower oesophageal musculature which normally guard against gastro-oesophageal reflux. Of the many mechanisms contributing to this (Fig. 27.6)–which are first the acute angle at which the oesophagus enters the fundus of the stomach, the 'pinchcock' action of the fibres of the right crus of the diaphragm, the formation of a 'rosette' of the lower oesophageal mucosal fold, and the intrinsic property of the lower oesophageal musculature in maintaining a tone—the balance of

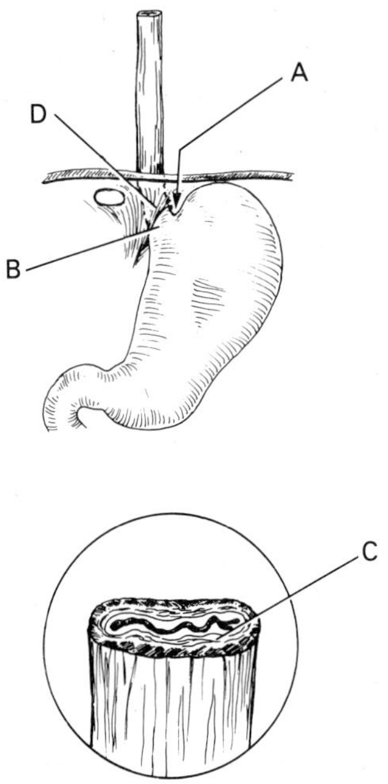

Fig. 27.6 The various factors which may contribute to the prevention of gastro-oesophageal reflux in normal health. (**A**) The acute angle between distal oesophagus and gastric fundus; (**B**) 'pinchcock' action of the crus of diaphragm; (**C**) The 'rosette' contact between mucosal folds at rest; (**D**) sphincteric action of the lower oesophageal muscle.

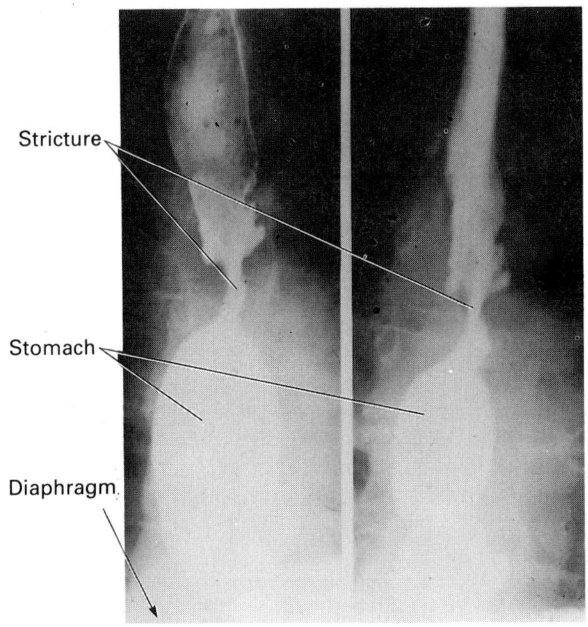

Fig. 27.7 Moderately large sliding hiatal hernia with benign fibrous stricture proximal to the hernia—the result of long-standing gastro-oesophageal reflux.

evidence indicates that the latter is the most crucial factor. Although it is not possible to identify a thickened muscular mass which can be described as an anatomical sphincter, there is abundant physiological evidence that the muscle fibres at the lower end of the oesophagus do truly act as a physiological sphincter. The efficiency of this zone is further assisted by its subdiaphragmatic location, where the hydrostatic pressure is greater than that within the thoracic cavity.

Clinical features

The dominant classical symptom is heartburn, a sensation of a gnawing, burning pain in the retrosternal region, aggravated by bending, stooping, large meals, or lying flat, particularly when turned to the right side. In addition there may be flatulence, water-brash, or even frank regurgitation of gastric content into the throat or mouth. Sometimes the symptoms may be accentuated by the act of swallowing, and if the symptoms persist for any length of time anaemia may result from repeated small blood loss from the inflamed mucosa.

In long-standing oesophagitis with subsequent stricture formation (Fig. 27.7), the additional symptoms of progressive dysphagia may follow. At first this may be to some extent intermittent, as a result of muscular spasm, but when fibrous tissue is deposited in the wall of the organ the difficulty in swallowing will be progressive.

Investigations

There are usually no obvious signs on simple clinical examination, and therefore one or more special investigations are required to ensure that the symptoms are truly arising from oesophagitis. First, testing of the stools may reveal positive occult blood, the result of small repeated bleeding from the inflamed eroded mucosa. It should be remembered, however, that there are other common causes of blood in the motions, such as peptic ulcer, tumours of both the proximal and distal segments of the alimentary tract, and where there are any grounds for suspicion of these other disorders the appropriate investigations will be required.

The principal investigations needed to confirm the presence of oesophagitis and/or reflux from the stomach are barium swallow and meal and endoscopy. In the former examination, as has been mentioned, the radiologist will look for evidence of regurgitated material from the stomach into the lower end of the oesophagus by one or other of a range of manoeuvres aimed at increasing intra-abdominal pressure. Oesophagoscopy will give the opportunity to assess the gross naked-eye appearances of the lining of the oesophagus, the presence of any erosions or ulcerations or strictures, and the opportunity should be taken to obtain multiple biopsies from any area which looks abnormal. Thus a microscopic assessment of the degree of any inflammatory changes can be made.

Where diagnostic doubt remains, one or other of the acid perfusion or pH profile tests may be helpful.

Once again it should be stressed that other common intra-abdominal disorders, notably peptic ulcer and gall bladder disease, may be accompanied by troublesome reflux symptoms, and appropriate examinations to detect these should be included, since these other conditions may require the appropriate treatment, and this may take precedence over measures to counteract the reflux.

Management

In the majority of patients with mild-to-moderate symptoms from gastro-oesophageal reflux, simple medical measures will prove effective. First of all, if the patient is clearly overweight the symptoms can often be brought completely under control solely by losing the excess weight. Furthermore a few simple physical precautions aimed at minimizing increases in intra-abdominal pressure are often helpful. These include sleeping with the upper part of the trunk slightly elevated, preferably by tilting the bed so that the upper end is higher than the lower end; strict avoidance of all tight, constrictive clothing; avoiding large meals, and eliminating bending and stooping as far as is possible. Furthermore, one of the commonly prescribed antacids, alginates and mucilagenous preparations frequently give symptomatic relief. Other agents such as carbenoxolone sodium and metoclopramide are also worth considering. Not surprisingly, the potent H_2-receptor antagonists such as cimetidine and ranitidine have been used to treat this condition, and clearly if the principal irritant to the oesophagus is regurgitated acid from the stomach, there is some rationale to giving these medicaments. It is worth spending some time discussing these various measures with the patient, and urging him or her to follow this regime.

If in spite of a good trial of these various measures troublesome symptoms persist, and in particular if there is sign of recurrent stricture formation, surgical treatment may then be required. Over the years a variety of operations have been described, all with the aim of reinforcing the various mechanisms known to defend the lower end of the oesophagus against regurgitation. Probably the most important objective which these various procedures achieve is the fixation of the lower end of the oesophagus in a subdiaphragmatic position, i.e. in the relatively higher pressure zone of the abdominal as opposed to the thoracic cavity. At present perhaps the most popular operation is Nissen's fundoplication (Fig. 27.8). Through an abdominal approach the lower end of the oesophagus and the proximal parts of both the lesser and greater curvature aspects of the gastric fundus are mobilized and then the freed greater curve aspect is wrapped around the

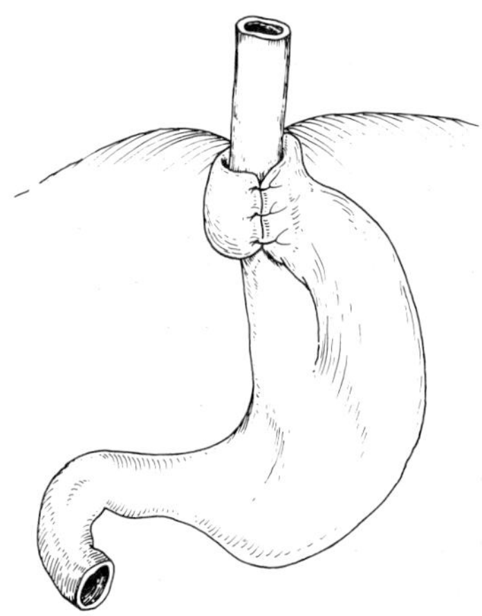

Fig. 27.8 Nissen fundoplication. The lower oesophagus and upper part of the gastric fundus have been mobilized, and a 'tongue' of the greater curve aspect of the fundus has been wrapped around the lower oesophagus and fixed by sutures, which pick up the anterior oesophageal wall. This procedure fixes the lower oesophagus below the diaphragm. If the hiatus is very lax, partial closure of the gap in the crus is also performed.

lower end of the oesophagus; the resulting cuff of stomach wall is fixed to the anterior oesophageal wall by a few interrupted sutures. This encircling gastric cuff then effectively anchors the lower segment of the oesophagus, thus preventing it from riding up towards and into the chest. The effectiveness of the lower oesophageal muscular zone is thereby strengthened.

HIATAL HERNIA

There are basically three types of anatomical defect under this heading, as illustrated in Figure 27.9. The first, and by far the commonest, is the sliding type of hernia in which the oesophagogastric junction lies above the diaphragm, a pouch of the gastric fundus being pulled or pushed up through the lax, widened hiatus in the right crus of the diaphragm. As a result the high-pressure lower 'sphincter' zone of the lower oesophagus has therefore to work at the disadvantage of being in the relatively subatmospheric pressure zone of the chest. The next type of hernia is the rolling, or paraoesophageal pattern in which the oesophagogastric junction is at its normal subdiaphragmatic level, but a pouch of the greater curve aspect of the gastric fundus rolls up through the hiatus in front of or to the left side of the lower oesophagus in the thoracic cavity. Finally, there is a mixed type which has both sliding and rolling components.

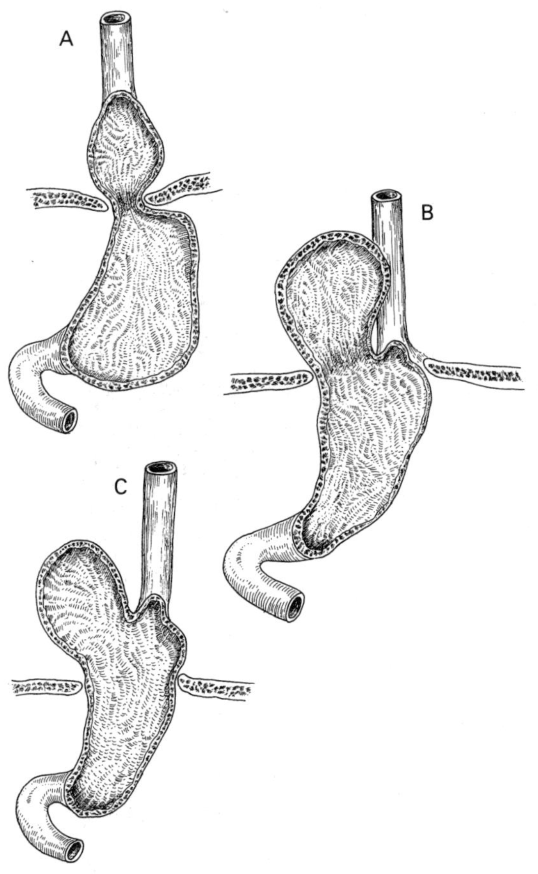

Fig. 27.9 The three main varieties of hiatal hernia. (**A**) Sliding; (**B**) paraoesophageal or rolling; (**C**) a combination of both sliding and rolling.

Clinical presentation

As the diagnostic procedures of endoscopy and contrast radiography have become increasingly accurate and more widely used it has been apparent that some degree of anatomical sliding hiatal hernia is common, therefore it must be emphasized that in many people this will not cause symptoms throughout life. It follows, therefore, that when a sliding hiatal hernia is demonstrated the clinician should be sure that it is truly the cause of any presenting symptoms. Many of the complaints relating to hiatal hernia are also features of other common disorders such as peptic ulcer, gallstones, pancreatitis, and even large bowel disease, and if there is reasonable doubt about the presence of such disorders the appropriate investigations should be performed.

Sliding hiatal hernia may present in infancy, is exceptional in childhood and young adult life, and the peak incidence falls in patients aged 50 years or more. In infancy the main presenting symptoms are forceful vomiting, with sometimes blood-stained content as well as regurgitated material, and aspiration of this material is fairly frequent, with consequent respiratory symptoms. If the reflux goes undetected fibrous strictures may occur in the oesophagus so that the infant has difficulty in swallowing any significant amount of feeds.

In adults the dominant symptoms of sliding hiatal hernia are those of oesophageal reflux, already described. Often the patients are obviously overweight, there is a clear history of heartburn, aggravated by lying prone or bending or stooping, and water-brash, reflux of bitter fluid up into the throat or mouth, persistent gnawing retrosternal pain and dysphagia which may persist if stricture formation occurs, are all classical features. Where the degree of reflux is great again there may be respiratory symptoms from aspiration of the regurgitated material, an occurrence which is particularly liable to take place when lying in bed.

The presenting symptoms in the much rarer pattern of rolling or paraoesophageal hernia are not those of reflux, since, with the oesophagogastric junction in its normal intra-abdominal location, competence of the lower oesophageal 'sphincter' usually remains intact. The principal symptoms fall under two headings. First are complaints related to mechanical pressure in the intrathoracic gastric pouch, all of which may be more noticeable after meals. These include a tight feeling of pressure in the chest, mainly on the left side, the awareness of gurgling noises in the same location, palpitation due to pressure on the heart, and tightness around the lower part of the chest. Patients may notice that these symptoms are improved by changes in posture, loosening tight clothing around the abdomen, belching, or simply with the passage of time following a meal. Secondly, these patients may present with anaemia, which is due to repeated chronic blood loss from mucosal ulceration in the region of the neck of the herniated portion of stomach. Rarely incarceration of the gastric pouch may occur and if this is not relieved either spontaneously or by surgical measures, strangulation may develop.

Investigations

X-ray after the swallowing of contrast medium (Fig. 27.10), and the employment of appropriate physical manoeuvres to fill the gastric fundus and exert slight increased pressure upon it, will usually demonstrate the hiatal hernia defect without difficulty. In addition oesophagogastroscopy should be performed to assess the degree of oesophagitis, and to inspect the mucosa of the area for erosions, ulcers, or other consequent or coincidental pathology.

As has already been mentioned, if there is any doubt that the hernia might be the sole cause of presenting symptoms other appropriate investigations should be arranged.

Treatment

Since the principal symptoms of a sliding hiatal hernia are those of gastro-oesophageal reflux, the

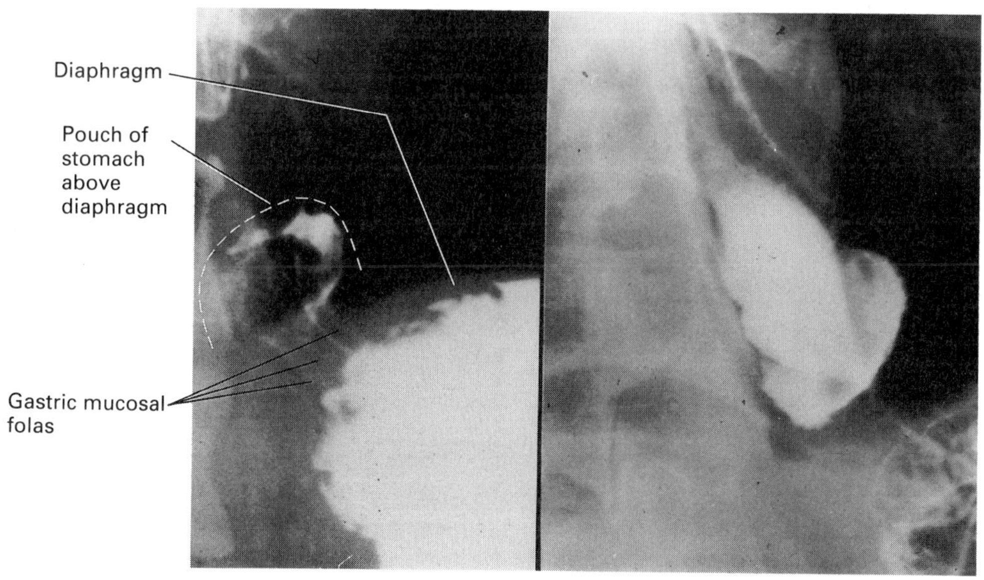

Fig. 27.10 Barium swallow appearances of a sliding hiatal hernia. A pouch of stomach is outlined clearly above the level of the dome of the diaphragm. The picture on the left, in which there is both air and barium, outlines clearly the gastric mucosal folds passing up through the hiatus into the chest.

measures to counteract this, already discussed, should be instituted at first, and in the great majority of instances these simple medical measures will be successful. Weight reduction in the obese is an important first step, and this alone may suffice. Advice regarding the various other measures to discourage reflux should be given, and the various medications which reduce acid or pepsin secretion and assist normal gastric emptying should be used.

Operation is reserved for those in whom these various conservative measures fail to control symptoms, where the hernia is particularly large, and where there are complications such as stricture formation or persistent bleeding. Although many techniques have been devised for the repair of sliding hiatal hernia, the procedures most popular at present are those which create some form of fixation of the oesophagogastric junction below the diaphragm, such as gastroplasties or fundoplication, e.g. the Nissen procedure described above. Where the anatomical defect in the right crus of the diaphragm is of appreciable size the opportunity is usually taken to narrow this at the same time. Satisfactory relief of the symptoms should be obtained in between 80 and 90% of cases.

The approach to rolling hernia is quite different (Fig. 27.11). Since the main symptoms are due to local mechanical factors, rather than reflux, there is no point in giving advice along the lines advocated for sliding hiatal hernia, and operative repair is the treatment of choice. The surgical approach may be either through the upper abdomen or via a left thoracotomy, and by either route the objectives are to reduce the hernia, excise the sac, and repair the defect in the diaphragmatic hiatus with non-absorbable sutures.

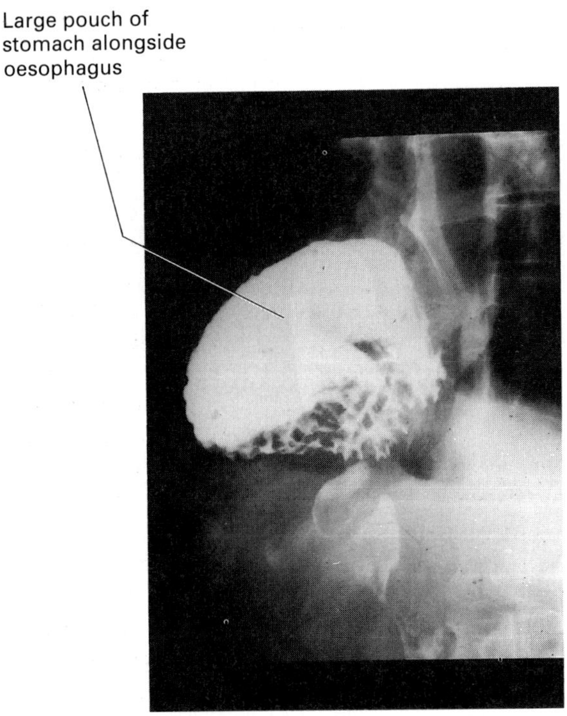

Fig. 27.11 A large paraoesophageal (rolling) hiatal hernia outlined on barium swallow/meal. Pressure has been applied on the abdomen to achieve good filling of the hernia.

COLUMNAR-LINED LOWER OESOPHAGUS (BARRETT'S OESOPHAGUS)

In this condition a variable length of the lower oesophageal mucosa comprises columnar epithelium instead of the normal stratified squamous pattern (Fig. 27.12). It was formerly believed that the true oesophagus was congenitally short, leading to a junction between squamous and columnar epithelium at an abnormally high level. However, the columnar epithelium at the lower end of the oesophagus is not true gastric-type epithelium, and there is considerable evidence that the change from a squamous type to a columnar variety is an adap-

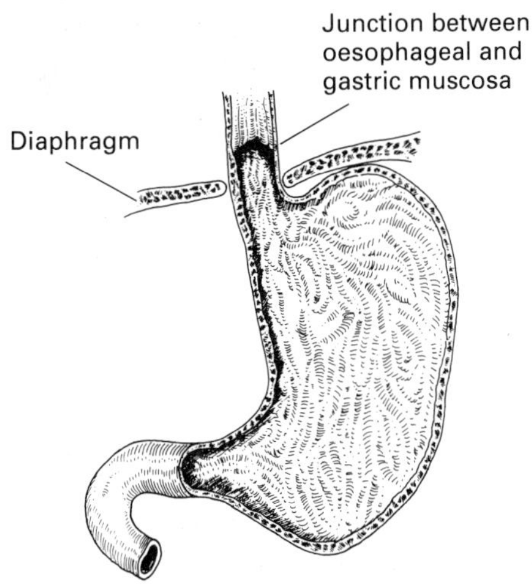

Fig. 27.12 Barrett's oesophagus. Gastric–type mucosa (columnar) has replaced the typical stratified epithelium of the lowermost segment of the oesophagus.

tive response to reflux from the stomach. It is therefore regarded as an acquired condition.

As a consequence of continued reflux, ulceration of the oesophageal lining usually at the junction between squamous and columnar epithelium may occur, as also may fibrous stricture formation.

The presenting symptoms are usually those of reflux oesophagitis, and if strictures develop there may also be some degree of dysphagia. The correct diagnosis may be established by a combination of barium swallow X-ray and endoscopy. Biopsies of the oesophageal mucosa at appropriate levels should confirm the difference in histological pattern.

Treatment should first be directed towards the control of gastro-oesophageal reflux, and if this fails an antireflux operation may be required.

FIBROUS STRICTURES OF THE OESOPHAGUS

The majority of these are the consequence of long-standing gastro-oesophageal reflux leading to erosion and ulceration of the mucosa and in turn the deposition of fibrous scar tissue which as it matures contracts, thereby constricting the oesophageal lumen. Strictures may also arise following mucosal damage as a result of accidental or intentional swallowing of corrosives. It follows, therefore, that a relevant previous history should be present.

The dominant symptom is, of course, dysphagia, which in the early stages may have an intermittent pattern, but as the stricture formation increases the dysphagia becomes progressive.

The diagnosis is established by a combination of barium swallow X-ray (see Fig. 27.7) and endoscopy and at the latter biopsies should be taken of the strictured area and above it, to exclude the presence of malignant disease. Since dysphagia is a common symptom to both conditions and they may coexist, it is important to achieve a precise histologically confirmed diagnosis. Furthermore, long-standing reflux slightly but significantly increases the risk of carcinoma developing in the mucosa.

The majority of benign fibrous strictures can be managed by a combination of dilatation through an oesophagoscope plus the measures outlined to control further reflux. Surgical measures, if required, should in the first instance be dilatation plus an antireflux operation, and this should be adequate in the majority of instances. Rarely, resection of the strictured area will be required, with either re-anastomosis of the proximal oesophagus to stomach, or interposing a segment of either small bowel or colon between oesophagus and the upper gastrointestinal tract. Such procedures should be reserved for only the most intractable strictures, since they are not altogether without the risk of further problems, including re-stricture.

TUMOURS OF THE OESOPHAGUS

Malignant

By far the commonest tumour to arise in the oesophagus is carcinoma, and since the oesophagus is lined by stratified squamous epithelium, the commonest histological type is a squamous carcinoma. However, at the lower end of the oesophagus adenocarcinoma arising primarily from the gastric mucosa at the upper end of the stomach may encroach on the oesophagogastric junction and present with clinical features exactly the same as those of the more common squamous carcinoma. Finally, adenocarcinoma can also arise occasionally in areas of abnormal columnar epithelium in the oesophagus itself.

The outlook in carcinoma of the oesophagus is still unfortunately very poor, and even when radical treatment either by surgery or radiotherapy is performed, 5-year survival without recurrence of the disease is to be expected in only about 10–15% of patients. In most countries it is predominantly a disease of the second half of life, with a peak incidence in the 60–80-year range, but occasionally it may be encountered at an earlier period of life. In the UK there is not much difference in the incidence between the two sexes, but there is a remarkable degree of variation in both the overall incidence and the sex distribution in other countries.

Some factors are believed to increase the risk of oesophageal carcinoma, for example, heavy cigarette smoking and alcohol consumption, the repeated ingestion of hot liquids and solids, the chewing of betel nut, and prolonged mucosal irritation or damage associated with gastro-oesophageal reflux, fibrous strictures, particularly when these are caused by swallowed chemicals, achalasia of the cardia, and the Plummer–Vinson (Paterson–Brown Kelly) syndrome.

Carcinoma may occur at any level within the oesophagus, but the middle and lower thirds are certainly more frequently involved than more proximal levels.

Two gross patterns of lesion are recognized: first a polypoid mass projecting from the mucosa into the lumen, soon ulcerating to produce a fungating, hard, irregular mass which progressively occludes the lumen, and secondly, a gradually stenosing infiltrative lesion spreading predominantly in the submucosal layer around the oesophagus to produce an irregular stenosing malignant stricture. If unchecked, further spread may be first by direct penetration of important neighbouring structures, by passage along the lymphatics to the appropriate nodes either proximally or distally depending on the primary location of the tumour, and lastly, but rarely, by blood spread.

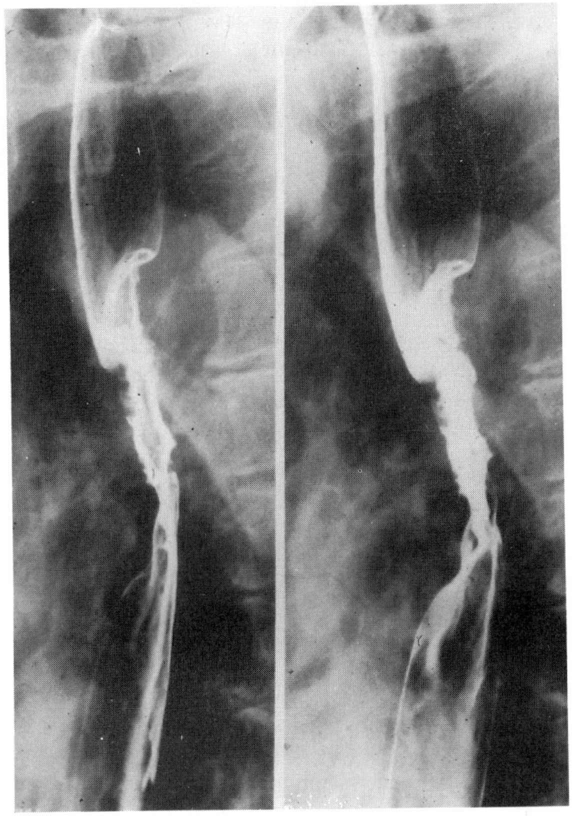

Fig. 27.13 Carcinoma of the oesophagus. Barium swallow outlining an irregular, constricting tumour in the middle third of the oesophagus.

Clinical features

The classical history is one of steadily progressive dysphagia. At first the patient may notice that only larger pieces of solid food, for example meat or fruit, are felt to stick somewhere in the retrosternal region on swallowing, and as the lesion progresses, difficulty is next encountered with smaller items of solid food, then semi-solids, and finally there may be difficulty even with liquids. The patient may also become anaemic from repeated small blood loss from the ulcerated tumour, and of course as dietary restriction ensues there will be loss of weight. As with other lesions which tend to obstruct the oesophagus, there may also be some spillage of material into the air passages and as a consequence, respiratory symptoms.

In early cases physical examination may reveal no abnormality, but later anaemia and signs of weight loss may be apparent. The supraclavicular areas should be palpated for enlargement of lymph nodes which may contain metastatic deposits from tumours in the proximal oesophagus, and careful examination of the abdomen may reveal masses arising either from the stomach, or as a result of gross lymph node enlargement around the coeliac axis.

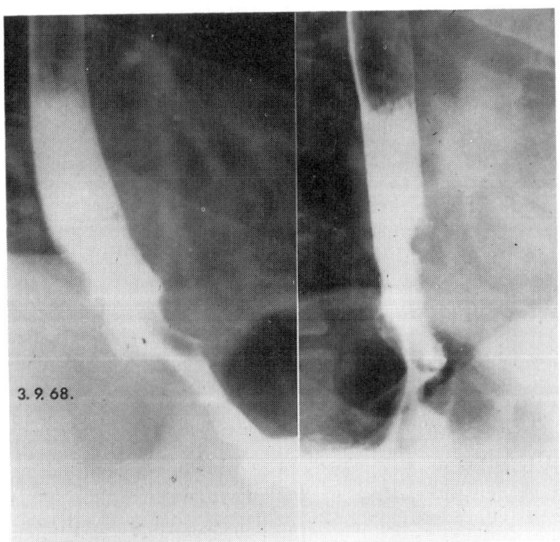

Fig. 27.14 Carcinoma of the lower end of the oesophagus—the irregularity reaching down to the oesophagogastric junction.

The two crucial forms of investigation are once

again radiological examination after barium swallow (Fig. 27.13), and endoscopy. The suspicious signs on X-ray are irregularity of the oesophageal outline (Fig. 27.14), with diminished or absent muscular movement on screening, raised ulceration or the clear delineation of a polypoid mass. There may also be signs of one or more of the predisposing disorders mentioned above.

All patients in whom there is a suspicion of carcinoma of the oesophagus on clinical or radiological grounds should have an oesophagoscopy. Even if the barium swallow examination is interpreted as essentially normal, oesophagoscopy should be performed if there is the slightest suspicion of this serious diagnosis from the symptom history. Through the endoscope one can obtain vital information regarding the level of the upper border of the gross lesion, the presence of other oesophageal abnormalities, e.g. oesophagitis, and most importantly, multiple biopsies can be taken, preferably from the main mass of the tumour and what appears to be its edge. If cytopathological expertise is available brushings from the surface of an ulcerated lesion taken by means of a special wire brush passed through one of the channels of the endoscope may give a satisfactory histological confirmation. If there is also suspicion of direct involvement of the air passages, bronchoscopy may also be advisable.

It is also wise to have plain X-ray examination of the chest seeking for any signs of segmental collapse which might point to bronchial occlusion, or paralysis of either dome of the diaphragm which would indicate phrenic nerve involvement.

Before embarking on treatment the blood should be examined for signs of anaemia and for indices of the nutritional state.

Management

The poor prognosis of carcinoma of the oesophagus, referred to at the outset of this section, is the consequence of several factors. First, the organ is of course deeply situated, and therefore inaccessible to simple physical examination. Second, by the time the patient presents with troublesome dysphagia, the tumour has often spread either to the lymphatics or directly to involve neighbouring structures. Third, as a result of the dysphagia many patients are ill-nourished and their capacity to withstand major surgery may be impaired. Fourth, anastomoses between the oesophagus and more distal parts of the alimentary tract are more prone to leakage and other problems of healing than are other gastrointestinal anastomoses.

The primary hope, of course, is to eradicate the disease by either surgical excision or radiotherapy or possibly in the future by some form of chemotherapy but even when complete cure is not possible every endeavour should be made to restore swallowing, at least of liquids. Complete dysphagia with regurgitation of even saliva is distressing in the extreme to the patient.

In keeping with squamous carcinoma at other sites of the body, squamous carcinoma of the oesophagus is on the whole sensitive to radiotherapy, but the chief difficulty is in delivering a satisfactory dose which will be lethal to the tumour but avoid serious damage to other normal structures. By and large, radiotherapy is preferred for lesions in the proximal part of the oesophagus, and surgical excision for more distal lesions.

For the resection of tumours at the lower end of the oesophagus the conventional approach is to use a combined thoracoabdominal incision opening up the left pleural cavity and the upper abdomen, dividing the diaphragm down to the oesophageal hiatus and dissecting the oesophagus several centimetres above the upper limit of the tumour and also freeing the proximal stomach. The lesser and greater omenta and often the spleen are also dissected free in continuity with the oesophagogastric junction. Continuity is then re-established by either direct anastomosis between the remaining oesophagus and the mobilized distal stomach, or between the oesophagus and a Roux loop of jejunum.

If resection of the middle third is undertaken this will involve removal of virtually the whole length of the oesophagus, usually through a right thoracotomy, and the stomach is mobilized in its entire length to allow it to be brought up through the thoracic cavity for anastomosis to the cervical part of the oesophagus (Fig. 27.15). This will require separate incisions in the abdomen, in the right chest, and possibly in the root of the neck.

In recent years there has been a tendency to employ more complete resection of the oesophagus for carcinomas at any level, since histological exami-

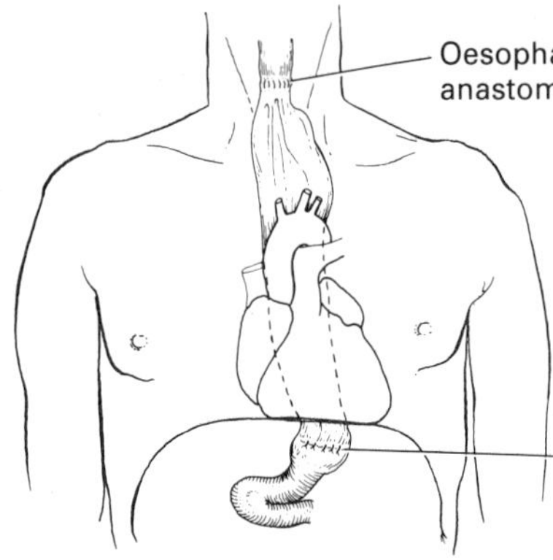

Fig. 27.15 Total oesophagectomy for carcinoma. The stomach has been mobilized completely, preserving an arterial blood supply from the right gastric and right gastroepiploic arteries. The proximal end of the stomach is then brought up through the mediastinum and anastomosed to the remaining oesophagus in the neck. Since the stomach will inevitably have been vagotomized, and emptying delayed, a pyloroplasty is also performed.

nation of excised specimens often reveals cellular infiltration longitudinally for quite some distance above the obvious tumour.

These surgical procedures are quite major, and as has been mentioned, there is always anxiety about the adequacy of healing of anastomoses between the oesophagus and other segments of the alimentary tract. Therefore, if the patient's nutritional status is impaired it is often worthwhile spending a few days improving the nutritional state by parenteral means before embarking on the operation. Correction of anaemia, replacing depleted protein stores and securing as good an electrolyte mineral and calorie balance as possible before surgery in such patients significantly reduces the risk of postoperative mortality and the incidence of early complications.

In addition to the fact that radiotherapy is the primary treatment of choice in proximal carcinomas in this organ, and may achieve their eradication, it may also be useful in lower lesions as a preoperative measure leading to substantial reduction in the size of the tumour and thereby making subsequent resection easier and more likely to succeed. Such an approach may well render operable a tumour which initially appears unsuitable for resection.

The role of chemotherapy in this disease is still unresolved, but here again it is possible that the judicious combination of radiotherapy and chemotherapy either as the total treatment, or used in an adjuvant way in addition to resection, may bring about a gradual overall improvement in results. It has to be stressed, however, that at the present time our ability to cure this tumour is very limited, and unfortunately most patients presenting with the disease will succumb to it.

Where for one reason or another it is impossible to remove a carcinoma of the oesophagus, useful palliation may be obtained by the insertion of one of the many patterns of rigid tube through the obstructing tumour mass. Rigid plastic tubes, e.g. the Mousseau-Barbin model (Fig. 27.16), may be introduced into the pharynx and oesophagus by

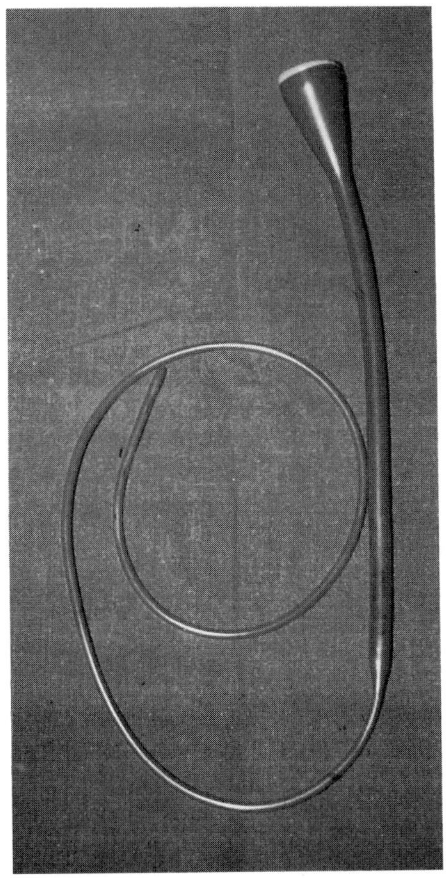

Fig. 27.16 Mousseau-Barbin tube. This is one of the patterns of rigid plastic indwelling tubes which may be passed through the obstructing tumour mass, and left in situ. At best it will allow the patient to swallow liquids and very 'sloppy' foods, but there is a risk of bolus obstruction and other severe complications. This one requires laparotomy to fix the lower end to the stomach.

the anaesthetist using a laryngoscope, and drawn distally by the surgeon through a small gastrotomy. The funnel-shaped proximal end of the tube can then be manipulated through the tumour mass and subsequently fixed in position. This will allow the patient to swallow liquidized food for some time. More modern patterns of tube can be inserted solely by endoscopic introduction, thus avoiding the laparotomy. There are, of course, hazards to these procedures which simply force the tubes in a somewhat blind fashion through the tumour mass, and understandably there is a risk of leakage, dislodgement, and yet further blockage. However, faced with the alternative of complete dysphagia their use is well worth considering as they can often give substantial if temporary relief for the most distressing symptom.

Even repeated simple dilatation through the tumour mass using either a rigid or flexible fibreoptic oesophagoscope may afford temporary relief.

Benign tumours

These are very rare in comparison with carcinoma, but leiomyoma, lipoma or fibroma may arise from the muscle, fatty tissue, or fibrous tissue respectively. Leiomyomata are encountered slightly more frequently than the others.

If these are large enough to cause symptoms, these symptoms will be predominantly dysphagia and a feeling of pressure or other discomfort behind the sternum. Diagnosis may be difficult, since both barium swallow and endoscopic appearances may to all intents and purposes be normal. The lesion which is in the wall of the oesophagus may be easily displaced by the passage of an endoscope, and of course the mucosa will be intact and of completely normal gross appearance. Larger lesions may show characteristic smooth indentation of the shadow on barium swallow, and there may be an obvious bulge or displacement of the mucosa on endoscopy. Biopsy of the mucosa will show a normal histological pattern.

For these soft-tissue benign tumours the newer techniques of computerized tomography scanning and nuclear magnetic resonance are much more promising, since these techniques are capable of outlining soft-tissue masses, and giving information on the consistency of the material in the tumour.

The treatment of these benign tumours, if they present with symptoms, is to excise them through an appropriately sited longitudinal incision directly over the lesion. Most are well encapsulated and therefore fairly easily enucleated.

PLUMMER–VINSON SYNDROME (PATERSON–BROWN KELLY SYNDROME)

In this uncommon condition there is an association between hypochromic anaemia and fairly widespread mucosal atrophy changes affecting the mouth, the pharynx and the oesophagus. In addition there may be cracks in the skin at the angles of the mouth, and signs of increased brittleness of the finger nails. The condition is more frequently met in women than in men, and if it remains undetected and untreated there is an increased risk of carcinoma developing in the oesophagus, particularly in the postcricoid region.

The clinical presentation is of anaemia and dysphagia. The pattern of the anaemia will be established by full blood count, and visualization of the pharynx and oesophagus both by barium swallow and endoscopy should be performed. Dysphagia may be due to either of two occurrences. First, as a result of the atrophic changes in the mucosa there may be stricture formation or the creation of crescentic mucosal webs partly encroaching on the lumen. Second, there is the increased risk of frank carcinoma developing, particularly when the condition has been present for many years.

If the condition is detected at an early stage, correction of the anaemia should result in a substantial return of the mucosal pattern towards normal, and it should also reduce the risks of both stricture formation and malignant change.

ACHALASIA OF THE CARDIA

This uncommon condition, basically due to some inco-ordination of the muscle movements in the oesophagus, affects men and women more or less equally, and the peak age of incidence is in the 30s and 40s.

The condition used to be known as 'cardiospasm', since it was believed that the principal defect was excessive spasm of the 'sphincter' muscles at the lower end of the oesophagus. It is now understood that the basic problem at this level is that the musculature of this high-pressure zone fails to relax in response to swallowing, and in addition there is an absence of distally sweeping propulsive movements down the oesophagus on swallowing. Debate continues as to whether there is a qualitative or quantitative abnormality in either the ganglion or plexus arrangement within the oesophageal wall.

As a result of this inco-ordination of motility, the oesophagus dilates, and if the condition is unrelieved may become as wide as half the diameter of the chest. Ingested materials and secretions may accumulate in the dilated organ, and a degree of oesophagitis arises in the mucosa. With increasing distension and dilatation some lengthening of the oesophagus may also occur so that the course of it through the mediastinum may become somewhat tortuous. There is also of course the risk of spillage of the oesophageal content over into the upper respiratory tree.

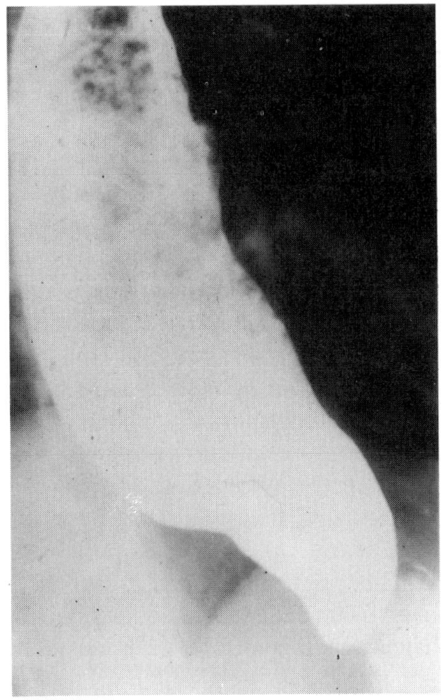

Fig. 27.17 Barium swallow of severe achalasia, with hugely dilated oesophagus, leading down to a narrow 'rat-tail' trickle passing distally into the stomach. The fluid level above the barium indicates the hold-up in oesophageal emptying.

Clinical presentation

Dysphagia is the chief complaint, although in this instance the pattern is somewhat different from those of the other complaints already discussed, e.g. fibrous stricture and carcinoma. At first the hold-up of both liquids and solids after swallowing may cause retrosternal discomfort for a few minutes and thereafter the symptoms ease off spontaneously. If the condition progresses, the dysphagia for both solid and liquid components will continue to occur after each swallowing act, and the patient may learn that certain specific changes in posture may allow the swallowed material eventually to pass through. If this is not possible he or she may regurgitate the recently ingested material. Ultimately there may be some weight loss from insufficient nutritional intake.

Diagnosis

Well developed achalasia of the cardia shows very typical signs on barium swallow X-ray examination, and an example is shown in Figure 27.17. The entire oesophagus is more or less uniformly dilated, and the mucosal pattern may be seen to be smoother than usual. Screening will demonstrate the absence of normal emptying waves. Turning to the lower end, the outline of the oesophagus gradually and smoothly narrows to a fine narrow channel, the so-called 'rat-tail' appearance. There may also be little or no gastric air bubble which one would normally expect in the absence of this condition. Sometimes in the most extreme cases even a plain anteroposterior film of the chest will outline the soft-tissue edges of the grossly dilated oesophagus (Figs 27.18 and 27.19).

Endoscopic examination should always be performed in patients even when the diagnosis is quite clear from both clinical and radiological assessments. The first main reason is to exclude the co-existence of a carcinoma at the lower end of the oesophagus, and as mentioned in the section on carcinoma, long-standing achalasia of the cardia is one of the known predisposing disorders to it. Secondly, endoscopy gives an opportunity to assess the degree of oesophagitis, and any other changes which might have arisen in the mucosa. Surprising-

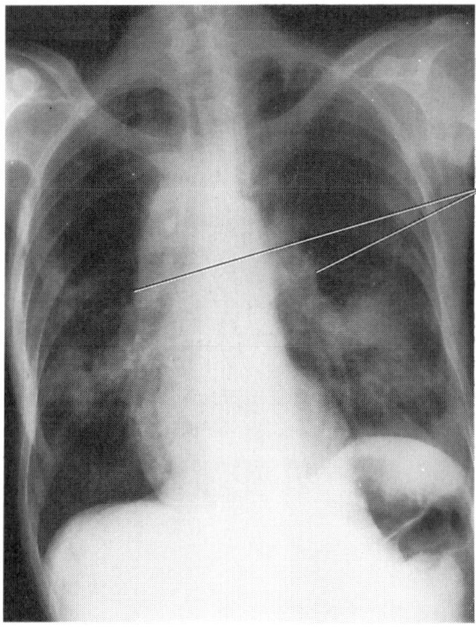

Fig. 27.18 Achalasia of the cardia. Straight anteroposterior X-ray of the chest showing the lateral edges of the shadow of the grossly dilated oesophagus.

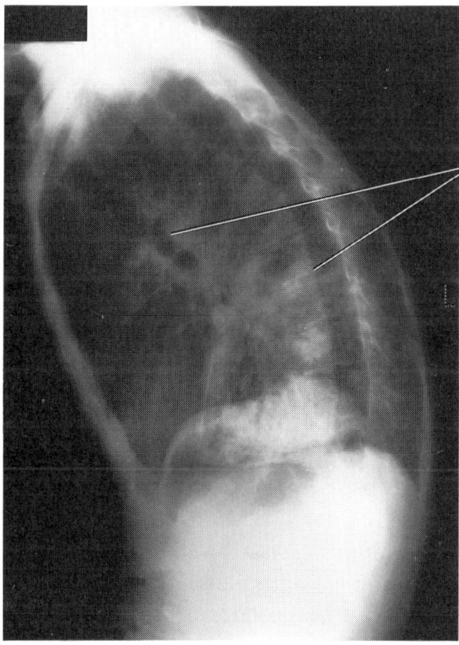

Fig. 27.19 Achalasia of the cardia. A lateral view of the chest showing a broad tubular faint opacity running down the posterior mediastinum. This is the grossly dilated oesophagus.

ly, it is quite frequently possible to coax the tip of the oesophagoscope through the narrowed lower end of the oesophagus, and thereby have the opportunity also to inspect the stomach and duodenum.

If the facilities for measuring pressures within the oesophageal lumen are available the incoordinated pattern of pressures may be recorded. In the past various tests have been advocated to get further confirmatory evidence, such as exaggerating the abnormal movements by a cholinergic drug, but it is probably unnecessary to give these.

Treatment

Although the basic defect in this disorder may be a generalized one affecting all the musculature of the oesophagus, it is possible to relieve all the symptoms by overcoming the resistance in the lower high-pressure zone of musculature by one means or another. The two main approaches are as follows.

The method of treatment most widely used is surgical division of the muscle fibres of the lower oesophagus (Fig. 27.20), similar to Ramstedt's operation on the pylorus in congenital hypertrophic pyloric stenosis. The operation can be performed through either an abdominal or a thoracic approach, the latter perhaps affording greater opportunity to extend the incision in the muscle layers for a sufficient length proximally. Once the lower end of the oesophagus is exposed it is usually a straightforward matter to make a longitudinal incision through the muscle only, but avoiding damage to the mucosa, from the oesophagogastric junction distally for several centimetres proximally.

The alternative approach is forcibly to stretch the tight musculature of the lower end of the oesophagus by means of a hydrostatic bag passed through the mouth, pharynx and oesophagus. The dilating device is carefully located across the lower end of the oesophagus and the diameter and maximal pressure of the stretch are preset. Although there is a slight risk of tearing structures other than simply the musculature, in expert hands good and lasting relief of symptoms has been widely reported.

A disorder with clinical features identical to those of achalasia of the cardia can result from infestation with a trypanosome most commonly encountered in South America, and called Chagas' disease.

Spasm of the oesophagus

On occasions chest pain and dysphagia may arise from unco-ordinated spasm at any level of the

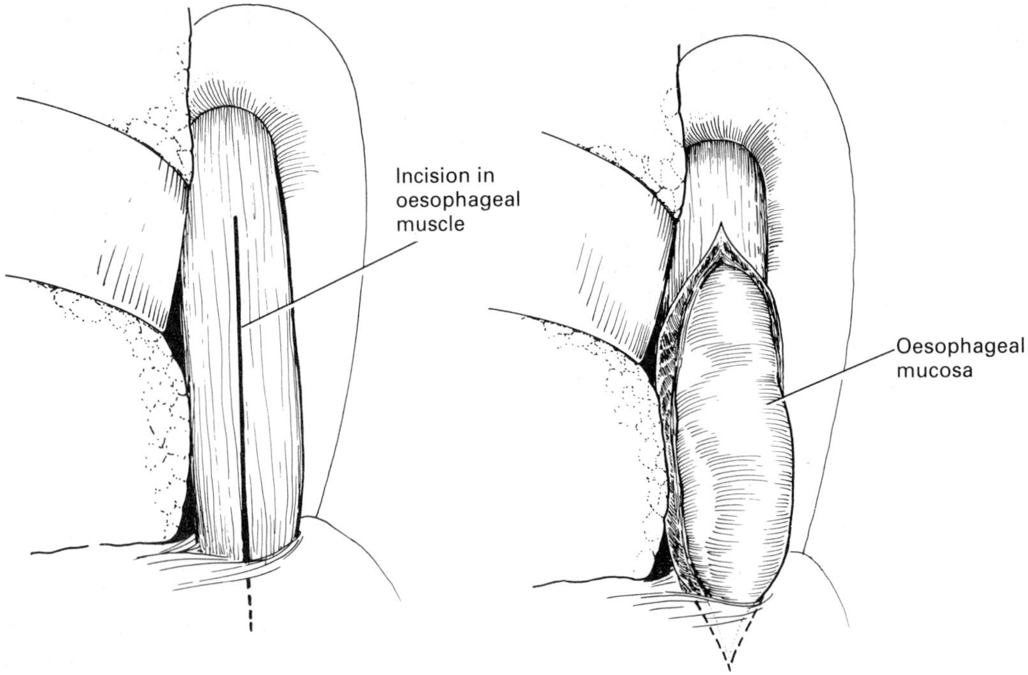

Fig. 27.20 Longitudinal myotomy for achalasia of the cardia (Heller's operation).

oesophagus, more frequently the lower end. Sometimes the symptoms are also relieved by nitrites, making it difficult to distinguish the pain from that of cardiac origin. Confirming that the symptoms are truly due to disordered oesophageal spasm usually requires the demonstration of manometry abnormalities during actual attacks of symptoms. The disorder usually proves quite difficult to control by medication, and on rare occasions relief may be sought from a long myotomy.

DIVERTICULA OF THE OESOPHAGUS

Rarely small congenital diverticula are encountered as coincidental findings during examination, and they are usually of no clinical significance.

Other diverticula may arise proximal to areas of increased pressure, e.g. proximal to achalasia or sliding hiatal hernia.

Pharyngeal pouch (Zenker's diverticulum; Fig. 27.21).

This is basically herniation of the mucosa at the junction between pharynx and oesophagus through an area of potential weakness between the oblique and transverse fibres of the inferior constrictor muscle. As the hernial pouch enlarges it passes usually to the left side of the neck descending towards the mediastinum. Swallowed material tends to go directly into the opening of the pouch rather than into the oesophagus proper, so that the pouch will continue to expand, and eventually become visible low on the left side of the neck anterior to the sternomastoid muscle.

Clinical presentation

The patient, usually elderly, may give a long history of some slight difficulty with swallowing, which will usually affect both solids and liquids. A soft swelling will next have been noticed, and the patient will usually be well aware that it comes up soon after starting to eat, there may be gurgling noises within it, and it may even be noticed that gentle manual compression will reduce it. In addition there may be respiratory symptoms from spillage of the stagnant contents within the pouch into the air passages. The two main risks of persistent pharyngeal pouch are local acute infection and carcinoma.

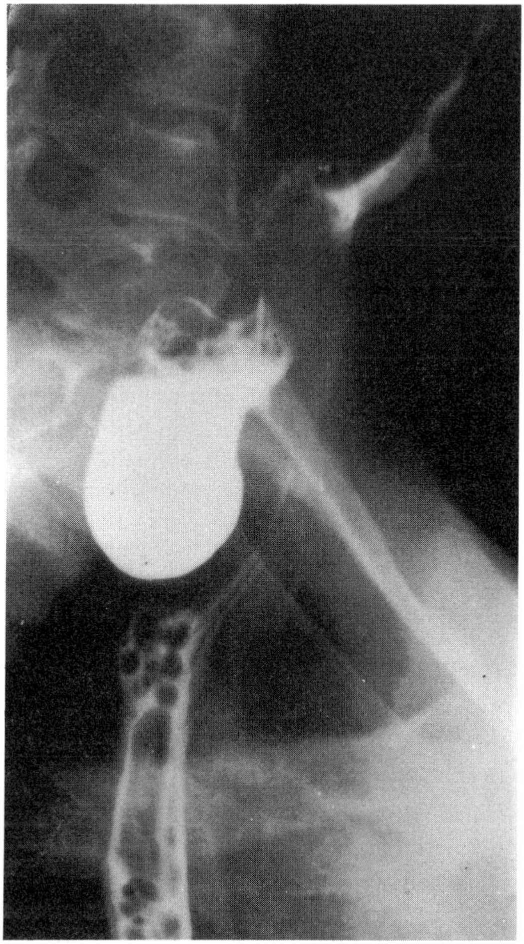

Fig. 27.21 Pharyngeal pouch outlined by barium, in the first few mouthfuls of a barium swallow.

Diagnosis

It is usually easy to demonstrate the outline of the pouch by X-ray after swallowing a mouthful or two of watery barium mixture. Great care should be taken on endoscopy, as the instrument will selectively enter the pouch, and unless the procedure is done with the utmost gentleness there is a risk of perforating the pouch.

Management

A single-stage resection operation is the treatment of choice, and since the majority of these appear on the left side this will involve an incision placed appropriately over the fundus of the pouch. It is often helpful to have the anaesthetist lightly pack the pouch with ribbon gauze or some other material as it is much easier to dissect it out if full rather than collapsed. Care should be taken not to narrow the pharyngo-oesophageal region too much after excision of the pouch, and the passage of a large-bore tube down into the oesophagus can be a helpful guide to this part of the operation.

TRAUMA TO THE OESOPHAGUS

This may be either physical or chemical.

Physical

Although the oesophagus may be damaged along with other structures in penetrating and other injuries of the neck and chest, this is somewhat unusual, and the commonest cause of physical trauma to the oesophagus is endoscopy. Although of very much less frequency with the modern flexible fibreoptic instruments than with the earlier rigid ones, damage to the lining of either the pharynx or oesophagus may occur once in every several thousand examinations. If perforation occurs in the postcricoid region the patient will complain of pain in the neck, and a lateral X-ray of the region may show air behind the oesophagus. If perforation is suspected or confirmed all further oral administration is withheld, and a broad-spectrum antibiotic should be prescribed. Observation for up to 24 h is reasonable where there is evidence that the tear is indeed a small one, and slow satisfactory healing may take place over the next few days. If, however, signs of improvement do not occur the appropriate segment of the oesophagus should be surgically explored through the neck, any escaped material carefully removed and the rent repaired by direct suture. It is wise to leave a small drain from the site for a few days.

Perforation may also occur in the lower oesophagus usually just above the diaphragmatic hiatus. In this case the patient will experience severe chest pain, and X-ray will show air either in the mediastinum or in the pleural cavity on the side of the perforation. Immediate thoracotomy is required to repair the tear, and this should be done under systemic antibiotic cover.

Trauma from forceful vomiting

Two very different but dramatic clinical presentations may result from tears in the oesophageal wall caused by sudden violent increases in intragastric pressure, usually when the stomach is particularly full. In the first, Mallory–Weiss syndrome, the tear involves the mucosa at or very close to the oesophagogastric junction, and presents as haematemesis; the second, Boerhaave's syndrome, involves a tear right through the entire wall of the distal oesophagus with spillage of gastrointestinal content into the left pleural cavity.

Mallory–Weiss syndrome. The history is usually of vigorous vomiting associated with much retching and straining soon after the ingestion of a large meal which often contains alcohol. If there is some form of anatomical weakness at this level, e.g. hiatal hernia, the occurrence is more likely. The vomited material obviously contains blood, sometimes in alarming quantities, and it is one of the differential diagnoses of haematemesis. If the condition is suspected, endoscopy is required to confirm the diagnosis, as barium meal will not demonstrate any gross abnormality. The torn veins are often just distal to the oesophagogastric junction on the proximal part of the fundus.

Conservative treatment with avoidance of further swallowing, replacement of lost blood if necessary, and the passage of time will usually result in control of the bleeding, but on rare occasions if blood loss continues operation may be required, at which the torn area is repaired under direct vision by suture after making a gastrotomy in the proximal stomach.

Boerhaave's syndrome. Again the immediately preceding history is generally violent vomiting acts soon after the ingestion of a heavy meal, and the vomiting act is suddenly followed by severe pain across the lower chest or epigastrium, restriction of breathing, which may amount to dyspnoea and cyanosis. The patient is obviously severely ill, and it may be difficult to differentiate the condition from other common acute abdominal emergencies such as perforated peptic ulcer, acute pancreatitis, or even myocardial infarction. Clinical or radiological signs of pleural effusion or pneumothorax are strong indicators of the syndrome, and later suspicious clinical signs include surgical emphysema in the root of the neck.

If there is genuine diagnostic doubt radiological examination after the swallowing of a small amount of gastrografin may clearly identify the tear.

As soon as the diagnosis is made operative treatment should be carried out. If it is less than 24 h since the accident occurred it should be possible to repair the tear by direct suture, followed by drainage of the pleural cavity. If, on the other hand, there has been some delay in establishing the diagnosis then primary repair may be exceedingly difficult and unwise, and surgical measures may be confined to securing adequate drainage of the pleural cavity, parenteral nutrition, and broad-spectrum antibiotic coverage. A later attempt at repair of the defect may then be made when the local tissue reaction and the general condition of the patient have improved.

Chemical

Corrosive damage

This is caused by the accidental or intentional ingestion of corrosives, which may be acid or alkaline. The mouth and pharynx are damaged to a varying extent. The brunt of the damage, however, is borne by the oesophagus. If the corrosive is very strong, the oesophagus may perforate and a fatal mediastinitis follow. If the patient survives, the natural processes of healing following the damage may result in the formation of a fibrous stricture, and the dysphagia will usually become apparent some weeks after the ingestion of the damaging chemical.

Following the ingestion of corrosives severe pain occurs in the mouth, neck and chest. First-aid treatment consists of rinsing the mouth and throat with copious amounts of water which is also swallowed. Although theoretically one might advocate simple alkalis for acid burns, and mild acids for alkali burns, this practice is not recommended. First, it may take some time to find the appropriate chemical, and secondly, a resulting chemical interaction between an acid and alkali might produce heat and therefore further damage. Water is readily available, and will rapidly dilute the effects of the offending agent.

Analgesics will be required, and it is wise to give broad-spectrum antibiotic coverage as well. It has also been conventional to prescribe cortisone with the objective of delaying and diminishing the deposition of fibrous tissue and therefore diminishing the risk of subsequent stricture formation. If the patient is reasonably comfortable and able to swallow, oral fluids are permitted after the first 12 h, and it is hoped that he or she will manage soft foods 2–3 days later. Barium swallow examination and gentle endoscopy are probably best deferred until about a week after the injury, as endoscopy might damage further the friable mucosa at an earlier stage, and barium swallow is unlikely to show any narrowing at this stage. If no stricture formation occurs a gradual return to normal diet is permitted, but if stricture formation does occur this may require repeated dilatation under direct vision through the oesophagoscope, or it may be managed by teaching the patient to swallow an oesophageal bougie threaded over a radiopaque string which has been previously introduced under radiological control.

While the majority of such corrosive strictures can be managed satisfactorily by one or other of these conservative means, occasionally in the most refractory cases a decision has to be taken to attempt operative repair. A preliminary period of nutrition either through a gastrostomy or via the parenteral route may be required to build up the patient's general strength for operation. For the most severe strictures bypass of the damaged area may be attempted using an isolated loop of intestine joined proximally to the cervical oesophagus, and distally to the stomach.

Foreign bodies

The majority of foreign bodies which become impacted in the oesophagus are swallowed accidentally, and this may happen in children who have a tendency to put various solid objects in their mouths, or again in adults who are mentally disturbed. Loose-fitting dentures may also become dislodged and accidentally swallowed during eating. The swallowed foreign object is usually held up at one of the areas in which there is narrowing, e.g. at the aortic arch or the lower end of the oesophagus. The history is usually apparent, and the patient is aware of the object being impacted and makes repeated swallowing attempts in an effort to dislodge it.

The problem should be dealt with urgently, and if the object is radiopaque a simple radiograph may help in locating the point of impaction. For those objects which are not radiopaque the swallowing of a small amount of contrast medium may identify it.

Many objects can be removed by special instruments passed through an oesophagoscope, and it is desirable to conduct the removal under direct vision to minimize the chances of further damage to the mucosa. At times considerable ingenuity is required to manipulate the object into a satisfactory position to allow safe removal, and on occasions all such attempts prove unsuccessful. If this is the case there are two further alternatives. First, it may be possible gently to propel the object distally into the stomach from which it may be removed by laparotomy and gastrotomy. The second alternative, if the object cannot be moved, is to explore the relevant segment of the oesophagus, usually through a left or right thoracotomy.

28. The stomach

Although the stomach is not absolutely essential for life, and reasonable health and satisfactory digestion can occur following total gastrectomy, it does perform the obvious physiological roles of accepting variable amounts of ingested material, mixing these, and delivering small, manageable metered quantities into the small intestine where the principal processes of digestion and absorption occur. Like other segments of the gastrointestinal tract there is a mucosa, a submucosa with a thin muscularis mucosa, an inner layer of smooth muscle which is predominantly circular, an outer layer which is predominantly longitudinal, and a covering of serosa. The gastric mucosa contains numerous simple tube-like glands lined and covered by a simple columnar type of epithelium, specialized cells in the fundic portion secreting hydrochloric acid and intrinsic factor, others producing pepsinogens, and others mucus. The mucosa of the antrum, on the other hand, produces no acid and pepsin, but among its glands are specialized cells which produce gastrin.

The main roles of hydrochloric acid are first to reduce the bacterial content of ingested substances, slightly to assist in the absorption of certain ions, e.g. iron and calcium, and to activate pepsinogens into active pepsin enzymes. A minor amount of both proteolytic and glycolytic digestion may take place in the stomach, but this is trivial compared to the digestion which occurs in the small intestine. The only essential secretory product is the intrinsic factor necessary for normal absorption of vitamin B_{12} in the distal small bowel.

The principal movements occurring in the stomach are well co-ordinated propulsive waves which start in the proximal stomach and sweep rhythmically distally to and beyond the pylorus three to four times per minute. By and large, parasympathetic stimulation via the vagus nerves increases both secretion and motility, and sympathetic activity inhibits both. Final mediation of nervous impulses, and integration of local reflex activity in the stomach wall occurs in the two fine plexuses in the submucosal layer (Auerbach's plexus), and between the main muscle layers (Meissner's plexus).

As has been mentioned, the hormone gastrin is released from specialized cells in the antral mucosa principally by the presence of food within the antrum, and in addition many of the functions of the stomach can be influenced by a variety of known gastrointestinal hormones.

The principal disorders of the stomach are first the congenital pattern of pyloric stenosis, peptic ulcer, carcinoma of the stomach, and various inflammatory forms of gastritis. Since most of the causes of haematemesis arise from the stomach, it is appropriate to discuss this major clinical problem also in this chapter.

CONGENITAL HYPERTROPHIC PYLORIC STENOSIS

This is the only significant congenital anomaly of the stomach to be encountered. It occurs much more frequently in boys than in girls, and classically the first-born is more likely to be affected than subsequent sibs. The pregnancy and birth are usually perfectly normal, and the symptoms become apparent in the second or third week of life. It is highly unusual for them to arise after the first six weeks of life.

Feeding during the first week or so has usually been quite normal, but thereafter the baby is seen to vomit forcefully immediately after feeding. Appetite is undisturbed for the baby is keen for a feed, and even after vomiting may want eagerly to feed again. If treatment is not sought the resultant loss of fluid and gastric secretion will rapidly cause weight loss, dehydration and possibly alkalosis.

Clinical examination while the baby is feeding will reveal the outline of the distending stomach, and it is usually possible to feel the typical rounded bobbin-like mass of the thickened pyloric musculature in the right upper abdomen.

The main risks of the condition are first the severe fluid and electrolyte depletion, and secondly the inhalation into the respiratory tract of regurgitated material.

Usually a firm diagnosis can be reached from a combination of the typical history and clinical findings, and no special investigations are required. If serious fluid and electrolyte depletion is suspected it is, of course, wise to assess these by measurement of serum electrolyte levels.

The condition is completely resolved by the operation of pyloromyotomy (Ramstedt's operation; Fig. 28.1), in which the thickened musculature at the pyloric region is divided longitudinally down to the mucosa which is left intact. This relieves the compression, and very shortly after the procedure the baby should be able to feed normally. It is unwise to delay the operative procedure or to administer any drugs which on theoretical grounds might be expected to reduce muscle tone as these are unlikely to succeed, and will serve only to delay the straightforward surgical correction of the abnormality. A normal life expectancy without further derangement of gastric function is expected.

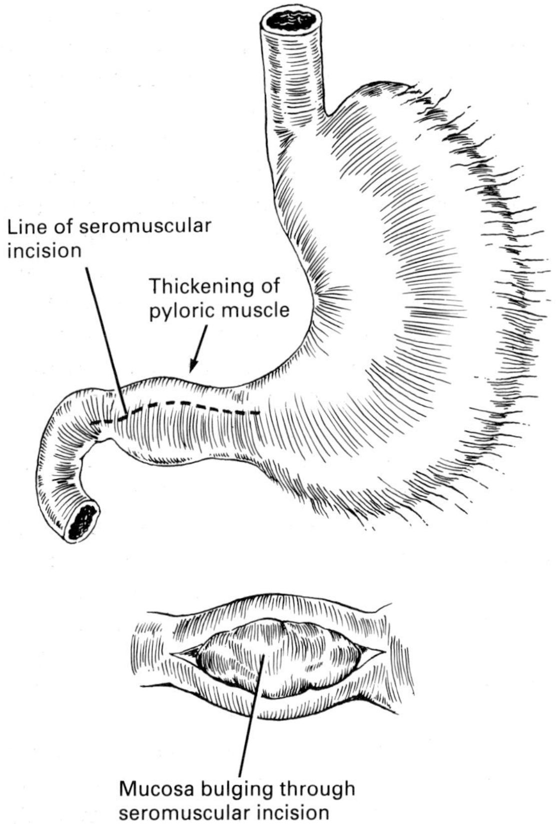

Fig. 28.1 Ramstedt's operation for congenital pyloric stenosis. A longitudinal incision is made through the serous and thickened bobbin-like mass of muscle, taking care not to damage the underlying mucosa of the distal antrum and proximal duodenum.

PEPTIC ULCER

Chronic peptic ulcer

Under this heading we are mainly concerned with the commonest types of ulcer which arise either in the duodenum or stomach. The vast majority of duodenal ulcers arise in the duodenal bulb—the 2–3 cm segment just distal to the pylorus. Gastric ulcers virtually all arise somewhere along the lesser curvature, the majority being in the antral region, i.e. in the distal one-third to one-half of the curvature.

Occasionally chronic ulcers can develop in the lower oesophagus as the result of long-standing gastro-oesophageal reflux, and again ulcers can arise at or just distal to anastomoses between the stomach and small intestine (anastomotic ulcers), and even more rarely they may arise in the distal ileum, for example in relation to a Meckel's diverticulum. The special clinical problems of these are discussed.

Aetiology

Although the exact cause or causes of chronic peptic ulcer are not known, much is known about the geographical distribution of the disease and of considerable changes in the pattern which have occurred in the last few decades in several countries. It is likely that the epidemiological observations contain important clues which are as yet incompletely understood.

Although peptic ulcer is still a common disease in most countries throughout the world, the incidence varies considerably from one country to another, and there are even marked differences within countries such as India from one region to another. There is much evidence from both North American and European data to suggest that the overall incidence and severity of the disease have diminished in recent years, and that these changes are not the direct result of improvements in medical or surgical treatment. While the disease is still commoner in men than in women, the order of difference has diminished so that the male preponderance is not as great as it was 20 or 30 years ago. Again, whereas duodenal ulcer remains more frequent than gastric ulcer, the ratio of the former to the latter has fallen steadily. A marked decrease in the occurrence of perforation of both duodenal and gastric ulcer has been recorded from several countries over the past 30 years, but whether this fall will continue or not is uncertain.

These few examples of the changing pattern of disease are quoted to emphasize that if the disease is changing our approach to the treatment may also require some modification as time passes.

Although we do not understand the precise mechanisms by which environmental factors directly affect gastric function, we can now list a number of factors which are known to lead to a greater than normal risk of ulcers developing: smoking cigarettes, chronic obstructive airways disease, renal failure, the taking of certain drugs such as salicylate, anti-inflammatory drugs and adrenocorticosteroids, and high levels of certain genetic markers, e.g. serum pepsinogen 1. While it has been known for some time that there is a higher incidence of duodenal ulcer in those of blood group O, this knowledge is of no significant clinical value with regard to prevention, diagnosis, or treatment.

Some relationship between the gastric secretion of hydrochloric acid and pepsin, and both gastric and duodenal ulcers clearly exists, for neither type of peptic ulcer can persist in the total absence of these secreted materials. Having noted this, however, there is a difference in this relationship between gastric and duodenal ulcers. Individual patients with either type of ulcer show considerable variation in their gastric outputs of acid under both resting and stimulated conditions, but on average duodenal ulcer patients produce twice as much as normal individuals both basally and following maximal stimulation, e.g. with pentagastrin. On the other hand, gastric ulcer patients have normal or even slightly reduced acid secretory levels to minimal and maximal stimulation. It is believed, therefore, that whereas in duodenal ulcer there is a direct or indirect aetiological link between the hypersecretion of acid and the ulcer, the principal defect in gastric ulcer is more likely to be a weakness in one or more of the defence mechanisms shielding the mucosa against the effects of the acid and pepsin. There is much less detailed knowledge concerning these defence mechanisms, e.g. the capacity of the mucosal cells to proliferate and repair, the adequacy of mucosal blood flow, the quantity and quality of mucus, and the bicarbonate content of the 'unstirred layer' within the mucus immediately adjacent to the epithelial cells. One hypothesis of the development of gastric ulcer suggests an impairment of one or more of these factors might permit the back-diffusion of a certain quantity of hydrogen ion from the lumen of the stomach into or across the gastric mucosa and the consequent damage to the latter by the local activation of proteolytic enzymes. This whole train of events could be initiated by the harmful effects of regurgitated material from the upper small intestine proximally through the pylorus.

The relative hypersecretion of acid in duodenal ulcer patients remains unexplained. It was formerly thought that various stresses arising in the central nervous system might be conveyed by the vagus nerves directly to the stomach, thereby increasing acid secretion, but there is remarkably little evidence to support this. Secondly, since the hormone gastrin is known to be a potent stimulant of the hydrochloric acid-producing cells in the gastric fundus, there might be some abnormal production of this hormone in duodenal ulcer. Again, there is no evidence to support this. The balance of available data suggests that for one reason or another duodenal ulcer patients have an excess number of acid-secreting cells in the stomach, and these cells are particularly sensitive to the various normal stimuli to acid secretion. Why these two factors should be present is not known.

While it is known that gross abnormalities of gastrin and other hormone production can result in ulcers which have the same pathological features as common peptic ulcer, and this observation is perhaps one of the strongest pieces of evidence pointing to a link between abnormal acid secretion and ulcer formation, it must be stressed that there is no evidence of abnormal hormone production in the common pattern of chronic peptic ulcer.

Clinical features

Although, as has been discussed, there are distinct differences between duodenal and gastric ulcer with respect to the basic pathophysiology, the clinical features of both are virtually the same, and it is not usually possible to distinguish them on clinical history alone. In both the principal symptom is epigastric pain, usually described as a gnawing or burning sensation, and the patient is usually able to localize this fairly accurately. The severity of the pain varies from one patient to another, and in any individual may vary considerably from time to time. It tends to occur when the stomach is empty, and therefore may be described as hunger pain, or it may be noted to appear fairly regularly at an interval following meals varying from 30 min to 2 h. The patient may also note that the further ingestion of food or liquid may temporarily relieve the pain. From this it is concluded that at least one of the factors contributing to the pain is exposure of nerve endings in the ulcerated area to acid gastric juice; the relief from further eating is then due to the dilution, neutralization or buffering of the acid with a consequent rise in intragastric pH. It is also common for the patient to be wakened from sleep, usually in the early hours of the morning, again probably due to the continuing secretion of acid after the last ingested material of the day has emptied from the stomach. The patient often discovers that taking a small snack will relieve the pain sufficiently to allow him or her to return to sleep.

If the severity of the pain gradually increases it may also radiate through to the back, and the patient's description is usually that he or she feels the pain boring directly from the front right through to a corresponding level in the back. This may indicate that the ulcer base has penetrated posteriorly into the retroperitoneal tissues.

It is absolutely characteristic of the disorder that over a period of time the patient experiences relapses of troublesome pain or discomfort over a few days or weeks, and then remissions totally free of symptoms. Both the relapses and the remissions may last for variable periods, and whereas there may appear to be environmental or emotional causes for some of the relapses, there is most often no obvious reason for the recurrences. This periodicity in the symptom history is so characteristic of the disease that an uninterrupted history of daily recurrent upper abdominal pain persisting without remission over many months is almost certainly not due to a peptic ulcer.

Vomiting is not a common complaint in peptic ulcer patients, but may occur occasionally in either duodenal or gastric ulcer. When vomiting does occur it is usually of recently ingested material and gastric secretions and it often relieves the pain. The onset of repeated vomiting of large amounts of stomach content in patients with duodenal ulcer suggests the onset of some degree of narrowing of the gastric outlet due to scarring and fibrosis at the duodenal ulcer site, referred to as pyloric stenosis.

Various other dyspeptic symptoms, e.g. heartburn, belching, and vague indigestion may also be present in patients with peptic ulcer, and it is not infrequent that they also complain of their symptoms being aggravated by fatty foods. Although it is customary to associate fatty intolerance primarily with gallbladder disease, this is by no means specific, as patients with peptic ulcer and indeed a variety of other intra-abdominal disorders not infrequently feel that fatty foods aggravate symptoms.

Clinical signs

On clinical examination the only physical sign which can normally be elicited is epigastric tenderness. This may vary considerably in severity from being detected on the lightest of pressure, and associated with some degree of muscle guarding, to requiring moderately deep pressure before it is demonstrated. In duodenal ulcer the tenderness is often distinctly to the right of midline in the epigastrium, whereas in gastric ulcer the site of tenderness is more variable.

Investigations

It is important to confirm the diagnosis of peptic ulcer before embarking on treatment as other important conditions may present with symptoms similar to those of peptic ulcer, and it is particularly important not to overlook early carcinoma of the stomach.

As for most disorders affecting the stomach, the two main investigations are barium meal X-ray and endoscopy. By the judicious use of either or both of these investigations a confident and accurate diagnosis of both gastric and duodenal ulcer should be made in virtually all instances. With the availability of modern, safe, flexible, manoeuvrable endoscopic instruments there is debate as to whether preliminary barium meal examination is necessary, and therefore that endoscopy should be the initial diagnostic procedure. In many centres, however, it is still usual to perform barium meal examination first, preferably by a double-contrast technique, which gives a clearer picture of the mucosal pattern. Typical examples of both gastric and duodenal ulcers are shown in Figures 28.2 and 28.3. In addition to the demonstration of the ulcer, the examination should give additional information, e.g. the presence of any significant gastro-oesophageal reflux, a simple estimate of the rate of gastric emptying, and the presence of any potential hazard to endoscopy such as marked osteoarthritic lipping of the cervical spine or oesophageal abnormality.

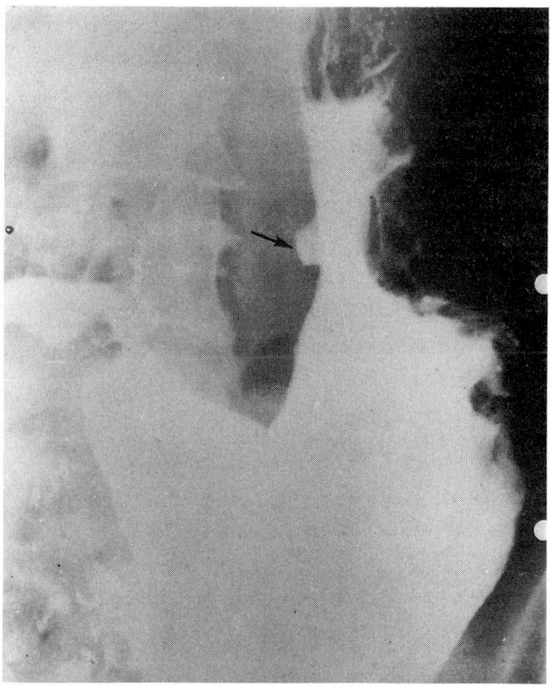

Fig. 28.2 Barium meal outlining a benign gastric peptic ulcer (arrowed). The crater is smooth and projecting outwards from the line of the normal lesser curvature of the stomach.

Endoscopy can be easily performed under light sedation and local anaesthesia, and permits the inspection of the entire oesophagus, stomach, and proximal duodenum (Fig. 28.4). It may be necessary to give an intravenous injection of a drug such as Buscopan to secure adequate relaxation of the pylorus, and thereby introduce the tip of the instrument into the duodenum. As well as visualizing the actual ulcer, the endoscopist is able to assess the degree of inflammatory change in the surrounding mucosa, to determine if there is any other coincidental abnormality, and to take small biopsies by a special forceps passed along one of the channels in the instrument (Fig. 28.5). It is particularly important to take biopsies of a gastric ulcer, as sometimes it is impossible to differentiate a benign gastric ulcer from an early ulcerating carcinoma solely on gross visual appearances.

Although a high degree of accuracy of diagnosis is expected from either barium meal examination or endoscopy, or a combination of both, a small number of peptic ulcers will be missed on either initial investigation, and if typical symptoms persist there should be no hesitation in repeating either or both. This will increase the accuracy of detection even further.

Other investigations

During phases of activity in either a gastric or duodenal ulcer there may be small amounts of blood loss from the ulcerated area, and therefore occult blood may be detected in the stools. It is also wise to check the haemoglobin level of ulcer patients from time to time, as more significant bleeding may lead to a degree of anaemia.

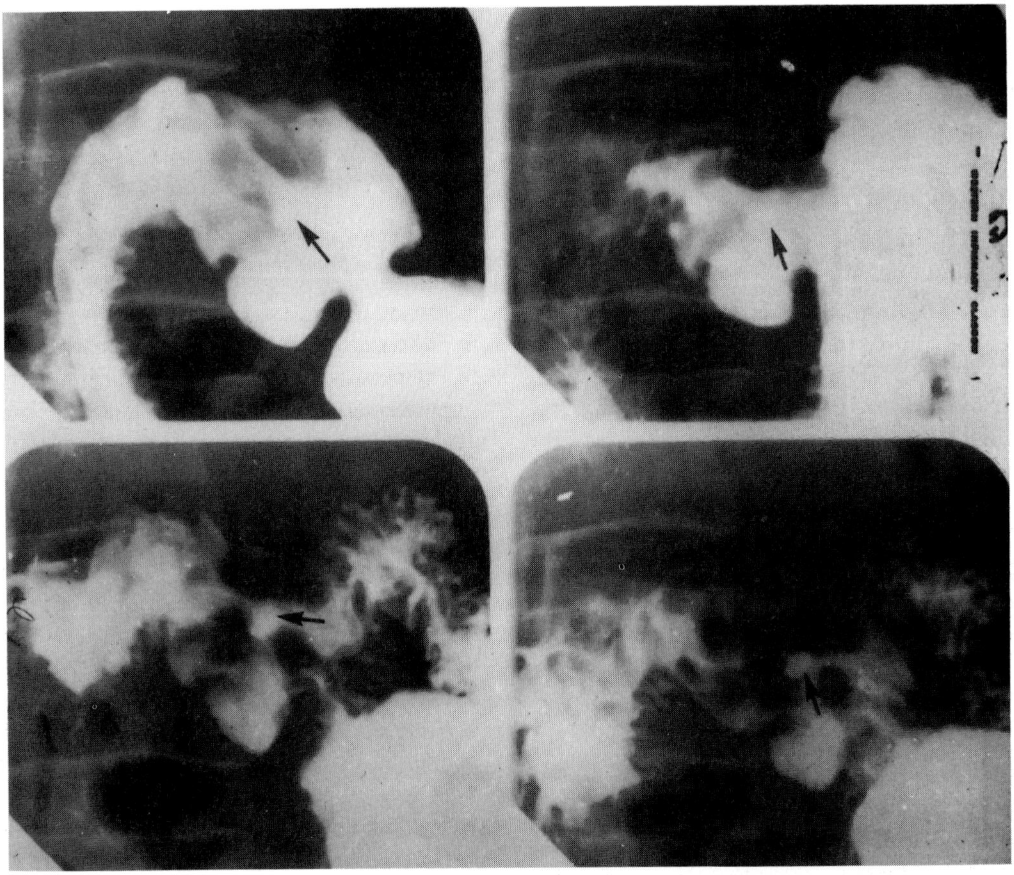

Fig. 28.3 Barium meal appearances in chronic duodenal ulcer. The ulcer niche is indicated by the arrow in these four different views of the barium-filled duodenal cap. Normally this cap should fill out smoothly as a triangular shadow with rounded corners. In the presence of the ulcer, scarring deforms this outline.

Acid secretion measurement

Although many studies have reported measurements of gastric acid secretion during basal conditions, overnight, and in response to a variety of test meals and pharmacological stimuli, any such measurements are of virtually no value in assisting diagnosis, or in deciding appropriate methods of treatment. As has been mentioned, duodenal ulcer patients generally secrete more acid under both resting and stimulated conditions, but there is such a wide overlap in the amounts of secretion in the different diagnostic groups that any diagnostic discrimination based on these measurements is extremely poor. There also appears to be little correlation between the amounts of gastric secretion and the severity of the ulcer disease.

The usefulness of tests of acid secretion are limited to three areas. First the very rare gastrinoma (Zollinger–Ellison syndrome) in which abnormally high levels of gastrin are released from the tumour is characterized by very high levels of basal acid secretion, and minimal further increase in response to maximal levels of a stimulant such as pentagastrin. Secondly, when a recurrent ulcer follows a previous operation for duodenal ulcer, this is usually the result of the first operation not having sufficiently reduced the capacity of the stomach to secrete acid, and higher than expected levels of acid secretion usually obtain. Thirdly, in the investigation of a recurrent ulcer following a previous vagotomy operation a significant acid-secretory response to insulin hypoglycaemia

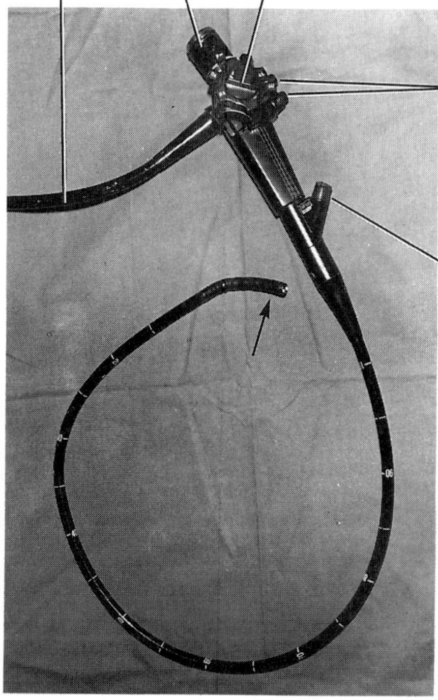

Fig. 28.4 Oesophagogastroduodenoscope. The fibreoptic cables transmitting the light and the images gives the instrument great flexibility and manoeuvrability. The tip can be moved in all directions and rotated to bring all parts of the stomach into view, and negotiated through the pylorus to inspect the proximal parts of the duodenum. Biopsies can be taken by passing a flexible wire carrying an open-and-close set of jaws at its distal end.

indicates the persistence of some residual vagal innervation of the stomach.

Apart from these three considerations most of the acid secretion tests on peptic ulcer patients are performed for research purposes to try and obtain further insight into the pathophysiology of the disease.

Medical treatment

The aims of treatment, medical or surgical, are twofold: to alleviate the symptoms, and to achieve healing of the ulcer with, hopefully, the prevention of further recurrence. The main objective of both conservative and surgical measures is to reduce either the production or the actions of hydrochloric acid, and by and large the means of achieving this objective are the most efficient at securing ulcer healing. This is basically true in the approach to both duodenal and gastric ulcer, in spite of the latter not being associated with hypersecretion of acid. Some of the drugs more recently used in the treatment of gastric ulcer do have actions which are believed to strengthen the mucosal resistance in one way or another, but these are usually used as a second line of approach, and they appear to be much less effective in the treatment of duodenal ulcer.

It is likely that many patients with relatively mild symptoms from peptic ulcers are able to obtain satisfactory relief and eventual ulcer healing by self-medication with one or more of the readily available proprietary antacid preparations and simple regulation of diet. A good number of others will be managed quite successfully by primary care doctors, and only the more troublesome and persistent will require medical or surgical specialist advice.

In addition to the specific measures about to be discussed, a few general pieces of advice should be given. First, since there is a clear relationship between cigarette smoking and the risks of peptic ulcer strong exhortation should be given to cigarette smokers to stop. Although there is no need to give strict dietary advice, it is reasonable to suggest that the patient should take modest meals on a regular basis and avoid long periods of fasting. It also seems common sense to advise that any foods which the patient feels are regularly followed by bouts of pain should be avoided.

Most patients presenting initially with uncomplicated peptic ulcer should be given a period of medical treatment in the first instance, and the majority will be satisfactorily controlled by these measures alone. Elective operation is required only for those who fail to respond to medical treatment, and those who are unfortunate enough to develop one of the complications of the ulcer.

Drugs

H_2-receptor antagonists

The first of this important group of drugs, cimetidine, became available in 1976, and this represented

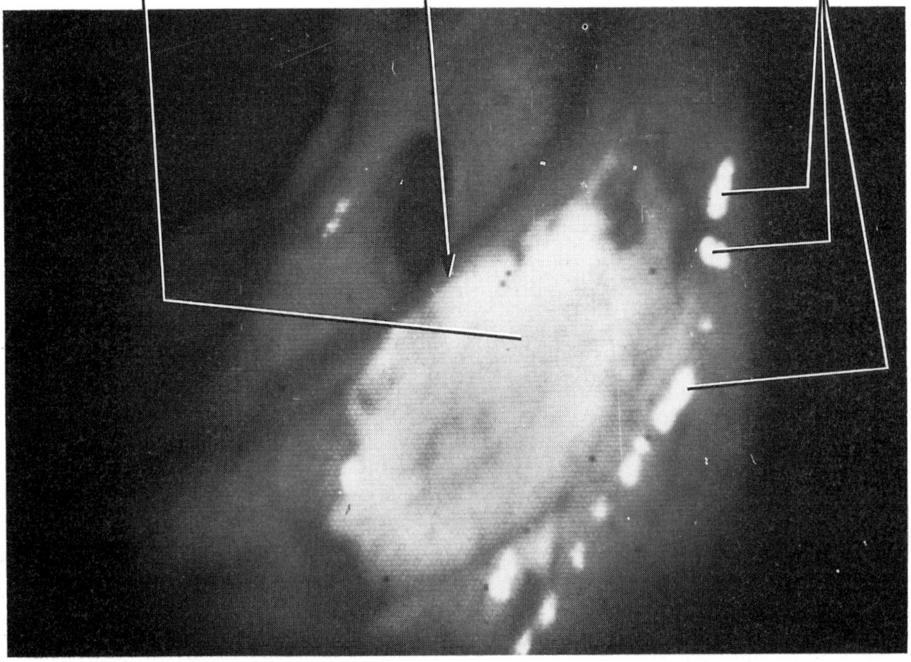

Fig. 28.5 Gastroscopic view of benign peptic ulcer in the distal segment—shallow, oval, clean-cut mucosal ulcer with a smooth edge *not* elevated from the normal mucosal level.

the first significant advance in the medical treatment of peptic ulcer for many years. It, and the more recently introduced famotidine and nizatidine are now in widespread use throughout the world as the first and strongest line of attack on both duodenal and gastric ulcer. This group of drugs was developed as the result of a deliberate search for molecules similar in structure to histamine, but which would block the histamine receptors on the acid-secreting cells of the stomach without displaying blockage of other histamine receptors or producing significant side-effects. It has been clearly shown that the H_2-receptor antagonists effectively suppress acid secretion in response to virtually all known stimuli. This does not necessarily imply that histamine is the final common path of all stimulation of the gastric acid cells. It is known that there are specific receptors on the acid-producing cells for not only histamine, but also gastrin and acetylcholine, and it is also known that activation of one type of receptor facilitates the action of the others. The action of H_2-receptor antagonists is therefore seen as impairing the effectiveness of these other linked receptors, and this explains the apparent effectiveness in suppressing responses to stimuli other than histamine-releasing ones.

Although there is some difference of opinion regarding the dosage and length of time of administration of the H_2-receptor antagonists, there is a general consensus that the first course of treatment at full dosage should be for approximately 6 weeks. Full dosage for cimetidine is of the order of 1 g/day in divided doses, and for ranitidine 150 mg twice a day. Symptom response to either of these agents is usually rapid, occurring within 1–3 days. The dosage should, however, be continued for the full 6 weeks even if symptoms remain completely under control during that time. Thereafter it is recommended that a reduced dosage of cimetidine 200–400 mg/day or ranitidine 150 mg/day be continued for a further period of approximately 3 months. If symptoms remain completely under control at the end of this period ideally the patient should be re-examined by endoscopy to assess the completeness of healing of the ulcer. If both symptoms and the ulcer have disappeared, the medication may be stopped and if symptoms recur at a later date the whole course of full dosage followed by reduced dosage may be repeated. Some medical specialists will continue H_2-receptor antagonist treatment for much more prolonged periods, particularly if there is any gastroscopic evidence of ulcer persistence. While the safety record of these drugs is very good, and the incidence of side-effects extremely small, many have reservations about prolonged periods of profound suppression of acid secretion in the stomach, and therefore feel that the more limited medication schedule outlined above is preferable.

Because the H_2-receptor antagonists have proved so effective in reducing acid secretion and controlling the symptoms of peptic ulcer disease there has been understandably the temptation to prescribe these drugs readily to all patients presenting with any type of upper abdominal discomfort or pain, dyspepsia or other digestive symptoms. This practice is to be condemned, for it is entirely possible that a short course of one of these agents will suppress symptoms which may prove not to be arising from peptic ulcer. It is particularly tragic if they are administered to someone who has an early carcinoma of the stomach, for it is entirely possible that the mild symptoms will be suppressed, and the tumour left to grow before a firm diagnosis is made. Such delay may make all the difference between an early operable lesion and a hopelessly inoperable one. It is therefore important to establish the diagnosis of benign peptic ulcer before starting treatment with one of these drugs.

Antacids

These preparations were the most widely used means of countering the effects of gastric acid before the H_2-receptor antagonists became available. From a long list of possible alkaline salts the more popular and effective contained various combinations of aluminium hydroxide, magnesium trisilicate, hydroxide or carbonate, or calcium carbonate. In earlier years it was common practice to advise patients simply to take modest doses of one or other of these preparations as and when symptoms were troublesome, and this regime often brought about satisfactory, if temporary, symptom control. If, however, the antacid preparation is given in frequently taken high dosage, sufficient to achieve reduction in intragastric acid equivalent to the effect of the H_2-receptor antagonists, a comparable degree of symptom control and ulcer healing may be achieved, so that if antacids are prescribed such a schedule should be used. This, of course, means taking the antacid preparation about every 1–2 h throughout the day, and this is exceedingly difficult if the patient remains normally active.

There seems to be some variation in the acceptance and apparent effectiveness of different antacid preparations and it is reasonable to take such preference into consideration.

Some antacids, for example those containing magnesium, have a mild laxative effect, whereas those containing aluminium hydroxide may have the opposite effect on the bowel. This is a factor which may to some extent influence the choice of a particular antacid for a particular patient. Most preparations are available in either liquid or tablet form, and usually the former are found to be more effective, although less convenient for usage in the ambulant patient. The possibility of calcium or magnesium overload should be kept in mind when large doses of antacids containing these substances are given. In the past there was considerable concern that alkalosis might occur from prolonged high dosage, but this was mainly a fear when sodium bicarbonate was used.

Other inhibitors of gastric secretion

One of the most interesting recent additions has been the development of omeprazole, a drug which interferes with the production of hydrochloric acid within the parietal cell. Impressive reduction in gastric acid can be achieved, and as well as it having considerable potential in treating peptic ulcer, it shows great promise of being of use in the long-term management of gross hypersecretory states, e.g. the Zollinger–Ellison syndrome (gastrinoma).

A large number of peptides, including some of the known hormones of the gastrointestinal tract, have the capacity to inhibit gastric acid secretion, but since these are all peptides they are only effective when given by systemic administration. There is, therefore, no realistic expectation of them having direct clinical application, particularly when such potent alternatives are now available. Evidence is accumulating that some of these may possess properties other than inhibition of acid secretion, which may have a beneficial effect on epithelial and fibrous tissue repair processes, and this is an avenue for further exploration.

Anticholinergic drugs

Theoretically agents which block the release or action of acetylcholine, the main mediator of vagal stimulation to the stomach, should be effective in the treatment of peptic ulcer. Not only should they reduce acid secretion, but also they should diminish the motility of the stomach which may also be of benefit to the patient. However, experience with a variety of conventional anticholinergic agents such as belladonna, atropine, hyoscine and probanthine has been on the whole disappointing. In order to achieve a sufficient anticholinergic effect on the stomach these agents have to be prescribed in doses which inevitably cause side-effects such as slight dryness of the mouth from a reduced flow of saliva, blurring of vision, and difficulty in emptying both the bladder and the bowel. Such side-effects constitute real risks to people whose work requires accurate vision, and to those with glaucoma, prostatic hypertrophy, and various other disorders. Until recently, therefore, these agents had largely fallen out of favour in the management of peptic ulcer.

A new generation of anticholinergic agents with much more specific activity against the gastrointestinal tract and appreciably less troublesome side-effects has recently appeared, and one of these, pirenzepine, shows more promise of being effective in the control of ulcer symptoms: its further evaluation is awaited with interest.

Carbenoxolone sodium

This is a synthetic material derived to resemble the structure of one of the components of liquorice. Evidence from trials based on a radiological control of ulcer size suggests that it has the ability to accelerate ulcer healing with a clearer effect on gastric than duodenal ulcer. It has no effect on acid secretion, and possibly its therapeutic benefit is the result of an increase in the amount and strength of mucus, a slight reduction in pepsin activity, and/or a direct effect on mucosal cells increasing their rate of maturation. In therapeutic doses it also has fluid-retaining properties resembling the action of adrenocorticosteroids. Indeed, spironolactone not only suppresses the sodium and water retention, but also blocks the healing effect of the carbenoxolone sodium, suggesting that in some way the two effects are related. Potassium loss from the kidney is increased by carbenoxolone sodium, so that caution must be exercised when prescribing this preparation, particularly in elderly patients and those with known renal disease. Where hypertension or cardiac embarrassment is present increased fluid retention from carbenoxolone sodium may also be undesirable. It seems wise to make frequent regular checks on body weight, blood pressure, and serum electrolyte concentrations of patients taking carbenoxolone sodium.

Deglycyrrhizinized liquorice

This is a purified extract of liquorice, and like carbenoxolone sodium, its beneficial actions may be mediated by similar mucosa-strengthening properties. It is free of fluid-retaining properties, so that there is no anxiety about this side-effect or hypokalaemia. However, the evidence of its effectiveness in securing ulcer healing is not so strong.

Other drugs

Various bismuth preparations have been used over the years in the treatment of peptic ulcer, in the belief that they may afford some physical protection of the mucosa against the ulcerative process. It is uncertain just how this protection might be achieved, but there is limited evidence that a particular liquid preparation containing tripotassium dicitratobismuthate (DeNol) may promote the healing of duodenal ulcer. The recommended dose is 5 ml diluted in water half an hour before each meal and at night. A tablet preparation is also available.

Other pharmacological agents demonstrated to have ulcer-healing properties, possible in mucosa-strengthening actions, include sucralfate, a complex of aluminium hydroxide and sulphated sucrose, and synthetic prostaglandin analogues, e.g. misoprostol.

In the past sedatives have often been prescribed for peptic ulcer patients; this practice has been prompted firstly by the theoretical view that stress and nervous tension have played a significant role in the aetiology of the ulcer, and secondly, on the argument that since a period of rest in bed usually results in remission of symptoms therefore mild sedation may be of value. As has been stated, there is no good evidence that nervous stress and tension are major factors in the causation of the ulcer, and therefore there seems no rational reason to sedate all ulcer patients. However, such drugs may well be helpful in a selected minority of peptic ulcer patients who show clear signs of hyperexcitability or anxiety, and for whom there would be good reason to prescribe such medication even in the absence of an ulcer.

In the past it was not uncommon for patients to be admitted to hospital for the medical management of their ulcer, but in present-day practice this is an exceedingly rare occurrence.

Surgical treatment

Here we are discussing only the elective planned surgical treatment of a chronic peptic ulcer and not the emergency operations which may be required for one or other of the complications.

The decision as to when to advise such an operation is basically a clinical one, taking into consideration a variety of factors in the overall assessment of the amount of disability suffered by the patient. The surgeon accepting a patient for surgical treatment should be satisfied that all the measures outlined under the section on medical treatment have been adhered to, and that in spite of these measures the ulcer persists and the symptoms remain troublesome enough to merit the operation. Generally this will imply that the patient has taken at least two full courses of one of the H_2-receptor antagonists at the proper dosage and that the various other pieces of advice have been carefully followed. On the whole patients coming to surgery will have had regularly recurring relapses over a period of several years, and will find that work and leisure activities have been interrupted by the symptoms. Other factors influencing the decision towards operation are interruption of sleep, a tendency for the pain to radiate through to the back, a strong family history of the condition, and any previous history of one of the complications of ulcer.

Since it is known that there is a very slightly increased risk of a gastric ulcer undergoing malignant change, there is a greater readiness to offer surgical treatment to a patient with a gastric ulcer if symptoms persist, and there is no clear gastroscopic evidence of complete healing.

Types of operation

Since the operations suitable for the treatment of duodenal ulcer differ from those for gastric ulcer, each will be considered separately.

Duodenal ulcer

Since the main aim of the operation is permanently to reduce the capacity of the stomach to secrete acid and pepsin, this can be achieved basically by one of three approaches:

1. The vagus nerves can be cut, interrupting the main nervous drive to the acid- and pepsin-producing cells.
2. The distal two-thirds to three-quarters of the stomach can be excised, thereby removing both the antrum which is the source of the hormone gastrin, and a proportion of the cells which produce acid.
3. A combination of vagotomy and antrectomy will remove the two main physiological sources of stimulation to the acid-secreting cells.

Vagotomy. The first operation introduced to achieve this objective in the 1940s was truncal vagotomy, i.e. simply dividing the main anterior and posterior trunks as they passed across the lower oesophagus to reach the stomach. It was soon discovered that this procedure not only reduced the acid secretion from the stomach, but also impaired gastric motility, leading to stasis within the stomach, and in some patients, troublesome vomiting. This latter problem could be overcome by the addition of a drainage procedure—either gastrojejunostomy or pyloroplasty (Fig. 28.6). Since a small number of troublesome unwanted sequelae following these

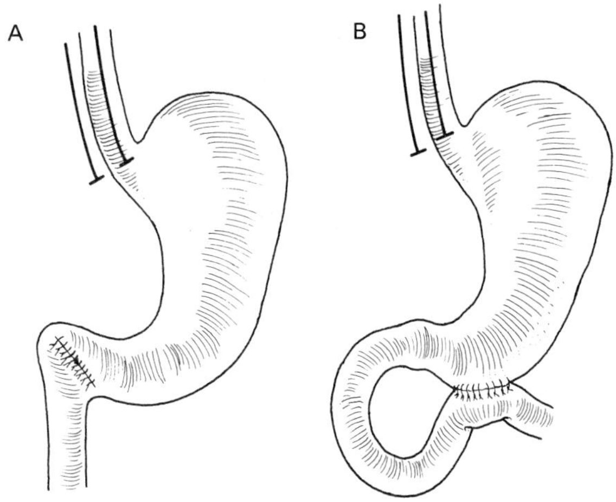

Fig. 28.6 Truncal vagotomy and (**A**) pyloroplasty—the simplest pattern being a longitudinal incision across the pylorus closed by suturing transversely (Heineke–Mikulicz) or (**B**) gastrojejunostomy, making an anastomosis between the greater curvature of the antrum and the proximal jejunum.

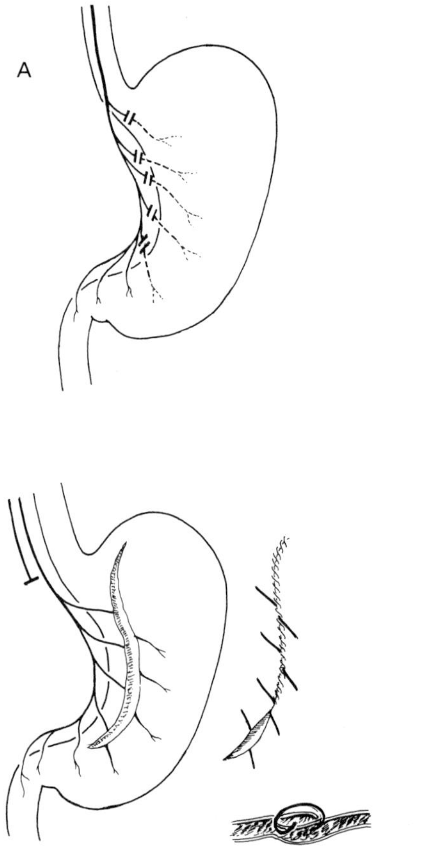

Fig. 28.7 (**A**) Highly selective (proximal gastric) vagotomy: in this operation the main anterior and posterior vagus nerve trunks (Latarjet) are left intact, and the individual terminal branches supplying the proximal acid-secreting part of the stomach are divided. (**B**) The combination of posterior truncal vagotomy plus anterior seromyotomy concentrates on preserving only the anterior vagal trunk. The limited denervation of the anterior proximal stomach is achieved by a long seromyotomy down to, but not including, the mucosal layer. Final closure involves overlapping the lesser curvature edge of this incision across the greater curvature edge, so that any attempt at regrowth of nerves is blocked by the serosa.

operations were thought to be due to the vagal denervation of upper abdominal structures other than the stomach itself, other techniques were introduced to limit the vagal denervation to the proximal segment of the stomach which produced the acid secretion. For this reason selective vagotomy, in which the vagal trunks, both anterior and posterior, were divided below the branches passing to the coeliac and hepatic plexuses, was introduced. This procedure still required the addition of either gastrojejunostomy or pyloroplasty.

A still more recent modification was the introduction of highly selective vagotomy (proximal gastric vagotomy; Fig. 28.7A) in which only the terminal branches of the anterior and posterior vagal trunks passing to the gastric fundus were divided along the lesser curvature. This technique preserved intact the main nerve trunks carrying the innervation to the pyloric antrum and all structures distal to it. Since motility was not substantially affected, it was not necessary in this operation to add a drainage procedure.

Since there is some evidence that the anterior vagal trunk is more important than the posterior one in regulating antral motility, it has been proposed that a combination of truncal posterior vagotomy and highly selective anterior vagotomy may be a satisfactory alternative (Fig. 28.7B), and further modifications of technique for achieving this objective have been devised and are under evaluation. It remains to be seen whether any of these will be a satisfactory substitute for highly selective vagotomy.

Gastrectomy. For the successful treatment of a duodenal ulcer and diminution of the risk of recurrent ulcer it is necessary to remove at least the distal two-thirds of the stomach, along with the mobilized ulcer in the proximal duodenum. The divided end of the duodenum is then closed by

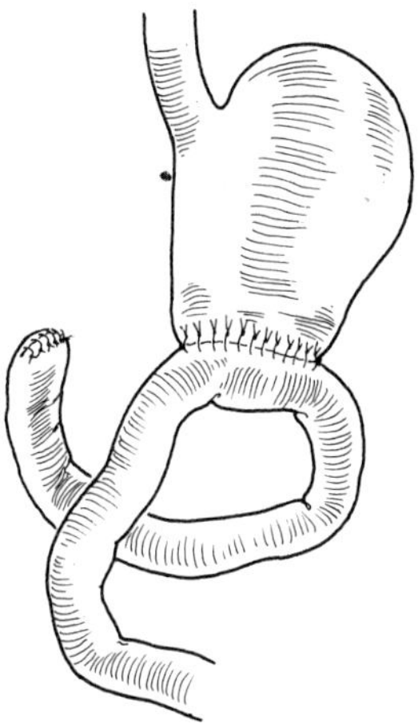

Fig. 28.8 Polya partial gastrectomy: approximately 70% of the distal stomach is resected, and the gastric remnant is anastomosed end-to-side to a loop of proximal jejunum.

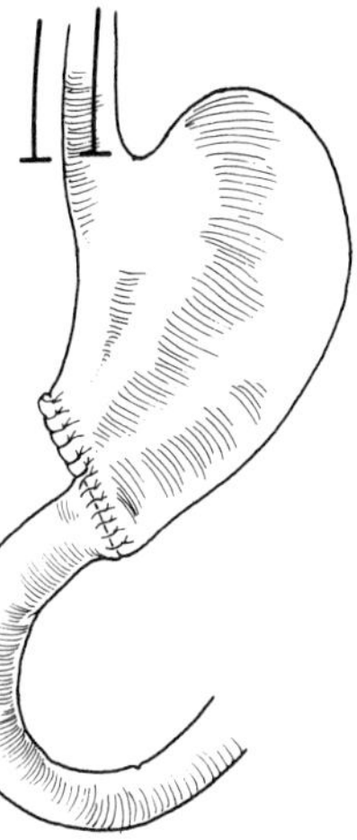

Fig. 28.9 Antrectomy plus truncal vagotomy: in this instance the gastric remnant is anastomosed either to the duodenum, as shown here, or to the jejunum, as shown in Figure 28.8.

sutures and left as a blind end, while the remaining proximal segment of the stomach is anastomosed to a loop of jejunum as near to the duodenojejunal flexure as is convenient. This is the Polya type of gastrectomy (Fig. 28.8). The jejunal loop can be brought up either in front of or behind the transverse colon through an opening made through one of the avascular areas of the mesocolon.

Antrectomy plus vagotomy. Since the antrum will be removed there is no virtue in attempting selective vagal denervation, and truncal vagotomy is usually performed. Excision of approximately the distal half of the stomach can usually ensure that all the antral mucosa will be removed, and since the antral type of mucosa usually extends more proximally on the lesser curvature than on the greater, the line of resection may accordingly be made obliquely. Once the resection is completed the surgeon has the option of either anastomosing the remaining stomach directly to the divided duodenum, after narrowing the lesser curvature end of the remnant with sutures, or performing a Polya type of reconstruction (Fig. 28.9).

When it comes to selecting an operation for an individual patient with duodenal ulcer there is thus a large range to choose from, and the decision is influenced by several factors. These are first of all the risk of immediate mortality from the operation itself; secondly the effectiveness of the procedure in preventing recurrent ulcer, and thirdly the chance of the patient being cured of the ulcer but developing one or more of the unwanted sequelae resulting from the surgical alteration of the gastrointestinal tract.

With regard to the most serious complication of all, operative mortality, the balance of evidence suggests that those procedures which involve the resection of a portion of stomach, and therefore anastomosis, carry a slightly but significantly increased risk of postoperative death. Although all the mortality figures are small, ranging from 0.5 to around 2%, even small differences in the figures should be considered important, bearing in mind that we are dealing with planned elective procedures in an essentially benign disease. For this reason, plus the finding that postgastrectomy sequelae tend on the whole to be more severe and difficult to treat than those following the non-resection procedures, partial gastrectomy and to a lesser extent antrectomy plus vagotomy have become less popular as the primary elective surgical procedures for chronic duodenal ulcer in recent years. Attention has therefore focused more on the comparison of the merits of the different patterns of vagotomy.

The second factor influencing the choice of operation is the degree of protection which each procedure gives against recurrent ulceration. Looking solely at this factor and ignoring all others, there is no doubt that the lowest recurrent ulcer rates follow antrectomy plus vagotomy, and this is in keeping with the fact that it removes the two main sources of stimulation to the acid-secreting cells. Polya partial gastrectomy is only slightly less protective against further ulcer, and it is not on account of this factor that the procedure has become less popular but, as mentioned, it is on account of the slightly higher mortality risk, and the various unwanted sequelae. Higher rates of recurrent ulcer follow truncal vagotomy plus either drainage procedure: average figures are between 5 and 7%. As time goes on the recurrences following highly selective vagotomy appear to be higher, some figures reaching between 15 and 20%. Unless these figures can be improved either by greater experience with present techniques, or modifications of them, they must give some concern regarding the adequacy of protection against recurrence.

The third factor in our comparison of the different procedures relates to the various unwanted postoperative sequelae: the main ones are listed in Table 28.1.

Table 28.1 The main unwanted postoperative sequelae for duodenal ulcer operations

Dumping
Postprandial hypoglycaemia
Reflux gastritis
Vomiting
Weight loss—malabsorption
Diarrhoea
Anaemia
Metabolic bone disease

These are discussed in slightly more detail later in this chapter but, in summary, taking all factors into consideration, the two operations currently most favoured for the elective surgical treatment of duodenal ulcer are truncal vagotomy with either pyloroplasty or gastrojejunostomy, and highly selective vagotomy. For reasons already mentioned, both Polya gastrectomy and antrectomy plus vagotomy are less favoured, and selective vagotomy with drainage has been supplanted by highly selective vagotomy. Both truncal and highly selective vagotomies have acceptably low operative mortality risks—well below 1%. On the one hand highly selective vagotomy appears at present to carry a higher risk of recurrence than truncal, but a lower incidence of unwanted sequelae such as dumping and diarrhoea.

Gastric ulcer

The standard operation of choice for gastric ulcer is Billroth I partial gastrectomy, involving removal of approximately the distal one-third of the stomach, and joining the gastric remnant directly to the first part of the duodenum (Fig. 28.10). Since the gastric ulcer is usually located on the distal part of the lesser curvature the ulcer itself is removed by this procedure. In the minority of occasions where the site of the gastric ulcer is higher, the lesser curvature dissection is taken more proximally to excise it along with the distal portion of stomach.

Since the secretion of gastric acid is not excessive in this condition there is no need to employ extensive resection of stomach, or to add other procedures aimed at reducing acid secretion. Having said this, some surgeons have sought to treat gastric ulcer by one or other of the vagotomy operations, with reasonable short- and medium-term results. There is a general feeling, however, that it is wiser to remove the gastric ulcer, particularly since there is a small risk of otherwise missing an early carcinomatous ulcer.

Overall the results of Billroth I partial gastrectomy for gastric ulcer are good; recurrent ulcer is extremely rare, and the incidence of the various

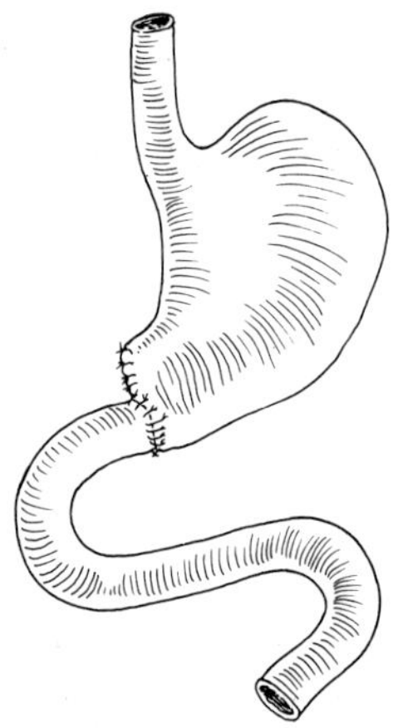

Fig. 28.10 Billroth I partial gastrectomy. The stomach remnant is anastomosed to the proximal duodenum, after excision of the ulcer and the distal portion of the stomach.

unwanted sequelae is distinctly less than when gastrectomy operations are used for duodenal ulcer.

Recurrent ulcer. It is always a matter of great disappointment to both patient and surgeon when a patient who has undergone an operation for a peptic ulcer develops a further one, usually at or just distal to the anastomosis or pyloroplasty. Most recurrent ulcers cause symptoms to appear within 2–5 years of the original operation, but a few do not become manifest until later years. The symptoms are similar to those of the first ulcer, being located mainly in the epigastric region, and showing periodicity. Some of the features may, however, be somewhat atypical; for example the site may be less precisely localized, and the relationship with food may not be so clear-cut.

When the symptoms are suggestive of recurrent ulcer both barium meal and endoscopy should be performed, and the latter examination is more likely to give an accurate diagnosis, since X-ray appearances are often distorted by the previous surgical procedure. Modern gastroscopes are extremely manoeuvrable, and it is possible to rotate the tip of the instrument through approximately 180° to allow clear inspection of the distal aspect of an anastomosis if this is necessary to view the ulcer.

Since virtually all recurrent ulcers follow procedures initially performed for duodenal ulcer, and are associated with insufficient diminution in the secretion of acid and pepsin, it is helpful to measure the gastric secretory responses. In the first place a measurement is made of 1-h basal secretion followed by a 1- or even 2-h response to a maximal dose of pentagastrin (0.6 mg/kg), and in most cases both measurements will be found to be higher than expected in a patient who has had an acid-reducing gastric procedure. Where the original operation has included vagotomy, it is also helpful to perform an insulin test. In this test basal secretion is again collected over a 1-h period, and then an intravenous injection of 0.2 u/kg of soluble insulin is given either as a single bolus injection, or as a continuous intravenous infusion over 1h. Acid secretion is collected continuously over a period of 2h following the insulin administration, and measured for volume, concentration and output every 15 min. Although it may seem more logical simply to measure the response to insulin stimulation on an absolute quantitative basis, it is conventional to regard a positive response, i.e. one indicating persistence of functioning vagal fibres, as an increase in acid concentration at any time within the 2-h postinsulin period of 20 mmol/l or more over the basal concentration. Should the basal secretion be totally anacid, then an increase in acid concentration of more than 10 mmol/l at any time within the 2h may also be regarded as a positive response.

Once the diagnosis of recurrent ulcer is made it is usual to start treatment with full dosage of one or other of the H_2-receptor antagonists, and in the majority of instances an initially good clinical response should be expected. While several series have been reported of continuous full or maintenance dosage of these agents achieving sustained control of the symptoms, many will relapse, and require further surgical treatment. On theoretical grounds it might be expected that where the main problem is clearly incomplete vagotomy, making this complete at the second procedure would suffice. However, experience has shown that when a second operation is required, regardless of the initial procedure the surgeon should aim to remove the antrum, as well as dividing any remaining intact vagal fibres. If complete vagotomy and antrectomy can be achieved, there appears to be little risk of a third ulcer developing.

Other unwanted postoperative sequelae. Although these will now be described under separate headings, it should be emphasized that patients often present with various combinations of symptoms and an attempt should be made to try and assess which are the most dominant and most troublesome features of the clinical presentation.

Dumping. This symptom complex is believed to be due primarily to rapid emptying of the gastric contents into the upper small intestine with often in addition an increased rate of transit through the small bowel itself right through to the colon. As a consequence a large volume of hyperosmotic fluid enters the small intestine and in an attempt to bring the osmotic tension back to a more physiological level, large amounts of fluid cross the intestinal mucosa from the rich blood supply, reducing first of all plasma volume, and secondly other parts of the extracellular fluid compartment.

There are, therefore, two sets of symptoms; the first arising from the gastrointestinal tract itself, and the second as a consequence of the vasomotor effect of the fall in plasma volume. The former include epigastric discomfort, nausea, a feeling of fullness, vomiting, increased abdominal noise, and possibly, following these other symptoms, an episode of diarrhoea. The vasomotor symptoms comprise general weakness, pallor, sweating, light-headedness, and palpitation.

The symptoms classically occur some 5–30 min after eating, and although they may be experienced after even modest intake, they are usually more marked if the meal is large, and particularly if it contains a substantial proportion of carbohydrate and liquid. Gradually with the passage of time the symptoms pass off, and they may subside more rapidly if the patient lies down immediately after eating.

Hypoglycaemia. This disorder, which also occurs in the early postprandial phase, has some clinical features which may resemble the symptoms of dumping, although their onset is usually delayed till 1–3 h after the meal. Again the basic defect is probably accelerated gastric emptying leading to the rapid absorption of monosaccharides from the jejunum, subsequent hyperglycaemia and an exaggerated insulin response, which in turn causes the hypoglycaemia. The symptoms of faintness, sweating, dizziness and mood change will last until the blood sugar returns gradually to normal levels. The taking of small quantities of glucose at the onset of symptoms may abort the attack. Attempts to try and prevent the initial hyperglycaemia by the administration of hypoglycaemic agents before meals are usually unsuccessful.

Bile reflux. Since all operations apart from highly selective vagotomy either bypass or widen the pylorus, it is not surprising that they permit the content of the upper small bowel to reflux more easily back into the stomach or stomach remnant. Some of the content, particularly bile, can cause a chemical irritation of the gastric mucosa. If in addition there is some degree of oesophagogastric regurgitation the result may be not only gastritis but also oesophagitis. This bile reflux may be responsible for upper abdominal pain, heartburn, and various other forms of dyspepsia. Gastroscopy may reveal evidence of free regurgitation into the stomach or stomach remnant, and will permit assessment of the degree of mucosal inflammation.

Vomiting. Some patients are troubled by bilious vomiting, which occurs approximately 30 min after a meal, and is characterized by bringing up only liquid which is obviously almost pure bile. The normal increased outpouring of bile from the liver, and gallbladder contraction in response to the meal, floods into the proximal small intestine after the meal has rapidly left the stomach, rapidly refluxes into the stomach, and is sufficient to induce nausea and vomiting. True bilious vomiting is much commoner when there is a direct anastomosis between the stomach and small bowel than it is after pyloroplasty.

Other patients are troubled by the occasional vomiting of partly digested stomach contents and secretions, sometimes as an isolated symptom, or more commonly associated with one or more of the other symptoms discussed in this section.

Weight loss—malabsorption. While a group of patients who have previously had any of the operations for peptic ulcer may on average be a little less heavy than a comparable group with no previous surgery, marked weight loss is usually encountered only after partial gastrectomy. In this group one of the obvious contributing causes is the diminution in gastric capacity leading to an inadequate caloric intake in the 24 h. All that may be required in this instance is to advise the taking of relatively high-calorie food at more frequent and regularly spaced intervals than the traditional two to three meals per day. On occasions true malabsorption with hypoproteinaemia and other indices of sub-optimal digestive transport may come to light following gastric surgery and if simple dietary adjustment does not bring about an improvement it is wise to check for small-bowel disease by appropriate tests of intestinal digestion absorption, including small-bowel mucosal biopsy.

Diarrhoea. It is not uncommon for there to be a transient period of bowel disturbance either towards constipation or more commonly diarrhoea after any of the gastric procedures outlined, but in most instances a return to a more or less regular pattern is usual in the following weeks. However, particularly after the various vagotomy operations, a tendency to looseness of bowel action may persist, either as a continuous pattern, or in an intermittent episodic fashion with varying intervals of relatively normal bowel action. There is no doubt that the frequency of either pattern of diarrhoea is much less following highly selective vagotomy than it is after the less selective procedures.

Various factors may contribute to the diarrhoea, such as the reduction in gastric acid secretion allowing proximal colonization by bacteria, alterations in digestive enzyme production or mucosal absorption following vagal denervation, and where drainage procedures are used, bypass of some of the physiological mechanism regulating function in the upper digestive tract.

In the majority of patients troubled by diarrhoea satisfactory control of the symptom may be achieved by one or more of preparations such as codeine phosphate, diphenoxylate hydrochloride, or loperamide hydrochloride. It is worth persisting with such preparations for some months, since in the majority of instances the frequency and severity of the diarrhoea will diminish with the passage of time, and eventually the patient may be able to do without these medications.

Very rarely, when all attempts to control the symptom by medical measures fail, and a specific cause of malabsorption has been excluded, a further operation may be considered. Occasionally considerable relief can be obtained by converting a gastrojejunal anastomosis into either a pyloroplasty, or if there has previously been a gastrectomy, a gastroduodenal anastomosis. An alternative approach, carrying a slightly higher chance of success, is the reversal of an approximately 10-cm segment of mid small bowel, as illustrated in Figure 28.11.

Anaemia. The commonest type of anaemia to develop after gastric surgery is an iron-deficiency type, and it is much more frequently encountered after gastrectomy than after the other procedures. It may develop gradually a few years after the operation, and the symptoms therefore present insidiously. The iron depletion may arise from a combination of insufficient intake in the diet, impaired absorption of the iron across the mucosa of the intestine, and excessive loss from the gastrointestinal tract from either increased speed of transit through the alimentary tract or recurrent small losses of blood from areas affected by inflammation.

It is probably wise, therefore, for patients with previous gastric operations, particularly gastrectomy, to have blood checked at regular and at least yearly intervals, and it is not unreasonable to offer postgastrectomy patients recurrent short courses

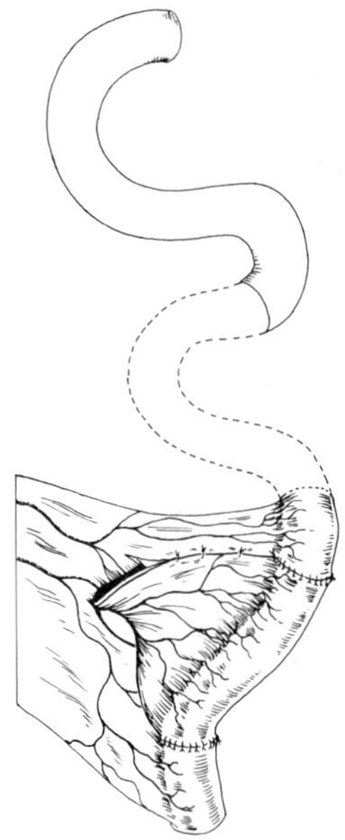

Fig. 28.11 Mid small bowel reversal: a 10-cm segment of small bowel, estimated at 100 cm distal to the duodenojejunal flexure, is reversed and re-anastomosed, along with its mesentery.

of a simple oral iron supplement once or twice a year as a prophylactic measure.

Anaemia due to vitamin B_{12} deficiency is occasionally encountered some years following partial gastrectomy, but is virtually unknown as a sequel to the various vagotomy operations. There are two possible mechanisms. First, the removal of a portion of the stomach plus mucosal damage to the remaining fundus by gastritis may impair the production of intrinsic factor. If this is the case the anaemia can be readily corrected by giving intrinsic factor, but in clinical practice this usually means giving monthly injections of vitamin B_{12}. Second, but even more rarely, the vitamin B_{12} deficiency may be the result of stagnation within a blind loop in which bacteria consume the combined intrinsic factor-vitamin B_{12} complex, thus preventing it from being available for normal absorption in the distal small bowel. This particular type of megaloblastic anaemia can usually be corrected by the appropriate surgical procedure for removing the blind loop.

The least likely type of anaemia to follow gastric surgery is folic acid deficiency, and it is only encountered on the rarest of occasions following a previous partial gastrectomy. If, as is likely, it is due to a diet deficient in folic acid, this can be given in tablet form to supplement the diet.

Metabolic bone disease. A troublesome complex of bone symptoms and biochemical changes may be seen usually many years after partial gastrectomy, but has not been reported after the other operations. Since the total number of gastrectomies has fallen in recent years the condition is now less frequently encountered. Some of the features of both osteomalacia and osteoporosis may arise in this condition, and the main complaints are of bone pain, pseudofractures, and various muscular pains. The condition is difficult to treat, and in spite of calcium supplements, vitamin D where osteomalacia is present, and various other preparations, it may prove quite refractory.

Management of disorders arising after gastric surgery

Various measures to prevent or control individual symptoms have been discussed under the appropriate headings. Generally these measures suffice for those whose symptoms are only mild or moderate, or where they are clearly improving with the passage of time. In a small proportion of patients, however, troublesome symptoms will persist, and seriously interfere with the patient's normal daily routine. Here there is a place for further revision operations. Not surprisingly, there is no uniform agreement as to precisely which procedure is preferred for different presentations of symptoms and, as has already been mentioned, patients present with varying groups of complaints, so that it is difficult to give simple, clear-cut advice on the procedures of choice.

There is, however, perhaps a general consensus of opinion that where the symptoms are predominantly due to an increased rate of transit through the upper gastrointestinal tract, the interposition of a jejunal loop between the stomach or stomach remnant and the duodenum is beneficial in having a slowing effect on transit (Fig. 28.12). On the other hand, where the principal disorder causing most of the symptoms is believed to be reflux from the small intestine into the stomach or oesophagus, a conversion to the Roux-en-Y configuration (Fig. 28.13), is recommended. These two procedures form the basis of most revision operations for

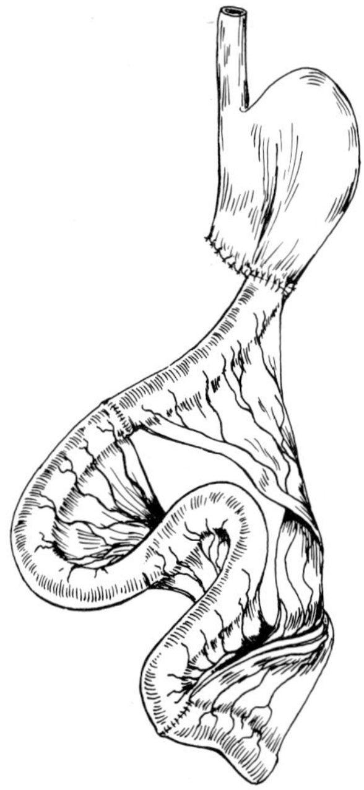

Fig. 28.12 Jejunal interposition: a segment of jejunum along with its mesentery is separated from its original site, and its proximal end is anastomosed to the stomach remnant, while its distal end is anastomosed to the duodenum.

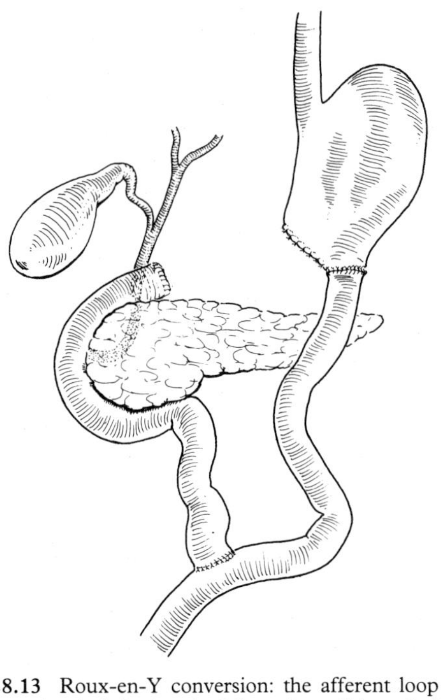

Fig. 28.13 Roux-en-Y conversion: the afferent loop of jejunum, previously bringing the bile and small intestinal content to the gastric anastomosis, has been disconnected and re-anastomosed end-to-side to a segment of jejunum at least 40 cm distal to the gastric stump.

the various sequelae. As has already been stated, reversal of a segment of mid small bowel is occasionally needed to control persistent postvagotomy diarrhoea.

Unfortunately, success can not always be guaranteed from these revisional procedures, but if patient selection is careful, a success rate of 60–75% should be obtained.

Complications of peptic ulcer

The three important complications are perforation, haemorrhage, and pyloric stenosis.

Perforation

In this complication the ulcerative process continues right through the entire wall of the stomach or duodenum, so that a hole is formed through which the contents of the stomach and duodenum, including air, escape into the peritoneal cavity. This causes a peritonitis which is at first chemical in response to the acid, enzymes, and bile, but which if untreated may be followed by infection as intestinal bacteria also escape into the peritoneal cavity.

Duodenal ulcers more commonly perforate than gastric ulcers, and in the former the situation of the duodenal ulcer is almost invariably on the anterior surface of the first part of the duodenum.

The clinical presentation is usually a most dramatic one, the patient being suddenly seized with acute severe pain which extends right across the upper abdomen, and soon spreads to the rest of the abdomen, with often radiation or referral through to the back and the shoulders. The pain is constant, unremitting and of great severity, and any movement of the trunk may exacerbate the pain. Characteristically the patient will be very reluctant to take any but the most shallow of breaths, since diaphragmatic movement accentuates the pain.

In most patients there is a clear previous history of typical peptic ulcer symptoms, but in perhaps 8–10% of patients the sudden perforation may be the first clinical presentation of the disorder, so that in these patients there may be no previous relevant history.

Although some nausea may be present, vomiting is not a dominant feature of the clinical picture, as the act of vomiting produces very severe pain. Patients who have perforated are usually pale, sweating and anxious, and some elevation of pulse rate is usually observed. However, this may remain within relatively normal limits in the first hour or two, and if the condition remains untreated for some hours the pulse rate may begin to increase, with a reduction in blood pressure.

The clinical signs are usually also quite dramatic. The patient lies very still and resists any movement, particularly of the abdominal muscles. Respiration is shallow. There is marked increase in the muscle tone throughout the abdomen, and any attempt to exert even gentle pressure, particularly in the upper abdomen, is resisted on account of the severe tenderness. Classically the findings on palpation of the abdomen are described as board-like rigidity. On percussion, if there has been a considerable escape of air through the perforation the area of liver dullness may be detectably diminished. On auscultation no bowel sounds are heard, since all gut motility has been reflexly inhibited by the peritoneal irritation. The diagnosis is usually straightforward on a combination of the history and clinical findings, particularly if there is a clear preceding history of peptic ulcer symptoms. The

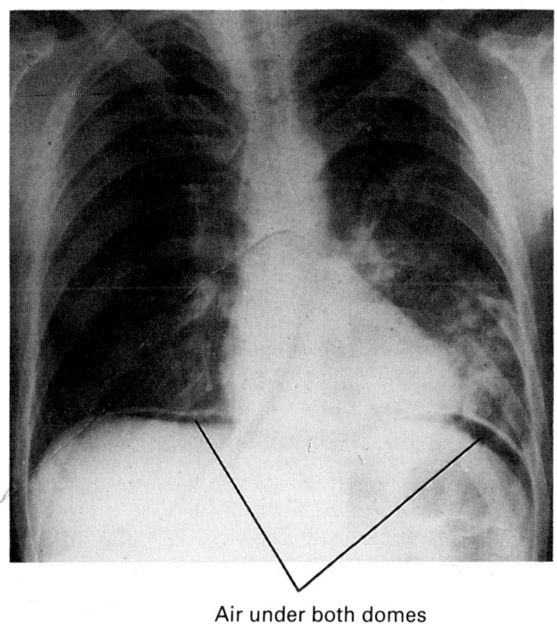

Fig. 28.14 An erect chest X-ray showing crescents of air collecting under both domes of the diaphragm.

most important conditions from which perforated peptic ulcer is to be differentiated are myocardial infarction and acute pancreatitis. In case of doubt, a plain X-ray of the chest taken with the patient in the upright position may show clear evidence of gas under the domes of the diaphragm (Fig. 28.14) and such a radiological sign is diagnostic of the escape of gas from the alimentary tract. In the absence of such a gas shadow, it may be helpful to perform an electrocardiogram if there is serious question about myocardial infarction, and serum amylase estimation if there is a strong possibility of acute pancreatitis. If these investigations are done it is essential to have the results speedily, so as not to delay the institution of the correct appropriate treatment.

Treatment

Once the diagnosis of a perforated peptic ulcer is established it is essential to undertake operative repair at the earliest possible opportunity. Morphine or pethidine by injection is usually required in sufficiently large dosage to give at least partial relief. It is wise to pass a nasogastric tube in order to empty the stomach of as much material as possible, thereby limiting further spillage into the peritoneal cavity. If the diagnosis is made promptly, i.e. within an hour or two of the occurrence of the perforation, the patients are usually not in a fluid and electrolyte depletion, but it is usual to establish an intravenous infusion line as fluid replacement may be required temporarily over the next 24 h or so.

At operation it is usually possible to close the perforation by a few sutures, and it is customary then to attach a tongue of greater omentum over the suture line (Fig. 28.15). All the obvious spilled material is aspirated from the peritoneal cavity, and if the spillage has been large in quantity the peritoneal cavity may be washed out repeatedly with saline. The abdominal wound is then closed, and it is usual to continue nasogastric aspiration and intravenous replacement until there is evidence of return of gastrointestinal activity as judged by the return of bowel sounds on auscultation.

This operation is usually a quick, simple, safe procedure, with a good immediate postoperative recovery rate. However, approximately 50% of patients treated in this manner will have a recurrence of chronic peptic ulcer symptoms after an interval of up to a few months or even a few years. For this reason, there has been a tendency in recent years to proceed at an operation for perforated peptic ulcer with a definitive operation, i.e. Billroth I partial gastrectomy for gastric ulcer, and one of the vagotomies with or without drainage for duodenal ulcer. This policy is reasonable for patients who had clear evidence of a long-standing troublesome ulcer before the incident of perforation; when the interval between perforation and operation is only an hour or two, and where the peritoneal contamination is minimal and the patient is otherwise fit to stand the somewhat longer procedure than simple closure. If all of these criteria are satisfied, an increasing number of surgeons advocate proceeding with the definitive operation at the same time as closure.

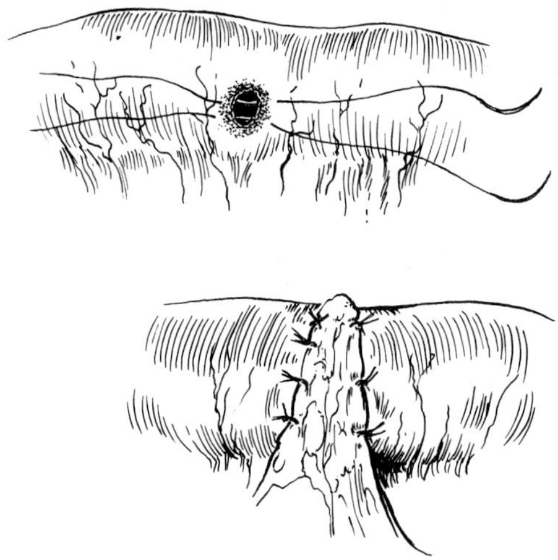

Fig. 28.15 Suture closure of perforated ulcer. Two or three sutures of absorbable material placed longitudinally are usually sufficient to give sound closure, and this is generally reinforced by fixing a tag of greater omentum over the closure with one or more sutures.

Bleeding—haematemesis and melaena

Since peptic ulcer is one of the common causes of acute bleeding from the upper gastrointestinal tract it is appropriate to consider the differential diagnosis and management of this dramatic and urgent clinical presentation at this stage. Chronic peptic ulcers of both the stomach and the duodenum can cause severe acute blood loss when the ulcerative process happens to erode the wall of a sizeable blood vessel in the base of the ulcer. In addition, other sources of major bleeding are:

1. Acute superficial erosions of the gastric mucosa which may be related to the ingestion of drugs such as salicylates, various anti-inflammatory agents, corticosteroids, and of course anticoagulants. Alcohol is sometimes another precipitating factor, and if it is taken in addition to one of the other drugs, the two together may potentiate the risk of erosive bleeding.
2. Oesophageal varices, the result of portal hypertension, which in turn is commonly a consequence of cirrhosis of the liver and less commonly of thrombosis of the portal or splenic vein.
3. The Mallory–Weiss syndrome, i.e. mucosal tears in the region of the oesophagogastric junction, the result of powerful mechanical forces exerted in this region by powerful retching or vomiting.

These account for the vast majority of acute bleeding from the upper gastrointestinal tract, but other rarer sources include various vascular anomalies, hiatal hernia, and carcinoma of the stomach.

The main clinical presentation falls into two groups of symptoms: first there is the vomiting of blood itself, which if copious or arising from oesophageal varices is quite obviously unaltered blood. If, however, it has lain in the stomach for any length of time before being vomited, it will have the darker colour from exposure to acid gastric juice which produces acid haematin. On the other hand the blood may not be vomited, but pass distally through the intestine to be noticed by the patient as melaena—stools which are significantly darker than normal—and may, in fact, if there is a large quantity of blood, be described as resembling tar or pitch. By and large, bleeding from oesophageal varices or gastric ulcers is more likely to present as haematemesis, while bleeding from distal erosions or duodenal ulcer is more likely to be the cause of melaena. However, free reflux of blood shed from a duodenal ulcer may well cause haematemesis, and it is therefore not an absolute rule.

The second group of symptoms are the general ones associated with a significant loss from the circulating blood volume, such as pallor, increased heart rate, increase in respiratory rate, sweating and anxiety. Clearly the greater the amount and rate of blood loss the more marked will be these symptoms, and since the various adaptive mechanisms to a decreased circulatory blood volume are generally less efficient with increase in age, the symptoms and signs may be more marked and of more serious import in older patients.

Management

Any patient who has clearly lost blood from the upper gastrointestinal tract or in whom the suspicion is strong from the indirect signs indicating blood loss should be admitted to hospital as a matter of urgency. In the majority of instances the bleeding will come under control at least temporarily with conservative measures, but there is always a risk of continued or recurrent bleeding, which may require urgent surgical intervention.

A record should be made immediately of the pulse rate, blood pressure and respiratory rate, and observations of these simple but important clinical measurements should be made regularly at least every half-hour. Blood should be taken for urgent grouping and cross-matching of at least 6 units of blood so that this is available in case of further severe blood loss. It is wise also to make baseline measurements of haemoglobin concentration and other haematological indices. These latter may be within normal limits just after the initial bleeding episode, but may show signs of considerable anaemia in the following hours or days. If there is any possibility of portal hypertension it is also desirable to have liver function tests performed without delay, and to include a profile of clotting factors.

If there is undue anxiety and restlessness a mild sedative such as diazepam may be given, by intramuscular injection, and morphine should probably be avoided. There is, after all, no significant pain associated with most episodes of haematemesis or melaena, and there is a risk to profound sedation which may encourage aspiration of further regurgitated material, and also make clinical assessment somewhat difficult.

Many advocate the passage of a nasogastric tube, with the aim of trying to empty further blood and other contents from the stomach, but this is often difficult in view of the blockage of the holes in the tube by clot. Another theoretical advantage of a nasogastric tube is that, if it remains patent, it may permit the detection of further episodes of fresh bleeding by simple inspection of the aspirated material.

The next step is to try and establish a firm diagnosis at the earliest opportunity, and this is most reliably achieved by endoscopy. It may be necessary to wash out the stomach content through a wide-bore gastric tube immediately before undertaking the examination, so that an adequate view will be obtained of all the important areas in the oesophagus, stomach, and the proximal duodenum. There need be little fear of the passage of the instrument provoking the recurrence of bleeding which has only recently stopped. There are far greater dangers in failing to identify the precise source of bleeding than of provoking further bleeding by the examination. Whereas a patient known to have a chronic peptic ulcer who presents with haematemesis or melaena is likely to be bleeding from that ulcer, it is always possible that he or she may, in fact, be bleeding from either erosions or varices which have silently developed, and similarly a patient known to have hepatic cirrhosis could develop either erosions or a peptic ulcer. It is important, therefore, to establish the source of the bleeding in each individual and not simply assume the source from the history and evidence from earlier investigations.

The indications for transfusing blood, which has been rapidly made available as soon after admission as possible, are mainly based on simple clinical observations. When a patient is admitted following an obviously massive haematemesis and is pale, sweaty, breathing rapidly, with a pulse rate over 100 beats/min and systolic blood pressure less than 100 mmHg, he or she will clearly need blood, and the rapid infusion of at least 2 litres of whole blood will be required. Where the blood loss is of this severity, or continues after admission it is very helpful to judge further blood replacement on the basis of measurements of central venous pressure through an appropriate catheter introduced through either the jugular or subclavian vein. This allows a much more accurate estimate of the rate of blood replacement required, and furthermore in elderly patients minimizes the chance of excessive transfusion which may overload the heart and precipitate cardiac failure. As the central venous pressure rises to the normal range the rate of further blood transfusion can be slowed and thus overload prevented.

As has been stated, the majority of patients will stop bleeding within a few hours of admission, and once the initial 24–48 h has elapsed it is reasonable to allow the patient to start taking a simple, semi-solid diet, and gradually return to normal dietary habits within a few days, provided that the simple clinical indices of pulse, respiratory rate, blood pressure and general well-being continue. Thereafter, any residual degree of anaemia due to the recent blood loss may be corrected by giving an oral iron supplement to the diet, and in addition treatment for the underlying disorder which led to the bleeding episode may be given on a longer-term basis.

Where the bleeding has arisen from either a gastric or duodenal ulcer, one of the H_2-receptor antagonists is commonly prescribed in full dosage as soon as the diagnosis has been established. However, there is no convincing evidence that these drugs given immediately after the episode of haemorrhage will overall influence the outcome of that particular occurrence, and there is even less reason to think of prescribing these for upper gastrointestinal bleeding from other disorders.

For the majority who safely recover from the episode of bleeding it is desirable to warn patients to avoid any of the drugs known to precipitate blood loss, e.g. aspirin and the various other anti-inflammatory agents for the rest of their lives.

Operative treatment

When the conservative management outlined above fails to stop the bleeding, or when there are repeated episodes of further bleeding, it may be necessary to take the patient to the operating theatre, sometimes with a degree of urgency. The surgical approach will differ depending upon the cause of the bleeding.

Peptic ulcer

Serious bleeding can occur from either a gastric or a duodenal ulcer, and there is a slightly greater risk of the former either continuing to bleed or bleeding in a repeated fashion. There is, therefore, greater readiness to operate on patients bleeding from gastric ulcer than from a duodenal one. Since older patients are more at risk from bleeding from either type of ulcer, there is also a tendency to operate sooner rather than later on older than younger patients. There are several other well known factors which increase the risk of mortality from upper gastrointestinal bleeding, listed in Table 28.1, and these can be useful guidelines in determining the likelihood of operation being required.

Table 28.1 Gastrointestinal bleeding — risk factors

Age
Site of ulcer—GU more likely to bleed than DU
Haematemesis more likely to rebleed than melaena
BP — systolic less than 100 mmHg on admission
Haemoglobin less than 10 g/dl on admission
Volume of transfusion
Repeated or continuous bleeding

Once the decision to operate has been taken, it is advisable to proceed with a Billroth I partial gastrectomy including the ulcer for gastric ulcer. For a bleeding duodenal ulcer the choice lies between removing the ulcerated portion of the proximal duodenum along with gastric resection of the Polya pattern, and opening the distal antrum, pylorus, and proximal duodenum longitudinally, thus exposing the bleeding ulcer, which is then underrun by several sutures to seal the vessels at the base of the ulcer, closing the incision transversely as a pyloroplasty and adding vagotomy. This latter approach has the merits of getting the bleeding under control at an early stage in the procedure, and involving an operation of lesser magnitude than the gastric resection. In many centres this is now the preferred approach to this serious problem, and the results are encouraging.

Gastric erosions

Every attempt should be made to avoid operation in this condition, since with perseverance and removal of the precipitating factors, it should be expected that the majority of these will heal. Very occasionally the stomach may have to be explored, and if the erosions are few these can be dealt with by under-running sutures. Even more rarely the segment of the stomach in which a group of erosions is concentrated may require to be resected. Rarest of all, there are isolated occasions in which oozing erosions are widespread throughout the entire stomach mucosa, and a total gastrectomy may be necessary.

Mallory–Weiss syndrome

In this condition one or more tears of the mucosa in either the oesophageal or gastric side of the oesophagogastric junction bleed. Once the diagnosis has been confirmed by endoscopy, the usual expectation is that these will heal with conservative management. Occasionally it is necessary to explore the stomach through an opening in the anterior wall, and repair the mucosal tears by direct suturing.

Oesophageal varices

Bleeding from this source can be one of the most alarming presentations since large amounts of blood may rapidly escape, and the patient may present with repeated vomiting of impressive quantities of freshly shed blood. A preceding history of one of the liver disorders known to lead to cirrhosis and in turn an increase in the portal venous pressure is often known. There will also frequently be clear evidence of liver disorder in the form of jaundice, ascites, liver palms, spider naevi, etc. However, the occurrence of a brisk haematemesis may on occasions be the first and dramatic clinical indication of the existence of liver damage and portal hypertension.

If the blood loss is large, rapid, and shows no sign of ceasing spontaneously, urgent measures may be required to try and stem the flow. The two principal measures are:

1. The passage of the triple-lumen Sengstaken tube (Fig. 28.16), the tip of which is introduced through the mouth down the oesophagus and well into the stomach. The rounded gastric balloon is then inflated, and the tube pulled firmly proximally to press on the gastric fundus. Immediately thereafter the oesophageal tube is inflated, and it is important to raise the pressure sufficiently to compress the varices and control the bleeding. If this is not achieved there is an

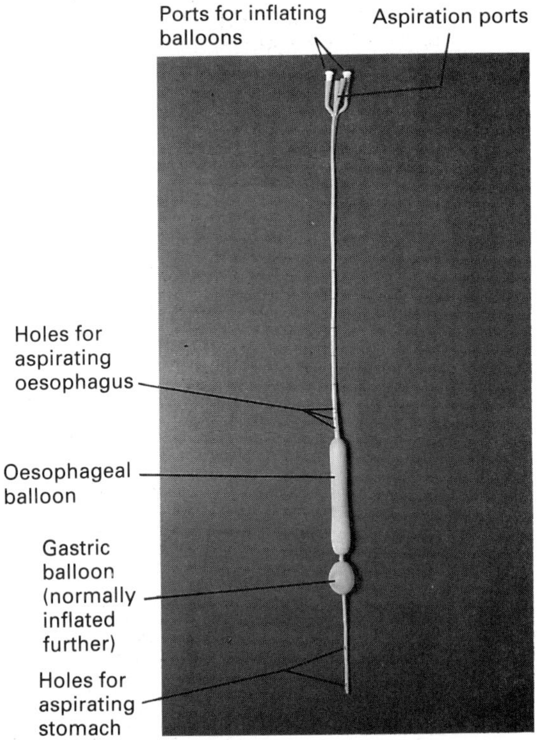

Fig. 28.16 Sengstaken tube, for temporary tamponade of bleeding oesophageal varices. With the distal end introduced well down into the stomach, the distal gastric balloon is dilated, pulled back to occlude the oesophagogastric junction and then the long oesophageal balloon is distended sufficiently to control the bleeding (but pressure not higher than 30 mmHg).

appreciable risk that continuing blood will pass proximally up the oesophagus and there is then the risk of aspiration into the air passages. This can be a fatal complication, so it is vital to ensure proper usage of this tube if it is required.

2. An intravenous infusion of the posterior pituitary hormone vasopressin or the synthetic analogue triglycil-lysine-vasopressin may be effective in reducing the portal venous pressure, allowing satisfactory clotting to occur at the site of the ruptured varix. This infusion should be given under carefully controlled conditions, as it has somewhat unpleasant side-effects, e.g. a powerful evacuating effect on the bowel.

Either or both of these measures are at best temporary ones to overcome the emergency loss of blood. If the Sengstaken tube is left fully inflated over a period of several days there is a risk of damage to the oesophageal wall simply from pressure necrosis. It should, therefore, either be deflated after 24 h or removed altogether after 48 h.

If after either of these two temporary measures bleeding continues or recurs, operative procedures have to be considered. These fall into two categories. First, a direct attack can be made on the varices themselves, the oesophagus being opened through either a thoracic or abdominal approach, and the obvious varices under-run by a series of sutures. Alternatively, the lower oesophageal region containing the varices can be resected and rejoined either by suture, or by one of the circular cutting and stapling devices now available (Fig. 28.17). Thirdly, it is possible to inject sclerosant materials through special needles introduced through an oesophagoscope (Fig. 28.17B), the aim being similar to the sclerosing of haemorrhoids and varicose

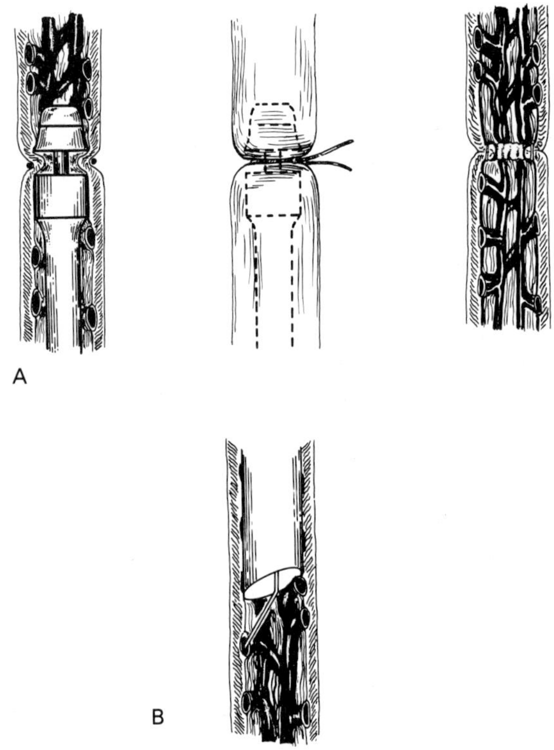

Fig. 28.17 (**A**) Simultaneous transection and re-anastomosis of the oesophagus by means of a circular stapling gun. This interrupts the transmission of the elevated pressure in the portal tributaries up into the systemic ones and therefore reduces the pressure in the varices. (**B**) Injection of sterile sclerosant into the varix (or into the submucosa at its base) under direct vision through an oesophagoscope.

veins—to precipitate a sterile thrombosis in the distended veins.

These procedures, of course, do nothing to bring about a reduction in the increased portal venous pressure which has after all been responsible for the oesophageal varices in the first place. Theoretically it would be more reasonable to perform an operation to reduce portal venous pressure (see Ch. 31). In the past a number of shunts have been employed by which the portal venous flow was diverted either wholly or partly to the relatively low pressure inferior vena cava, but in patients with severe liver dysfunction this diversion of the portal venous blood carries a relatively high risk of serious complications, notably portasystemic encephalopathy, with impairment of consciousness, tremors, and profound interference with cerebral function, and also an aggravation of the already impaired hepatic function. For this reason, and the relatively high mortality rate, there has been less enthusiasm for portasystemic shunting operations in recent years.

Pyloric stenosis

Although this term has been used for many years to describe this clinical condition, the stenosis really occurs in the most proximal part of the duodenum, being the result of fibrous scar tissue laid down by the reparative response to a long-standing duodenal ulcer. Gradually the lumen narrows, with the result that there is considerable delay in emptying of the stomach. The stomach may gradually dilate until the greater curvature lies well down in the pelvis (Fig. 28.18).

There is usually a long history of typical peptic ulcer symptoms over many years, and as the stenosis develops there is the additional symptom of the vomiting of large amounts of stagnant food and gastric secretions often towards the end of the day. Before vomiting the patient may feel that the stomach is full and uncomfortable, and directly after vomiting usually feels very much relieved, and indeed may be hungry. Patients will sometimes notice that among the material they have vomited there are particles of food which they remember swallowing many hours previously.

A striking physical sign in a patient with established pyloric stenosis is the presence of a succussion splash (Fig. 28.19). This is elicited by having the patient lie completely relaxed, and with a hand laid against each loin, gently rocking the patient's trunk from one side to the other. A characteristic splashing sound is heard from within the abdomen as the mixture of fluid and gas is rocked backwards and forwards. It is only of real clinical significance when some hours have elapsed from the patient's last meal, since occasionally in normal individuals it is possible to hear such a splash if it is within half an hour of a large meal.

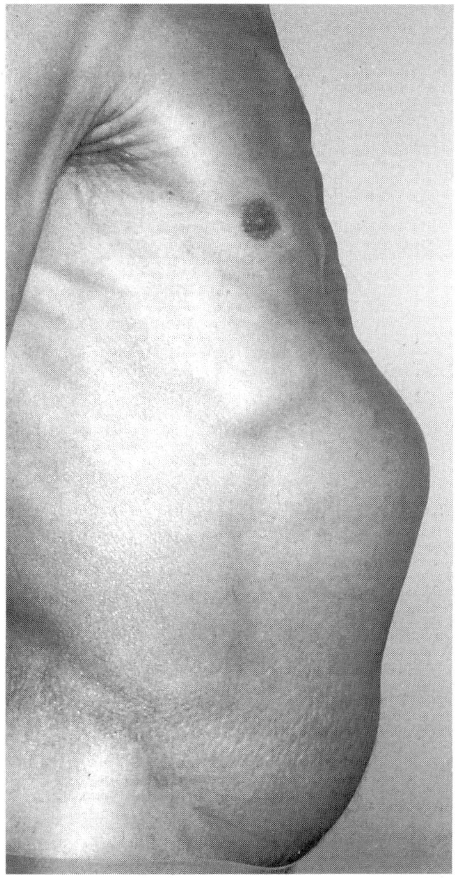

Fig. 28.18 Gross pyloric stenosis which has led to enormous distension of the entire stomach, the outline of which is visible as it stretches the overlying skin. Normally a diagnosis should be reached long before this degree of dilatation is present.

If the stenosis has been present for some time, the patient may lose substantial volumes of liquid which contains relatively high concentrations of both hydrochloric acid and potassium. There is, therefore, a risk of hypokalaemic alkalosis which, if severe, may require correction by intravenous

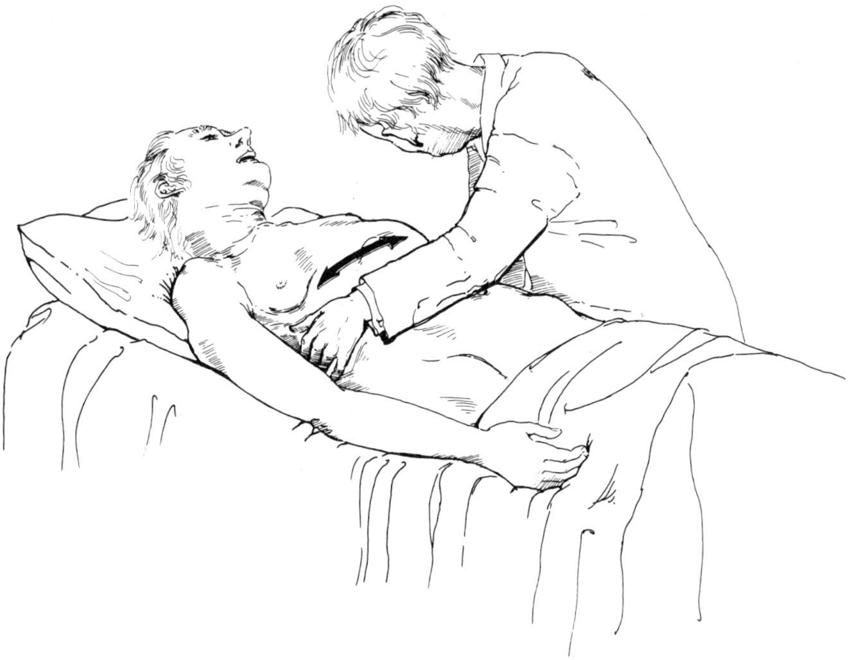

Fig. 28.19 Method of demonstrating a succussion splash in pyloric stenosis.

saline or Ringer lactate solution with added potassium supplements.

Patients with pyloric stenosis require operation, and in view of the often considerable gastric dilatation it seems logical to suggest truncal vagotomy plus a drainage procedure, with a preference for gastrojejunostomy. As an alternative, those who favour highly selective vagotomy may combine this procedure with dilatation of the pyloric region either with the finger or some form of dilating instrument.

Gastrinoma (the Zollinger–Ellison syndrome)

This is an exceedingly rare disorder, characterized by peptic ulcer usually in the duodenum, but sometimes in unusual sites, and associated with very grossly increased levels of gastric acid secretion. The latter is in turn due to the excessive production of the hormone gastrin from tumours in either the pancreas or ectopic sites alongside the upper gastrointestinal tract. The gastrin-producing cells, unlike the normal G cells in the pyloric antrum, become quite autonomous and release into the circulation quantities of gastrin which are greatly above the physiological range. In most cases the tumour cells are malignant, but the order of malignancy may be relatively low, so that with proper treatment prolonged life expectancy is the rule.

Where the disease is suspected the diagnosis can be confirmed by the direct measurement of gastrin, preferably in a fasting sample of plasma, by radioimmunoassay.

Fortunately the H_2-receptor antagonists, e.g. cimetidine and ranitidine, or the newer omeprazole, are usually effective in controlling the gross hypersecretion of gastric acid, and the dosage of these agents will often require to be pushed to higher levels than those used in common duodenal ulcer. Many gastrinoma patients are now satisfactorily controlled by continuing indefinitely on these preparations.

Since the majority of these tumours are either multicentric or malignant, there is generally little hope of excising all the tumour tissue responsible for the excessive production of gastrin, so that tumour excision is unlikely to be successful. On a few occasions there appears to be a solitary isolated tumour in the pancreas, in which case local resection of the involved segment of the pancreas may be successful.

Prior to the introduction of the H_2-receptor antagonists the only alternative of controlling the massive hypersecretion was to perform total gastrectomy, and this may still be required should the drugs be unable to prevent persisting or recurrent ulceration which may bleed or perforate.

In approximately a quarter of patients presenting with gastrinoma there is evidence of other endocrine-producing tumours in the parathyroids, the pituitary, or the adrenals.

GASTRITIS

Although gastritis is not regarded primarily as a surgical condition, it is relevant to mention it briefly for two reasons. First, acute gastritis is a very common condition, and its symptoms may mimic those of other conditions of interest to the surgeon. Commonly acute gastritis arises from the ingestion of irritant material or a variety of dietary indiscretions, and the main symptoms are disturbance of appetite, nausea, epigastric discomfort or pain, and perhaps retching and vomiting. Unless a careful history is taken there may be confusion with peptic ulcer or gallbladder disease. The diagnosis will usually be established by gastroscopic examination, and treatment is directed towards removing any obvious irritants with the expectation that symptoms will resolve within a few days.

The term chronic gastritis refers more to definite histological changes within the gastric mucosa, and again the diagnosis requires not only visual inspection through the gastroscope, but also the histological examination of mucosal biopsies. Chronic gastritis is relevant to diseases which involve surgeons for two reasons. First, there is evidence that the presence of chronic gastritic changes, particularly where there is atrophy of the villi and metaplasia, increases the risk of carcinoma of the stomach. Secondly, as has been discussed, reflux of small-bowel content into the stomach or oesophagus following various gastric operations may be responsible for some of the symptoms in postgastric surgery disorders, and measures may be required to remove the source of this chronic gastritis.

TUMOURS OF THE STOMACH

Malignant

Carcinoma is the commonest and most important tumour of this organ. Unfortunately, it has a bad reputation, since the early symptoms and signs are usually vague, and by the time the diagnosis is made the patient may not be able to be cured of the disease. One encouraging feature, however, of the last 20–30 years is that there has been a significant reduction in the incidence of carcinoma of the stomach in many countries where reliable statistics are available. The widespread variation in the prevalence of the disease in different countries throughout the world is well known: some countries, e.g. Japan and Chile, have had for many years among the highest incidences, whereas North America has a much lower incidence.

Although the causes of this sinister disease have not been discovered, there is much evidence from many good epidemiological studies that environmental factors are of considerable importance, and among the substances under suspicion are the various nitrosamines.

The great majority of malignant tumours in the stomach arise from the mucosa, and since this is glandular epithelium, the tumour will nearly always be an adenocarcinoma. Very rarely other malignancies, for example lymphosarcoma or leiomyosarcoma, may arise primarily in the stomach, but the clinical presentation and gross appearances will suggest the presence of the usual type of adenocarcinoma, and the precise diagnosis will be made on histological examination of biopsy specimens.

The commonest site in which carcinoma of the stomach arises is the pyloric antrum; the next most common is the mid-portion, and the least common the cardiac area. However, it may develop at any point where gastric mucosa is present.

On gross inspection the majority are proliferative, fungating, ulcerative growths which project into the lumen of the stomach, with ill defined edges extending into the neighbouring tissues. Commonly there are obvious areas from which small amounts of blood are seen to ooze and irregular necrotic areas where ulceration has occurred. In one particular pattern of tumour—fortunately rare—there is very widespread infiltration of the malignant cells, chiefly in the submucosal layer, spreading extensively and perhaps completely along the length of the stomach wall. As a result, there is rigidity of the stomach—the so-called 'leather-bottle' stomach.

All carcinoma of the stomach unfortunately carries a bad prognosis, and most people will succumb to the effects of extension or metastases. The prognosis is particularly bleak in those who develop the 'leather-bottle' variety.

Spread of the tumour

There are four ways in which carcinoma of the stomach may involve other tissues and organs.

1. As the tumour continues to grow at its primary site it penetrates through the entire thickness of the stomach wall and may then erode into neighbouring structures, e.g. the undersurface of the liver, the portal vein, the major vessels in the posterior abdominal wall, the pancreas, or the transverse colon.
2. In common with most other adenocarcinomas, invasion of the draining lymphatic vessels occurs, and these may carry cells in the first instance mainly to the local lymph nodes in both the greater and lesser omenta. From these nodes there may be further lymphatic spread to para-aortic nodes, and rarely via the thoracic duct to the left supraclavicular nodes. This latter is, however, a rare finding in clinical practice.
3. Carcinoma of the stomach also has a tendency to spread by the venous outflow which, of course, will be in the first instance via the portal vein to the liver. The liver is therefore the commonest site of blood borne metastases, but if cells pass through the hepatic circulation they may then be disseminated widely to many sites in the body, even to subcutaneous tissues.
4. Metastases from carcinoma of the stomach may be deposited in the pelvic pouch, and in the female on the surface of the ovaries. There is debate as to whether the deposits of cells simply travel downwards through the peritoneal cavity, or whether they are transported in either lymphatic or blood vessels to these pelvic sites.

Clinical features

In the vast majority of patients there is no significant preceding history of other gastric symptoms, although very rarely indeed a benign gastric peptic ulcer may eventually undergo malignant change.

Early symptoms are mild, vague and gradual in onset, and for this reason there may well be delay before the patient seeks medical advice. The disease mostly affects those over 50 years of age, but can also arise in younger patients.

Early symptoms fall into two main categories: first those related to the digestive tract, and secondly those of a more general nature.

The gastrointestinal complaints may include any one or more of the following; slight diminution or alteration in the appetite, vague discomfort in the upper abdomen, a feeling of fullness after taking even small amounts to eat, excess belching of unpleasant gas, or a bad taste in the mouth.

Of the more general symptoms, the first to raise suspicion of the disease are loss of body weight, and any symptom suggestive of anaemia, such as tiredness, increasing breathlessness on exertion, pallor of the facial skin, and a general feeling of weakness and uninterestedness. In older patients with some degree of cardiac inefficiency the anaemia may aggravate previous symptoms and perhaps cause swelling of the feet and ankles which is more noticeable towards evening. The anaemia usually develops gradually and is the result of the repeated loss of small quantities of blood from the ulcerated tumour.

It should be stressed that when a patient, particularly a middle-aged or elderly male, presents with the clinical picture of an otherwise unexplained anaemia, the possibility of carcinoma of the stomach should be borne in mind, and the appropriate investigations arranged.

Unfortunately, a minority of patients will either ignore these early symptoms or be unaware of their significance, and present with the tumour at a relatively advanced stage. The presenting complaint may then be the presence of an obvious mass in the upper abdomen, or gradually increasing abdominal distension due to the accumulation of ascitic fluid in the peritoneal cavity as a result of the presence of multiple metastases within the abdomen.

If widespread metastasis to the liver has occurred before the patient comes to the doctor, the clinical presentation may be dominated by jaundice, partly due to hepatic damage, and partly due to the obstruction of bile ducts by the tumour tissue.

Some nausea and vomiting may occur, but are not usually an early sign of the disease. However, if the tumour happens to arise close to the pylorus it may cause partial obstruction of the gastric outlet and in this case recurrent vomiting comparable to that of the pyloric stenosis of peptic ulcer may be present. This can sometimes be a favourable feature, since it may bring the patient to surgical treatment before the tumour is too advanced.

Clinical examination

Anyone presenting with symptoms suggestive of carcinoma of the stomach should have a thorough examination of the abdomen, searching for any palpable mass in the region of the stomach, and also checking for hepatic enlargement and the presence of ascites. A rectal examination should also be performed in a search for any evidence of hard metastatic deposits in the pelvis. A sample of stool should be tested for the presence of occult blood, which is an almost constant feature of the disease. The rest of the general examination should include palpation of the various lymph node areas, particularly the left supraclavicular fossa, although as already stated, it is rare to find such deposits. A sample of blood should be taken to determine whether anaemia is present, and if so whether the pattern is compatible with chronic blood loss.

Confirmation of the diagnosis of carcinoma of the stomach requires gastroscopy, and the histological examination of multiple biopsies taken from any suspicious area. Often the initial investigation is a barium swallow and meal, preferably with a double-contrast technique, and certainly a very high order of suspicion can be obtained in the case of moderate-sized to large tumours which show classical signs such as those shown in Figures 28.20–28.22. However, even when the X-ray points

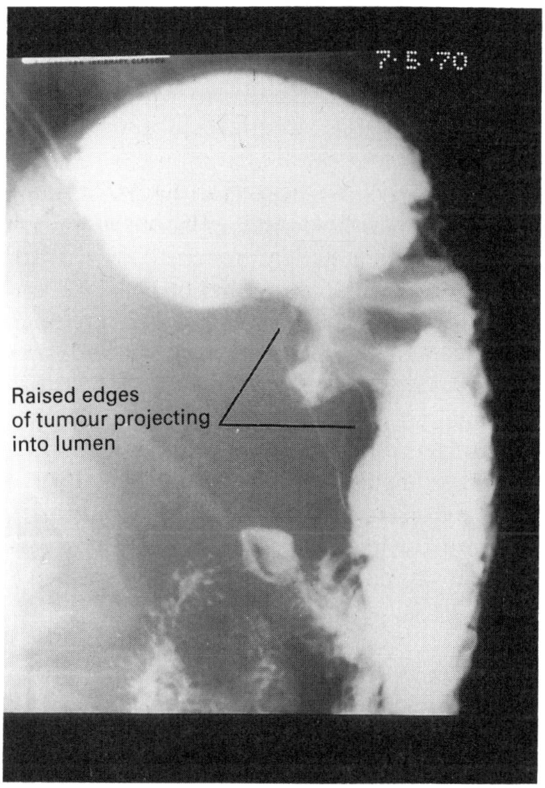

Fig. 28.20 A fungating, ulcerated carcinoma of the stomach, arising from the lesser curvature, shown on barium meal examination. Here, in contrast with Figure 28.2, the line of the lesser curve is apparently pushed in towards the luminal side by the radiotranslucent edges of the tumour, and its summit has necrosed to cause an irregular ulcer crater.

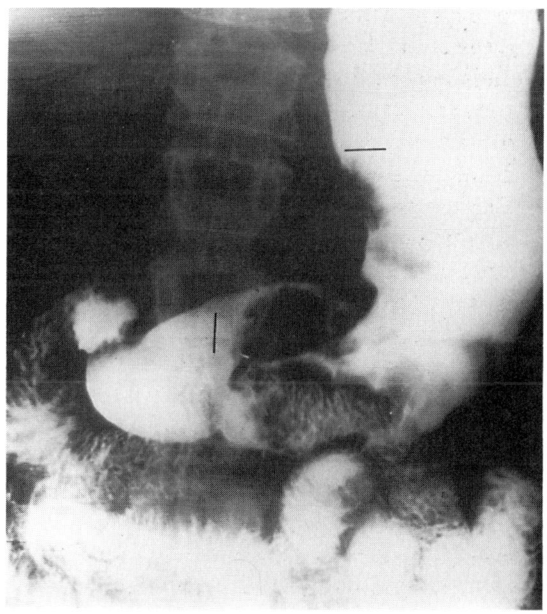

Fig. 28.21 Barium meal showing a large proliferative carcinoma, with outgrowths into the lumen from both the lesser and greater curvature aspects. Although the most bulky masses of tumour are in the antrum, lesser nodules distort the barium outline for some distance proximally along the lesser curvature. The lines mark the limits of the obvious tumour, but almost certainly microscopic extension beyond these lines is present.

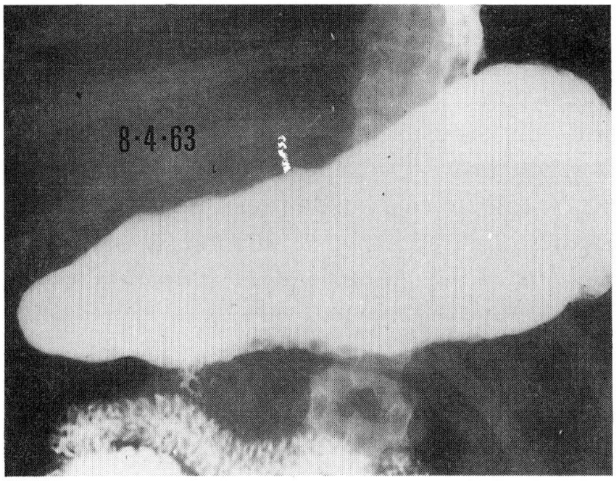

Fig. 28.22 The characteristic appearances of linitis plastica or 'leather-bottle' stomach on barium meal. In this rare variety of carcinoma of the stomach there is widespread submucosal extension converting a large part or the entire organ into a rigid, cone-shaped tube. When repeat views are taken at intervals no gastric movements are seen and the gastric outline remains constant. On the greater curvature there is some nodularity of the mucosal pattern due to the underlying tumour deposits.

to the correct diagnosis, it is advisable to proceed with endoscopic examination, which can achieve certain histological confirmation, and can also permit assessment of the extent of the tumour with somewhat greater accuracy. Endoscopy should also be undertaken where, in spite of an apparently normal X-ray appearance on barium meal, the clinical picture is still suspicious of the possible diagnosis (Fig. 28.23).

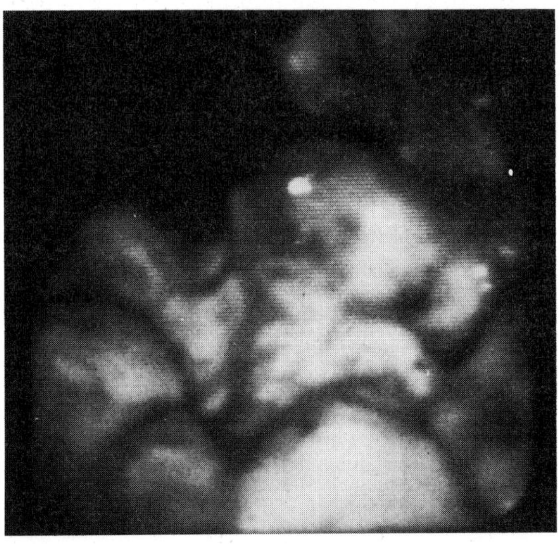

Fig. 28.23 Endoscopic appearances of a proliferative gastric carcinoma. Irregular heaped-up nodules and ulcerated areas are seen. Multiple biopsies would be taken from different segments of the lesion, especially at the edges.

Treatment

At present the sole hope of curing a patient who has a carcinoma of the stomach is if the tumour is early enough for it to be removed surgically. The tumour is not responsive to radiotherapy, and although evaluation of various cytotoxic drugs will continue, there is no good evidence to date that these give useful benefit in this particular form of malignancy.

Once a histological diagnosis has been confirmed, and there is no gross evidence of metastases in the liver, pelvis or elsewhere, exploratory operation is advised. Any significant anaemia may be corrected by blood transfusion preoperatively. After opening the abdomen a thorough exploration of the entire abdominal cavity is made, so that an assessment of the feasibility of removing the tumour may be made. Particular attention is paid to the size of the tumour, the presence or absence of direct invasion of neighbouring organs, and the presence or absence of suspicious or definite deposits of malignant tissue in lymph nodes, omenta, and other structures. Unfortunately, it is usually found on exploration that approximately one-third of tumours are either too firmly fixed to neighbouring important structures or are accompanied by such widespread metastases that no form of resection can be safely and usefully undertaken. In approximately another one-third there will be evidence of metastases, for example in the liver or elsewhere, although it is technically possible to remove the primary tumour and anastomose the proximal segment of the apparently uninvolved stomach to a segment of the proximal jejunum (a Polya-type partial gastrectomy). Under these circumstances it is wise to proceed with this resection, even though it is known that the metastases will remain. Such a course of action will give worthwhile palliation, and in particular spare the patient from many of the unpleasant symptoms arising from the primary tumour. In the remaining third of patients coming to operation for carcinoma of the stomach the tumour will appear to be confined to the stomach itself, and there appears to be no evidence of involvement of neighbouring structures or metastases, and there is therefore hope that all the malignant tissue may be removed. The objective is to excise the primary tumour with a wide margin of stomach both proximal and distal to the tumour mass, and also to remove as much as possible of both the lesser and greater omenta in the hope that any microscopically involved draining lymphatics will also be excised. This involves a distinctly more radical partial gastrectomy than that described under the section on Polya partial gastrectomy for duodenal ulcer earlier in this chapter, and the remnant of proximal stomach is usually quite small.

When the tumour arises in the proximal part of the stomach and is still operable, it may be necessary to remove a portion of the lower end of the oesophagus and the greater part of the proximal stomach to achieve satisfactory clearance. In this situation it is then possible to mobilize the remaining portion of the antrum sufficiently to bring it up to anastomose to the divided lower oesophagus.

Even less frequently total gastrectomy may be required in a particularly bulky tumour of the stomach which may still appear not to have metastasized beyond that organ itself. If this procedure is undertaken, the divided end of the proximal duodenum is closed by sutures, and a segment of upper small bowel is brought up either as a loop, or as a single end in the Roux-en-Y fashion for anastomosis to the divided oesophagus, as illustrated in Figure 28.24.

Both the proximal gastrectomy and total gastrectomy operations may require the left pleural cavity to be opened by extending the abdominal wound across the costal margin and through the left chest wall.

In the past total gastrectomy was performed for carcinoma of the stomach much more frequently than nowadays, and indeed for a while there was a vogue for advocating total resection for all cases including small early ones. However, the overall mortality and morbidity figures were so high that this more radical approach has receded.

In patients presenting with a carcinoma in the distal segment of the stomach, but which proves at exploration to be unresectable, it seems not unreasonable to perform a proximal gastrojejunostomy, in the hope of bypassing the tumour. Although

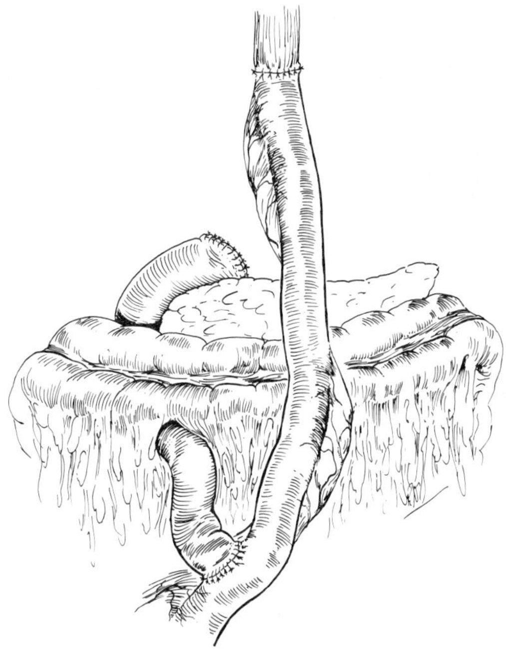

Fig. 28.24 Total gastrectomy: the proximal duodenum has been closed by sutures, and a length of jejunum has been freed and along with its mesentery brought up to be anastomosed to the severed lower oesophagus. Finally the proximal divided end of the jejunum is anastomosed end-to-side well down from the oesophageal anastomosis, to prevent regurgitation of digestive juices.

theoretically this would seem to be a good attempt to achieve palliation, particularly when the patient has been troubled by increasing eructation and vomiting, it is often very disappointing to find that the patient may not be significantly relieved of these symptoms. There is, however, an understandable tendency to try to do something which might help, rather than nothing at all.

As mentioned before, the overall prognosis in this sinister disease is poor, and as one would expect, those who have obvious metastases at laparotomy, or in whom only a palliative procedure is possible, are unlikely to survive more than a few months at best. It is also disappointing to find that even in those who have a wide resection of what looks like an operable tumour, there is a high incidence of recurrence of disease either locally or at metastatic sites in the following 1–5 years. As a result, a 5-year survival rate of somewhat less than 10% is achieved in this resectable group.

These gloomy figures raise the question as to

whether better cure rates might be obtained if we were able to diagnose the condition at a much earlier stage than when the firm diagnosis is usually made. The answer to this question appears to be 'yes', for there have been in recent years many reports of substantially better 5- and indeed 10-year survival rates in groups of patients in whom the diagnosis was made before the tumour had penetrated completely through the wall of the stomach and had the chance to spread to other tissues. The only known way of making a significantly greater number of truly early diagnoses is by the widespread application of good-quality endoscopy services, which enable the repeated screening of large numbers of patients at risk to the disease, and there are obvious practical difficulties to securing such a programme.

It is nonetheless worth emphasizing that any middle-aged or elderly patient presenting with a short history of mild or vague digestive upset, slight unexplained weight loss, or symptoms of anaemia should be referred for gastroscopy and biopsy of any suspicious mucosal area, since there is only a reasonable chance of cure if the disease is caught at a truly early stage.

29. The gallbladder and bile ducts

DEVELOPMENT

The liver, gallbladder and pancreas develop from a ventral diverticulum of the foregut which appears when the embryo is about 3 mm in size in the third week of gestation. The liver develops from the cranial part of the diverticulum, the gallbladder from the middle, and the pancreas from the caudal part. In the course of development the tube destined to form the biliary apparatus becomes blocked by the proliferation of cells, but becomes recanalized during the second and third months. Failure of recanalization gives rise to atresia of the biliary apparatus.

ANATOMY

Bile canaliculi are spaces between liver cells which join to form interlobular ductules. Several interlobular ductules unite to form lobar ducts which drain in turn into the right and left hepatic ducts. The two hepatic ducts unite at the porta hepatis to form the common hepatic duct which is joined at a distance of 4 cm from its commencement by the cystic duct from the gallbladder to form the common bile duct. The common bile duct traverses the free margin of the lesser omentum, lying on the right side of the hepatic artery and in front of the portal vein. These three structures, enclosed in the fold of peritoneum forming the free margin of the lesser omentum, constitute the anterior boundary of the foramen of Winslow. The posterior boundary of the foramen is formed by the peritoneum covering the inferior vena cava. Bleeding from the area during operations on the gallbladder and liver can be effectively controlled by digital compression of the free margin of the lesser omentum.

The common bile duct opens into the second part of the duodenum in close association with the pancreatic duct. In about 80% of cases, the two join together in the ampulla of Vater which is surrounded by the sphincter of Oddi.

The gallbladder lies in a fossa on the inferior aspect of the liver at the junction of its right and left lobes. It has a capacity of about 70 ml, and is pear-shaped. It is supplied by the cystic artery, which is a branch of the right hepatic artery. The venous drainage is into the portal vein. It receives its secretomotor nerve supply from the vagus, and the sensory fibres pass through the coeliac ganglia to the splanchnic nerves of the sympathetic system.

FUNCTION

The chief function of the biliary apparatus is the transport of bile from the liver to the duodenum. The mucous glands in the ducts and the gallbladder secrete small quantities of mucus, which is added to the bile. The gallbladder concentrates the bile by absorbing water and electrolytes. It contracts intermittently under the influence of the duodenal hormones, cholecystokinin and pancreozymin, which cause simultaneous contraction of the gallbladder and relaxation of the sphincter of Oddi. These hormones are liberated from the duodenum when its mucosa is stimulated by the entry of gastric contents. Starvation and gastric aspiration, therefore, help in providing rest to the gallbladder in acute cholecystitis.

Morphine causes strong contraction of the sphincter of Oddi when given alone as an analgesic in acute cholecystitis or gallstone colic. This may worsen the patient's condition.

SYMPTOMS OF BILIARY DISEASE

The most frequent symptoms of disease of the gallbladder and biliary passages are upper abdominal pain, jaundice, nausea, vomiting and flatulent dyspepsia. The last term denotes a combination of symptoms of a feeling of fullness after meals, heartburn and belching. When, as often, there is an infective element, there is fever also. Any or a combination of some of the above symptoms should arouse the suspicion of biliary disease.

In the majority of patients with suspected disease of the gallbladder or biliary ducts some form of imaging is employed, and good-quality scans or radiological pictures generally provide the most critical decision-making information with regard to precise diagnosis and the most appropriate treatment.

Ultrasound

Increasingly the initial imaging investigation is ultrasound scanning. This has great advantages for the patient, since he or she has to take no drugs, the procedure is comfortable and completely non-invasive and therefore totally safe. Although the quality of pictures obtained and their interpretation are influenced by the skill and technical expertise of the radiologist, the general standard of scan should be satisfactory for many clinical decisions to be made on this information alone. The probe is passed over the right upper quadrant of the abdomen, using a film of oil to make direct contact between the probe and the skin. The echo pattern is watched continuously during the procedure and appropriate prints are taken for permanent recording.

Ultrasound will normally give measurements of the size and contour of the gallbladder, the thickness of its wall, the size and number of any stones, and the size of the bile ducts, both extra- and intrahepatic. It may also detect abnormalities in nearby structures, e.g. the liver, pancreas or aorta. This form of examination is particularly useful in patients with jaundice, in whom the various types of contrast radiography would be contraindicated.

A few false-negative scans and even fewer false-positive ones still may occur, but with increasing experience a high degree of accuracy can be obtained.

Oral cholecystography

This is the visualization of the gallbladder by radio-paque dye which is excreted by the liver into the bile. Oral or intravenous routes may be used. In the former a dose of usually 6 tablets of a proprietary iodine-containing preparation are swallowed, and 12–16 h later, X-ray films of the abdomen are taken. If a gallbladder shadow is visualized, a fatty meal is given and approximately 1 h later, another radiograph is taken to see if the gallbladder has contracted normally in response to the fatty meal. A healthy gallbladder shrinks to about one-third of its normal relaxed size after a fatty meal.

The cholecystogram may show:

1. A normal gallbladder shadow which shrinks normally after a fatty meal, and in most cases this is evidence that the gallbladder is healthy.
2. No gallbladder shadow. If the clinician is sure that the patient has taken the tablets, and he or she is not suffering from any gastrointestinal disorder causing intestinal hurry thereby not allowing time for proper absorption to take place, then non-visualization means a non-functioning, diseased gallbladder.
3. Filling defects in the form of translucent areas in the opaque shadow of the gallbladder. This signifies the presence of gallstones.
4. A gallbladder which does not contract to one-third of its size in response to the fatty meal. This points to some malfunction of the organ, and often this is associated with stones.

Intravenous cholangiography

When the intravenous route is used the entire biliary tree is usually visualized. Biligrafin (Iodipamide) is generally used for this purpose: 20 ml of the dye is slowly injected intravenously after a sensitivity test has been carried out by giving 1 ml of the drug by intravenous injection a few hours before the full dose is given. If any signs of sensitivity occur, e.g. fall in blood pressure, stertorous breathing, cyanosis or incontinence of urine, the intravenous cholangiography is not undertaken, and reliance is placed on other techniques of visualization.

The main indications for intravenous cholangiography are:

1. to visualize the biliary tree after a previous cholecystectomy to ascertain the presence or absence of any obstruction to the flow of bile;
2. to visualize the gallbladder and ducts in patients in whom oral cholecystography has been unsuccessful for one reason or another;
3. in combination with oral cholecystography, to visualize both the gallbladder and the intra- and extrahepatic biliary apparatus where this appears strongly desirable on clinical grounds. For this purpose, 12 h after the patient has taken the contrast tablets, he or she is given the intravenous injection of biligrafin, and 1 h later X-ray pictures are taken.

Both oral and intravenous cholangiography are contraindicated in the presence of jaundice, as in this condition the liver cells do not excrete the dye in sufficient concentration to produce radiological shadows.

Percutaneous transhepatic cholangiography

This examination can be carried out in the presence of gross jaundice. A long, fine, flexible needle is introduced into the liver substance, usually through an intercostal space, and as the needle is slowly withdrawn gentle aspiration is applied. Bile coming back into the aspirating syringe indicates that the tip lies in a bile duct and then the biligrafin is injected to outline the duct system. The chances of success are, of course greater when the ducts are grossly dilated due to distal obstruction. If the first pass of the needle fails to locate a duct, then one or more repeat insertions are permissible. There is a small risk of leakage of blood or bile into the peritoneal cavity and this procedure is done in the knowledge that an operating theatre and surgeon are available in case laparotomy is required.

Endoscopic retrograde cholangiopancreatography (ERCP)

ERCP is an important method of investigation under certain well defined clinical circumstances, and is by no means a first-line examination. A flexible side-viewing endoscope is passed into the duodenum, the papilla is identified on the medial wall of the second part, and a fine plastic cannula is inserted under direct vision, into either the common bile duct or the main pancreatic duct. Radiopaque fluid is then introduced to give contrast radiograms of the ducts and their tributaries.

This approach is appropriate when stones, tumours or strictures are suspected within the duct system. Additional advantages are that tumours may be biopsied, stones may be extracted, if necessary after enlargement of the orifice at the ampulla of Vater by diathermy, and various specially designed devices and palliative tube stents may be introduced through malignant or other strictures, all endoscopically.

In addition to the normal unpleasantness and discomfort associated with protracted endoscopic procedures, there are risks of bleeding and damage to the duct wall, and the precipitation of pancreatitis following ERCP, therefore there should be very strong indications for undertaking it, and of course, the availability of someone with the necessary high degree of skill to do the examination.

Radionuclide scan

This is another modern method of visualizing the biliary tree. A technetium 99m-labelled derivative of aminodiacetic acid is given by intravenous injection and a gamma-camera image is obtained. As the chemical is excreted by the liver cells in high concentration into the biliary tree, the entire biliary apparatus can be visualized. This technique, not generally available, is still under critical evaluation, and its role in diagnosis of the commoner biliary tract problems is not defined as yet.

CONGENITAL ATRESIA OF THE BILE DUCTS

As already mentioned, the primitive biliary buds are canalized and contain bile when the embryo is about 12 weeks old, but if recanilization does not occur, or is incomplete, varying degrees of atresia may result. This may involve the extra, intrahepatic or both parts of the biliary tree. It is a rare anomaly and females are affected more frequently than males.

Obstruction to the biliary outflow leads to hepatomegaly and cirrhosis. Histologically there is fibrosis, proliferation of the hepatic ductules, infiltration with leukocytes and accumulation of bile pigments within the liver cells. In many cases there is lymphadenopathy in the porta hepatis and enlargement of the spleen. If the latter is present, there is usually portal hypertension.

Clinically , the picture is that of painless, progressive, afebrile jaundice, and the baby passes clay-coloured stools. Jaundice is not present at birth, but appears a few days later. In rare instances it takes as many as 3 weeks to appear. It is progressive, though a few cases have been reported in which it was intermittent in the beginning. The liver is enlarged and feels hard with rounded borders. The urine is dark and contains bile pigments. Liver function tests show no characteristic changes apart from a raised serum alkaline phosphatase and the serum bilirubin is, of course, also raised.

The diagnosis is established by excluding other causes of neonatal jaundice, e.g. congenital spherocytosis, erythroblastosis fetalis, jaundice of haemolytic sepsis, homologous serum jaundice and neonatal hepatitis.

Surgery is the only hope for these infants. Cholangiography by injecting the dye directly into the liver is usually carried out on the operating table, to reveal the site of the atresia.

In intrahepatic atresia nothing useful can be done, but in extrahepatic atresia, various operative procedures are available for the anastomosis of the distended and patent part of the biliary passage to the small intestine—either duodenum or jejunum.

CHOLEDOCHUS CYST

This is a rare congenital anomaly affecting the supraduodenal part of the common bile duct. In this condition, there is cystic dilatation of the duct like an aneurysm (Fig. 29.1). Occasionally the dilatation involves the hepatic or cystic ducts. The wall of the cyst is usually thin and translucent, but in some cases it may be thick and fibrotic. Inflammatory changes may develop in the cyst wall which, in places, may become ulcerated. Ascending cholangitis and biliary cirrhosis are the complications most likely to develop and prove fatal in untreated cases. In about 1% of cases, stones develop in the cyst. The cyst may rupture causing biliary peritonitis.

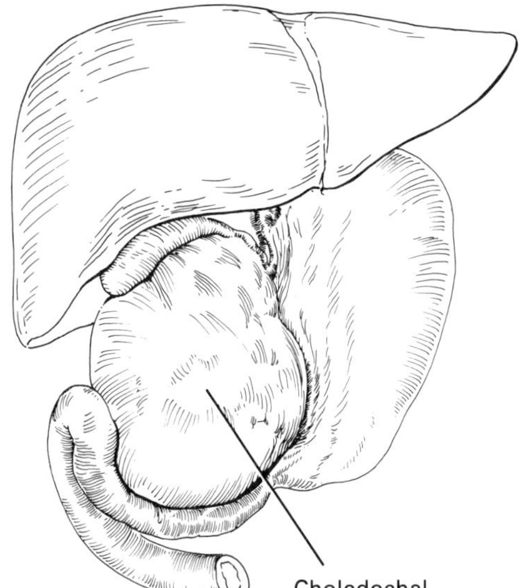

Fig. 29.1 Large choledochal cyst arising from the common bile duct, displacing and compressing the stomach, proximal duodenum and gallbladder.

Females are affected more often than males. Approximately half present in childhood, but in the others symptoms do not appear before the age of 20 years.

Abdominal pain, jaundice and epigastric mass are the main clinical manifestations. The diagnosis is usually established by an intravenous cholangiogram. The preferred surgical approach is to excise the cyst, and anastomose the proximal divided duct to a Roux-en-Y loop of jejunum, but if this is not feasible, then simple anastomosis of the wall of the cyst to either the duodenum or jejunum is an alternative.

GALLSTONES

Stone formation is the commonest of all biliary disorders. It is estimated that about 20% of all women of child-bearing age, and 20% of all persons, male and female, above the age of 40 years develop gallstones.

Aetiology

Although the precise mechanism of calculus formation is not known, some factors which encourage stone formation are as follows:

1. Inflammation of the gallbladder may lead to the formation of pus or epithelial debris. This may form a nucleus for the deposition of solid materials, e.g. cholesterol, bile pigments and calcium salts. Moreover as a result of inflammation, more bile salts are absorbed by the mucosa of the gallbladder than normally. This decreases the solubility of cholesterol, which may be thereby precipitated. Normally the ratio of bile salts to cholesterol is 25 :1. A threshold is reached when this is reduced to 13 :1 and beyond this point, cholesterol is precipitated.
2. Biliary stasis occurs during pregnancy under the influence of hormones which tend to inhibit the musculature of the gallbladder. Due to this stasis, the incoming bile comes into contact with the bile already present, which is more concentrated and so of different specific gravity. When layers of bile of different specific gravity come into contact with each other, some of the solutes may be precipitated.
3. Bile pigments may be precipitated whenever there is excessive production of these, as occurs in haemolytic anaemias, e.g. congenital spherocytosis, and in malaria.
4. The reabsorption of bile salts which normally takes place in the distal small bowel is hampered in some intestinal diseases, and of course is reduced after resection of large segments of small bowel, or after bypass procedures. There is evidence that the incidence of gallstones in patients suffering from these conditions is higher than among normal subjects.
5. It has been shown that women who use stilboestrol either as a contraceptive or as a substitute after the menopause are more liable to form gallstones than non-users, and similarly persons who take clofibrate may also have an increased tendency towards stone formation.

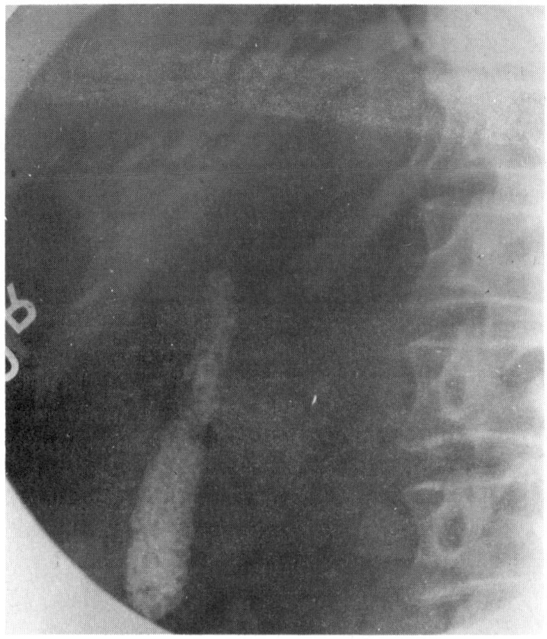

Fig. 29.2 Multiple radiopaque gallstones, packed within a narrow gallbladder.

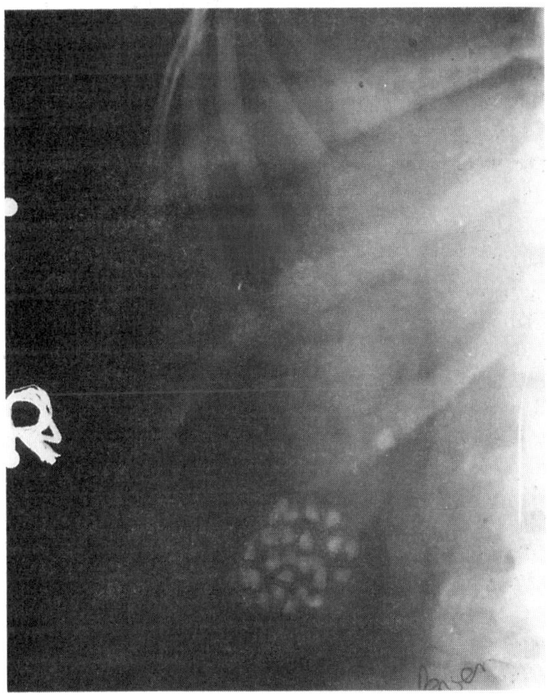

Fig. 29.3 Oral cholecystogram showing multiple faceted gallstones in the fundus of the gallbladder, and one located in Hartmann's pouch. There is only a faint shadow outlining the gallbladder, indicating that function is impaired.

Pathology

Three main types of gallstones are encountered:

1. Mixed stones, which constitute about 80%

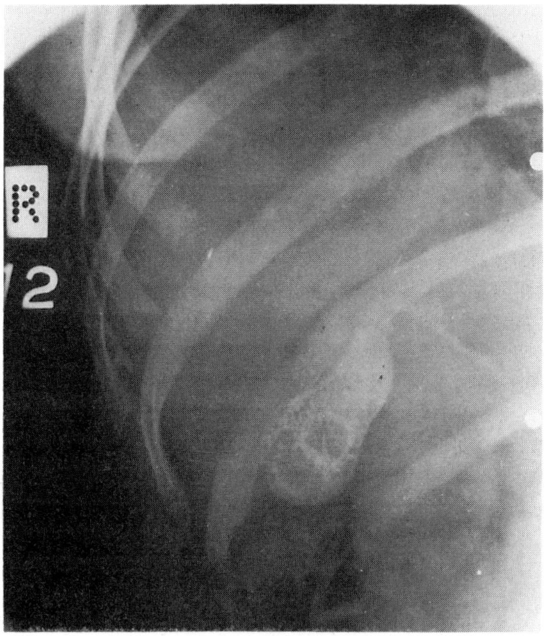

Fig. 29.4 Two large gallstones, plus numerous very small ones, all radio translucent, and being shown up by the contrast medium in an oral cholecystogram. The cystic duct is also shown, emptying in turn into the common bile duct.

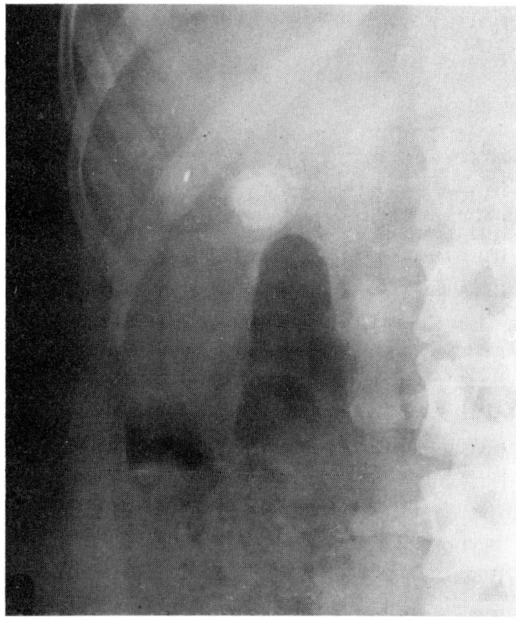

Fig. 29.5 A large solitaire gallstone, shown in an asymptomatic patient, as an incidectal finding. Note the concentric ring shadows representing growth in size as new layers of calculus material have been laid down. There is less risk of this large solitary stone causing obstruction or other serious consequences than is the case with smaller stones which can more easily become displaced.

of all gallstones (Figs 29.2–29.4). These are multiple, of varying sizes and may have either a whitish cholesterol, or brownish pigment coating. On section, the stones are laminated like sections of an onion, the laminae consisting of alternate layers of cholesterol, bile pigments and calcium salts.

2. Pigment stones, which are the second most common stones, consist of calcium bilirubinate. These are multiple, dark, and vary in size from small particles to about 5 mm in diameter. Often they are so small that they form what is called biliary mud. These stones may easily find their way into the common bile duct.
3. Cholesterol stones, which are usually single and constitute about 6% of all gallstones, are light in weight and, in pure form, of light yellow colour and faintly translucent. On section, cholesterol crystals are usually found to radiate like spokes in a wheel. A single cholesterol calculus often lies in Hartmann's pouch, and is then referred to as a solitaire.

Only about 10% of all gallstones are radiopaque.

Complications of gallstones

1. The most common complication of gallstones is cholecystitis, which may be acute or chronic. It is estimated that at least 90% of cases of cholecystitis are associated with stones. In most instances the episode of acute infection will settle down after a few days, but on occasions further severe consequences may complicate the illness even more. First, if there is profuse pus formation and blockage of the cystic duct outlet by a stone or stones an empyema of the gallbladder may form, the tense gallbladder being transformed into a bag of pus. Second, if this remains unrelieved and a portion of the wall becomes necrosed, pus escapes into the peritoneum to cause a very severe form of peritonitis. Thirdly, a localized abscess may arise at the point of rupture of the gallbladder. A fourth possibility is the formation of a fistula between the inflamed dilated wall of the infected gallbladder fundus and the duodenum, against

which it comes in contact. Through such a fistula one or more gallstones may pass, and if a stone is large enough it may cause intestinal obstruction, most likely in the ileum, the narrowest segment of the small intestine. This rare form of intestinal obstruction is called gallstone ileus. A fifth serious complication of infection in the gallbladder and biliary tree is the extension of the infective process up the proximal bile ducts into the liver—ascending cholangitis.

2. Chronic cholecystitis is also a common sequel of gallstones. This often takes the form of repeated episodes of acute cholecystitis, with perhaps also a background of continuing dyspeptic symptoms and signs between attacks.
3. If a stone obstructs the cystic duct and there is no gross superadded infection, the bile in the gallbladder may be absorbed and its cavity filled with mucus secreted by its epithelium. This mucus-distended gallbladder may become clearly palpable, being referred to as a mucocele of the gallbladder.
4. A serious complication of gallstones is the impaction of one or more in the common bile duct, resulting in obstructive jaundice. If, for one reason or another, the obstruction remains prolonged, liver cell damage results, giving the pattern of biliary cirrhosis.
5. In many cases of acute pancreatitis gallstones are found to be a precipitating cause.
6. Almost all cancers of the gallbladder are associated with stones in that organ. On the other hand, it is estimated that carcinoma develops in only about 1% or less of patients suffering from gallstones, so that the risk of patients who have gallstones developing cancer is indeed very small.

Clinical features

Gallstones may be silent, i.e. cause no symptoms and may only be discovered accidentally during either radiography or laparotomy for some other condition. It has been estimated that in post-mortem examination, about 8% of individuals who have died of causes unrelated to gallstones are found to harbour stones in their gallbladders.

In previous years it was taught that the most typical sufferer from gallstones was a middle-aged, overweight woman who had had several children. Although gallstones are frequently encountered in such individuals they may also be seen in both sexes and in a wider age range from the early 20s to the elderly, and many of the patients are well within the normal weight range or are even quite slim.

Flatulent dyspepsia is a common manifestation of gallstone disease. The patient complains of a feeling of fullness after meals, and may also experience heartburn and belching. On examination, there may be some tenderness in the right hypochondrium. If a mucocele has developed this is felt as a round mass moving up and down with respiration.

If, in someone presenting with such a history, gallstones or diminished or absent function of the gallbladder is demonstrated on ultrasound or cholecystography examination, then the usual advice is to undergo cholecystectomy, or if the stones are suitable and the methods available, one or other technique to dissolve or disintegrate the stones may be recommended.

ACUTE BILIARY PAIN

Biliary colic and acute cholecystitis

Gallstones and some degree of infection usually coexist. Acute severe pain can therefore result from either a stone becoming impacted in the neck of the gallbladder or cystic duct, or an acute inflammation episode due to the infection.

Where the main problem is temporary mechanical blockage of the gallbladder outlet by one or more stones, and there is a negligible inflammatory flare-up the condition is predominantly that of biliary colic, whereas when the inflammation is greater and dominates the clinical picture, the episode is referred to as acute cholecystitis. In practice, it is generally very difficult clearly to differentiate one from the other, and in any event the so-called biliary colic rarely presents with the clear-cut rhythmic pattern so characteristic of gut or renal colic, and is more by way of a continuous pain, persisting throughout the duration of an attack.

Since the majority of attacks of acute cholecystitis start with partial or complete obstruction of the gallbladder outlet by stones it is largely a matter of degree and timing whether the attack is short-lived, i.e. over an hour or two, and resolves with the spontaneous falling back of the occluding stones into the gallbladder and is described as biliary colic, or it goes on to a more prolonged episode of acute cholecystitis.

Biliary colic

The pain is of sudden onset, located in the right hypochondrium and epigastrium, and often radiates to the back or between the shoulder blades. It may cause the patient to double up, or to roll about in bed, and it is often accompanied by nausea, retching and vomiting. It often passes off as suddenly as it started, after lasting for a few hours.

On examination during the attack there is usually marked tenderness in the gallbladder region, and a strong analgesic, e.g. pethidine 100 mg, is usually required to obtain relief. There has been a convention also to administer an anticholinergic antispasmodic to reduce muscular contraction and spasm of the gallbladder wall, but this consideration is probably more theoretical than of real practical importance.

Acute cholecystitis

This condition is usually more gradual in onset, but otherwise is the same as that of biliary colic. However, since progressive inflammatory changes develop, e.g. oedematous thickening of the gallbladder wall, increased vascularity, and pus formation, not only does the localized right hypochondrial pain persist and steadily worsen, but nausea and vomiting tend to become more troublesome and systemic symptoms and signs develop. These include malaise, sweating, fever, tachycardia, and maybe signs of diaphragmatic irritation such as shoulder pain and restricted depth of respiration.

The commonest organism involved is *Escherichia coli*, but other organisms which may be responsible are streptococcus, *Bacterium typhosum* and *Clostridium welchii*. The infection is believed to reach the gallbladder most commonly through the bile from the liver. Adhesions develop between the inflamed gallbladder and the neighbouring structures such as the greater omentum and loops of intestine, and thus a gallbladder mass is formed. Sometimes the interior of the gallbladder becomes filled and distended with pus, to form an empyema of the gallbladder.

Usually the acute phase eventually subsides and the oedema becomes less marked. In such cases, the stone obstructing the cystic duct may become loose and fall back into the cavity of the gallbladder. Once obstruction to the flow of the contents has been removed, the infected bile is passed into the duodenum via the common bile duct. As the inflammatory changes subside all the signs and symptoms of the disease disappear but the gallbladder probably never returns to its normal state.

On examination at the height of an attack of acute cholecystitis, in addition to the general signs of toxicity, fever, sweating and tachycardia, there is marked tenderness in the right hypochondrium, and often muscle guarding. The gallbladder tenderness may be most dramatically demonstrated by the traditionally hallowed Murphy's test—a positive response is the sharp halting of inspiration on account of pain, when a deeply placed examining finger is placed directly below the costal margin at the level of the ninth costal cartilage.

A palpable mass at this area may represent either the adherent omentum or small bowel loop wrapped over the swollen gallbladder, or an empyema.

The diagnosis is supported by the presence of a gross leukocytosis—15 000–20 000/mm^3 or more.

Occasionally jaundice may develop during the attack, and this may be due to a stone in the common bile duct, or to pressure on the latter by oedematous swelling of the grossly inflamed neck or Hartmann's pouch, or more rarely to cholangitis.

The main conditions which may at times be difficult to differentiate from acute cholecystitis are:

1. Acute pancreatitis—although slight elevation of serum amylase levels may occur in acute cholecystitis, gross elevation to over 1 000 u/dl clearly points to acute pancreatitis.
2. Perforated peptic ulcer—an erect film of the chest may show gas under the diaphragm, confirming the perforation.
3. High retrocaecal appendicitis—although the principal site of tenderness should be lower than the costal margin, this can sometimes prove a difficult clinical judgement.

4. Myocardial infarction—depending on the duration of the symptoms either elevation of cardiac enzymes or the appropriate electrocardiogram changes may give the lead.
5. Basal pneumonia—reduced breath sounds, advential sounds and opacity on chest X-ray are helpful indicators.

Management of an acute attack

The vast majority of acute attacks of biliary colic or cholecystitis will spontaneously settle after a few hours to a few days, and therefore primary measures are directed at encouraging this process. Rest in bed, avoidance of food, a strong analgesic, and if there is concern regarding the infective element, a broad-spectrum antibiotic are advised, and if vomiting is profuse and troublesome a nasogastric tube may give relief. When the symptoms and signs subside a gradual return to fluids, semi-solids and then full diet can be made. The patient is closely and repeatedly examined several times each day to detect any signs of impending complications, e.g. an expanding gallbladder mass, signs of spreading peritonitis, high fever and chills suggesting cholangitis, rising pulse rate and temperature. Suspicion of any of the complications mentioned on page 294 may cause the conservative treatment outlined above to be abandoned in favour of operative exploration.

Ultrasound examination is usually quite possible without causing additional distress to the patient, even during the acute attack, and of course often gives useful information, identifying stones, and assessing the state of both the gallbladder and the biliary ducts. A straight film of the abdomen rarely provides much help, since the chance of revealing gallstones is only about 1 in 10, and the interpretation of various vague shadows can be difficult.

Once the presence of gallstones is confirmed in a patient with such an acute presentation, sooner or later he or she should have them removed, by one method or another. Until recently this always meant cholecystectomy. As far as the timing of the surgical procedure is concerned there are two main options. Either the patient can be allowed to recover from the acute attack and a few weeks later, when the inflammatory reactions have subsided, the operation is scheduled as an elective procedure, or the surgeon can proceed with cholecystectomy without delay. If the latter policy is pursued, the operation should be done within 48–72 h of the onset of the attack, and by a surgeon experienced with biliary procedures; antibiotic cover is wise. The general hesitation in recommending early operation is in case the oedema and other inflammatory reactions obscure the anatomy at the important area of the bile ducts and blood vessels, and as a result there may be more risk of damaging these structures, with devastating results. If delay is undue, i.e. more than 48–72 h, then there is an increased likelihood of such technical difficulty, but provided the procedure is done early enough (usually on the first available operating list), there should be little or no problem in identifying the anatomy clearly. Obviously if the surgical removal of the source of trouble can be achieved at the initial admission this saves time and is more convenient for the patient. It also removes the chances of recurrent attacks arising before the delayed, planned elective operation.

One further operative procedure which rarely is the only safe option is cholecystostomy, the opening of the gallbladder fundus, evacuation of all contained stones, and insertion of a wide drain into its lumen. This approach would only be recommended in patients who are grossly unfit for more major surgery, and in situations where dense adhesions around the gallbladder, particularly in the neck region, would make dissection difficult or hazardous. Once the patient's fitness improves and the acute inflammatory reaction has subsided, cholecystectomy can be performed electively weeks later.

Non-operative treatment of gallstones

The idea of dissolving stones has been entertained for a long time, and some success is sometimes possible in selected groups of patients, with stones in which the main constituent is cholesterol. A bile salt is given orally—either chenodeoxycholic or ursodeoxycholic acid. These substances increase the total bile acid pool and in turn desaturate the bile of cholesterol, so that some of the cholesterol in the stones may return into the liquid bile. This process takes some time to achieve gross reduction in stone size; also the bile salt preparations often provoke diarrhoea and other unpleasant side-effects. Their use is generally confined to those in whom operation is risky. Contraindications include large stones, the presence of a non-functioning gallbladder and calcium stones. There is also, of course, the risk of further stones reappearing after cessation of treatment.

Lithotripsy is a technique of delivering accurately focused narrow beams of shock waves to the stones. The technique is similar to that described in Chapter 39 for the disintegration of urinary calculi. The shock waves may pass safely through soft tissues without causing any effect, but whenever they come in contact with any solid object they cause it to disintegrate. It is important therefore to ensure that the waves are directed solely through soft tissue and that no bony structures intervene. Various instruments have become available recently, primarily for the disintegration of urinary tract stones, and some of these are also capable of focusing on gallstones. Again, only certain patients are suitable candidates for this form of treatment. The stones should not be numerous, arbitrarily less than five, there should be good gallbladder function so that the fragments can be expelled, and the patient should be capable of remaining still for up to 40–60 min. As with dissolution methods there is, of course, once more the question of the formation of further stones after the initial ones have been successfully broken down and cleared.

The role of this new method has still to be evaluated. Certainly the possibility of a completely non-invasive form of treatment would be greatly welcomed by patients and further improvements in this and other techniques are likely in the future.

Chronic cholecystitis

This describes the situation in which the patient usually has had several bouts of biliary colic or acute cholecystitis, and between the attacks has continued to complain of various dyspeptic symptoms, e.g. upper abdominal discomfort often precipitated by meals; belching; heartburn, and a feeling of abdominal distension. Although it has been traditionally maintained that fatty foods are the main triggering factors and that this is fairly specific to gallbladder disease, this is not borne out in practice, for such a complaint is not uncommon in a wide variety of digestive disorders, from peptic ulcer to irritable colon. However, some degree of fatty intolerance is often volunteered in chronic cholecystitis.

With the increasing inflammatory reaction the gallbladder usually becomes thick-walled, loses its contractility and may shrink in size. Function is lost and it ends up as a passive container of stones and infected material.

Tenderness in the gallbladder region may or may not be detected, depending on whether any gross inflammation is present at the time of the examination.

Once the diagnosis is established and any other possible causes of the symptoms are excluded, the only reasonable recommendation is cholecystectomy. In this condition there is no realistic expectation that one or other of the non-operative approaches will help.

Rarely chronic cholecystitis occurs in the absence of stones, and the possibility of the patient being a carrier of typhoid bacilli in the organ should be borne in mind.

Cholecystectomy

The operation, one of the commonest abdominal procedures in most countries, can be done through either an upper vertical incision, either midline or right paramedian, or through an oblique incision running parallel to and about 3 cm below the right costal margin (Kocher's incision). The cystic duct is first exposed and traced to its junction with the common hepatic duct to form the common bile duct. Most surgeons will next routinely perform peroperative cholangiography by introducing a fine catheter (e.g. an umbilical catheter) into an opening made in the cystic duct and passing its tip into the common duct (Fig. 29.6). The catheter is then held firmly in position by a thread suture tied round the cystic duct distal to the opening, and X-ray films are exposed after the injection of first 2–4 ml, and then 10–15 ml contrast medium. Thus a good outline of virtually all the main branches of the extrahepatic biliary duct tree is obtained and any stones lying in these passages should be detected. Once satisfactory pictures have been obtained, the cystic duct is divided and the stump ligated. The cystic artery is located, divided and

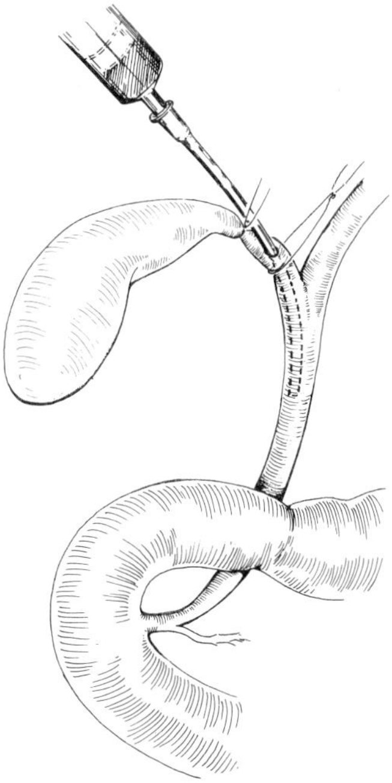

Fig. 29.6 Peroperative cholangiography: once the tip of the cannula is in good position in the common bile duct, the ligature around the distal part of the cystic duct is tightened to keep the cannula secure and prevent leakage of the injected contrast medium.

ligated, and then the gallbladder is removed from its bed in the under-surface of the liver. Any accessory ducts or blood vessels are also divided and ligated or sealed as the removal proceeds.

An alternative technique, which may be used where dissection near the cystic duct–porta hepatis region proves difficult, is to do a retrograde removal, starting the dissection around the fundus of the gallbladder and working gradually towards the neck, leaving identification of the cystic duct and artery to the last steps in the procedure.

Whichever method is employed, once the gallbladder has been removed and haemostasis has been secured, a drain is generally left down in the gallbladder bed, and brought out through a separate small stab wound in the lateral abdominal wall. This will allow any blood or bile leakage from the raw bed in the liver to escape, and also permit the early detection of any gross bleeding should a ligature slip from a divided vessel.

Laparoscopic cholecystectomy

In the last few years many centres throughout the world have acquired the skills of dissecting out and removing the gallbladder under vision which is either direct along the laparoscope, or transmitted to a videocamera. The retracting, cutting, clipping, ligating or suturing instruments are introduced through separate small stab or puncture wounds, and their actions are controlled by external handles. X-ray procedures, e.g. cholangiography, can be performed during the procedure. The procedure requires general anaesthesia, but postoperative recovery is rapid, the wounds are very small, and often the patient can eat later the same day, return home within 24 h, and resume normal daily activities immediately. Needless to say, these factors make this particular approach very popular with the patients, and can result in very large savings of beds and other resources.

On occasions this technique will be unsuitable, e.g. when there are stones impacted in the cystic duct, gross anatomical abnormalities, etc., but it is likely to prove completely satisfactory for many — probably the most—gallstone patients.

Common bile duct stones

The vast majority of stones which are encountered in the hepatic or common bile duct originate in the gallbladder and have passed through the cystic duct. Although they must, of course, have been small enough at first to pass through this rather narrow channel, they may enlarge once they reach the relatively wider space in the common duct. The diagnosis is made when the stones obstruct the flow of bile, usually at the narrowed lower end as it approaches the ampulla of Vater. In the Far East they may occasionally arise primarily in common ducts which are infested with liver flukes or roundworm.

The clinical picture is therefore that of obstructive jaundice. An attack of typical biliary colic often precedes the jaundice and pain in the right hypochondrium may continue to be troublesome as the pigmentation increases in depth. The amount of pain is, however, variable, and it is possible for an occasional patient to present with painless, deep jaundice which proves to be due to a stone impacted in the duct. For the first few days the jaundice becomes progressively deeper, but after that may diminish, only to deepen again after an interval. Classically as the jaundice appears the urine passed becomes increasingly darker, containing bile pigments but no urobilinogen, and the stools become lighter in colour due to the absence of bile pigments. Body itching frequently occurs, and can be most distressing to the patient.

On examination, in addition to the obvious jaundice, and often visible scratch marks on account of the itch, there is frequently tenderness in the gallbladder region. It should not be possible to feel the gallbladder for, as a result of previous damage by the inflammation, its wall is thickened and inelastic. This conforms to Courvoisier's law, which states that in the presence of obstructive jaundice, if the gallbladder is palpable the jaundice is due to a cause other than stone. Like all laws this is generally true, but not infallible. The blood profile of liver function tests shows a characteristic pattern, the main features of which are a grossly elevated serum bilirubin and alkaline phosphatase accompanied by slight elevation of the transaminases serum glutamic oxaloacetic and pyruvic transaminase. Where the obstruction is prolonged and more back-pressure damage arises to the liver cells, these latter enzymes may continue to rise, but virtually never to the same extent as the alkaline phosphatase —a predominantly duct enzyme.

If obstruction in the common duct is prolonged, further complications are likely to arise. The ducts proximal to the occlusion may greatly dilate and back-pressure on the hepatocytes may stop bilirubin secretion, with the leading result that only mucus is present within the ducts—the so-called white bile. Ascending infection may give the full-blown picture of cholangitis, with pain, fever and tachycardia in addition to the jaundice. Vitamin K deficiency may follow, giving rise to bleeding problems. Acute pancreatitis may be precipitated.

Treatment

Every patient with a common bile duct obstructed by a stone requires urgent relief of the obstruction and removal of the stone. Until recently the most widely applicable method of achieving this has been by open operation, cholecystectomy plus exploration of the common duct. Vitamin K or K_1 is given prophylactically before operation in all patients with obstructive jaundice to minimize the chances of operative or postoperative bleeding. Removal of the stone or stones may be a simple matter of combined suction through the opening in the duct and gentle pressure from below, or the insertion of a balloon catheter, Dormia basket, or specially designed forceps, e.g. Desjardin's. It is helpful to have had a preliminary outline of the ducts by peroperative cholangiography, and further visualization of the ducts once it is thought that all the stones have been removed. It is all too easy to overlook one or more small ones, and every attempt should be made to ensure complete clearance. The most direct evidence is visual inspection of the lumen both proximally and distally through a flexible choledochoscope (Fig. 29.7). A clear view right down to and through the ampulla of Vater should be obtained. Failing this, it should at least be demonstrated that a probe or catheter can be easily passed right down into the duodenum and the tip seen through the duodenal wall on tenting this over it. The operation is conventionally completed by leaving the short arms of a plastic T-tube in the

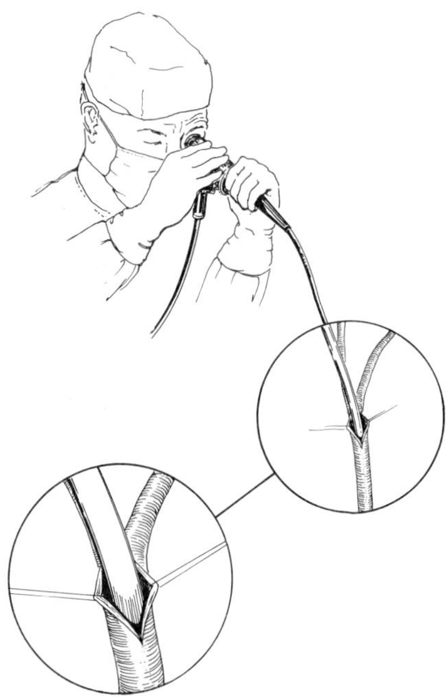

Fig. 29.7 Choledochoscopy: direct inspection of the inside of the common bile duct at operation via a fibreoptic instrument.

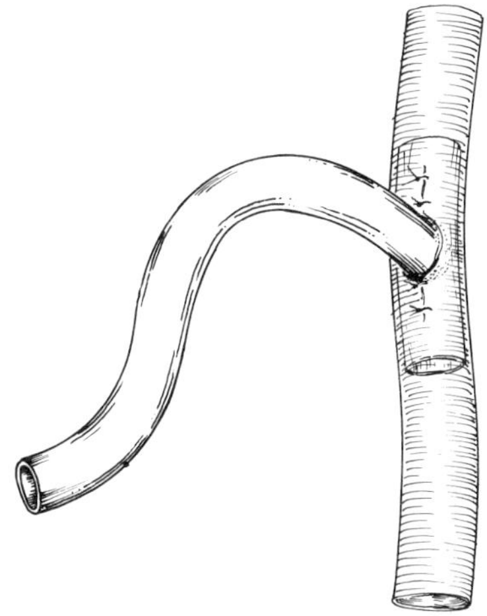

Fig. 29.8 T-tube: the short limb is inserted into the opening in the common bile duct, which is then closed with absorbable sutures around the emerging long limb; the latter is brought out through a small stab wound in the abdominal wall.

duct (Fig. 29.8), and closing the incision in the duct snugly around the tube, bringing the long end out through a separate stab wound.

Approximately 1 week after the operation further cholangiograms are taken after injecting contrast medium down the T-tube, and if there is no sign of any residual stone or other duct problem, the tube can be clamped for increasing lengths of time during the day, and then removed. Of course any remaining stones or the presence of pain or leakage on clamping the tube will necessitate appropriate further steps to deal with the matter, and leaving the tube in situ until it has been resolved.

Endoscopic removal of stones

Increasingly skilled endoscopists are able to extract stones from the common bile duct by ERCP, and if necessary the ampullary outlet of the duct can be divided vertically by a diathermy knife passed through a side-channel in the endoscope: the procedure is done under direct vision. Various specially designed instruments can be passed through the widened duct opening to manipulate stones within the duct system and pull them down through the ampulla and into the duodenum. This is increasingly becoming the treatment of choice for this problem.

The main groups of patients in whom this ERCP approach should be considered are those who are

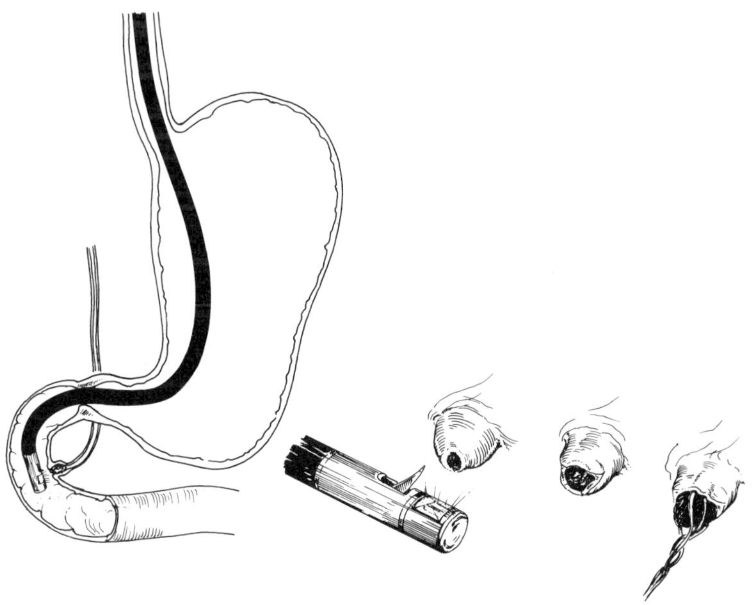

Fig. 29.9 Endoscopic removal of a stone from the lower end of the common bile duct. After visualizing the ampulla of Vater, as shown in the inserts, the opening can be sufficiently enlarged by a manoeuvrable knife or dïathermy to allow the stone to pass, or the stone may be grasped by a basket device and extracted.

at high risk for a general anaesthetic and open operation, and those with retained stones in the common bile duct after operation. It may also be argued that in patients who present with deep jaundice, the initial relief of this may render them less at risk of a subsequent operation to remove the gallbladder and any other non-obstructing stones.

If ERCP is not available, or if it fails to remove residual duct stones following cholecystectomy and exploration of the common duct, it sometimes may be possible to coax them out via the T-tube track, using a variety of basket snare on a fine flexible wire under X-ray control, or by flushing saline or other solutions through the tube (Fig. 29.9). If all these methods fail, then there is no alternative to proceeding with a repeat exploration and clearing of the stones via open laparotomy.

JAUNDICE

At this point it is relevant to discuss briefly the various other patterns of jaundice which have to be differentiated from obstructive disease. Often the discrimination is easy, but on occasions considerable difficulty may arise and the skilful interpretation of various signs and investigation results may be required to reach the correct conclusion. This is important, for just as obstruction needs urgent surgical relief, so other forms may be aggravated by unnecessary surgery.

Jaundice is the yellow discoloration of skin, sclera and mucous membranes due to an increased concentration of bile pigments in the plasma. The main bile pigments, bilirubin and biliverdin, are produced by the breakdown of haemoglobin released from dead erythrocytes by the cells of the reticuloendothelial system. Haemoglobin is split into iron, globin and haem. The iron is stored in the body, mainly in the liver, and is used again for the synthesis of further haemoglobin, globin is added to the protein pool for further metabolism, and haem is converted into biliverdin. Bilirubin is the reduced form of biliverdin. Both of these pigments are not soluble in water and remain bound to serum albumin. In this form they cannot be excreted by the normal kidneys. In the liver, bilirubin and biliverdin are conjugated into cholebilirubin with the help of a microsomal enzyme, transferase. Cholebilirubin is water-soluble and is excreted in the bile and then converted into stercobilinogen in the intestines, the bulk being excreted in the faeces. A part of the stercobilinogen is absorbed into the circulation and excreted by the kidneys in the form of urobilinogen.

A simple classification of jaundice is into three main categories—prehepatic, hepatic and posthepatic.

Prehepatic jaundice

Two varieties of prehepatic jaundice are of importance to surgeons, one from a therapeutic point of view and the other being largely a preventable condition. Congenital spherocytosis belongs to the first category and haemolysis resulting from incompatible blood transfusion belongs to the second category.

Congenital spherocytosis is a disease of the red blood cells in which their fragility increases and haemolytic anaemia develops. The liver cells cannot fully conjugate the excess of bilirubin produced by the increased haemolysis, and so unconjugated bilirubin circulates in the blood. Unconjugated bilirubin cannot be excreted by the kidneys and so in this form of jaundice bile pigments are not present in the urine and this is called acholuric jaundice. In this disorder gallstones are apt to form due to the excess of bilirubin.

Clinically, if jaundice is apparent, it is generally only mild and the spleen is enlarged. Blood examination reveals anaemia and reticulocytosis; the increased fragility can be demonstrated by exposing the cells to solutions of increasing osmotic tension. There are no bile pigments in urine and the stools are usually dark brown. This is almost the only condition in which gallstones may develop in children.

Splenectomy is the prescribed treatment. It neither prevents the spherocytosis nor lessens the fragility of the red blood cells, but reduces the rate of their destruction in the spleen, thereby correcting the anaemia.

Transfusion with incompatible blood is the preventable type of haemolysis which may lead to prehepatic jaundice. Even when the principal blood groups are matched, as should always be the case, there is the possibility of other forms of incompatibility, the first manifestation of which may be a reaction to the transfusion and then the appearance of jaundice.

Hepatic jaundice

Hepatic or hepatocellular jaundice is that which results from direct damage to the hepatocytes. A large number of agents may bring about this damage, e.g. bacteria in leptospirosis (Weil's disease); viruses — hepatitis A and B, infective mononucleosis, yellow fever; drugs — alcohol, halothane; toxins—carbon tetrachloride, phosphorus, and certain plant alkaloids.

Those most commonly encountered in clinical practice are viral hepatitis and cirrhosis. Various disordered mechanisms contribute to the overall jaundice picture, e.g. diminished transport of the bilirubin to the conjugating sites, reduced secretion into the bile duct radicles, leakage of a proportion of the secreted bile pigments back into the hepatocytes. There may also be present some haemolysis and bile stasis.

Both bilirubin and urobilinogen may be detected in the urine, even before jaundice becomes clinically apparent, and further increase in quantity as the condition deepens. With greater damage to the liver cells both bile pigments may disappear from the urine, and a good indication of subsequent improvement is the reappearance of urobilin in the urine.

In the blood both conjugated and unconjugated bilirubin are present.

Posthepatic jaundice

Posthepatic jaundice is due to obstruction to the flow of bile, either in the extrahepatic duct system or in the intrahepatic ducts. The commonest cause is obstruction of the common bile by a stone or tumour. The latter may be carcinoma of the head of the pancreas or of the bile ducts themselves, or metastatic deposits in lymph nodes in the porta hepatis pressing on the bile ducts. Other causes are congenital atresia, fibrous strictures, usually due to previous surgical trauma, and in eastern countries impaction of parasites, e.g. flukes and roundworms. The rarer intrahepatic variety arises from damage and occlusion of the finest radicles of the duct system, e.g. from chlorpromazine poisoning.

The main clinical features, methods of investigation and biochemical abnormalities have already been considered (see p. 299). Deep jaundice, pale stools and dark urine, body itching, and gross elevation of serum bilirubin and alkaline phosphatase levels, with much lesser proportional increase in other liver enzymes, are the salient features. Whereas with stone in the bile duct there may be fluctuation in the degree of the jaundice and associated changes, the typical pattern in duct obstruction due to malignant tumours is steadily progressive painless jaundice, and steadily climbing biochemical levels.

In all forms of extrahepatic obstruction the liver will enlarge and there is dilatation of the duct system. Eventually the back-pressure can stop bile secretion, when a pressure of around 350 mm of water is reached. However, bile duct mucus may still be produced at this or higher pressures, and therefore the ducts may be filled only with this mucus—the so-called white bile.

While, of course, the main object of operation in obstructive jaundice is to remove the cause, sometimes in the case of tumour this is not technically possible, but still useful palliative relief of the jaundice can be achieved by making a bypass between either the distended gallbladder or the supraduodenal portion of the common bile duct, and either the duodenum or a loop of jejunum.

Postcholecystectomy problems

Although the majority of patients undergoing this very commonly performed operation have an uneventful convalescence and return to completely normal health, there are occasional problems either in the early postoperative period, e.g. bleeding from the gallbladder bed, or from a ligature slipping from the cystic artery stump', localized infection and subphrenic abscess formation; undue bile leakage from divided accessory ducts in the gallbladder bed, or later, e.g. stricture formation in the bile ducts due to damage at the operation, or retained stones in the extrahepatic duct system. Each will require appropriate surgical or endoscopic treatment.

Bleeding from the cystic artery requires urgent re-exploration, identification of the vessel and the

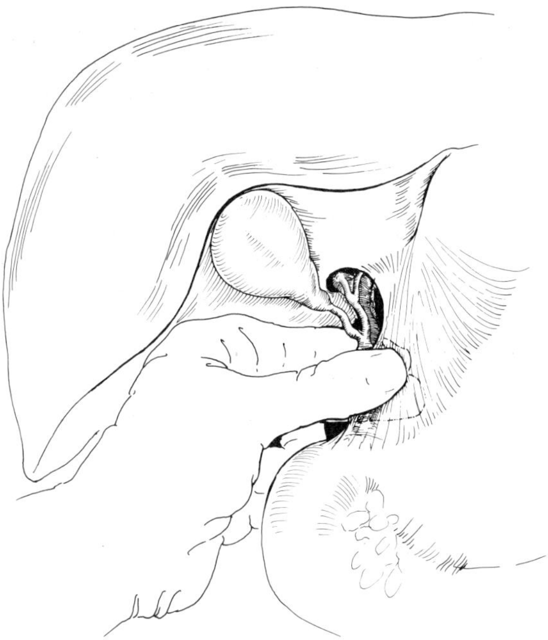

Fig. 29.10 Pringle's manoeuvre to control bleeding from the porta hepatis, e.g. from the cystic artery. The index finger can usually be easily inserted into the foramen of Winslow: thumb pressure applied against this finger will temporarily occlude both the portal vein and the hepatic artery. This can be helpful in allowing identification of the precise source of bleeding.

application of a further secure ligature (Fig. 29.10). An abscess will need to be drained, either by surgical incision or by the introduction of a catheter under ultrasound or other imaging control. Bile leakage which does not diminish spontaneously may need coagulation or other sealing of the ducts at further laparotomy. Strictures will usually require dissection of a patent proximal segment of duct and anastomosis, usually by Roux-en-Y to jejunum, or some other reconstructive procedure. Retained stones are managed as discussed on page 301.

In addition to these specific complications, there is a group of patients who present, some time after cholecystectomy, with various symptoms, e.g. flatulence, upper abdominal pain or discomfort, indigestion, fat intolerance. When it has been possible to exclude causes such as retained stone, gastro-oesophageal reflux, peptic ulcer and pancreatitis, the patient tends to be labelled as having the postcholecystectomy syndrome. Attributing the complaints to a long cystic duct stump, sphincter dysfunction, etc. rarely appears convincing, and it is doubtful if a specific syndrome truly exists. Treatment, often not too successful, is along symptomatic lines.

CANCER OF THE GALLBLADDER

The gallbladder is not a common site for cancer, and almost all cancers in this organ are associated with gallstones (Fig. 29.11). However, the incidence of cancer in persons harbouring gallstones is very small—estimated to be much less than 1%. Beyond this, nothing is known about the aetiology of these cancers.

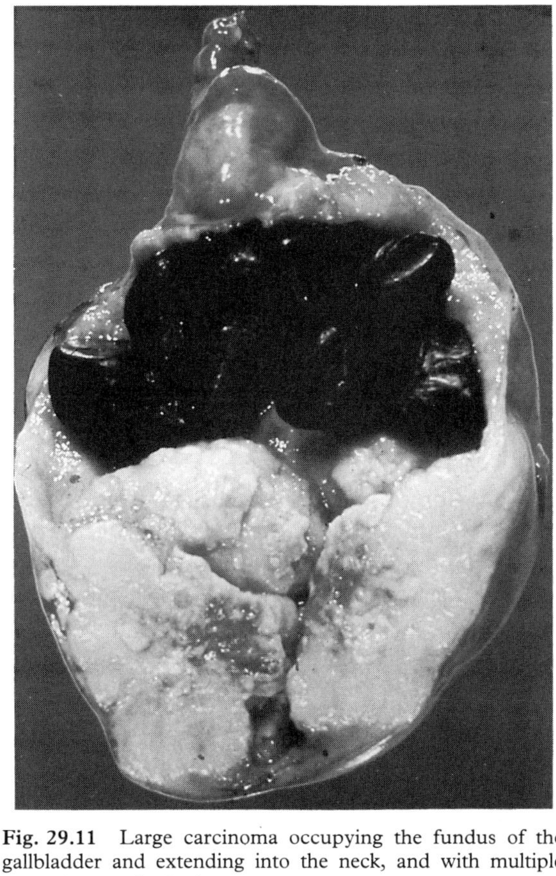

Fig. 29.11 Large carcinoma occupying the fundus of the gallbladder and extending into the neck, and with multiple faceted stones in the lumen.

Pathology

In the early stages, the cancer may appear as a nodule or localized area of induration, or later as a more proliferative growth, occupying the greater part or all of the gallbladder.

Microscopically, most of the tumours are adenocarcinomas, but rarely squamous cell carcinoma may arise in areas of metaplasia, developing as a result of chronic irritation of the mucosa by gallstones.

The tumour spreads by local infiltration to the adjoining part of the liver, and lymphatic spread through the vessels running along the cystic and hepatic ducts may produce secondaries in the glands in the porta hepatis, causing obstructive jaundice. Sometimes the tumour spreads by dissemination throughout the peritoneal cavity. The patient usually succumbs before distant metastases have time to appear.

There are no specific pathognomonic clinical features of carcinoma of the gallbladder. In many cases the diagnosis is established at laparotomy performed for recurrent attacks of acute cholecystitis, gallstones, jaundice, or a mass in the abdomen.

Treatment is unsatisfactory. Cholecystectomy with excision of adjacent liver tissue, including about 3 cm of healthy tissue all round, may be possible. In most cases, however, by the time advice is sought, the disease is too far advanced for any treatment. Best results are obtained when the cancer is reported by the histologist on the examination of a gallbladder removed for an apparently non-malignant condition. The overall 5-year survival is only about 2%.

30. The pancreas

DEVELOPMENT

Dorsal and ventral pancreatic buds develop from the lower part of the foregut in the region of the duodenum during the fourth week of intrauterine life (Fig. 30.1). These buds form the pancreatic ducts around which the pancreatic tissue is laid down and the organ is formed by the fusion of the dorsal and ventral parts. A part of the head and the uncinate process develop from the ventral bud whereas the rest of the gland develops from the dorsal one.

ANATOMY

The pancreas is a pyramid-shaped organ situated in the upper part of the abdomen behind the stomach and the lesser sac, opposite the first and second lumbar vertebrae. It consists of a head portion, which is enclosed in the C-shaped space formed by the first, second and third parts of the duodenum; a body which lies over the vertebrae and in front of the abdominal aorta covering the origin of the coeliac and superior mesenteric arteries, and the tail, which lies in close relation to

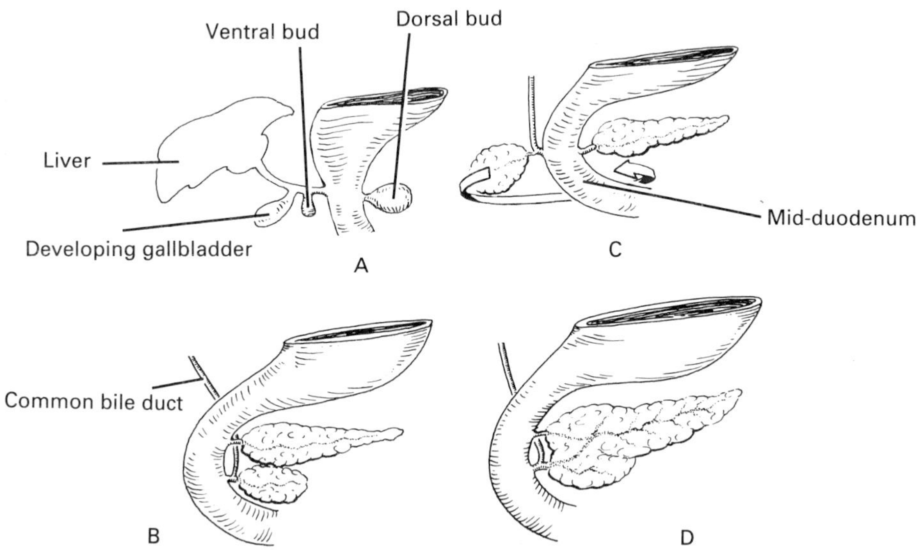

Fig. 30.1 Embryological development of pancreas from two buds arising from the mid-duodenum—a ventral and a dorsal bud. The diagram shows progressive stages of growth and rotation of the ventral bud to fuse with the dorsal one (**A–D**). Normally the fully developed organ drains through the more distally placed duct developed from the ventral bud, but sometimes a portion of the dorsal bud duct also persists, giving an accessory duct.

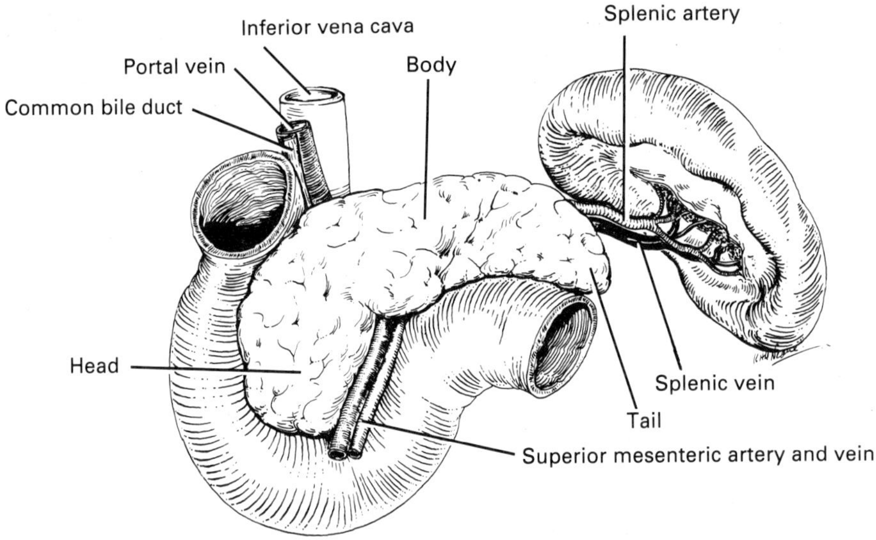

Fig. 30.2 Principal relations of pancreas. The tip of the tail of the pancreas normally lies more snugly in contact with the hilum of the spleen, but is drawn slightly displaced to show the position of the splenic blood vessels.

the hilum of the spleen (Fig. 30.2). The splenic vein forms a posterior relation to the body, and the splenic artery runs along its superior border. The superior mesenteric artery crosses the uncinate process, which is a projection of the head of the pancreas near the third part of the duodenum.

The main pancreatic duct comes to lie very close to the terminal part of the common bile duct, and joins it in the substance of the duodenal wall to form the ampulla of Vater before opening in the duodenum. The opening is guarded by the sphincter of Oddi. The accessory pancreatic duct, when present, opens into the second part of the duodenum about 2.5 cm above the opening of the main duct. The pancreas derives its arterial supply from the splenic, hepatic and superior mesenteric arteries. The veins drain into the splenic, portal and superior mesenteric veins. Lymphatics go to the pyloric, the coeliac and the splenic groups of lymph nodes. Secretomotor fibres are derived from the vagi and the sensory supply comes from the sympathetic via the splanchnic nerves and the coeliac plexus. Scattered throughout the pancreas are its units of endocrine secretions called the islets of Langerhans, which number between 500 000 and 1 000 000.

PHYSIOLOGY

The exocrine secretions of the pancreas constitute the pancreatic juice which is delivered to the intestine through the pancreatic duct. The pancreatic enzymes are trypsinogen, which is activated into trypsin by enteropeptidase secreted by the duodenum, lipase and amylase, which take an important part in the digestion of proteins, fats and carbohydrates respectively. The exocrine secretion of the pancreas is mostly under humoral control, though a minor part of the control is neurally exercised through the branches from the vagi.

The hormonal stimuli are secretin and cholecystokinin (pancreozymin), which are produced in the duodenum in response to food and gastric secretion. The juice secreted in response to secretin is rich in bicarbonate, and that in response to cholecystokinin is rich in the digestive enzymes.

Surgical excision of the pancreas or its destruction by disease results in a profound disturbance in the digestion of protein and fat, whereas carbohydrate digestion is not so greatly affected because of the existence of other saccharolytic enzymes in the small intestine.

Insulin, glucagon and somatostatin are produced

in the pancreatic islets of Langerhans in health. In rare diseases characterized by proliferation or tumour formation of islet cells, various other peptide hormones can be produced, sometimes in very large quantities. The best known of these is the gastrinoma (Zollinger–Ellison disease), which releases large amounts of gastrin into the circulation and manifests itself clinically as a severe and persistent peptic ulcer diathesis.

Insulin, which is secreted by the beta cells of the islets of Langerhans, helps in the utilization of glucose for energy production and for the synthesis of glycogen in the liver and muscles. It is an anabolic hormone and also helps in the synthesis of fatty acids in the liver, proteins in the muscles, and glucose and fatty acids in the adipose tissue. It prevents glycogenolysis, gluconeogenesis and ketogenesis.

Glucagon is secreted by the alpha cells and it causes glycogenolysis in the liver and acts on fats by activating lipase present in both the liver and adipose tissue, producing fatty acids. On the whole glucagon acts as an antagonist to insulin.

Somatostatin is produced by the delta cells of the islets of Langerhans.

CONGENITAL DISORDERS

Congenital diseases of the pancreas are not usually of surgical importance. However, rarely mucoviscidosis (fibrocystic disease) gives rise to meconium ileus on account of the very viscid stools and this may come to surgical attention as one of the causes of neonatal intestinal obstruction. Also rarely duodenal obstruction can be caused by an annular pancreas, in which an encircling mass of pancreatic tissue compresses the second part of the duodenum (Fig. 30.3).

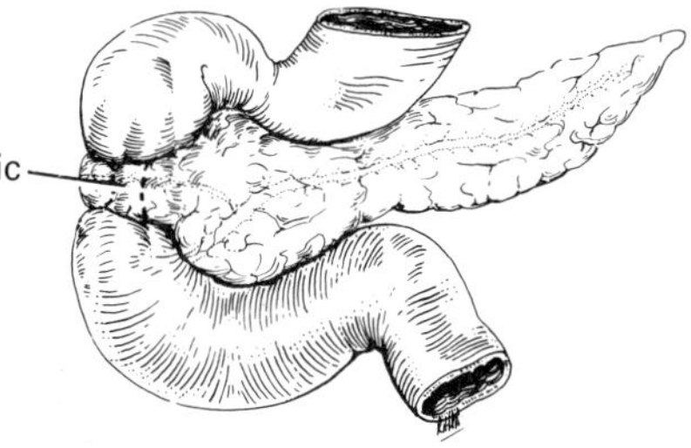

Fig. 30.3 Annular pancreas: a congenital abnormality in which a completely encircling ring of pancreatic tissue is laid down around the mid-duodenum.

INFLAMMATORY DISEASE OF THE PANCREAS

Pancreatitis can present in an acute and/or chronic form. Several clinical courses are possible:

1. An acute attack may resolve completely and the patient may remain healthy and free of further trouble.
2. There may be recurrent acute attacks at intervals; the patient returns to full health between the attacks.
3. With repeated episodes of acute pancreatitis pancreatic function becomes progressively impaired, ending with a chronic pancreatitis picture.
4. The clinical presentation is that of chronic pancreatitis from the start.

ACUTE PANCREATITIS

Acute pancreatitis is a disease of unknown aetiology but apparently increasing frequency in western communities. It is characterized by varying degrees of disruption of the normal structure of the pancreas, and the escape of pancreatic enzymes into the retroperitoneal space and the peritoneal cavity.

Although, as has been stated, the precise aetiological mechanisms initiating the disease are not known, there are significant associated factors in the majority of cases. Biliary disease and high alcohol consumption account for at least 70%, and other less common precipitating conditions include viral infections, e.g. mumps or coxsackie virus hyperparathyroidism, hyperlipidaemia, cancer of the pancreas—especially ampullary—drugs, e.g. steroids, and following operations on the pancreas or other abdominal organs, following blunt or penetrating trauma to the abdomen, or endoscopic retrograde choledochopancreatography (ERCP).

However, in approximately 20% of patients there is no obviously related factor, and these are simply labelled as idiopathic.

With regards to how these associated factors may initiate damage to the pancreas, some may act by blocking segments of the duct system, others by permitting or encouraging reflux of infected or toxic material up the ducts, others by direct chemical damage to duct or acinar cells, and yet others by diminishing the local blood supply to the active exocrine tissues. All hypotheses have some, often indirect, evidence in support of them but the real contribution of these and other mechanisms remains uncertain.

Most of the damage in acute pancreatitis is done by the pancreatic enzymes lipase and trypsin escaping from the acini and ducts into the surrounding tissues. Normally these digestive enzymes are prevented from inflicting damage on the pancreas itself by being aggregated within the cells in zymogen granules; being secreted in an inactive form, e.g. trypsinogen, and requiring activation by enzymes found normally in the small bowel lumen, and as there are several inhibitors of the exocrine enzymes both in the pancreas and the plasma. In acute pancreatitis these protective mechanisms are overcome. It has recently been suggested that the abnormal production or action of enzymes like phospholipase A and elastase may be aetiologically related to the disease.

Pathology

Varying degrees of changes occur in the pancreas. In mild cases there is only oedema of the gland; in more severe ones there is patchy necrosis with extravasation of blood, and in the most extreme cases there is considerable haemorrhage and massive necrosis of the gland.

As a result of the initial damage to the pancreas, further enzymes escape into the surrounding tissues. Trypsinogen is converted into active trypsin by contact with the inflamed tissues, and acts on the walls of small blood vessels, allowing the escape of blood. This phenomenon is seen not only in relation to the pancreas itself but also may rarely occur at a distance, e.g. in subcutaneous vessels in the loin (Grey Turner's sign), or the anterior abdominal wall (Cullen's sign).

Lipase acts on fat in the neighbourhood of the pancreas as well as at a distance in the abdominal cavity and elsewhere. Triglycerides are converted into monoglycerides, which are split into fatty acids and glycerol. Fatty acids combine with calcium to form insoluble soaps. These soaps are deposited on the omentum, the peritoneal surfaces of the viscera and the parietal peritoneum and the deposits are called areas of fat necrosis.

In rare instances, areas of fat necrosis may develop in the bone marrow also. This is due to release of extra lipase into the circulation.

Clinical features

Pain is the leading symptom. It is felt in the epigastrium and from there may spread to the rest of the abdomen. It often radiates to the back. In mild cases, it is usually of gradual onset, increasing to a steady plateau after some time. In severe cases it is often of sudden onset and extreme severity. It is constant and *not* colicky in nature. However, it may on occasions be minimal in a few patients in spite of severe damage to the organ.

Nausea and vomiting are also almost invariable features, though the frequency of vomiting is variable. Often there is more retching than actual vomiting.

The general systemic effects vary from slight tachycardia in mild cases to profound shock in fulminating cases. In the latter the patient sweats, has a low blood pressure and cold extremities. Cyanosis and rapid respiration may also be present.

In mild cases, tenderness in the upper abdomen can usually be elicited by deep and firm palpation and in severe cases there is extreme tenderness and marked muscle rigidity throughout the upper abdomen.

A faint degree of jaundice may appear on the second day. In some cases abdominal distension occurs due to ileus.

It is sometimes difficult to make a diagnosis of acute pancreatitis on clinical grounds alone. However, a single estimation of the serum amylase concentration is usually all that is required to confirm or exclude the condition. The main conditions which usually come into the differential diagnosis are perforated peptic ulcer, biliary colic, high intestinal obstruction, myocardial infarction and leaking aneurysm of the aorta. In most of these the serum amylase may be slightly raised from the normal range of 100–300 to 300–500 iu/dl, but levels in excess of 1000 iu/dl signify acute pancreatitis.

The elevation of the amylase usually starts within 4–6 h of the onset of the attack and after reaching a peak starts to subside in about 48 h. If the patient is not seen until that amount of time has elapsed it may be more helpful to measure the amylase content of the urine, since increased levels persist after the serum concentration has returned to normal. It may also be worth checking urine amylase levels in those in whom the clinical suspicion of acute pancreatitis remains high in spite of apparently normal serum values, as false-negative results may appear in 1–5% of cases.

Another method of using amylase estimations is to compare the clearance of amylase to that of creatinine. Elevation of the ratio of amylase: creatinine clearance above the normal range of 1–3% suggests acute pancreatitis. However, in fulminating cases of acute pancreatitis, renal failure may develop, in which case an accurate estimation may not be possible. In severe cases the serum calcium concentration may fall from the normal level of 9–11 mg/dl to as low as 7 mg/dl. Tetany often develops in such cases. A low serum calcium level is usually of grave significance.

Plain X-ray of the abdomen may show one or two distended loops of small intestine in the upper abdomen, but it is mainly taken to help in the differential diagnosis from perforated peptic ulcer, i.e. to look for free gas under the diaphragm. Occasionally, in spite of all the physical signs and laboratory results it is not possible to rule out perforated peptic ulcer or intestinal obstruction and in such cases the diagnosis is established at laparotomy. However, laparotomy is to be avoided as far as possible, especially in poor-risk patients.

Management

As the cause of the disease is not known, the aims are to give general supportive treatment, alleviate pain, reduce stimulation of the pancreas, and watch carefully for any signs of important organ failure until the episode resolves, usually over the course of several days.

The patient should rest in bed—preferably in hospital—be given potent analgesics, e.g. pethidine, in adequate dosage, given nil by mouth and have continuous gastric aspiration to minimize the release of secretin and cholecystokinin from the duodenum, and should have an intravenous line set up. It is advisable to monitor the haematocrit, haemoglobin level, serum calcium and protein levels, urine output and blood–gases initially, and at regular intervals—daily, or more frequently if clinically indicated.

Various drugs have been advocated in the past, mainly on theoretical grounds that they should decrease the amount of or activity of the exocrine pancreas, e.g. anticholinergics, corticosteroids, the kallikrein inhibitor Trasylol, and glucagon. None, however, has been convincingly beneficial and they are not recommended. Likewise there is little evidence that antibiotics are worthwhile in this disorder. Peritoneal lavage with isotonic fluid may sometimes accelerate clinical improvement, and at times may indeed be a helpful diagnostic procedure.

In moderate and severe cases the loss of fluid and protein in and around the inflamed pancreas and into the peritoneal cavity can be very great indeed, necessitating the infusion of large volumes of crystalloid and/or plasma or dextran. Adequate replacement of lost fluid is the best protection against renal impairment. Blood transfusion may also be required in the grossly haemorrhagic pattern of the disease.

Damage to the lungs may lead to the need for oxygen administration, and a watch should be maintained for cardiac irregularities, consumptive coagulopathy, and frank pleural effusion.

Acute pancreatitis is a serious disease, and although with a high standard of medical care most episodes will gradually resolve, there is still a mortality rate of around 10%. It is possible to give more accurate prediction of risk by scoring for various biochemical and other measurements during the attack (Table 30.1). Generally, alcohol-related acute pancreatitis carries a worse prognosis than other cases.

Once the acute episode has subsided, investigations for biliary disease, i.e. ultrasound and/or cholecystography, are undertaken, and if gallbladder disease is detected, cholecystectomy is advised to diminish the chances of recurrent pancreatitis. This operation is usually performed 1–2 months after the episode. However, some surgeons advocate ultrasound at the earliest opportunity, proceeding to cholecystectomy if gallstones are found during

Table 30.1 Unfavourable prognostic factors in acute pancreatitis

Factor		Unfavourable range
Leukocytosis (white blood cell count)	>	15 000/mm^3
Blood glucose	>	10 mmol/l
Blood urea	>	16 mmol/l
Partial pressure of arterial oxygen	<	60 mmHg
Serum lactate dehydrogenase	>	600 iu/l
Serum GOT/GPT	>	100 u/l
Serum calcium	<	2 mmol/l
Serum albumin	<	32 g/l
Age	>	55 years

If three or more unfavourable factors are present within 48 h of admission, it is judged that the disease is severe, with a mortality risk of about 20%. In those with less than three present (the majority), the mortality risk is nearer to 1%. GOT = Glutamate oxaloacetate transaminase; GPT = glutamic pyruvic transaminase.

the same admission for the acute pancreatitis once the signs and symptoms have settled.

PSEUDOCYST OF THE PANCREAS

This is a collection of fluid in the neighbourhood of the pancreas, usually in the lesser sac. It arises either as a sequel of acute pancreatitis, or as a result of blunt trauma to the organ. It is called a pseudocyst because its walls are made up of fibrous tissue laid down in response to the inflammation, rather than epithelium which would comprise the wall of a true cyst. In the case of injury the cyst may develop within a few days or may not appear till weeks or even months after the injury. Whatever the origin of the cyst, blood and pancreatic secretions collect either in the lesser sac or between its posterior layer and the pancreas. The foramen of Winslow is sealed because of oedema and a localized cyst develops, most commonly in relation to the head of the pancreas. The fluid is usually rich in pancreatic enzymes, though sometimes these may be in an inactivated form or absent altogether.

The cyst usually protrudes between the stomach and the liver, but sometimes it is situated between the stomach and the transverse colon. A cyst of the head of the pancreas may press on the common bile duct giving rise to obstructive jaundice. If it becomes secondarily infected it will be converted into an abscess.

Clinical features

Many smaller cysts remain asymptomatic and spontaneously resolve. Larger ones may cause local upper abdominal discomfort or actual pain, and by displacing the stomach interfere with appetite, eating and digestion. The patient may become aware of fullness or may feel the swelling by pressing with the hand on the abdomen.

If the cyst is of sufficient size to cause symptoms it is usually palpable on clinical examination, and the smooth, even contour is often apparent. Most frequently it occupies part or all of the epigastrium

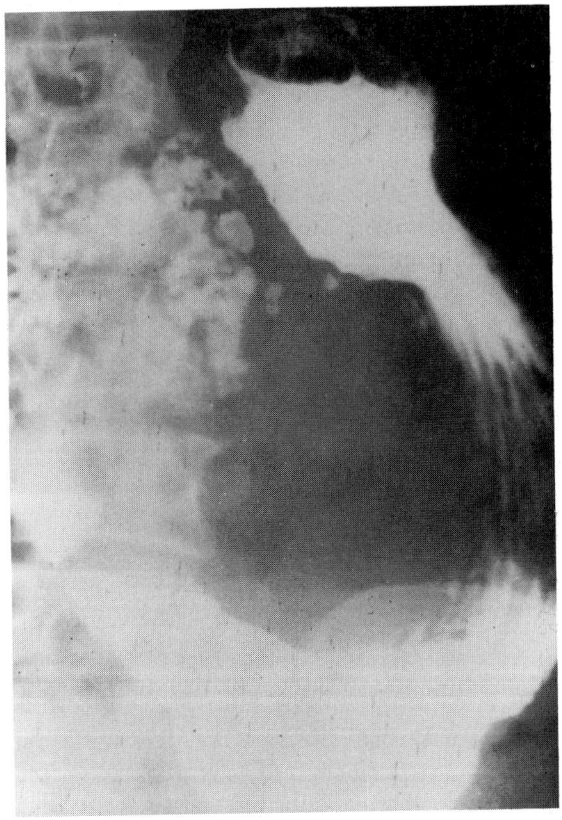

Fig. 30.4 Pancreatic pseudocyst demonstrated by barium meal. There is a large rounded radiotranslucent area with displacement of the stomach shadow anteriorly and to the left. The stomach itself is normal, but stretched. There are also several mainly rounded opacities lying in the upper prevertebral region; these are calcified deposits in and around the pancreas, from previous episodes of acute or chronic pancreatitis.

and the left hypochondrium. Confirmation of the cyst by ultrasound is usually straightforward and rarely is any other investigation required. If barium meal is performed a characteristic rounded indentation of the outline of the stomach is usually seen (Fig. 30.4). Computerized tomography (CT) scanning will also outline the cyst, but it is an unnecessarily expensive method of achieving the objective.

Treatment

Since a proportion of pseudocysts spontaneously disappear, any which are asymptomatic can simply be observed over a few days until it is apparent that resolution is occurring. However, if troublesome symptoms persist or if there are clear signs of further enlargement of the pseudocyst then operation is advisable. It is as well to try to allow 4–6 weeks to elapse before surgery in the hope that a good tough wall will have developed, because it should be strong enough to hold sutures.

The operative procedure of choice is internal drainage of the pseudocyst into the stomach or a segment of small intestine (Fig. 30.5). Cystogastrostomy is accomplished by opening the stomach through its anterior wall, making a circular incision through the combined thickness of the posterior gastric wall and anterior wall of the pseudocyst, evacuating all the contents, and suturing around the circular opening to approximate firmly the two walls. Curiously the cyst, even if large, very rapidly become obliterated and indeed it is difficult to detect the scar in the posterior wall of the stomach.

If an abscess develops, it should be drained like any other abscess.

CHRONIC PANCREATITIS

This disorder, less common than acute pancreatitis, is characterized by significant destruction of the pancreatic tissue and varying degrees of fibrosis. In milder forms the gland may become firmer and rubbery in consistency, but in more severe cases it becomes hard and nodular, and widespread deposits of calcification may be laid down in the areas of parenchymatous destruction. The fibrosis usually also involves the duct system giving rise to distortion, strictures, partially obstructed segments, and the process may also extend to the lower end of the common bile duct, causing obstructive jaundice. Plugs of protein material are often present in these damaged ducts, and indeed intraduct calculi can be formed, further obstructing the ducts. The islets of Langerhans may also be destroyed, and if sufficient of them are lost the patient may become diabetic, though usually in a mild form.

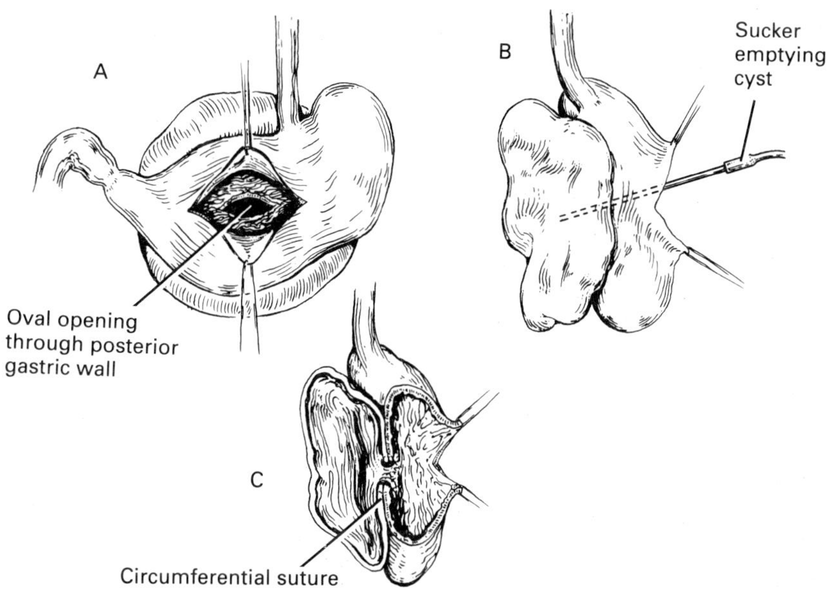

Fig. 30.5 Cystogastrostomy: see text for the steps of the procedure.

The condition may arise as the ultimate outcome of repeated damage by recurrent attacks of acute pancreatitis, but in most cases of chronic pancreatitis there is no clear history of such preceding episodes, and the precise initiating mechanism of the disease remains unknown. Most patients in western countries are men in middle age, and there is a strong aetiological link with excess alcohol consumption and a lesser one with gallstones. In the African and Indian continents there is often an association with malnutrition, and the condition is seen in younger patients.

As the glandular tissue is destroyed there is a deficiency of pancreatic digestive enzymes in the pancreatic juice. The deficiency of lipase greatly impairs the digestion of fat, leading to the excretion of large amounts of fat in the stools. This increase in fat content leads to an increase in both the frequency and bulk of bowel motions, and as a consequence greater loss of colonic bacteria, which mainly consist of protein. This factor, plus the reduction in the output of proteolytic enzymes, is responsible for protein deficiency.

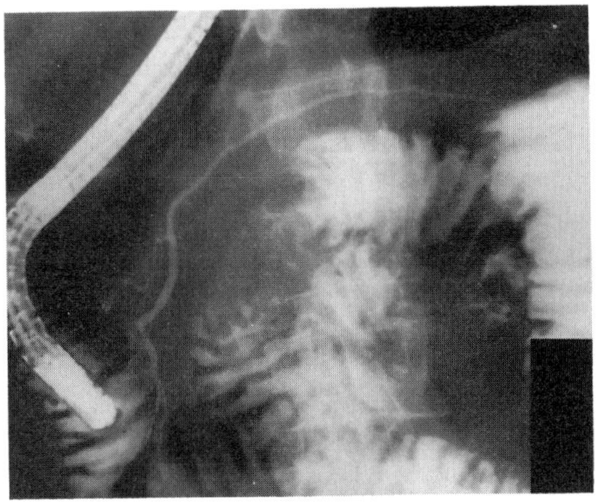

Fig. 30.6 ERCP showing normal outline of pancreatic duct.

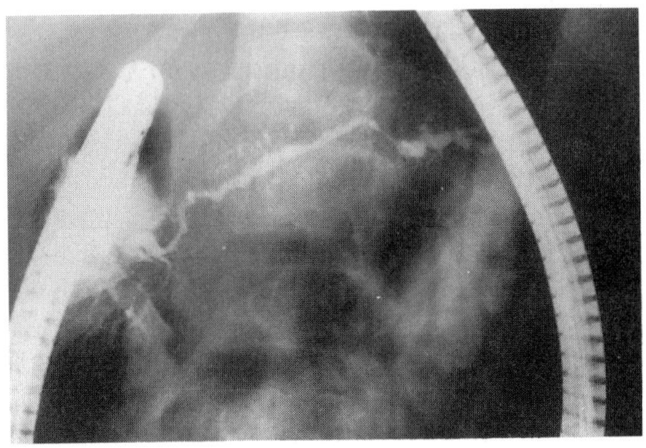

Fig. 30.7 ERCP showing strictures and dilatation of the main pancreatic duct in a patient with chronic pancreatitis.

Clinical features

The main symptoms of chronic pancreatitis are abdominal pain, loss of weight and jaundice. All of these are not present together in all patients. In some, upper abdominal pain radiating to the back may be the predominant feature. In others, jaundice or weight loss with diarrhoea are the main complaints. In still others, all three symptoms may be present.

Abdominal pain is of constant type and many patients get some relief by sitting in bed and leaning forward over a pillow. The pain may be aggravated by eating, so that a disinclination to eating develops. Nearly every patient will have some weight loss, and in some it is striking. It is frequently associated with the clear complaint that the bowel motions have become bulky, pale, offensive, greasy and difficult to flush away in the lavatory.

Confirmation of diagnosis

This is sometimes quite difficult. The objectives of investigations are to show evidence of structural damage to the organ and impairment of exocrine pancreatic function.

Under the first heading, first a straight X-ray of the abdomen may show areas of calcification within the pancreatic substance. If ERCP is available this may permit outlining of the duct system and reveal strictures, dilated segments, absence of tributary ducts and other irregularities (Figs. 30.6 and 30.7).

Under the second heading accurate measurement of the faecal fat loss over a 3–5-day period will give clear evidence of steatorrhoea. Direct estimation of the pancreatic secretion of bicarbonate and digestive enzymes after stimulation by secretin and cholecystokinin may be useful. It does require precise technique and good supervision, preferably in a unit experienced in such measurements. One tube is carefully positioned with its tip in the second part of the duodenum and a second tube, or the second limb of a double-lumen tube, is placed to aspirate the stomach contents, so that it does not interfere with the pancreatic juice collections. A variety of other provocation tests have been described, and each has its advocates. However, the degree of diagnostic discrimination is not high.

If glycosuria is present and therefore significant damage to the islets of Langerhans is suspected, it will be advisable to measure fasting blood sugar levels and perhaps also perform a glucose tolerance test.

Management

Medical

All patients are advised to avoid alcohol completely. As far as diet is concerned encouragement is given to take plenty of carbohydrate and protein, but to restrict fat intake to between 80 and 100 g/day, and to avoid bulky meals. Pancreatic enzyme preparations are commercially available and the addition of these during meals may improve digestion and absorption. Since these extracts are vulnerable to be broken down and inactivated by acid gastric juice, they are most effective if taken after the first few mouthfuls of the meal.

Pain relief will usually require one of the more potent analgesics, but there is a real risk of inducing addiction if the opiates are prescribed. On occasions, however, no less powerful agent appears to suffice. One approach to pain relief which is worth considering if it is difficult to achieve satisfactory relief by oral medication is a coeliac plexus block.

Surgical

The main indication for considering operative intervention is relief of intractable pain, but the operation will be helpful only if it achieves satisfactory drainage of blocked ducts or resects the segment responsible for the pain. If neither of these objectives is attainable the patient will undergo an exploratory laparotomy and perhaps some unnecessary empirical procedure. Good demonstration of the pancreatic and ductal anatomy is therefore of prime importance before or during operation, and a logical procedure is then based on these findings.

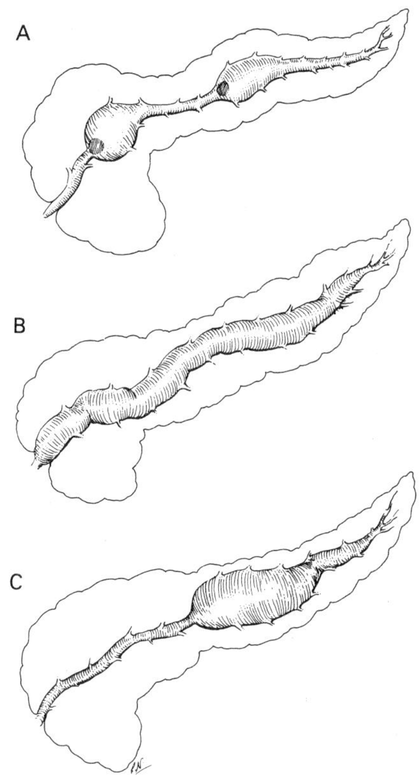

Fig. 30.8 Various patterns of distortion of the pancreatic duct as a result of pancreatitis. (**A**) Two separate strictures and segments of proximal dilatation; (**B**) dilatation of the entire length of the main duct on account of a single stricture at the ampullary region; (**C**) dilatation only of the body and tail segments.

Several different approaches to drainage of the damaged duct system are available, and choice of a particular method depends on the site and number of the strictures (Fig. 30.8). With a single lesion near to the ampullary end of the main duct, amputation of the tail of the pancreas and anastomosis of the severed body of the organ to a Roux-en-Y loop of jejunum may be appropriate, but when there are multiple strictures and segments of obstructed dilated ducts, it may be necessary to open up the anterior wall of the entire length of the main duct by filletting the gland, and making a longitudinal anastomosis between this opened-out duct and the opened-out end of a Roux-en-Y loop (Fig. 30.9).

If none of the duct drainage procedures is feasible, a further radical possibility is resection of all but a small rim of the head of the pancreas within the concavity of the duodenum (Fig. 30.10). The

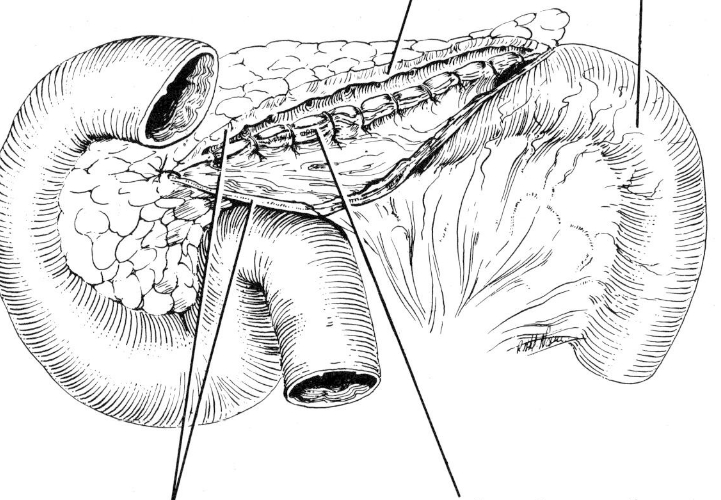

Fig. 30.9 Almost the complete length of dilated pancreatic duct is split anteriorly and laid open. The flap of a Roux-en-Y loop of jejunum is prepared and shaped to a suitable length and the edges sutured snugly to the lower and upper edges of the divided pancreatic duct, or more correctly, to the divided edge of the pancreatic incision.

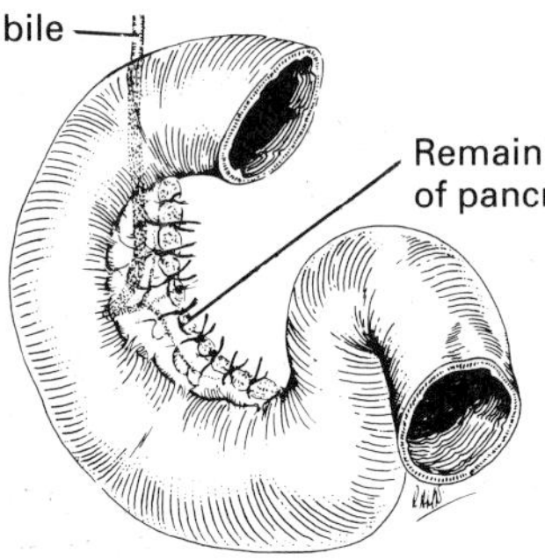

Fig. 30.10 Subtotal pancreatectomy for chronic pancreatitis. All of the pancreas apart from a small rim in the concavity of the duodenum has been excised.

retention of even the smallest crescent of pancreatic tissue may be sufficient to prevent frank deficiency and malabsorption, though this of course depends on how badly the residual glandular tissue is affected.

Any benefit obtained from these surgical procedures can be completely abolished if the patient continues to drink alcohol, and lifelong abstinence from this harmful agent is essential.

TUMOURS OF THE PANCREAS

The majority arise from epithelial exocrine glandular or ductal tissue, but rarely endocrine-producing tumours may arise from the islet cells. Benign neoplasms, adenomas or cystadenomas are rare, seldom cause symptoms, and if they present clinically may require removal either by enucleation with the capsule, or local resection of the portion of pancreas from which it arises.

Clinically the most important and frequently encountered tumour of the pancreas is adenocarcinoma.

Adenocarcinoma of the pancreas

Although this is still less common than cancers in other parts of the alimentary tract, e.g. stomach and colon, there are indications that it is increasing in incidence in many western countries. It is commoner in men, particularly in the over-55 age group, and there may be an association with tobacco-smoking and excessive drinking of coffee.

Most often the tumour arises in the head of the pancreas, but this may be partly the simple consequence of there being a greater amount of glandular tissue in this part of the organ. The malignant process soon involves the neighbouring structures, e.g. stomach or duodenum, and also spreads to the local lymphatics and via the blood to the liver and eventually to many other tissues and organs throughout the body. Malignant ascites not infrequently occurs. If the tumour arises close to the ampulla of Vater it may at a relatively early stage occlude the lower end of the common bile duct, causing obstructive jaundice. Since this usually leads promptly to seeking medical advice, and appropriate investigation, there may be a somewhat greater chance of diagnosing the tumour when it is still small and localized enough to resect with some hope of cure. However, in the majority of cases of adenocarcinoma of the pancreas, by the time symptoms develop and the diagnosis is confirmed there is no realistic prospect of ridding the patient of the disease.

Clinical features

In the absence of obstruction to the common bile duct, the initial symptoms tend to be vague and non-specific. There is often some upper abdominal discomfort, or even pain, sometimes radiating to the back, and almost invariably some weight loss, and perhaps some signs suggesting pancreatic insufficiency, e.g. bulky fatty stools. The onset of mild diabetes in this age group should alert one to this possible diagnosis, as should the development of either single or recurrent episodes of superficial thrombophlebitis (thrombophlebitis migrans).

The obstructive jaundice which occurs when the common bile duct is involved is characteristically steadily progressive in depth, the motions becoming increasingly pale and the urine increasingly dark with the passage of time. These symptoms are usually accompanied by intense itching. Occasionally, however, there may be a temporary diminution in the severity of the jaundice when the tumour is at the ampulla and a small necrotic portion separates and allows the temporary escape of some of the retained bile.

On examination in the absence of jaundice, there may be no obvious physical signs. On the other hand there may be clear evidence of weight loss, and either tenderness or a palpable mass in the epigastrium. Search should be made for hepatomegaly due to secondary deposits or ascites. It is also worthwhile performing a rectal examination to determine whether there are palpable secondaries in the pelvic pouch. In the jaundiced patient the gallbladder may be palpable, in keeping with the oft-quoted Courvoisier's law, but this sign is not totally reliable.

Investigations

Procedures to outline the pancreas for irregularities, e.g. ultrasound and CT scanning, may be helpful but usually do not give accurate identification of small, hopefully operable tumours. Where, however, a mass is located, it may even be possible to obtain material for histological examination by guiding a fine aspirating needle into the area under scanning control. More detailed information can usually be obtained at ERCP (Fig. 30.11). By this examination ampullary tumours may be biopsied, juice may be obtained from the pancreatic duct for cytological examination, and contrast outlining of the duct system can be performed.

In the past barium meal outlining of the stomach and duodenum has been advocated to detect deformity caused by the pancreatic tumour, but this is an outmoded means of investigation which is

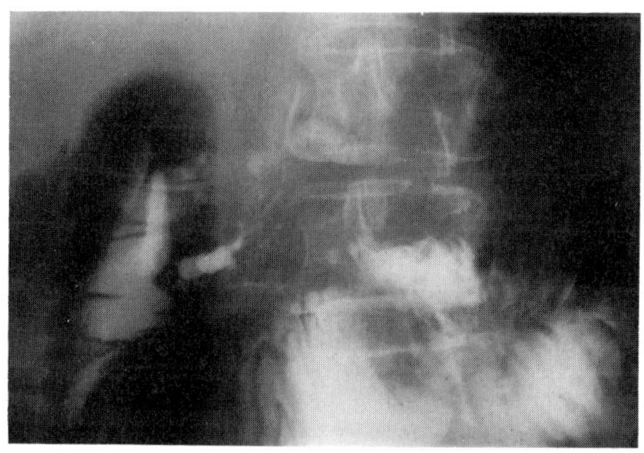

Fig. 30.11 ERCP showing complete blockage of the pancreatic duct at the site of an adenocarcinoma.

only really capable of detecting large, grossly invasive lesions.

In the presence of obstructive jaundice percutaneous transhepatic cholangiography may visualize the exact site of bile duct blockage.

Treatment

This is on the whole unsatisfactory and since there is as yet no sign of a significant response to non-surgical measures, the only real hope at present is from resection. However, as mentioned, by the time the patient seeks advice the growth is usually inoperable. In the very few cases where the tumour is confined to the head of the pancreas, is well lateral to the portal vein and not already clearly metastasized to other sites, pancreaticoduodenectomy (Whipple's procedure) can be performed (Figs 30.12 and 30.13). This involves removal of the entire head of the pancreas, the distal stomach, all the duodenum, and a few centimetres of proximal jejunum, and the lower end of the common bile duct. In turn the bile duct, the pancreatic remnant and the residual stomach are anastomosed to the divided jejunal segment. This is a major procedure, with multiple anastomoses subject to the danger of leakage, and carries a relatively high mortality and morbidity. It has a significantly better chance of success when done for truly ampullary lesions, rather than for tumours arising more within the substance of the head of the pancreas.

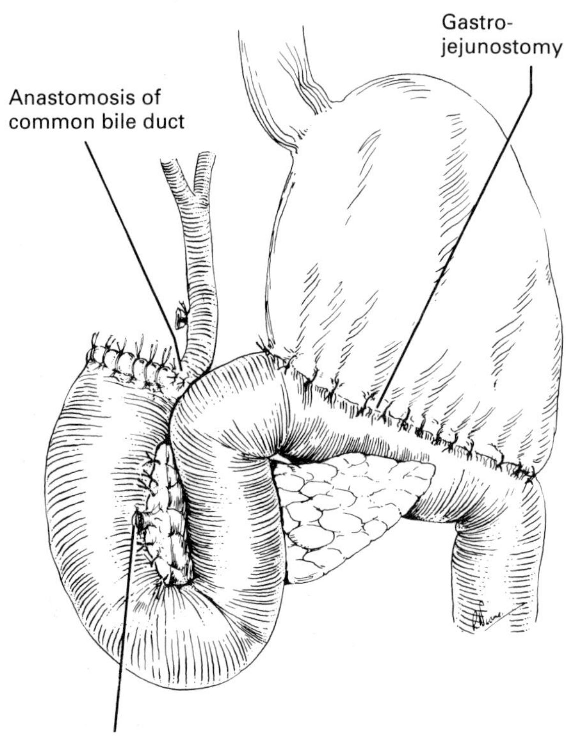

Fig. 30.12 Whipple's procedure: the head of the pancreas, the distal portion of the stomach, the entire duodenum, proximal few centimetres of jejunum, and the lower end of the common bile duct have been removed en bloc. Continuity has been restored by anastomosing the cut end of the common bile duct to the narrowed end of the jejunum, the severed pancreas to the side of this segment a few centimetres distally, with precise end-to-side anastomosis of the pancreatic duct to jejunal mucosa, and the proximal gastric remnant is anastomosed end-to-side to the jejunal loop still further distally.

Only too often either nothing useful or at best only palliative measures can be done at operation in this disease. Obstructive jaundice can be relieved either by performing a cholecystojejunostomy (Fig. 30.14), if the gallbladder is distended but otherwise apparently healthy, or preferably a choledochojejunostomy (Fig. 30.15). If duodenal obstruction by tumour seems imminent some surgeons also advocate the creation of a gastrojejunostomy. Unfortunately the prognosis in cancer of the pancreas is very poor indeed, and during terminal care the severity of pain caused by eroding tumour may justify the neurosurgical division of pain-carrying nerves or spinal tracts.

Endocrine-secreting tumours

Although these are rare they provoke great interest. The least uncommon are insulinomas arising from the B-cells and gastrinomas from the G cells of the islets of Langerhans. Rarest of all are various lesions producing glucagon and other polypeptides, such as vasoactive intestinal peptide.

Insulinoma

In all, 90% of these tumours are benign and although occasionally they are very small, the majority are single adenomas about 1–3 cm in diameter. When multiple they may be accompanied by functioning tumours in other organs—they form part of a multiple endocrine neoplasia picture.

The clinical manifestations result from the inappropriate high levels of circulating insulin, pro-

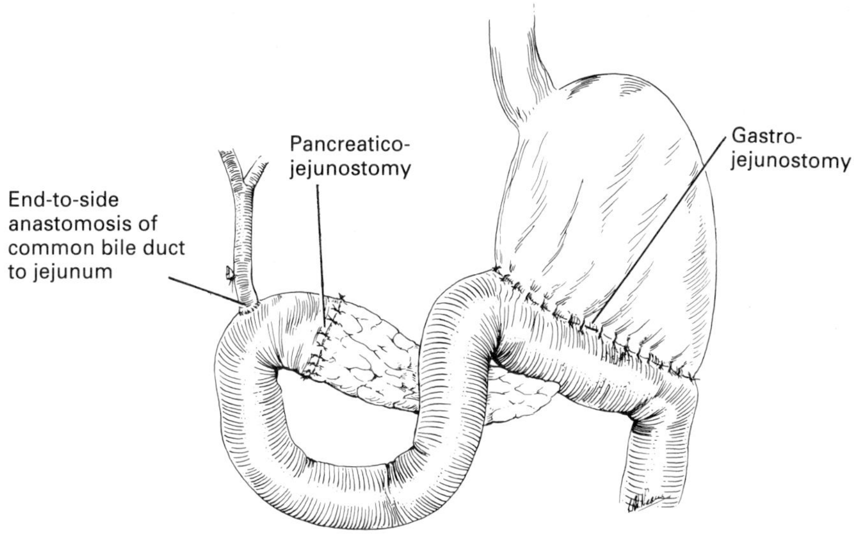

Fig. 30.13 Whipple's procedure, with alternative reconstructions. In this instance the severed end of the pancreas is anastomosed, capsule to jejunal edge, with no need to anastomose the actual pancreatic duct. The common bile duct is joined end-to-side to the jejunum distal to the pancreaticojejunostomy, and a gastrojejunostomy is performed as in the other procedure.

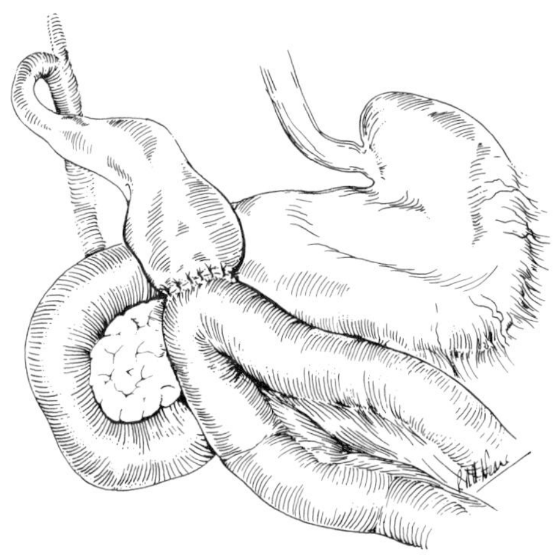

Fig. 30.14 Palliative cholecystojejunostomy to relieve jaundice when the tumour is not resectable. A simple side-to-side anastomosis is made between the fundus of the previously distended gallbladder and a convenient loop of proximal jejunum. If there is a possibility of obstruction of the duodenum by the tumour, it is wise also to add a gastrojejunostomy.

ducing hypoglycaemic symptoms. These are often episodic, and include at first sweating, hunger, palpitations and minor mood changes. When more severe there may be profound psychological disturbance, tremor, even epileptiform seizures and loss of consciousness. On recovery from an episode

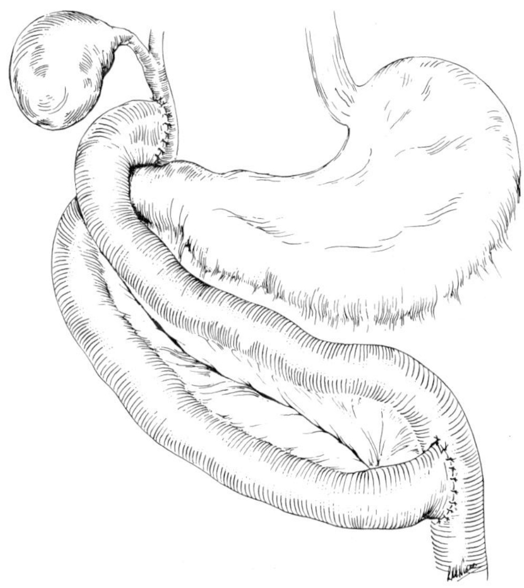

Fig. 30.15 Palliative choledochojejunostomy. An anastomosis is made either, as shown in this diagram, between the anterior wall of the common bile duct, or between the proximal end of the divided duct and the end of a long Roux-en-Y jejunal loop. This is preferable to a simple loop of jejunum: the chance of regurgitation of infected material into the bile ducts, and consequent cholangitis, is greatly reduced.

memory of the events may be lost. At first the patient may discover that eating or drinking sweet liquids will improve the symptoms, and if recourse to this is taken frequently there may be noticeable weight gain.

The diagnosis is often made quite late in the course of the disease, mainly because of the delay in considering the possibility when faced with predominantly psychological symptoms.

Confirmation comes from the finding of a low fasting blood sugar concentration—below 2.2 mmol/l—and the direct detection of elevated insulin levels in the blood, by radioimmunoassay. Preferably several measurements should be made at intervals during a 12 h fast.

Attempts to localize the tumour by ultrasound or CT scanning are usually unsuccessful in view of the relatively small size of most adenomas.

The treatment is surgical excision of the insulinoma. At laparotomy the pancreas is mobilized and thoroughly explored by inspection and palpation. If a discrete tumour is identified it is locally excised. If, however, no localized lesion is discovered at operation selective sampling of the veins draining different segments of the pancreas is advisable to determine where the elevated insulin levels are arising from. The previous practice of blindly resecting the tail and part of the body of the pancreas is not advised, since this has only about 50% chance of removing the responsible lesion.

Excision of a solitary insulinoma will completely cure the condition.

Gastrinoma

This rare tumour is associated with intractable peptic ulceration due to secretion of a gastrin-like hormone which causes hyperacidity and an enormous increase in the volume of the gastric juice. Most of the tumours are situated in the tail of the pancreas and nearly half are malignant. Occasionally, the tumour is situated not in the pancreas but in the neighbouring retroperitoneal tissues or in the wall of duodenum.

Clinically, the tumour gives rise to Zollinger–Ellison syndrome, which is characterized by an enormous increase in the volume and acidity of the gastric juice, resulting in severe peptic ulceration and diarrhoea. Sometimes a benign or malignant tumour or hyperplasia of other endocrine glands like the parathyroid, pituitary, or adrenal cortex may also be present, in which case it is regarded as part of a multiple endocrine neoplasia.

Suspicion of the syndrome is aroused in all cases of repeated peptic ulceration in spite of what should be effective medical and surgical treatment.

The diagnosis is confirmed by finding grossly elevated levels of gastrin in fasting serum. Rarely a provocation test with secretin or calcium will be required to stimulate a further gastrin release. Again ultrasound or CT scanning may help to localize the tumour or several tumours.

In the past the only effective way of dealing with this disorder was excision of the tumour if it was single and total gastrectomy to prevent life-threatening complications of the peptic ulcers. Nowadays many gastrinoma patients can be controlled for many years by prolonged large doses of antisecretory drugs such as H_2-receptor antagonists or proton pump inhibitors, e.g. omeprazole. When surgery is required, a less radical acid-reducing procedure plus continued antisecretory drugs may be sufficient. Occasionally in the most severe instances, however, total gastrectomy may be needed as the only effective way of preventing recurrent ulceration, bleeding or perforation. The postoperative course and outlook when total gastrectomy is performed in this situation are much better than when the procedure is done for carcinoma of the stomach.

31. The liver

DEVELOPMENT

The liver develops from the cranial part of a ventral diverticulum of the foregut which grows into the mesoderm of the septum transversum. The mesoderm gives rise to the capsule of the liver, its ligaments, and the Kupffer cells which belong to the reticuloendothelial system.

ANATOMY

The liver is the largest solid organ in the body, occupying the major part of the right hypochondrium, the upper part of the epigastrium and a small part of the left hypochondrium. In adults, only the part in the epigastrium has its lower edge normally below the costal margin; the rest is covered by the thoracic cage and not able to be palpated. Even although the central part does project a small amount below the margin, the tone of the overlying rectus abdominis muscles makes it virtually impossible to feel the lower edge at this site normally. In the newborn, however, the lower edge of the liver is palpable.

The liver consists of right and left main lobes, the division corresponding to a line passing vertically through the gallbladder fossa (Fig. 31.1). The caudate lobe on the posterior surface to the left of the inferior vena cava and the quadrate lobe on the posteroinferior surface to the left of the gallbladder and below the porta hepatis belong to the left lobe of the liver. Further subdivision into eight segments is based on the distribution of the branches of the left and right hepatic arteries, portal veins and hepatic ducts.

The portal vein carries two-thirds of the blood supply to the liver, and the hepatic artery the remaining one-third. The smallest branches of the two drain their blood into liver spaces called the sinusoids, where the two streams mix. The sinusoids are drained in turn by the tributaries of the hepatic veins which carry the blood to the inferior vena cava. The hepatic veins are arranged in two groups—the upper, comprising two or three large veins, and the lower, consisting of smaller veins numbering from six to 20.

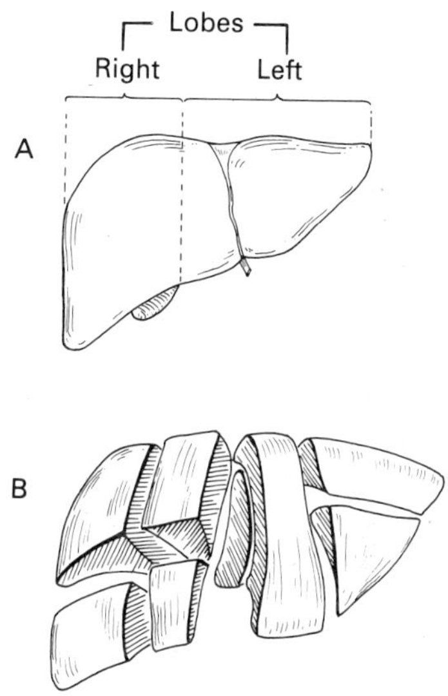

Fig. 31.1 Anatomical subdivision into (**A**) right and left main lobes, and (**B**) eight segments: see text.

Lymphatics of the liver mostly drain into the nodes in the porta hepatis. The porta hepatis is the hilum of the liver, situated on its posteroinferior aspect, enclosed between two layers of the peritoneum derived from the upper part of the lesser omentum. It transmits the hepatic ducts, the hepatic artery and its branches and the portal vein and its branches, situated in that order from before backwards, together with lymphatics and nerves. A number of lymph nodes are situated within the porta hepatis.

The nerves are derived from both the vagus (parasympathetic) and the coeliac plexus (sympathetic).

PHYSIOLOGY

The liver serves as a store-house for glycogen, which is a ready source of energy; it plays an important part in the metabolism of protein, carbohydrates and fats; it is the centre for the production of enzymes and for detoxication of endogenous and exogenous substances; it is the source of bile which plays an important role in the digestion and absorption of fats, and through which the products of haemoglobin metabolism are excreted.

The liver also produces fibrinogen, prothrombin and other factors responsible for blood coagulation. Of these, factors II, VII, IX and X are dependent on the availability of vitamin K, a fat-soluble vitamin. When fat absorption is grossly impaired due to the absence of bile salts in the intestine in obstructive jaundice, lack of absorbed vitamin K thus causes a haemorrhagic tendency.

The liver is the only site for the formation of albumin and therefore the albumin concentration in the blood tends to fall in extensive liver damage.

Many enzymes are formed in the liver. Alkaline phosphatase, which is predominantly of ductal origin, passes from the liver into the intestine via the bile. In obstructive jaundice this flow is interrupted with the result that the enzyme spills over into the blood in larger quantities than normal. Gross elevation of the serum alkaline phosphatase concentration is therefore a sign of duct obstruction.

Transamination signifies the transfer of amino radicals from amino acids to other compounds. Enzymes responsible for this process are called transaminases. The one which helps in the amination of oxaloacetic acid from glutamic acid is called glutamic oxaloacetic transaminase (GOT), and the transaminase which helps in the amination of pyruvic acid is called glutamic pyruvic transaminase (GPT). When estimated in the serum these enzymes are expressed as SGOT and SGPT. The normal values are SGOT 5–17 u; SGPT 4–13 u. Both are intercellular enzymes and are found in many tissues as well as the liver, e.g. the heart, kidneys and skeletal muscles. SGPT, however, occurs mainly in the liver and a rise in its value is pathognomonic of liver damage.

Detoxication is carried out by conjugation, destructive oxidation, or a combination of the two processes. In extensive liver diseases the process of detoxication becomes very much diminished and several hormones which are normally detoxified in the liver remain in the system in excess of their normal values. Thus, the level of serum oestrogen increases in cirrhosis of liver, and may give rise to gynaecomastia. Similarly, the aldosterone level may also increase; this is probably a contributory factor in the development of ascites in cirrhosis of liver due to retention of sodium and water.

DISORDERS OF THE LIVER

Liver abscess, hydatid cyst, portal hypertension and neoplasms of the liver are the main liver disorders of surgical importance and this large friable, vascular organ is also prone to injury in both penetrating and blunt abdominal trauma. Hydatid cyst is discussed in Chapter 16. The other conditions will be considered here.

Liver abscess

Two types of abscess are encountered in the liver: the first specific due to infestation with *Entamoeba histolytica*, and the second from invasion by pyogenic organisms, reaching the liver substance by the biliary ducts (ascending cholangitis), the portal vein from abdominal sepsis, or via the hepatic artery from an infective process elsewhere in the body.

Amoebic liver abscess

Entamoeba histolytica reaches the liver via the portal vein from lesions in the large intestine. The

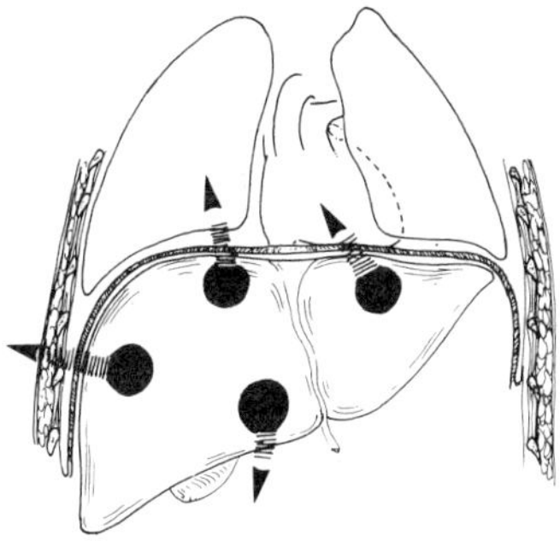

Fig. 31.2 Amoebic abscess: various routes of extension to and through neighbouring tissues: see text.

right lobe of the liver is most often affected. In the majority of cases there is only one abscess, but occasionally there may be multiple abscesses.

The parasite causes destruction of the liver tissue, and the surrounding areas of inflammatory response (Fig. 31.2). The involved part may become adherent to the diaphragm or to other abdominal viscera, or to the parietes. The abscess, which is most often situated in the superior part of the right lobe, may cause secondary inflammation of the pleura, giving rise to a pleural effusion. It may burst into the pleural cavity, thereby producing empyema. Sometimes the abscess may penetrate even into the lung and the pus may be expectorated through the bronchial tree. Very rarely, it may burst into the pericardium, causing cardiac tamponade, or more commonly it may burst into the peritoneal cavity, producing peritonitis. Other possibilities include rupture into the colon or to the skin surface.

In the early stages of infestation, spontaneous resolution may sometimes occur. Alternatively, fibrosis of the walls of the abscess cavity may isolate it from the rest of the liver and no harmful effects are produced over a period of many years. The pus is usually of chocolate colour due to a mixture of dead liver cells and both white and red blood cells. It may also have a greenish tinge due to the presence of bile pigments. The abscess may furthermore become secondarily infected with pyogenic bacteria. Toxins are liberated from the dead tissue, giving rise to toxaemia.

Clinical features

Men are affected more often than women. Though the abscess develops far more frequently in tropical countries, where infestation with *E. histolytica* is common, the disease is not unknown among the people of Europe and the USA.

General symptoms and signs are more prominent than local ones. Loss of appetite and weight and fever are common, and a dull pain in the right upper abdomen or lower chest is felt. It is usually constant and becomes worse on movement. Sometimes it radiates to the right shoulder.

On examination, the patient is generally anaemic and has a peculiar earthy complexion. There may be tenderness in the right upper abdomen or lower chest. Enlargement of the liver may be felt on abdominal examination, but more commonly the enlargement is upwards, and is detected by percussion of the chest. On auscultation, crepitations and rhonchi may be heard over the base of the right lung.

X-ray of the chest may show elevation of the right dome of the diaphragm, immobility of the dome, and pleural effusion.

Stool examination is of value only in persons living away from the tropics. In such persons, in the presence of the signs and symptoms described above, if *E. histolytica* can be demonstrated in the stool, a confident diagnosis of amoebic liver abscess can be made. On the other hand, a negative stool report does not rule out the possibility of amoebic abscess. In the tropics, amoebiasis is so endemic that a positive stool report is of little value in arriving at a diagnosis.

Management

Where amoebiasis is confirmed by stool examination, but local signs and symptoms in the liver region are absent, antiamoebic treatment is given with 100 mg metronidazole three times daily for 10 days. Alternatively, chloroquine is given in a dose of 600 mg/day for two days, to be followed by 300 mg/day for 12 days. In early cases, these measures are curative.

If local signs are present, the abscess is aspirated under local anaesthesia in the operating theatre, using a wide-bore needle. All the pus is evacuated and a swab is sent for culture and sensitivity test. Antiamoebic treatment is continued. Broad-spectrum antibiotics like Terramycin or Chloromycetin 250 mg four times daily may be prescribed to combat secondary infection. The antibiotics may be changed according to the sensitivity report.

In cases where exploration with a needle is not successful, or if the abscess has burst into the peritoneal cavity, laparotomy is required. In the former case, the liver is re-explored under direct vision with a wide-bore needle, and the pus is aspirated completely. In the event of peritonitis, thorough peritoneal toilet is carried out, and all pus from the liver abscess is removed.

The insertion of a drainage tube is discouraged by some surgeons, as it may lead to severe amoebiasis of the skin, which is a serious complication and very difficult to treat. In the opinion of others the adequate drainage of the liver abscess is more important than the risk of skin complications, which may have been exaggerated.

Pyogenic liver abscess

A pyogenic abscess develops in the liver as a result of infection reaching it from a septic focus usually within the abdomen, e.g. appendicitis, cholecystitis or diverticulitis. Occasionally the infection is blood-borne, from a more distant site. The most common causative organism is *Escherichia coli.*

The abscess may be single or multiple and the condition in which multiple abscesses develop in the liver is called portal pyaemia or pylephlebitis. It is thought that an infected thrombus becomes detached from a vein draining the primary infected focus, and this embolus becomes fragmented and lodges in various parts of the liver, giving rise to multiple small abscesses.

Multiple abscesses may also develop in the liver as a result of inflammation of the biliary apparatus, i.e. as a complication of cholangitis. Most often these abscesses are associated with bile duct obstruction, usually due to stones, but sometimes to tumour. These are called cholangitic abscesses.

Clinical features

In pylephlebitis there is usually a history of acute appendicitis, diverticulitis, acute cholecystitis or other intra-abdominal infection. General signs and symptoms are again usually more prominent than local ones. High fever, chill and rigors are the chief symptoms. Sometimes there is diarrhoea also. On examination, there is slight jaundice with a palpable, tender liver and ascites may be present.

Management

The primary focus of infection should be treated along accepted lines. When an abscess is suspected on clinical grounds useful information can be gained by either ultrasound or computerized tomography scanning. Either may give precise localization and dimensions of any collections. Whereas multiple small abscesses may resolve under treatment with antibiotics alone, solitary ones and large ones, whether solitary or multiple, are better drained to avoid further spread and fatal septicaemia. Blood samples are sent for culture and sensitivity test, and a broad-spectrum antibiotic like tetracycline is started pending the sensitivity report. This is given parenterally till the toxaemia is brought under control. Later on the drug can be given orally and continued for 10 days after the disappearance of all signs and symptoms. In very ill patients, blood transfusion may be needed.

Drainage may be achieved either by guiding a fine catheter into the abscess cavity under direct ultrasound scanning control and leaving it in place—repeated checking can be performed at intervals to ensure that complete emptying is obtained—or by open operation and the insertion of a wide-base drainage tube, which is then brought out through the abdominal wall. The adequacy of drainage can then be checked by repeated X-ray after the gentle injection of a suitable contrast medium along the drainage tube.

Portal hypertension

Portal hypertension is the term used to describe a state of increased pressure in the portal vein and its tributaries, usually due to obstruction to the flow of portal blood. The obstruction may be posthepatic, hepatic or prehepatic. In the posthepatic variety, which is the least common, there is an impediment to the flow of blood from the hepatic veins to the inferior vena cava. This occurs in

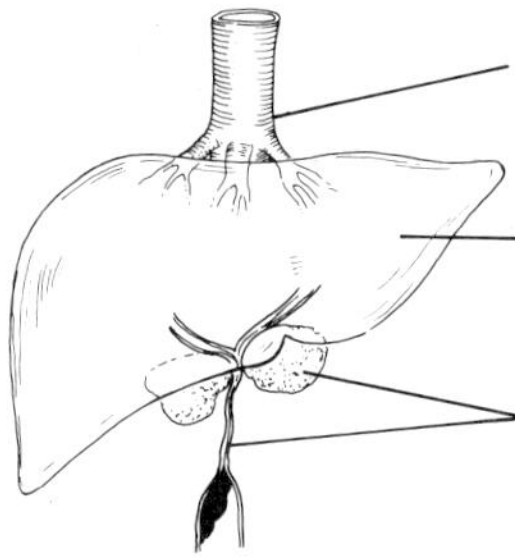

Fig. 31.3 Various causes of portal hypertension: see text.

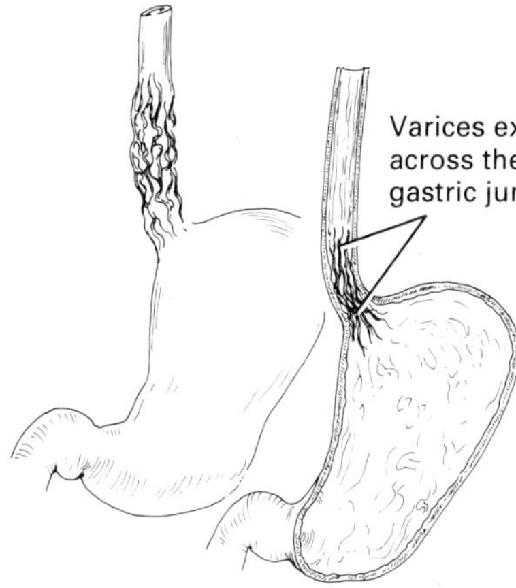

Fig. 31.4 Oesophageal varices: the veins on both the outer and inner aspects of the oesophageal wall become grossly dilated, tortuous and thin-walled. Dangerous bleeding occurs when one or more of the luminal veins ruptures—most often at the lower end, near the oesophagogastric junction—or even in the most proximal part of the gastric fundus.

constrictive pericarditis, tricuspid incompetence, congenital occlusion or thrombosis of the hepatic veins, and pressure of neoplastic tissues on the hepatic veins or inferior vena cava.

Hepatic obstruction is most commonly due to cirrhosis of the liver and, in endemic areas, to schistosomiasis.

Prehepatic obstruction may be due to congenital abnormalities of the portal vein, the most common variety of which is replacement by a cavernous plexus of veins; thrombosis of the portal vein, e.g. from umbilical sepsis in infants, or in portal pyaemia, or pressure by diseased lymph nodes in the porta hepatis.

As a result of the portal hypertension, communications between the portal and systemic circulations which are normally present but remain insignificant enlarge and indeed some become quite engorged. There are four sites at which this venous communication exists: behind and around the retroperitoneal viscera; around the umbilicus; in the anal canal, and at the lower end of the oesophagus and oesophagogastric junction (Fig. 31.4). The latter are the most dangerous as they often become varicose and bleed easily and dramatically.

Engorgement of the veins round the umbilicus, described as caput medusa, is rarely found clinically but if present is a strong pointer to the disorder.

Although theoretically one might expect haemorrhoids to be a frequent manifestation of the portal hypertension picture, they are in fact very rarely encountered as a problem in the syndrome.

The spleen becomes congested and enlarged and hypersplenism develops in many patients, giving rise to pancytopenia, i.e. anaemia due to haemolysis, neutropenia and thrombocytopenia.

There are also changes in the structure of the walls of the portal vein and its tributaries, including irregularity of the intima, and thrombosis occurs in many cases due to the slowing of the circulation.

Damage to the liver cells occurs if the obstruction is postsinusoidal. In prehepatic portal hypertension, liver functions should be normal, and if the hypertension is relieved, the patient can expect to lead a normal life. In cirrhosis of the liver, on the other hand, there is both pre- and postsinusoidal venous obstruction due to fibrosis and pressure of the regenerated liver cells. Hence in these cases, the prognosis should be guarded.

Ascites is a common feature of portal hypertension associated with cirrhosis of the liver (Fig. 31.5). Many factors are thought to contribute towards its development. Firstly, there is engorgement of the lymphatics on the surface of the liver and in its ligaments. Lymph escapes from these vessels. Secondly, if there is gross damage to the liver, hypoalbuminaemia develops, as the liver is the only site for the manufacture of albumin. This leads to a fall in the colloid osmotic pressure of the capillaries, and this is a contributory factor to the escape of fluid into the interstitial spaces throughout the body. Thirdly, aldosterone which is normally metabolized in the liver is not metabolized as effectively, and its level in the blood rises. This causes retention of sodium and leads to oedema. However,

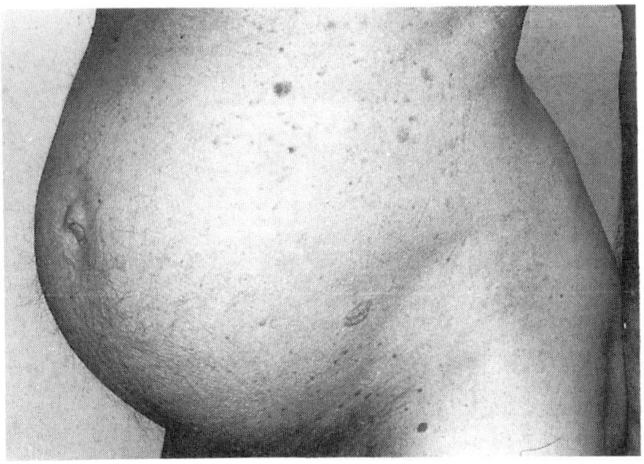

Fig. 31.5 Gross central abdominal distension due to ascites in a patient with cirrhosis of the liver.

hypoalbuminaemia and excess of aldosterone do not explain the localization of the fluid in the peritoneal cavity.

Clinical features

Patients are referred to surgeons mainly because of haematemesis or melaena. Sometimes patients known to be suffering from cirrhosis are referred for treatment to prevent massive haemorrhage from oesophageal varices. On examination the patient may have one or more of the systemic manifestations of liver disease, e.g. slight jaundice, anaemia, spider naevi or 'liver palms'. There may also be present the prominent veins at the umbilicus, and some ascites may be present. Palpable liver enlargement may be detected in early cirrhosis, but in more advanced disease the liver often shrinks and becomes impalpable. The spleen nearly always becomes palpable and sometimes is very grossly enlarged.

Identification of oesophageal varices is best made under direct vision by endoscopy, although evidence of gross varices can also be obtained on barium swallow. One of the flexible fibreoptic endoscopes is preferable to the rigid instruments and, even in the presence of recent bleeding suspected as coming from varices, oesophagoscopy should be performed. The risk of precipitating further bleeding by the passage of the instrument, though present, is very much less than was formerly feared, and the accurate knowledge obtained by the examination is extremely important. As well as inspecting the oesophagus, the opportunity is taken to examine the stomach and upper duodenum, to determine whether any other lesion, e.g. gastric or duodenal ulcer, or erosion may be present.

Management of acute bleeding from oesophageal varices

On suspicion that a patient presenting with an upper gastrointestinal bleed may have varices, immediately after the clinical examination and before any other diagnostic procedures, the following should be rapidly completed:

1. Take blood for grouping and urgent cross-matching of at least 6 units.
2. Blood should also be sent for haemoglobin, haematocrit, and coagulation factors, particularly platelet count and estimation of prothrombin time.
3. It is also helpful to have baseline liver function tests.
4. A bladder catheter is inserted to monitor urinary output.
5. Vital signs of pulse and blood pressure are recorded every 15 min.
6. A good central venous line is established.

The next step is to arrange urgent endoscopy, for the sooner the source of the bleeding is established the better. Resuscitative measures can be continued during the examination if necessary. Any blood within the lumen can be gently aspirated to obtain a reasonably clear view. Unless the bleeding is occurring at a torrential rate, there is an approximately 50% chance that it will come under at least temporary control with rest in bed, gentle sedation, and transfusion if indicated. When the active bleeding shows no sign of ceasing or recurs then one or more of the following procedures will be necessary—balloon tamponade, vasoconstrictors or injection.

Sclerotherapy balloon tamponade

Either a Sengstaken, or preferably a four-lumen Minnesota pattern tube (Fig. 31.6) is passed via the mouth through the oesophagus until its tip and distal balloon are well down into the stomach. This

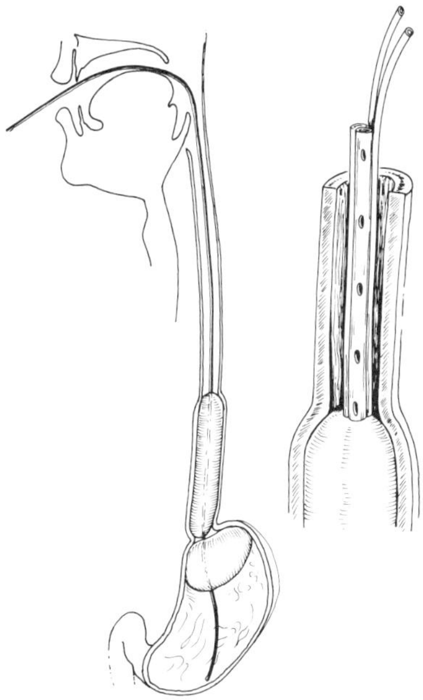

Fig. 31.6 Minnesota oesophageal tamponade tube: this is passed with both balloons deflated. The gastric tube is inflated first and then pulled up to occlude the oesophagogastric junction. The oesophageal balloon is then inflated. A third lumen permits aspiration of the stomach. The fourth tube connects with holes proximal to the oesophageal balloon (**inset**), thus allowing aspiration of any blood or other fluid above it and preventing aspiration into the respiratory tree.

distal rounded balloon is then inflated, ideally with a radiopaque contrast medium, for future X-ray confirmation of position, and traction is applied to bring the inflated balloon snugly up against the gastric fundus, where extension of the varices may well occur. Then the longitudinal proximal balloon is inflated. The pressure in this balloon is critical, for it must be enough to stop the bleeding by compressing the veins, and yet not too high or it may lead to pressure necrosis of the oesophageal wall. Generally a pressure of around 40 mmHg is adequate. If the four-lumen tube is used any blood or saliva which collects above the oesophageal balloon can be readily aspirated by applying suction to the fourth proximal lumen. When the Sengstaken variety is used repeated suction is required to the back of the mouth and pharynx. If adequate clearance of all this material is not achieved there is, of course, a considerable risk of aspiration into the air passages, and pneumonia. Either continuous or regularly repeated suction through the gastric lumen is also instituted, both to ensure an empty stomach and to detect any further or continuous bleeding which fails to be controlled by the balloons. Some means of fixing the tube as it emerges from the mouth is desirable, to prevent any chance of it slipping distally.

If successful control of the bleeding is achieved by the balloon device, it should be left inflated for no more than 24 h, otherwise the risk of pressure necrosis becomes significant. The balloons are deflated, but the tube left in situ in case repeat inflation is required for rebleeding within the following few hours.

Vasoconstrictors

Vasopressin, the posterior pituitary hormone, is known to reduce portal venous pressure, probably by constricting splanchnic arterioles, and there have been several reports of effective control of bleeding from oesophageal varices, when it has been given intravenously, either as a bolus of 20 u over a period of 10–20 min, or as a continuous intravenous infusion at a rate of 0.4–1.5 u/min.

The actions of vasopressin, however, are not restricted to the splanchnic vessels and other cardiovascular and smooth muscle effects may cause distressing and at times dangerous side-effects. Slowing of the heart rate and diminution of coronary artery flow may result, and systemic blood pressure may become elevated. Increased gut contraction may cause cramps and even infarction, and emptying of both bowel and bladder may arise urgently after infusion.

Other drugs which have also shown promise in achieving reduced portal vein pressure and control of variceal bleeding are an analogue of vasopressin, glypressin, which has much less action on cardiac function, dosage 2 mg intravenous 6-hourly, and somatostatin, the polypeptide hormone with numerous actions on various gastrointestinal functions, among them the capacity to reduce splanchnic blood flow. A suggested dose schedule is 50 μg intravenous as a bolus, followed by a continuous intravenous infusion of 250 μg/h, increasing if necessary to 500 μg/h.

Injection sclerotherapy

A sclerosant, such as sodium morrhuate or ethanolamine oleate, can be injected directly into the varix or into the submucosa just proximal to it, by means of a specially designed long guarded needle which is passed through either a rigid or flexible oesophagoscope. Temporary compression immediately following the injection is achieved either by the end of the endoscope or a specially designed cuff or balloon. One or more injections may be made at a single session. If the bleeding is initially controlled but later recurs, a repeat injection of sclerosant is always possible. Indeed it can be argued that as many sessions as are required to obliterate all identifiable varices should be arranged.

This approach to the treatment of oesophageal varices, presenting either with bleeding or electively, has become increasingly popular in recent years.

Operations for the control of bleeding

When bleeding continues or recurs in spite of the above measures, surgical control is usually required, and several options present:

1. Direct exposure of the oesophagogastric junction, dissection of the varices and ligation/division under direct vision (Fig. 31.7).
2. Transection of the oesophagus just above the oesophagogastric junction, and re-anastomosis (Fig. 31.8).
3. Devascularisation of lower oesophagus and proximal stomach, by division/ligation along greater and lesser curvatures (Fig. 31.8).
4. The use of a circular stapling gun, introduced through the anterior stomach wall, to divide and immediately rejoin the lower oesophagus.
5. Some form of portacaval shunt.

For the specific clinical problem of acute bleeding the first four options are preferred to the fifth, because experience has shown clearly that portacaval shunts carry a high risk of mortality and morbidity in the survivors, and have been largely abandoned in this situation.

The objective of each of these operations is to interrupt the transmission of the raised pressure in the tributaries of the portal vein across the junction with the systemic venous drainage of the oesophagus, and the quickest and easiest way of achieving this is the ring stapler.

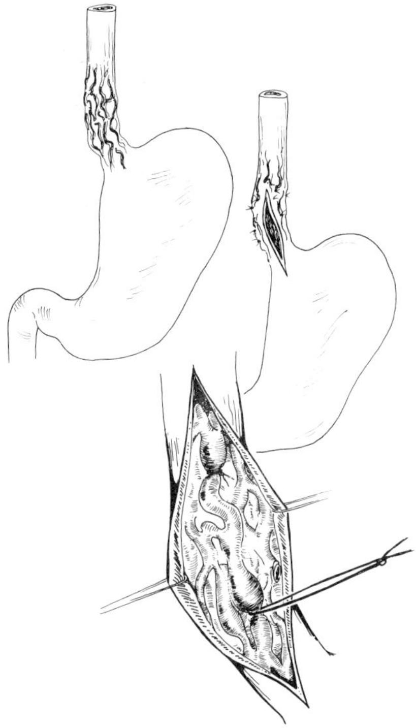

Fig. 31.7 Direct under-running and ligation of the intraluminal varices through an incision in the anterior wall of the oesophagus.

Prevention of further bleeding

The main consideration under this heading is whether the patient is a candidate for an elective procedure permanently to reduce the portal venous pressure, i.e. portacaval shunt, or whether reliance is placed on repeated sclerotherapy prophylactically.

Although shunts have been largely abandoned in the immediate control of bleeding there is still a definite place for them in carefully selected patients with certain patterns of portal hypertension. The first requirement is that liver function is not too grossly deranged, for if it is there is a high risk of the shunting of large amounts, or all of the portal venous blood directly into the vena cava, of portasystemic encephalopathy. This condition, which can range in its milder forms from slurring of speech, dysarthria or flapping tremor to gross mental disturbance and even coma in the most extreme, may develop spontaneously as liver disease causes progressively more damage, and is worsened by either spontaneously developing shunts or those created surgically. The absorption of large amounts of

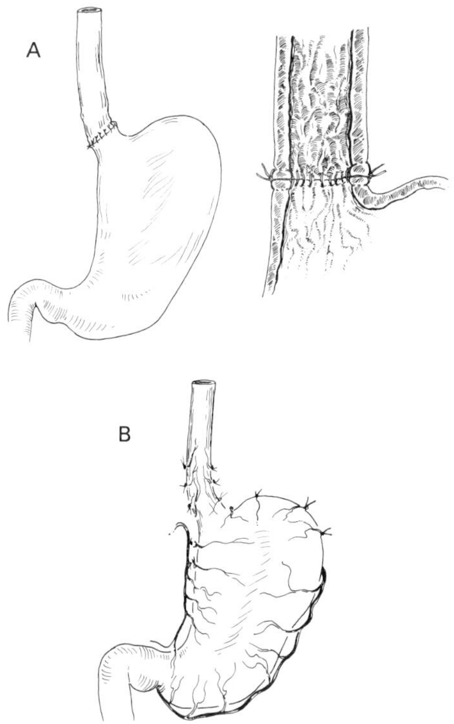

Fig. 31.8 (**A**) Transection of the lower oesophagus (to interrupt transmission of the elevated venous pressure from below) and immediate re-anastomosis. (**B**) Devascularization by dissecting out, ligating and dividing the vascular pedicles for several centimetres along the distal oesophagus and proximal gastric fundus.

protein, e.g. from blood in the gastrointestinal tract, will often precipitate the picture of encephalopathy or aggravate any pre-existing manifestations of it in those at risk. If a patient does show such symptoms and signs as a result of a bleed, subsequent shunt surgery should be avoided. Likewise the presence of jaundice or ascites are generally contra-indications. Careful follow-up analyses have shown that the prognosis is markedly worse when either the serum bilirubin is greater than 34 μmol/l or the plasma albumin is less than 35 g/l. Any sign of gross malnutrition also adversely affects the outcome.

If the patient satisfies these criteria for acceptance as a reasonably low risk for a shunt operation it is next necessary to outline the portal venous tract to determine whether a shunt is feasible on anatomical grounds. This is usually determined by percutaneous splenoportography, by which a needle is introduced directly into the splenic pulp and contrast medium is injected to outline as much of the tributaries and main trunk of the portal venous system as possible. The opportunity should also be taken to measure the splenic pulp pressure.

If suitably patent vessels are displayed, the next consideration is the pattern of portasystemic shunt to recommend.

Types of portasystemic shunt

The various main alternative procedures are shown in Figure 31.9. First, the main portal vein itself may be anastomosed to the inferior vena cava, either by complete division and end-to-side union, or by side-to-side anastomosis. Second, a segment of the superior mesenteric vein may be drained into the distal vena cava by a short Dacron graft—the so-called H-graft. Third, after removal of the spleen the proximal divided end of the splenic vein may be joined end-to-side to the left renal vein. Fourth is a combination of interruption of the lesser and greater curvature of stomach venous channels plus separation of the distal part of the splenic vein

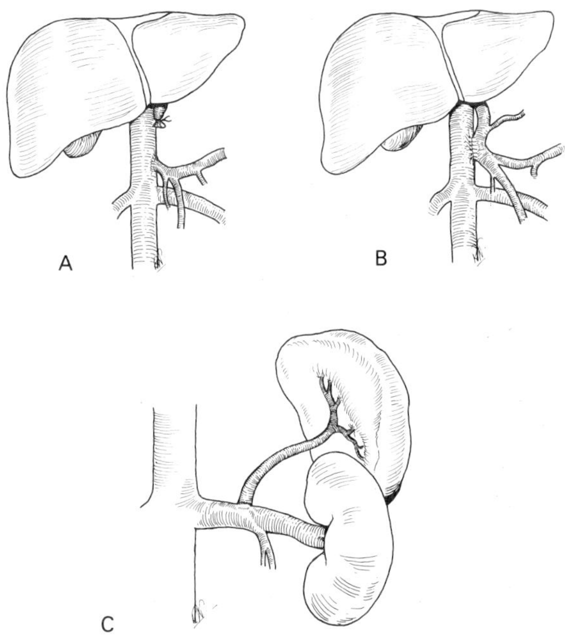

Fig. 31.9 Various types of portacaval shunt. (**A**) End-to-side, in which the portal vein is completely divided and anastomosed to the side of the inferior vena cava; (**B**) side-to-side anastomosis between these two great vessels; (**C**) end-to-side anastomosis between the splenic vein and the left renal vein.

from the inferior mesenteric vein and end-to-side anastomosis to the left renal vein. The aim of this procedure (Warren shunt) is more selectively to reduce the portal venous pressure in only the proximal stomach and lower oesophagus. Other variants of shunts have also been advocated. The development over the years of the latter more limited diversion of the portal venous blood has been prompted by the hope that their legacy of post-shunt sequelae, notably portasystemic encephalopathy, might be reduced. Some degree of reduction probably has resulted, but possibly at the price of some increase in the risk of rebleeding, variously estimated at up to 10%.

If encephalopathy develops it should be managed by a combination of colonic wash-outs to remove as much protein material as possible, dietary restriction of proteins, and antibiotics, e.g. neomycin, to reduce bacterial activity in the colon.

TUMOURS OF THE LIVER

Benign tumours are rare, the least rare being cavernous haemangioma. Small ones are usually discovered as an incidental finding during laparotomy. Larger ones may cause local discomfort or swelling or may bleed and local resection may be required.

Malignant tumour tissue in the liver is most frequently metastatic deposits from a primary lesion in stomach, pancreas or colon, or from non-gastrointestinal origin, e.g. breast, bronchus, ovary or kidney. Most often the deposits are multiple, affecting both lobes, and no treatment is possible. Very rarely a solitary accessible metastasis may justify resection of the involved segment or lobe. Attempts have been made to reduce metastases by ligation of the hepatic artery, or by radiotherapy or chemotherapy, but no convincing evidence of lasting benefit has been produced.

Primary malignant tumours of the liver fall generally into one of two categories—hepatocellular carcinoma (hepatoma) and cholangiocarcinoma. Both are relatively uncommon in Europe and North America, but less rare in Africa and the Far East.

Hepatocellular carcinoma

As its name indicates, hepatocellular carcinoma arises from the hepatocytes, the primary liver-cell element, and predisposing conditions include cirrhosis of the liver, viral hepatitis and a fungal aflatoxin found as a contaminant on maize and nuts. Unfortunately the tumour is usually far advanced before significant clinical symptoms and signs are apparent. These include abdominal discomfort or pain, distension, general malaise and weight loss and pyrexia. Marked deterioration in well-being in a known cirrhotic should alert the attendant to the possibility of a superimposed tumour. The detection of alpha-fetoprotein in the serum is often a useful marker, particularly in African patients.

Clinically there is often gross hepatomegaly, and scanning by ultrasound or computerized tomography or radionuclide scintiscanning will usually outline the extent of the tumour and its relation to important structures.

If the tumour is confined to one lobe it may be amenable to lobectomy, but this is rarely feasible. Chemotherapy with Adriamycin or methotrexate or 5-fluorouracil may give some palliation, as may hepatic artery ligation.

Cholangiocarcinoma

Cholangiocarcinoma arises from some part of the biliary duct system, and it has an association with long-standing parasitic infestation of the biliary tree, particularly in the Far East. Since it is primarily ductal in origin, not surprisingly obstructive jaundice is the commonest presenting feature. The diagnosis is usually reached by a combination of ultrasound revealing enlarged obstructed ducts proximal to the lesion, endoscopic retrograde cholangiopancreatography (ERCP) and perhaps also fine-needle percutaneous transhepatic cholangiography. If the tumour is still small there is a possibility of surgical resection along with the segments or lobe involved, and anastomosis of the divided duct or ducts to a suitable Roux-en-Y loop of jejunum. If not resectable, palliative relief of the jaundice may be obtained by the passage of a tube stent through the tumour mass. This can often be achieved at ERCP.

Although the outlook for patients with primary malignant tumours of the liver is still very poor, with few long-term survivors, more radical resections based on better understanding of the detailed segmental vascular anatomy and using improved techniques permit more adventurous attempts at resection, with better immediate survival. Such procedures are, as yet, best confined to units with special expertise in this branch of surgery.

INJURY TO THE LIVER

This large, vascular friable organ is, not surprisingly, vulnerable to damage from both blunt injuries, e.g. road traffic accidents, and penetrating wounds, e.g. stab and gunshot wounds. It should be borne in mind that penetrating injuries of the lower chest may also involve the liver, e.g. in a stab wound the knife may have gone through the diaphragm and entered the liver. The damage can range from a small tear at one part of the thin capsule to gross disruption of a large part of the organ (Fig. 31.10). The main presentation is that of gross interabdominal haemorrhage. The local signs and symptoms are abdominal pain, perhaps diaphragmatic irritation and increasing abdominal girth, with reduced or absent bowel sounds, and the systemic signs of reduced circulating blood volume, e.g. rapid pulse, hypotension, facial pallor and sweating, and rapid respiration.

On occasions immediately after injury a subcapsular haematoma may form, and this may in turn rupture some hours or even 1 or 2 days after the injury. The important clinical signs may be delayed in onset. Where there is doubt as to whether the liver is damaged or not peritoneal lavage may be helpful. After running 500—1000 ml of lavage fluid into the peritoneal cavity, the bag is placed on the floor and gross blood-staining of the returned fluid confirms the presence of significant damage, and the need for laparotomy.

At operation all that may be required for the smallest tears is suture of the torn capsule, if necessary using fibrin buttons to avoid cutting out of the suture material. Subcapsular haematomas should be evacuated. More severe lacerations may need exploration, identification of torn vessels and ducts and ligation of these. Still more extensive damage may be best dealt with by finger-fracture across residual bridges of liver substance and removal of obviously damaged portions, or formal excision of one or more segments after identification of the appropriate segmental vessels. Resection of an entire lobe may even be necessary. These procedures demand a detailed knowledge of the anatomy if they are to avoid the risk of compromising the blood supply to the remaining segments.

Where bleeding from the torn liver is profuse, temporary reduction in loss may be obtained by

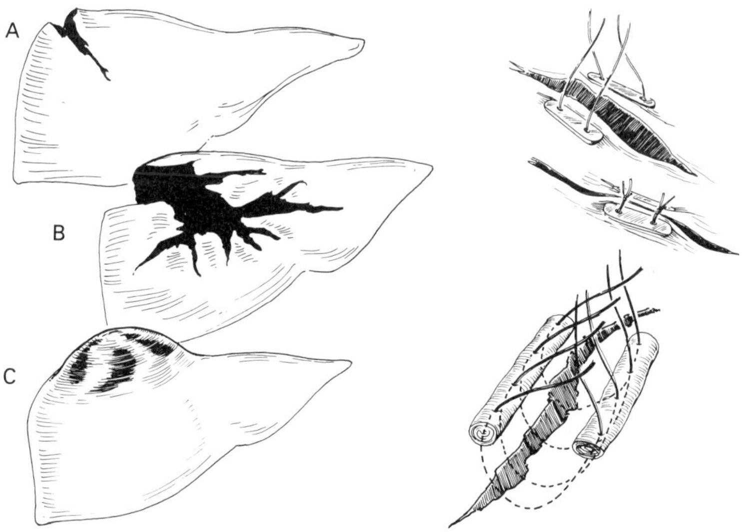

Fig. 31.10 Different patterns of liver injury. (**A**) Small linear tear; (**B**) large stellate disruption; (**C**) subcapsular haematoma. On the right are shown two techniques for achieving suture repair, using either manufactured collagen buttons, or rolls of fibrin material to help the stitches to hold without cutting through.

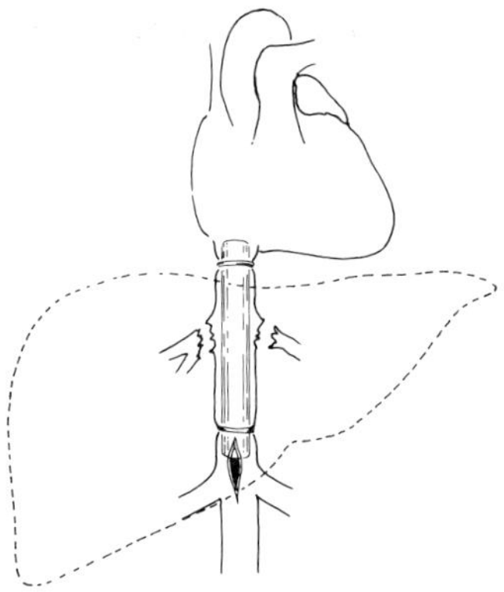

Fig. 31.11 Drastic measure to try to control bleeding from torn hepatic veins: total bypass of the hepatic venous drainage by the insertion of a wide-bore tube from the supradiaphragmatic segment of the inferior vena cava down to the infrahepatic segment, and firm ligation around this tube both proximally and distally.

compressing between fingers and thumb the vessels in the porta hepatis, introducing the fingers through the foramen of Winslow (Pringle's manoeuvre). This effectively occludes both the portal vein and hepatic artery, and if the bleeding is not controlled the inference is that it is coming from tears in the hepatic veins. This is much more difficult to control, but a drastic means of attempting it is by opening the chest, isolating the suprahepatic segment of the inferior vena cava and passing a large-bore tube shunt from the lower vena cava to above the upper exposed segment and firmly ligating around it both above and below (Fig. 31.11). This effectively shunts blood past the hepatic veins and permits exploration to find and repair the tears.

Rarely, if direct repair or resection is not feasible, packing of a rupture in the liver may be the only way of securing life-saving control. Subsequent cautious removal of the packs in the operating theatre 48–72 h later may allow one of the above approaches to be performed, if further bleeding persists.

32. The spleen

DEVELOPMENT

The spleen develops from the dorsal mesogastrium in the embryo, and can be identified at the 8-mm stage of embyronic development. It is essentially lobular in origin, and indeed in several other species it retains this characteristic in adult life. The notch often palpable on the anterior inferior border of the grossly enlarged organ is probably a remnant of this essentially lobular origin.

ANATOMY

In adult life the spleen is a comma-shaped organ situated under the left dome of the diaphragm opposite the eighth, ninth, 10th and 11th ribs (Fig. 32.1). Its visceral surface is related to the stomach, the left adrenal gland, the left kidney, the tail of the pancreas and the splenic flexure of the colon.

Its arterial blood supply is provided by the splenic artery, which in turn arises from the coeliac axis. The splenic vein joins the superior mesenteric vein to form the portal vein. Both the splenic artery and vein are contained in the lienorenal ligament.

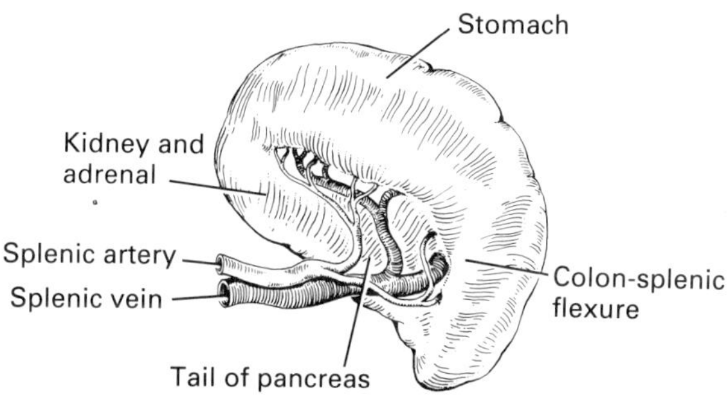

Fig. 32.1 Gross structure of normal spleen and its relations with immediately neighbouring organs.

The gastrosplenic ligament contains the short gastric vessels which, though arising from the main splenic vessels, are of course destined to contribute to the blood supply of the proximal portion of the stomach.

The nerve supply of the spleen comes mainly from the greater splanchnic nerves via the coeliac plexus, and their main function is probably of a vasomotor nature.

Underneath its peritoneal covering the spleen is enclosed in a fibrous capsule from which trabeculae pass into the substance of the organ (Fig. 32.2). Branches of the splenic artery, called trabecular arteries, lie in very close association with these trabeculae, and these terminal branches end either in the red pulp blood spaces, or in the white pulp lymph spaces. This provides a sieve-like arrangement through which particulate matter, including living cells, passes. Cells which lose their elasticity with age or disease, e.g. spherocytes, are trapped

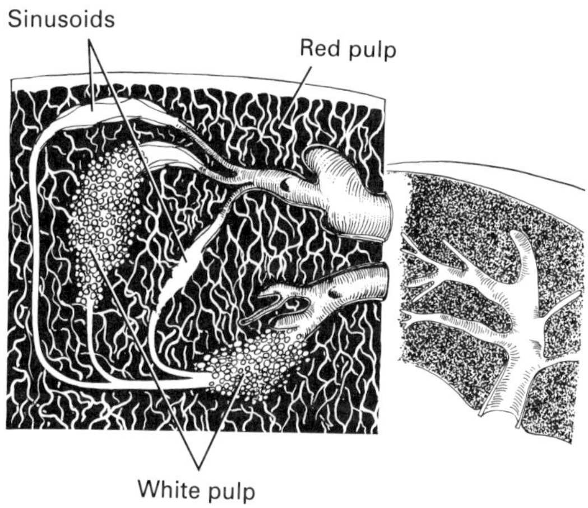

Fig. 32.2 Diagrammatic representation of the fine structure of the spleen.

by this sieve-like process, and are retained to undergo phagocytosis.

PHYSIOLOGY

The two main functions in which the spleen participates are regulation of the blood and the defence mechanisms against infection and other disease processes.

Haematological roles

The spleen is mainly concerned with the cellular and particulate elements of the blood, and its relatively large overall blood supply and the fine structure of the meshwork of vascular channels in the substance of the organ already outlined make it eminently suitable for this function. It seems that there is a finely tuned system of vascular pathways which will permit either fast or slow passage through the red pulp substance of the spleen, so that some cells may be allowed swift passage without significant alteration, whereas other, mainly faulty, elements will be more slowly passed through a grid of macrophages capable of removing damaged cells. In this way the spleen exercises a fine quality control over the red blood cells and others passing through the organ. In normal health, the spleen will tend to remove any nuclear fragments, or red cells containing obvious residual nuclear material, and therefore, although these are not normally seen in circulating blood, they may in fact be present following splenectomy.

Although the spleen may in other species act as a store for blood capable of augmenting the circulating volume on contraction of the organ, no such role has been demonstrated in the adult human. However, some storage of platelets, iron, and factor VIII does take place in the normal human spleen.

In fetal life the spleen is one of the main sources of haemopoiesis, but in adult life such a role may only be manifest where there is destruction of the bone marrow.

Defensive role

The spleen contributes to defence mechanisms in two ways. Since it is the seat of elements of the reticuloendothelial system, it is useful in removing potentially harmful particulate elements in the circulating blood, including bacteria. Its second defensive role is its contribution to the immune system. Relatively large amounts of lymphatic tissue are present throughout the organ, and particularly in aggregates of white pulp, and it is noteworthy that at least 50% of the lymphocytes in the spleen take part in recirculation to other sites in the body and are not stationary. In addition to this important role of participating in the life-cycle of lymphocytes, the spleen is probably responsible for the production of antibodies, both specific and non-specific. These latter factors have an effect on the actions of opsonins and complement.

When the spleen has to be removed for one reason or another it might therefore be expected that the overall efficiency of defence against disease, and in particular infection, would be impaired, and there is some evidence that this is so, particularly in children, but less importantly in adult life.

DISORDERS OF THE SPLEEN

The commonest operation required is splenectomy, and this may be indicated either as an urgent matter when the organ is damaged, or as an elective planned procedure because the spleen is responsible for or contributing to troublesome symptoms.

Into this latter category fall a large variety of disorders. There are first of all a group of haematological abnormalities, e.g. congenital spherocytosis, thrombocytopenic purpura, in which splenectomy may give substantial lasting benefit. In these conditions the decision to offer splenectomy is usually fairly clear-cut. In other groups of diseases mostly associated with splenomegaly, the surgeon's advice may be sought as to whether splenectomy would be beneficial, and often this will present a more difficult decision, requiring close consultation with other colleagues involved in the overall management of the patient. Some of the diseases in which splenomegaly is often a feature are listed in Table 32.1. Briefly these fall into three main categories:

1. A substantial increase in the immunologically active elements.
2. Neoplasia of either the Hodgkin's or non-Hodgkin's pattern.

Table 32.1 Various causes of splenomegaly

Infective	Metabolic
Typhoid and paratyphoid	Storage disorders, e.g. Gaucher's disease
Tuberculosis	Porphyria
Septicaemia	Amyloid disease
Splenic abscess	Still's disease
	Felty's syndrome
Syphilis	
Glandular fever	
Malaria	
Kala-Azar	
Hydatid cyst	
Blood Disorders	
Leukaemia—lymphatic and myeloid	
Myelofibrosis	
Polycythaema vera	
Pernicious anaemia	
Congenital spherocytosis	
Haemolytic anaemias	
Thrombocytopaenic purpura	
'Hypersplenism'	
Sickle-cell anaemia	
Neoplasia	
Lymphoma—Hodgkin and non-Hodgkin	
Lymphosarcoma	
Fibrosarcoma	
Angioma	

3. Secondary enlargement due to some primary haematological disorder.

Clinical features of splenomegaly

Even the lower pole of the normal spleen cannot be palpated after the deepest of inspirations, and therefore the detection of a palpable spleen indicates that there is substantial enlargement of the organ (Fig. 32.3). The degree of enlargement, however, varies enormously, the least being encountered usually in the non-specific splenic enlargement associated with some infections and anaemias, and the greatest degrees being seen in parasitic diseases, e.g. malaria, leishmaniasis, and schistosomiasis (Fig. 32.4).

Typically the presence of splenomegaly is detected by palpating a smooth, firm mass in the left hypochondrium, the lower edge of which moves downwards medially and slightly forwards when the patient takes a deep inspiration. It is important in examining for splenic enlargement to start the palpation of the abdomen with the right hand low down in the right iliac fossa and, moving the examining fingers progressively upwards towards the left costal margin, asking the patient to take a succession of deep breaths (Fig. 32.5). The left hand placed around the lower left ribs posteriorly assists in bringing the lower pole of the spleen into greater prominence (Fig. 32.6). If a distinct notch is felt on the lower medial border of the organ this is further suggestive evidence that it is truly the spleen that is enlarged, but the notch may not always be apparent. The enlarged spleen will be dull to percussion, and here again it is wise to start the percussion well below the estimated lower border of the organ, so that the transition from resonance to dullness will be clearly detected. Percussion should

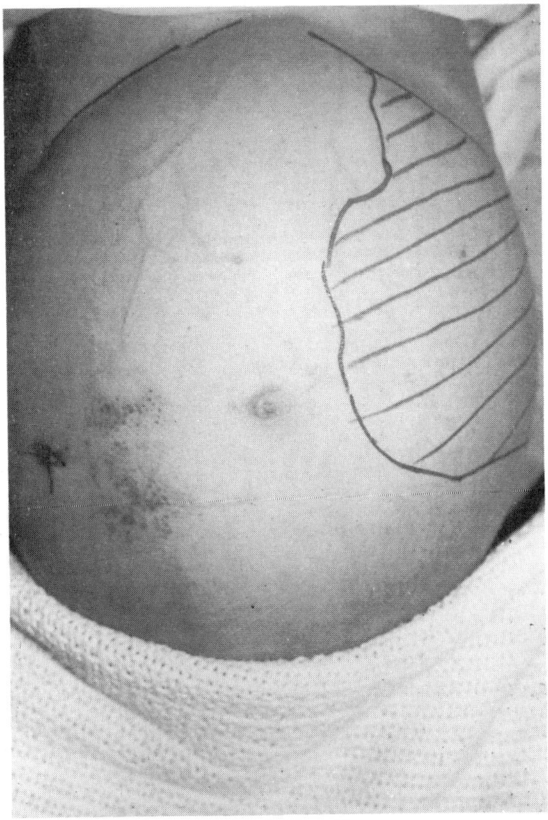

Fig. 32.3 Gross splenomegaly—outlined by hatched area—in a patient with myelofibrosis. Ascites is also present.

continue upwards and to the left costal margin posterolaterally.

Although it is usually possible to be fairly confident about a grossly enlarged spleen, there may sometimes be difficulty in distinguishing splenomegaly from a mass in the kidney, colon, or stomach. The direction of a renal mass is more directly up and down with respiration, as distinct from downwards, medially and forwards, and masses in either the colon or stomach tend to be much less mobile, and it may be possible to get partly or completely above them with the examining fingers.

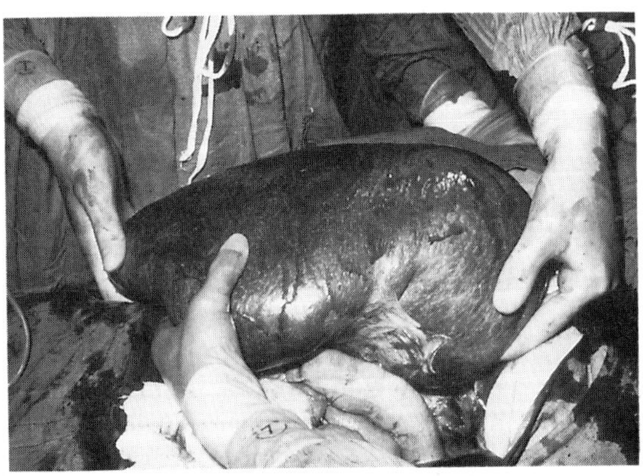

Fig. 32.4 Hugely enlarged spleen mobilized at operation.

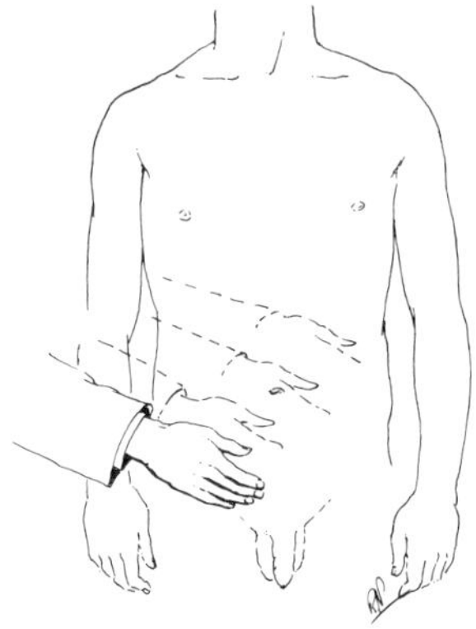

Fig. 32.5 Palpation to detect enlargement of the spleen starts low in the right iliac fossa, and progresses upwards and to the left, towards the left costal margin.

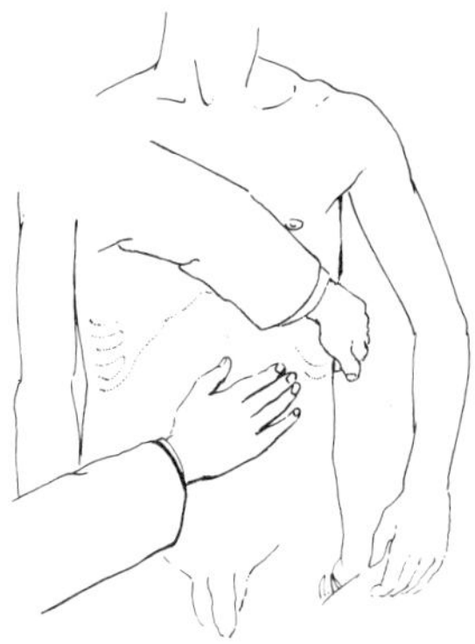

Fig. 32.6 Where the splenic enlargement is relatively slight, pressing the posterior lower ribs with the left fingers passed round the back of the patient may displace the spleen somewhat forwards, and thus make the lower pole palpable to the fingertips of the right hand, when the patient takes a deep inspiration.

RUPTURE OF THE SPLEEN

The spleen may be injured by either blunt or penetrating trauma. The enlarged diseased spleen is more liable to be injured than a normal one, which is well protected by the left lower ribs. In

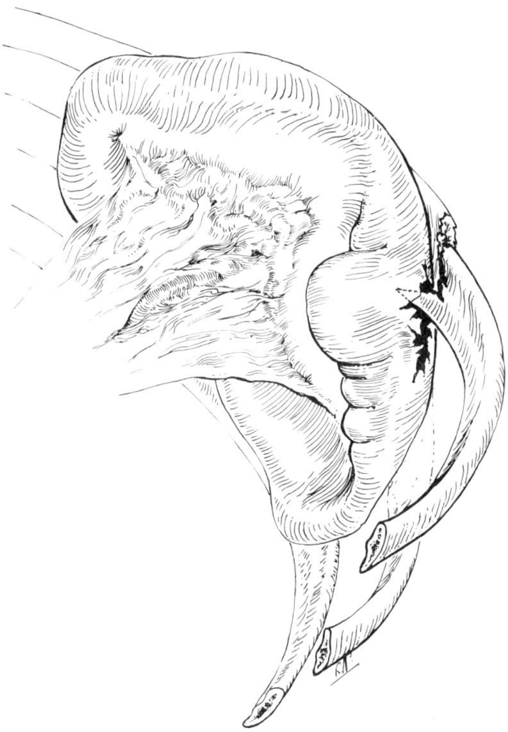

Fig. 32.7 A tear in the splenic capsule caused by fracture of an overlying rib.

accidents, splenic injury is often associated with injuries to the left side of the chest, especially involving fracture of lower ribs (Fig. 32.7), or with other intra-abdominal injuries (Fig. 32.8). The diagnosis may be very difficult in patients with multiple injuries, as the attention of the patient and the clinician may be diverted to the more obvious injuries, like compound fractures. The diagnosis is also very difficult in the unconscious.

The spleen is also occasionally injured in abdominal operations, most commonly in those performed on the stomach or other upper abdominal structures. Injuries of the spleen are rarely fatal immediately but of course pose a severe threat to life if the profuse haemorrhage from the tear is not recognized and promptly treated. Usually, the patient survives and the signs and symptoms of intraperitoneal haemorrhage follow either straight away or may be delayed for a considerable period, sometimes measured in hours or days, but very occasionally in weeks (Fig. 32.9). This latter may arise because extravasated blood may remain confined within the splenic capsule if this has not been torn, as can happen in blunt injuries. This, combined with spasm of the splenic vessels, may delay the

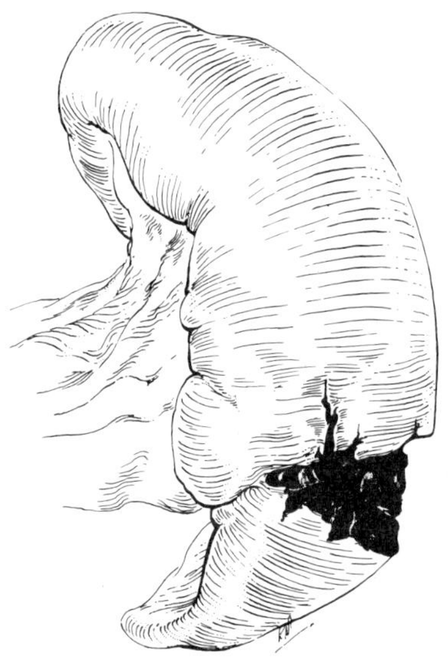

Fig. 32.8 Traumatic rupture in a closed abdominal crush injury. The tear has almost severed the lower pole from the remainder of the organ. This injury might be treatable by formal excision of the damaged lower pole and suture of the divided capsule, using collagen buttons, or other means of supporting the sutures passed through the capsule. Failing this, splenectomy would be required.

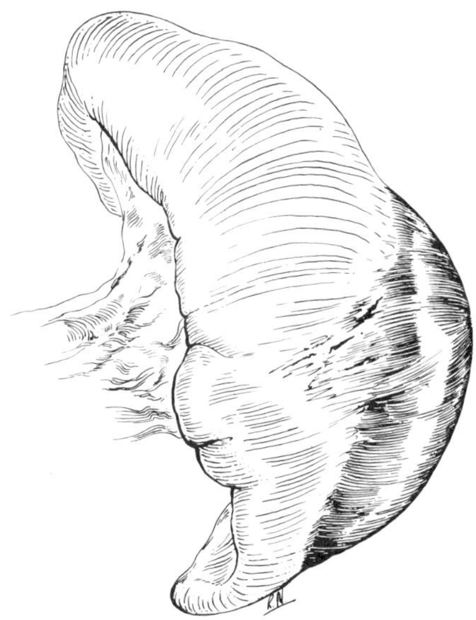

Fig. 32.9 Traumatic disruption of a segment of spleen, but without rupture of the capsule. The contained subcapsular haematoma may give way hours, days, or occasionally weeks after the injury, leading to the delayed onset of signs of blood loss and/or peritoneal irritation.

spilling of blood into the peritoneal cavity. Later, when the capsule gives way under the pressure of the contained blood, haemoperitoneum occurs and the signs and symptoms become apparent. Another factor which may delay haemoperitoneum is the formation of blood clot which blocks the opening in the torn vessels for some time.

With the onset of intraperitoneal haemorrhage, the pulse becomes rapid and the blood pressure falls. Untreated, the patient will die from the resulting hypovolaemia and hypoxia of the vital centres.

Clinical features

In the overwhelming majority of cases, there is a clear history of trauma, but this may not be available in the patient who is presenting unconscious. Occasionally a spleen, usually one grossly enlarged by disease, apparently ruptures spontaneously. Possibly the very fragile organ has been damaged by a minor injury, which has not been sufficient to be noticed or recalled by the patient.

The cardinal symptoms are abdominal pain, and those of severe blood loss. The pain is constant and increases on movement. On examination, the general condition of the patient does not always give a clear indication of the injury to the spleen. Classically there is pain, with a rapid pulse, low blood pressure, abdominal tenderness, muscle guarding, and an absence of bowel sounds on auscultation of the abdomen. In some there are obvious bruises on the left side of the abdomen and chest, and there may be evidence of fracture of the left lower ribs.

If all of these signs and symptoms are present the diagnosis of rupture of the spleen is fairly straightforward. However, few signs may at first be apparent, and if any question of damage to the organ arises, there should be no hesitation in re-examining the patient after a short interval.

Additional physical signs, which if present may be helpful, but on which less reliance can be placed in comparison to the main ones already noted, include pain referred to the left shoulder by blood irritating the diaphragm and the combination of fixed dullness to percussion in the left hypochondrium due to clotted blood around the spleen, and shifting dullness in the right hypochondrium, due to unclotted blood free in the peritoneal cavity.

Straight X-ray films of the lower chest and abdomen may show any fractures in the ribs, and may also show obliteration of the psoas shadow on the left side or indeed on both sides.

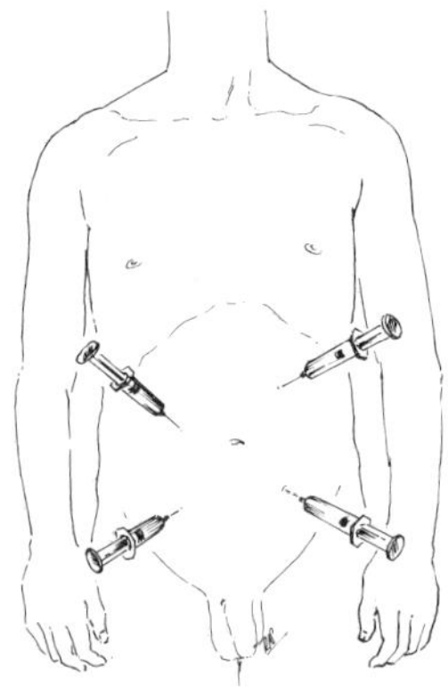

Fig. 32.10 Where clinical suspicion of intraperitoneal bleeding persists in the presence of few gross signs, confirmation of free blood within the peritoneal cavity may be obtained by inserting a needle into one of the quadrants of the abdomen, and needling the remaining three in turn if the first tap finds no blood.

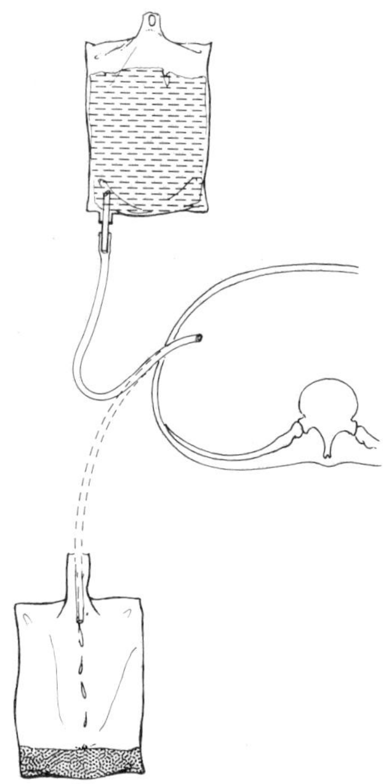

Fig. 32.11 Perhaps a more satisfactory method of determining whether there is free blood in the peritoneal cavity is the insertion of a peritoneal dialysis cannula into a lower quadrant, running in a litre of dialysis fluid and then allowing the washout to run back into the bag, by placing it at floor level.

In doubtful cases, paracentesis of the peritoneal cavity may be undertaken under local anaesthesia (Figs 32.10 and 32.11). If blood is aspirated from the peritoneal cavity this is positive proof of haemoperitoneum. This test is of particular value in the unconscious patient and in those with multiple injuries.

Management

Laparotomy should be undertaken even if there is a suspicion of rupture of the spleen, and if the diagnosis is confirmed splenectomy is carried out as a life-saving measure.

There are occasions when there are no significant signs of intraperitoneal haemorrhage, but rupture cannot be ruled out because of the history of injury. In such cases, the patient should be kept under strict observation in a hospital, where a record of pulse and blood pressure is maintained. At the slightest suggestion of intraperitoneal haemorrhage, laparotomy is undertaken without hesitation.

In recent years some surgeons have advocated a more conservative approach to the injured spleen in view of the increased recognition of its important role in the defence mechanisms of the body, particularly against infection. Clearly where the organ is very grossly damaged there is no alternative to removal of the entire spleen, but where there is only a short capsular tear, or the damage is confined to one pole, it is technically possible to repair the defect and secure sound haemostasis in many cases (Fig. 32.12). However, clinical judgement of a high order, considerable experience, and facilities to keep the patient under close postoperative supervision are necessary to select appropriate patients for this approach.

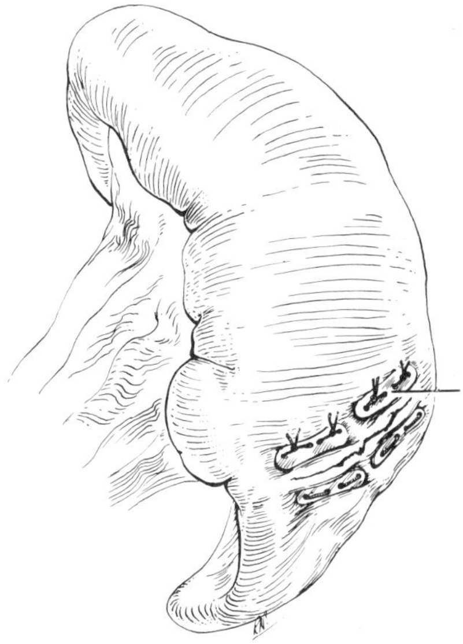

Fig. 32.12 Surgical repair of a small linear tear in an accessible part of the splenic capsule. Several horizontal absorbable mattress sutures have been inserted through the holes in firm collagen 'buttons', which take and distribute the tension, thus apposing the torn edges. If the sutures were simply inserted directly through the delicate capsule they would tear out on being tied sufficiently tightly to control bleeding.

Disorders for which elective splenectomy may be performed

The three haematological disorders for which splenectomy is of value are congenital spherocytosis, thrombocytopenic purpura and hypersplenism. These will be discussed individually. There then follows a group of other diseases in which splenectomy may have a more limited application.

CONGENITAL SPHEROCYTOSIS

This is a rare inherited disorder in which the fragility of the red blood corpuscles is greatly increased. Normal red cells are biconcave (Fig. 32.13), whereas those in congenital spherocytosis are biconvex or spheroidal, as the name of the disease suggests. The cause of this abnormality is not known, but it may be due to some defect in the development of the enzymes concerned with the synthesis of adenosine triphosphate.

The disease is transmitted as a Mendelian dominant from either parent to children of either sex. Clinically it manifests itself in several ways. The baby may be born with mild jaundice which persists, but with no other signs or symptoms. In other cases, the baby is not jaundiced at birth but later there are episodes of acute haemolysis, which are characterized by attacks of abdominal pain, nausea, vomiting and extreme pallor, followed by the appearance of jaundice.

In some patients vague symptoms of weakness and fatigue, with or without jaundice, the intensity

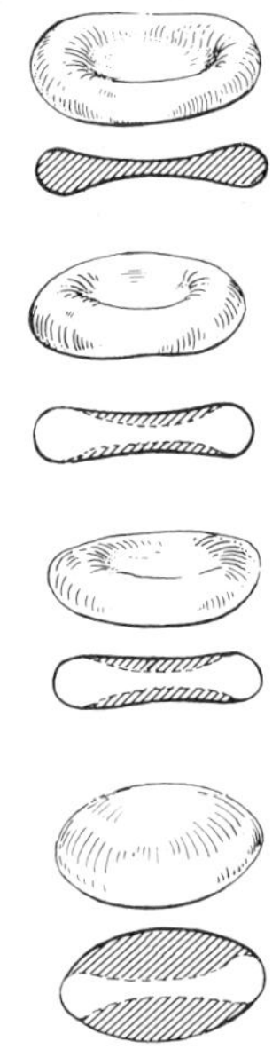

Fig. 32.13 Diagrammatic representation of appearance and cross-section of red blood corpuscle ranging from normal (**top**) to spherocyte (**bottom**). The more progressive the change in shape from above down, the more fragile is the red cell.

of which varies with the severity of the symptoms, may develop in early adult life.

Gallstones are liable to develop in these patients on account of the increased output of bile pigment produced by the liver from the haemoglobin released by the haemolysis. Gallstone colic may, therefore, be a leading symptom in many patients. Congenital spherocytosis is almost the only condition in which gallstones develop in childhood.

On examination, jaundice, if present, is usually mild. In non-jaundiced patients, pallor is often a striking feature and the spleen may be palpable. Occasionally, the liver is also palpable.

The diagnosis is established by the demonstration of abnormal red blood corpuscles in a blood film, by the absence of bile pigments in the urine and by the presence of excessive stercobilinogen in the stools. Coombs test, in which the red blood corpuscles of the patient are tested against sensitized rabbit serum, is negative. In a positive test haemolysis of the red blood corpuscles occurs, as abnormal globulins remain adherent to the washed red blood cells and combine with the antigen in the rabbit's serum. In congenital spherocytosis, the test is negative as there is no abnormal globulin.

Splenectomy is the treatment of the disease. It does not abolish the spherocytosis but diminishes the number of abnormal red blood cells and returns their lifespan towards normal.

THROMBOCYTOPENIC PURPURA

This disease of unknown origin is characterized by a tendency to develop spontaneous haemorrhage into the skin, into mucous surfaces, and within the skull. There is a reduction in the platelet count of the blood.

Many theories have been advanced to explain the phenomenon, among them the following:

1. that there is excessive destruction of platelets in the spleen;
2. that the spleen elaborates a specific hormone which restrains the formation of platelets from the megakaryocytes of the bone marrow;
3. that the primary defect is not in the platelets but in the fragility of the capillaries.

None of these hypotheses has been clearly substantiated.

Clinically the disease manifests itself in a number of ways. There is a tendency for wounds to bleed excessively. Small cuts, which should normally stop bleeding after a few minutes, continue to bleed for a long time. The patient also complains of being easily bruised. Often there is epistaxis, haematuria, gastrointestinal haemorrhage and menorrhagia. Very rarely, submucosal haemorrhage in the intestine may be a cause of intestinal obstruction, either by direct occlusion, or by it being a starting point of an intussusception. Bleeding into joints, however, is rare.

On examination, there may be petechial haemorrhages, especially on the extensor aspects of the limbs. If a tourniquet of a sphygmomanometer is applied to one of the arms and the pressure in it is maintained between diastolic and systolic pressure for about 5 min, petechial haemorrhages appear distal to the tourniquet and under cover of it. As mentioned above, the spleen is enlarged in about 25% of cases. The enlargement, however, is not massive.

Examination of the peripheral blood demonstrates the thrombocytopenia: figures are much below the normal of between 250 000 and 500 000 mm^3.

Since purpura may arise as a secondary phenomenon to a number of conditions, e.g. drug sensitivity, septicaemia, tuberculosis, aplastic anaemia, leukaemia, carcinomatosis of bone, X-ray therapy and allergic reaction to some foods, the diagnosis of idiopathic purpura should only be considered as established if secondary purpura has been excluded.

The treatment of idiopathic thrombocytopenic purpura is empirical. Corticosteroid therapy is successful in about half the cases. In the remainder, especially in adults, the disease is not controlled by these measures, and in these cases splenectomy is recommended. The results of this operation are excellent in the majority of cases.

HYPERSPLENISM

In certain diseases involving the spleen there is excessive destruction of one or more of the formed elements of blood and these diseases have been grouped under the term hypersplenism.

Clearly if the excess destruction is of red blood cells the presentation will be that of anaemia; of white cells it will be recurrent infection, and of platelets, purpura. If all elements are affected there may be a pancytopenia.

The hypersplenism may be primary, the spleen overacting in response to an increased load of abnormal cells, or secondary from splenic function disturbed by disease, e.g. malaria, leishmaniasis, bilharziasis, portal hypertension, splenic vein thrombosis, myelofibrosis or the lymphomas.

It is possible, by a variety of isotope and other scanning techniques, to measure the rate of red cell destruction within the spleen, and also to assess bone-marrow activity. These tests, if available, should help in determining the likelihood of a good response to splenectomy. Since the removal of a large spleen may be hazardous and difficult, and there is reluctance further to impair resistance against infection, the operation should only be undertaken when there is good evidence that the spleen is truly the source of the abnormal blood changes.

OTHER DISORDERS FOR WHICH SPLENECTOMY IS OCCASIONALLY PERFORMED

Removal of the spleen in these other disorders is usually to relieve the local discomfort caused by gross splenomegaly.

Myelofibrosis

This is characterized by abnormal proliferation of tissue of mesenchymal origin in the bone marrow, liver, lymph nodes and spleen. The patients often need repeated blood transfusions in view of marrow function suppression. Splenectomy can reduce the frequency of transfusion as well as relieve discomfort from local pressure by the enlarged organ.

Lymphomas

In both Hodgkin's and non-Hodgkin's types of lymphoma splenectomy may be required, but for essentially different reasons. In Hodgkin's disease splenectomy is part of the staging procedure carried out at laparotomy in order to plan the most appropriate programme of treatment. In the various non-Hodgkin's varieties splenectomy may be indicated for either hypersplenism or for local pain or discomfort, e.g. arising from a splenic infarct.

Removal of the spleen is also occasionally required in amyloid disease, sarcoidosis, cysts or tumours of the spleen, and splenic artery aneurysm. Rarely abscesses arise in the spleen and either drainage or splenectomy is needed—the latter may prove exceedingly difficult.

POSTSPLENECTOMY COMPLICATIONS

First there is a risk of early postoperative bleeding, either from one or more of the delicate vessels in the vascular splenic pedicle, or more likely from the splenic bed, particularly when the spleen has been very grossly enlarged.

Second, any collection of blood in the subdiaphragmatic area may become infected, leading to the formation of a subphrenic abscess.

Third, since there is always a brisk increase in the number of circulating platelets following splenectomy, there is an increased risk of deep venous thrombosis, and appropriate prophylactic measures should be taken, e.g. early mobilization, support stockings, leg exercises, antiplatelet agents such as aspirin or dipyridamole, and even anticoagulants if the thrombocytosis is prolonged.

As has already been mentioned, there is also some evidence of a reduced resistance to infections following removal of the spleen, so that a careful watch for any such infections and prompt treatment of them with appropriate antibiotics is needed in the months and years which follow.

33. The small intestine

DEVELOPMENT

The small intestine extends from the pylorus to the caecum. The first and second parts of the duodenum down to the entry of the common bile and pancreatic ducts develop from the foregut, and the rest from the midgut. At first, the entire gut is a midline structure, but as a combination of differentiation of the various segments and rotation takes place, the caecum and the terminal ileum come to lie at first in the left hypochondrium and subsequently move to the right side, at first below the liver and finally descending to the right iliac fossa. This process may become arrested at some stage, leaving the ileocaecal region at a higher than usual location.

ANATOMY

The small intestine is divided into three parts—the duodenum, which is mostly a retroperitoneal structure, the jejunum, which is the proximal two-fifths of that part of the gut which is mobile because it possesses a mesentery, and the ileum, which becomes continuous with the caecum. The ileum can be distinguished from the jejunum on inspection because of the presence of many arterial arcades in its mesentery, whereas there are fewer in the mesentery of the jejunum.

The main artery supplying the small intestine is the superior mesenteric artery, the artery of the midgut, which crosses the third part of the duodenum soon after its origin from the aorta. As the proximal part of the duodenum develops from the foregut it receives branches from the coeliac axis via the superior pancreaticoduodenal branch of the hepatic artery.

The main venous drainage is provided by the superior mesenteric vein which joins the splenic vein to form the portal vein.

Branches from the vagus nerve supply the fibres which stimulate the motor and secretory activity of the small intestine. These effects are further mediated and regulated by two intrinsic nerve plexuses within the gut wall, the first (Meissner's plexus) in the submucosal region, and the other (Auerbach's plexus) between the longitudinal and circular layers of muscle.

Pain sensation is carried via the splanchnic nerves and the sympathetic trunk to the posterior root ganglia of the spinal nerves.

PHYSIOLOGY

The small intestine is, of course, the main site of digestion and absorption of fat, carbohydrate and protein by the pancreatic enzymes. Bile salts facilitate fat digestion, and there are a few enzymes arising from the intestinal mucosa itself which may minimally contribute to various digestive processes. Fats are broken down into fatty acids and glycerol, carbohydrates into monosaccharides and proteins into amino acids. The major part of this process takes place in the lumen of the bowel but the final stages are carried out by enzymatic action at the brush border of the mucosal cells, or within these cells. Monosaccharides and amino acids are absorbed into the portal circulation, while fatty acids and glycerol re-combine inside the mucosal cells to form small particles of triglycerides which then receive a coating of lipoprotein to become chylomicrons. Some of these then pass into the lymphatic lacteals, from where they are carried via the thoracic duct into the systemic circulation.

Peristaltic waves are generated in the small intestine mostly by an intrinsic pacemaker situated in the periampullary region of the duodenum, from where they are propagated distally. The co-ordinating mechanism for this may involve the longitudinal muscle or the intrinsic nerve plexuses. Although cholinergic activity will increase the frequency and force of these movements, normal propulsion continues after vagotomy.

CONGENITAL ABNORMALITIES

Among the variety of congenital defects in the small intestine which are of clinical importance surgically are the following:

1. Atresia and stenosis.
2. Malrotation, causing volvulus and intestinal obstruction.
3. Meconium ileus.
4. Meckel's diverticulum.

Atresia and stenosis

Atresia and stenosis of the small intestine are the commonest causes of small bowel obstruction in the newborn. The duodenum is the most frequent site of the lesion; the second most common is the ileum, and in a few cases, jejunum or colon alone may be affected.

The essential pathology in atresia is the failure of the lumen to develop in the intestine. In stenosis, the lumen, though present, is very narrow. The blood vessels supplying the distended portion of the gut above the affected segment may be stretched. This may cause ischaemic necrosis of the bowel, which may in turn lead to perforation and peritonitis.

In both atresia and stenosis, the infant is born with intestinal obstruction. Clinically, the baby starts to vomit shortly after birth. The vomitus may or may not contain bile, depending on the site of obstruction in relation to the duodenal papilla. In atresia or stenosis of the duodenum there is very little abdominal distension, whereas if it occurs in the ileum, abdominal distension may be considerable. If the lesion is confined to the small intestine some meconium may be passed per rectum.

A plain X-ray of the abdomen may give helpful information in that it may show a single gastric air bubble but no gas shadows in the rest of the gut in duodenal atresia, and distended loops of bowel with multiple fluid levels in the more distal lesions.

Surgery offers the only hope for these infants. In duodenal atresia, duodenojejunostomy, bypassing the involved segment, is usually performed. For ileal lesions, a Paul–Mikulicz type of operation may be required: the affected part is excised and the adjacent distended and collapsed segments of the bowel are brought out of the abdomen as separate openings. After a few days, the spur between the loops may be gradually crushed by applying a crushing clamp or the two ends may be anastomosed at a second operation.

Malrotation

Malrotation of the gut is a rather infrequent cause of neonatal intestinal obstruction. In the majority of cases, the caecum lies in the left upper abdomen and a band of fibrous tissue (called the band of Ladd) passing from the left to the right side may cause obstruction of the second part of the duodenum. In addition to the obstruction produced by the band of Ladd, a second potential cause of obstruction is the malrotated gut which is liable to undergo volvulus. In a few cases, there is only obstruction due to the band without any volvulus.

The symptoms are those of intestinal obstruction, i.e. vomiting and abdominal distension. The diagnosis is established at laparotomy, which should not be delayed in the presence of vomiting and abdominal distension. The band is divided and the volvulus, if present, is reduced.

Meconium ileus

Meconium ileus is one of the complications of fibrocystic disease of the pancreas. In this condition, the pancreatic secretion is very thick and does not contain any trypsin. As a result, masses of inspissated, putty-like material occlude the lumen of the intestine, and the infant is born with intestinal obstruction. Vomiting, constipation and abdominal distension are the main symptoms. X-ray examination of the abdomen shows no particular diagnostic sign. The condition can, however, be diagnosed if a piece of an exposed X-ray film is dipped in the vomitus. In the case of meconium ileus, digestion of the film, which will take place on exposure to normal intestinal content, does not occur.

At laparotomy the sticky gelatinous material is removed from the intestine by opening an appropriate loop. Its removal may be assisted by irrigation with 1% hydrogen peroxide. After all the meconium has been removed, the wound in the intestine is sutured and the abdomen is closed.

Further long-term treatment for the basic underlying abnormality of pancreatic enzyme deficiency will be required, with, among other measures, oral supplements of enzyme preparations.

Meckel's diverticulum

Meckel's diverticulum is a remnant of the vitello-intestinal duct. Normally, this duct is completely obliterated by the time the baby is born. However, it partially persists in about 2% of people. It is then usually situated on the antimesenteric border of the ileum at about 60 cm from the ileocaecal junction, and can vary in length from a slight bulge to a well developed blind pouch of several centimetres (Fig. 33.1). In the vast majority of cases it does not produce any symptoms. In a few, however, it comes to clinical notice because it becomes the seat of certain complications, namely:

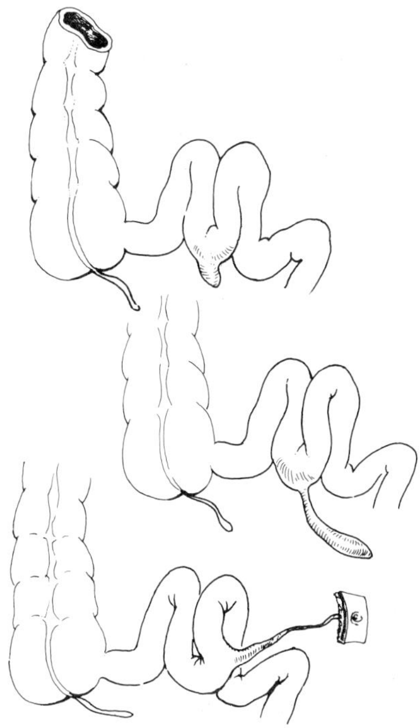

Fig. 33.1 Meckel's diverticulum. This is usually situated about 60 cm proximal to the ileocaecal valve and varies from a small bulge on the antimesenteric aspect of the ileum to a long appendix-like pouch, or even, more rarely, a smaller pouch which continues as a fibrous cord to the umbilicus.

1. Meckel's diverticulitis, in which the diverticulum is infected, possibly obstructed, and may even perforate. This condition is clinically indistinguishable from acute appendicitis, and is usually only recognized at laparotomy.
2. Intussusception, in which the diverticulum may become invaginated to form the apex of the intussusception. The pathology, clinical features and treatment of this condition are described later.
3. A chronic peptic ulcer occasionally develops when, as occasionally happens, there is ectopic gastric type mucosa in the diverticulum. These ulcers may be prone to bleed, and therefore the clinical presentation may be that of a young patient with repeated episodes of unexplained loss of blood from the gastrointestinal tract.
4. Intestinal obstruction may occur in one of a number of ways. If a fibrous band remnant of the vitellointestinal duct persists, passing from the apex of the diverticulum to the umbilicus, this band may either become an axis for volvulus of the small intestine, or trap a segment of the bowel, in both cases producing intestinal obstruction.

At operation, required for any of the above reasons, it is usually possible simply to excise the diverticulum and close the incision in the ileum by sutures in a transverse direction to avoid any narrowing of the lumen. On occasions it may be necessary to remove a short segment of the intestine from which the diverticulum arises if the neck is wide or if there is doubt about the integrity of the immediately adjacent ileum.

If a symptomless Meckel's diverticulum is encountered during an operation for another condition, and the patient is otherwise fit, it is reasonable to remove it to minimize the chances of later complications.

INJURY TO SMALL INTESTINE

Traumatic lesions of the small intestine may be encountered in both civil and military practice. Penetrating wounds by bullets, knives or pointed fragments of metal or glass may damage any segment in the path of the injuring agent, and blunt force applied to the abdomen is more likely to rupture intestine which is firmly fixed to the posterior abdominal wall, especially the duodenum. The mesenteric blood vessels are also liable to damage by both types of injury, leading to gross haemorrhage into the peritoneal cavity.

The signs and symptoms are those of peritonitis, i.e. pain in the abdomen, general abdominal tenderness, muscle guarding and, when intraperitoneal bleeding is significant, the signs of systemic blood loss. The abdomen may be silent to auscultation. An X-ray taken with the patient in the upright position may show gas under the right dome of the diaphragm. These signs have to be specially looked for in patients with multiple injuries, and the diagnosis is particularly difficult in unconscious patients.

If there is any suspicion of injury to the intestine, arrangements should be made for early laparotomy. A nasogastric tube should be inserted to empty the stomach as far as possible, cross-matched blood should be obtained, an intravenous line established, and an antibiotic likely to cover organisms, particularly Gram-negative ones, from the gastrointestinal tract started. At operation if the tear in the gut is small and clean-cut it may be possible simply to repair it with sutures. More extensive damage may require resection, exteriorization, or the creation of a tube fistula and bypass procedure or the insertion of a feeding enterostomy. The latter is more likely for severe injuries to the duodenum than for more distal lesions.

It is important always to examine thoroughly all other intra-abdominal structures to ensure that there are no other damaged organs.

INFLAMMATORY LESIONS

There are three types of inflammatory lesions of the small intestine which are of surgical importance. These are tuberculosis, regional ileitis, and typhoid ulcers.

Tuberculosis

Tuberculosis of the intestine may be primary or secondary. The former is due to the ingestion of infected milk, and the latter occurs when a patient suffering from pulmonary tuberculosis swallows his or her own sputum. In both cases, tubercle bacilli survive the antibacterial action of the gastric juice.

Tuberculosis is primarily a disease of the lymphatic system and therefore in the intestine it is primarily the submucous lymphatics which are involved. Two patterns of presentation are encountered clinically.

Ulcerative form

An ulcerative form arises secondary to disease in the lung, and is characterized by multiple ulcers lying transversely to the intestine. The serous coat overlying the affected part shows considerable thickening and many small tubercles. These ulcers heal by fibrosis, producing strictures which may be multiple.

In the active stage of the disease, which is commonly in young women, diarrhoea is the main complaint. There is loss of weight and there may or may not be obvious signs and symptoms of pulmonary tuberculosis. The patient is usually referred for surgical advice when intestinal obstruction develops, and the pattern is often of recurrent episodes of acute or chronic obstruction. An awareness of multiple swellings appearing in the abdomen at the time of pain and the observation of visible peristalsis on inspection give further support to the diagnosis. An X-ray of the chest and bacterial examination of the sputum will often confirm the presence of obvious active pulmonary disease, but sometimes the results are apparently normal.

The primary treatment is to give a regime of antitubercular drugs, and manage the obstructive symptoms, if these are not complete, expectantly. An intravenous infusion and gastric suction are instituted and the attack may pass off in a few hours. If it becomes clear that the symptoms are not resolving, or obstruction becomes complete, surgical exploration will be necessary and the exact procedure to be undertaken depends upon the operative findings. If only a small segment of the bowel is involved, containing one or more strictures, this segment is excised. If, on the other hand, there are scattered strictures involving a large segment, these may be bypassed by side-to-side anastomosis. Postoperatively, antitubercular treatment is continued for at least 18 months.

Hyperplastic ileocaecal tuberculosis

Hyperplastic ileocaecal tuberculosis is a primary infection of the small intestine, and is less common than the ulcerative variety of the disease. It results from the ingestion of infected material, mainly milk, and the terminal ileum is usually involved. Considerable granulomatous thickening of the bowel wall occurs and this may cause obstruction either by obliteration of the lumen, or by the adherence of adjacent loops of intestine.

Clinically, the patient complains of attacks of abdominal pain and diarrhoea. Some present with symptoms of intestinal obstruction. On examination, a tender mass is palpable in the right iliac fossa. Barium meal and follow-through X-ray examination may show a longitudinal filling defect on the right side in the region of the terminal ileum.

Antitubercular treatment is started, and laparotomy is usually required, at which it is best to excise the involved segment and perform a right hemicolectomy. In severely ill patients with symptoms of intestinal obstruction, bypass of the lesion by an ileotransverse colostomy is performed simply to relieve the obstruction. In some, later resection of the bypassed segment can be done, if the mass continues to give symptoms or the effects of a 'blind loop' develop. In some, if there is a satisfactory response to the antitubercular drugs, no further operation will be required. In any case these drugs should be continued for at least 18 months.

Regional ileitis

Under this heading there are two separate conditions, each with its own characteristic clinical presentation, natural history and management. On gross superficial examination of the segment of bowel affected there may be some apparent similarity, but they are quite distinct entities.

Acute ileitis

The usual presentation resembles that of acute appendicitis, with a history of some hours or up to 2 days of central abdominal pain settling into the right iliac fossa; nausea; perhaps vomiting, and either mild diarrhoea or constipation. There is often mild pyrexia and loss of appetite. The main clinical sign is tenderness in the right iliac fossa, and there may also be a vaguely defined mass in this area.

Not surprisingly the preoperative diagnosis is suspected appendicitis, and the correct diagnosis is made at exploration of the abdomen. On opening the peritoneal cavity the appendix is found to be normal, but there is a short segment of reddened thickening of the terminal ileum. The adjacent lymph nodes are enlarged and fleshy, and there may be a small quantity of free, straw-coloured fluid lying in the peritoneal cavity itself. The remainder of the intestine appears completely normal. This is a self-limiting disease, which can be expected to resolve completely without recurrence, and therefore no interference with the inflamed segment, apart from excision biopsy of an easily accessible lymph node, is indicated. Histological examination of the node, will show only non-specific inflammatory changes. The aetiology is unknown, but possibly some cases are due to infection with *Yersinia*, or another uncommon organism. Formerly there was reluctance to remove the normal appendix but since there is no significant risk of subsequent complications if this is done, it is quite reasonable to excise it, since appendicitis is a common disorder, and this prevents any future attack of it.

Chronic regional ileitis (Crohn's disease)

The cause or causes of this disease also remain unknown, but among the various thoughts on aetiology are some disturbance of an immune response to ingested foreign material, or of autoimmunity, or a modified response to tubercle or other bacilli. These ideas have arisen from the gross and microscopic pathological pattern which features thickening, mainly in the submucosal layer, round cell infiltration, the presence of giant cells, and the formation of granulomas. However, no specific organisms or foreign particles have been isolated from excised samples of the disease. In Crohn's disease typical lesions may arise at any level in the gastrointestinal tract, from mouth to anus, but the commonest location by far is the terminal ileum. It is typical of the disorder to affect multiple sites in the intestine, with intervening segments of varying length, which appear to all intents completely normal, and for this reason these multiple diseased areas are referred to as 'skip' lesions. More such lesions may develop with the passage of time, and thus a chronic recurrent illness, with increasing involvement of more and more parts of the gastrointestinal tract, is not unusual.

Segments of the disease have a great tendency to adhere to any neighbouring structures, and to form abscesses and fistulas, e.g. to the overlying skin, to other portions of small or large intestine, to the urinary tract, or if the anal region is affected, to the perianal region (Fig. 33.2).

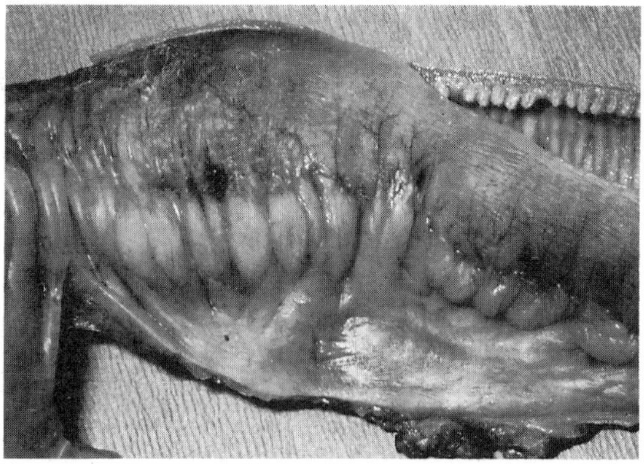

Fig. 33.2 Crohn's disease: resected specimen, showing typical gross appearances of thickened bowel wall and mesentery, fleshy lymph nodes and general tube-like characteristics.

Clinical features

Patients with Crohn's disease may present to surgeons mainly because of a painful mass in the right iliac fossa, intestinal obstruction, or the presence of fistula. There will, however, nearly always be a preceding history going back weeks, months or years, of general malaise, recurrent diarrhoea, abdominal discomfort and maybe weight loss and anaemia, thus distinguishing it from more acute causes of these problems. On palpation of the abdomen the thickened segment of intestine is usually felt as a tender, elongated mass, and since the ileum is the commonest seat of the disease, the mass generally lies in the right iliac fossa. When early operation is not required, e.g. for complete obstruction or abscess, X-ray barium meal and follow-through examination may show the characteristic narrowing and irregularity of mucosal pattern illustrated in Figure 33.3 (the so-called string of Kantor). In the presence of obstruction there will, of course, be gas–fluid levels in the proximal bowel. There is often occult blood present in the stools, and the patient may be anaemic.

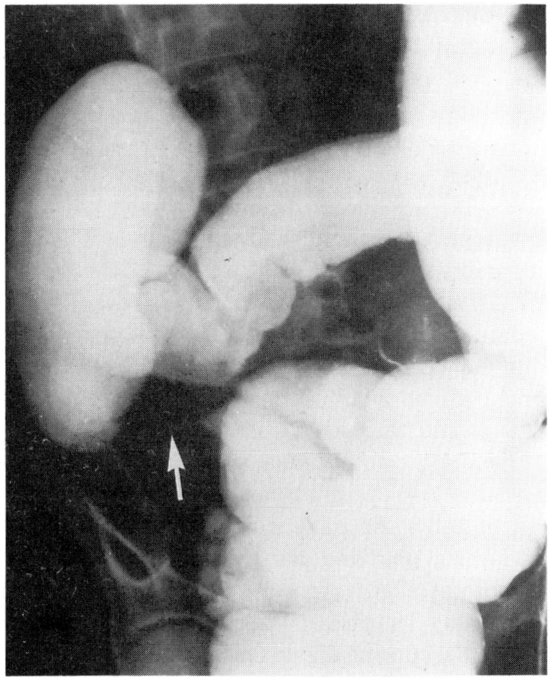

Fig. 33.3 String-sign of Kantor (arrowed): the typical narrow line of barium passing through grossly narrowed segment of terminal ileum in Crohn's disease. This is the most frequently involved part of the intestine. Proximal to the narrowed diseased segment the small bowel appears dilated because of the partial obstruction.

Treatment

Patients presenting without complications needing surgical treatment are started on either corticosteroid drugs or sulphasalazine, or both, and in many this will diminish symptoms and improve general health. The drugs may be continued for months or years, and there is suggestive evidence that prolonged administration may decrease the chances of recurrence of the disease in later years.

Operation may be required urgently for the drainage of an associated abscess, or for the relief of obstruction. The usual principle of incision and drainage is appropriate for such an abscess, but there is quite a high chance that in this case it will be followed by fistula formation. At exploration for obstruction, resection of the diseased segment may be possible, with direct end-to-end anastomosis, but if this is technically difficult or there is considerable distension of proximal bowel, it may be safer to perform an appropriate bypass procedure, leaving possible resection for consideration at a later date, when the patient's condition has improved.

Apart from these emergency indications, elective surgery is advocated when troublesome symptoms fail to come under control with medical measures and where fistulas are present. These latter are unlikely to heal without operation. After bowel preparation, the abdomen is explored, and hopefully the diseased segment is freed, mobilized and resected, with end-to-end anastomosis. The surgeon aims to divide bowel—both proximal and distal to the involved portion—through normal tissue, but at the same time avoiding the removal of excess lengths of apparently normal gut. The reason for this is that functioning mucosa for digestion/absorption may be damaged by future disease, or lost if a later additional resection is required.

If resection proves excessively difficult or hazardous to other important structures, it is permissible instead to bypass the diseased segment, but the subsequent progress is better if resection can be performed.

It is debatable whether treatment with either corticosteroids or sulphasalazine following resection reduces the risk of recurrence in the remaining bowel. It is wise to give a guarded prognosis in Crohn's disease, as recurrence frequently appears even many years after an initially encouraging response to either medical or surgical treatment.

Typhoid ulcers

These ulcers are mostly situated in the terminal ileum with the long axis lying parallel to that of the bowel. Occasionally, paratyphoid ulcers may be found in the large intestine. Perforation, usually occurring in the third week of the illness, declares with the symptoms and signs of peritonitis, i.e. abdominal pain, nausea and vomiting, and on examination there is muscle guarding and an absence of sounds to auscultation. It is a grave complication of typhoid, and its treatment is unsatisfactory. The patient is usually so toxic that laparotomy for the closure of perforation is seldom successful. Expectant treatment with intravenous fluids, gastric suction and administration of parenteral chloramphenicol probably offers the best hope of recovery.

TUMOURS OF THE SMALL INTESTINE

Both benign and malignant tumours occur much more rarely in this organ than in the other parts of the digestive tract.

Benign

Occasionally small adenomas or benign connective tissue tumours such as lipomas, leiomyomas or angiomas can be encountered as coincidental findings during an abdominal operation for some other disorder. Since these are usually quite asymptomatic, there is no need to remove them.

When larger benign tumours cause symptoms, the usual clinical presentation is either as intestinal obstruction from intussusception starting at the lesion itself and drawing the proximal segment of intestine distally, or as a result of anaemia due to repeated small blood loss from ulcerated mucosa overlying the tumour.

In either of these clinical situations local resection of the segment of small intestine bearing the tumour is required.

Peutz–Jeghers syndrome

This is a rare hereditary condition, transmitted by a Mendelian dominant gene. It is characterized by the occurrence of multiple adenomatous polyps containing highly differentiated epithelial elements identical with these of normal mucosa, most frequently in the jejunum, but occasionally also arising in either the stomach or colon, and melanosis of the skin and mucous membranes, chiefly affecting the lips, the mucosa of the mouth, the fingers, or perianal region. Of these various areas the commonest and most easily recognizable is the presence of scattered small areas of brown pigmentation along the edges of the lips.

As far as the intestinal polyps are concerned, these may remain asymptomatic throughout life, or they may present by bleeding into the gastrointestinal tract, or intestinal obstruction due to intussusception. If either of these complications arises it will be necessary to excise the involved segment, but unless the polyps are confined to a relatively short segment of the bowel, it will be impossible to remove them all.

If the condition is suspected, it may be possible to outline the polyps by a double-contrast barium follow-through X-ray examination, but it is unlikely that a complete and accurate assessment of the total number and distribution of the polyps will be achieved.

Malignant change occurring in one or more of these congenital polyps is an extremely rare occurrence.

Malignant

Of the relatively small number of malignant tumours which arise in the small intestine, the two least uncommon are lymphoma and adenocarcinoma. Although there appears to be some variation in the relative incidences of these two types of malignant disease from one country to another, the overall frequencies seem to be about the same. Both types usually come to light clinically by the presentation of either subacute or complete intestinal obstruction.

Malignant lymphoma

Patients affected by this disease are often young adults, and some may give a preceding history of coeliac disease with its characteristic malabsorption picture, since this disorder is known to predispose to the development of lymphoma. It is believed that many of these tumours initially arise from the B lymphocytes or plasma cells. The tumour often infiltrates a segment of the bowel wall without initially producing substantial narrowing of the lumen, and sometimes multiple segments may be involved. Sometimes perforation of the diseased intestine may occur, and as a result the patient presents with peritonitis. Spread occurs to the regional lymphatic nodes, and may subsequently become widespread throughout other areas of the lymphatic system. The converse is also true, in that systematized malignant lymphoma may secondarily involve the intestine.

At operation, required for either obstruction or perforation, the diseased segment or segments should be excised widely, along with the appropriate segment of the mesentery, if this is technically feasible. Subsequent treatment with either radiotherapy or a combination of chemotherapeutic drugs is usually advised. In spite of these various therapeutic endeavours, however, the prognosis is poor.

Adenocarcinoma

Although this may arise at any level in the small intestine, it is more frequent in the jejunum than at a more distal site. Often it grows circumferentially around the bowel, so that sooner or later it causes obstruction. Prior to this episode, however, there may be a history of vague indigestion, and of anaemia from repeated blood loss, but by the time the diagnosis is established, there is frequently spread to the mesenteric lymph nodes or to more distal sites. If the diagnosis is suspected prior to an episode of obstruction, it may be possible to outline it by double-contrast barium follow-through examination.

The main hope of cure for adenocarcinoma of the small intestine is wide resection of the tumour-bearing segment and its associated mesentery, but unfortunately most have advanced beyond the limits of resection by the time they come to laparotomy.

Carcinoid tumour

This interesting but rare group of tumours arises almost exclusively in the region of the terminal ileum and the appendix. Basically those which occur in the appendix behave in a benign fashion and are rarely a threat to life, whereas those of ileal origin display more malignant tendencies, albeit of a low grade.

The tumour arises from the argentaffin cell of the intestinal mucosa, hence the alternative name argentaffinoma. These cells normally produce small quantities of 5-hydroxytryptamine (serotonin), and tumours arising from them retain their capacity to secrete this material and possibly other hormones, so that carcinoid is regarded as an endocrine-secreting tumour. It may belong to the class of tumours designated as arising from the APUD (amine precursor uptake and decarboxylation) system of cells.

5-hydroxytryptamine is normally detoxicated in the liver, but if that organ is extensively infiltrated with secondary deposits, the 5-hydroxytryptamine is released directly into the radicals of the hepatic veins, and therefore enters the systemic circulation. Under these circumstances the patient may present with symptoms due to this excess level of circulating 5-hydroxytryptamine—the carcinoid syndrome. The main features are pulmonary hypertension, due to spasm of the pulmonary arterioles; subsequent pulmonary artery stenosis and right-sided heart failure; diarrhoea; excess borborygmi, and attacks of flushing of the skin over the face and upper trunk, especially after the ingestion of food or alcohol (Fig. 33.4).

Since, as has been noted, carcinoid tumours arising in the appendix are benign and therefore rarely metastasize, manifestations of the carcinoid syndrome do not usually accompany appendiceal lesions. If the syndrome is present it implies that the lesion has primarily arisen in the ileum, and that it has already metastasized to the liver (Fig. 33.5).

The diagnosis of carcinoid affecting the appendix is usually made either as an incidental finding during abdominal exploration, or when it causes symptoms similar to those of acute appendicitis. In either event suspicion of the true nature of the tumour arises from gross inspection, since it is often a bright yellow in colour. Appendicectomy is

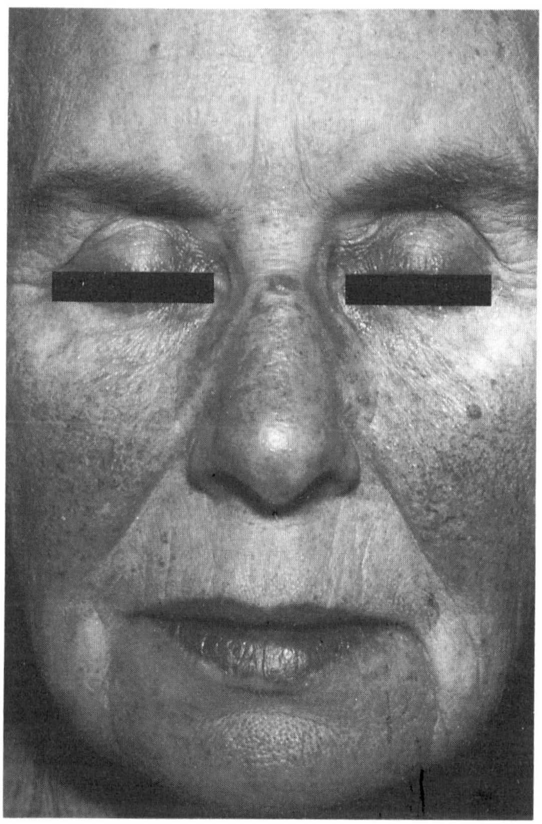

Fig. 33.4 Carcinoid syndrome: the characteristic facial flush, most prominent on the cheeks.

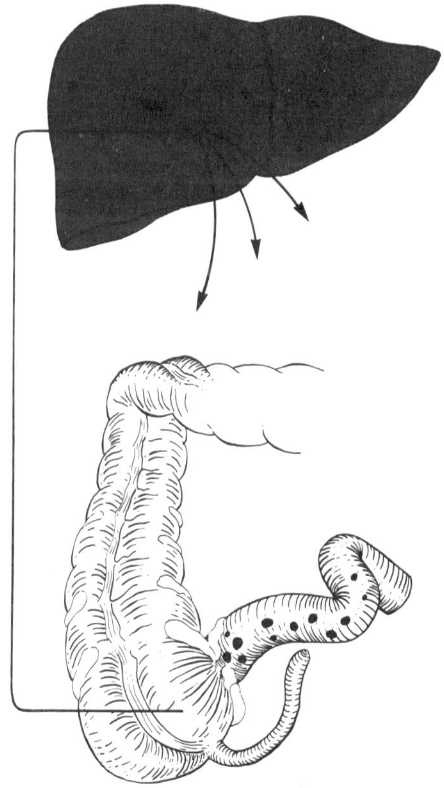

Fig. 33.5 Carcinoid syndrome. When primary tumour arises in the ileum it is often malignant, spreading via the portal blood to the liver. The 5-hydroxytryptamine released from these metastases is responsible for the endocrine manifestations of the syndrome. Any 5-hydroxytryptamine released from the ileal tumour would be inactivated by passage through the liver.

sufficient in most cases, unless it arises at the base of the appendix, when a slightly more extended resection may be necessary.

Ileal carcinoid may present either with some or all of the features of the carcinoid syndrome, or as the result of local symptoms of an obstructive nature. When the condition is suspected a measurement of the urinary excretion of 5-hydroxyindoleacetic acid (5-HIAA), which is a metabolite of 5-hydroxytryptamine, may confirm the diagnosis. An output of more than 10 mg 5-HIAA in 24 h is confirmatory.

Wide resection of the involved segment of ileum, usually involving a right hemicolectomy, is the treatment of choice, and this is still a worthwhile procedure even when there is evidence of metastases in the liver. The tumour tends to be very slow in its further growth, and long survival is still possible.

Although there are some drugs which can act to antagonize the effects of 5-hydroxytryptamine, most of these have troublesome, and indeed serious, side-effects which limit their usefulness. It may therefore be preferable to treat any persistent symptoms of the carcinoid syndrome by appropriate medication, e.g. antidiarrhoeal agents.

34. The appendix

ACUTE APPENDICITIS

Acute inflammation of the appendix is one of the commonest diseases of the abdomen treated surgically (Fig. 34.1). Appendicectomy is one of the commonest operations performed in many countries throughout the world, though in some western countries it is being overtaken by gallbladder operations. The exact cause of the disease is not known. It is thought to be more common in the industrial areas of Europe and North America and this has been attributed to the large intake of meat in these regions. However, total vegetarians are not immune to the disease, and it is difficult to implicate a particular type of diet with appendicitis. Possibly the disease is as common in the developing countries, but the facilities for early diagnosis may not be as good as in the industrially developed countries.

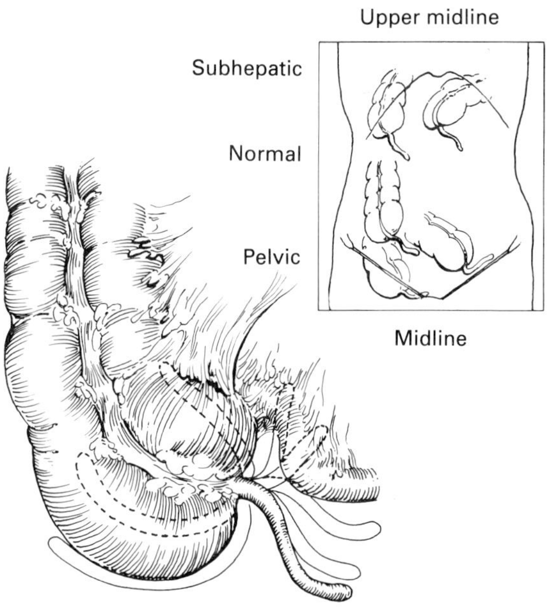

Fig. 34.1 The appendix may lie descending from the caecum and pointing towards the pelvis, or in front of or behind the terminal ileum, or in a retrograde position up alongside or behind the caecum.

Both sexes and persons of all age groups are liable to develop the disease. This is an important fact to remember as it is often difficult to diagnose the disease in the very young and the very old. At both extremes of age the symptoms may be quite difficult for the patient to describe clearly, and the natural defence mechanisms against infection may be deficient. Furthermore, the progress of the disease may be very rapid in these two age groups. There is therefore greater risk of complications and mortality in the very young and very old. The peak incidence is between 15 and 30 years of age.

The common causative organisms are *Escherichia coli*, enterococci, non-haemolytic streptococci, anaerobic streptococci and *Clostridium welchii*. The exact route by which the infection arrives at the appendix is not generally clear. Probably there is more than one way, e.g. the bacteria may come from the lumen of the appendix, especially in cases where the lumen is obstructed; from the blood stream, or via the lymphatics.

Two forms of appendicitis are usually described. In the more common type there is inflammation of the appendix without any obstruction of its lumen. In the less common but more dangerous variety, there is obstruction of the lumen in addition to the inflammation of the organ. It is more dangerous because the pent-up products of inflammation cannot escape into the caecum, and so there is greater danger of gangrene and perforation of the organ. The lumen of the appendix is occluded most commonly by a faecolith, but occasionally the blockage is by a foreign body, or even worms.

Inflammatory changes start in the mucosa, which may then ulcerate, and become the seat of pus formation. If the disease progresses further, thrombosis of the appendicular artery or its branches may lead to generalized or localized gangrene of the organ. The tip of the appendix is more likely to become gangrenous, as the terminal branches of the appendicular artery are likely to be thrombosed earlier than the main artery.

As the inflammation proceeds the organ becomes oedematous and adhesions may develop in which the greater omentum and coils of the small intestine become adherent to the inflamed appendix and caecum. The parietal peritoneum of the region also shows evidence of inflammation and becomes adherent to the inflamed bowel, thus forming an inflammatory appendicular mass (Fig. 34.2).

Infection from an inflamed appendix may spread to the peritoneal cavity, even in the absence of perforation. This may give rise to local abscess formation, generalized peritonitis or the development of an abscess in the pelvis, or more rarely in the subdiaphragmatic region (Fig. 34.3). Pyelophlebitis and liver abscess are extremely rare complications of this disease.

In a proportion of patients spontaneous resolution occurs, and over a number of days all the signs of inflammation disappear. However, it is impossible to predict with certainty when resolution will occur or when any one of the dangerous complications listed above may develop.

Clinical features

The illness usually starts with the patient feeling generally unwell and with reduced appetite, plus perhaps nausea and even vomiting. A dull, ill-localized central abdominal colicky pain builds up, and after an hour or so pain moves into the right iliac fossa, changing in nature to a more severe, sharper, more constant pain, which steadily increases in severity. At this stage the patient usually wants to lie still, with the right hip slightly flexed. There is most often mild constipation, e.g. the bowel

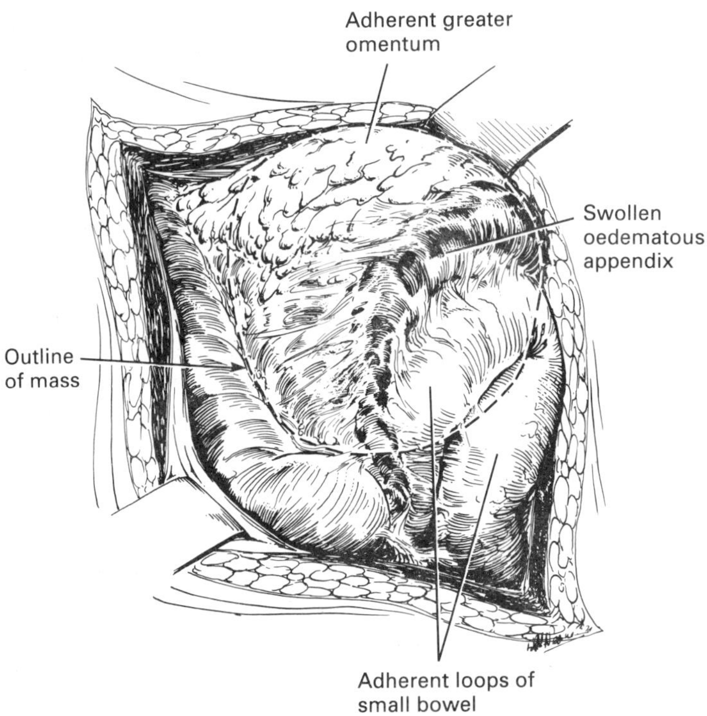

Fig. 34.2 A palpable tender mass in the right iliac fossa may form from a combination of the swollen, oedematous appendix plus adherent tongues of the greater omentum and adjacent loops of small intestine.

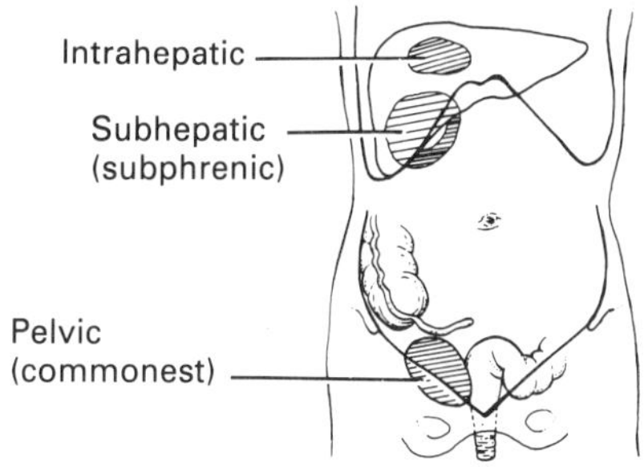

Fig. 34.3 Various possible sites for an abscess to form as the result of spillage of infection from the inflamed appendix.

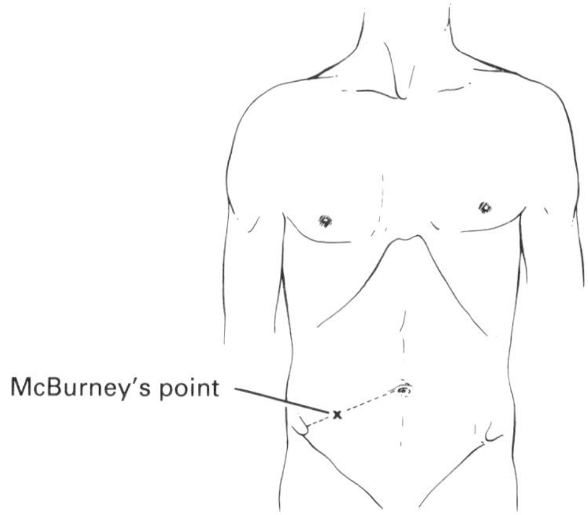

Fig. 34.4 McBurney's point—two-thirds of the way along a line drawn from the umbilicus to the anterior superior iliac spine.

may not have been opened for 1–2 days. Occasionally, however, if the inflamed appendix is lying down in the pelvis, in contact with the sigmoid colon or upper rectum, there may be diarrhoea.

Although it is claimed that there is more colic, nausea and vomiting in the obstructive type of acute appendicitis than in that not associated with obstruction, this is not a clear-cut differential feature, and it is not really possible to make a confident classification into these two patterns—nor is it important as far as management is concerned.

On examination, the patient looks generally unwell, the tongue is usually coated and there is foetor. A moderate degree of tachycardia arises, between 80–90 beat/min, and the temperature also increases by 1 or 2°. In children the tachycardia and pyrexia may be even greater.

On abdominal examination the most reliable sign is localized tenderness in the right iliac fossa, usually at or near McBurney's point (Fig. 34.4), i.e. two-thirds of the way along a line drawn from the umbilicus to the right anterior superior iliac spine. However, when the appendix lies in the retrocaecal position the point of maximal tenderness may be at a higher level, and when it lies low in the fossa it may be at a lower level. For each individual the accurately reproducible, constantly situated local tenderness is the clearest confirmation of the clinical diagnosis. Certainly the presence of one or more of the following signs is helpful as further pointers to the disease, but these are not essential or as reliable indicators.

First, there may be rebound tenderness, i.e. a sharp stab of pain across the abdomen immediately after the sudden release of pressure by the examiner's hand, which has previously been pressed slowly but firmly down on the abdominal wall away from the tender area. This is such a painful experience that it is wise to leave the examination to detect this sign until the end of the physical examination. Next, it may be possible, in a proportion of patients, to elicit pain in the right iliac fossa by deep pressure with the examining hand in the left iliac fossa. This may be attributed either to back pressure along the colon to distend the caecal area, or to simple stretching of the abdominal wall irritating the inflamed area of parietal peritoneum over the appendix.

In the majority of cases the diagnosis is straightforward on the history and physical findings, and no special investigations are required to establish it. However, in a small number of cases there may be difficulty in differentiating acute appendicitis from the following conditions.

It may be difficult to distinguish between acute appendicitis and non-specific mesenteric adenitis. In the latter condition, almost exclusively found in children from 5 to15 years of age, the patient does not look ill, and is generally completely free from pain between bouts of colic. On turning the patient to the left side, tenderness may also shift towards the left. These are some of the features which help in diagnosing mesenteric adenitis. However, if the child does not show marked improvement in the next few hours, it is best to diagnose and treat the condition as acute appendicitis.

In acute salpingitis, the onset of abdominal pain

usually follows menstruation. A history of vaginal discharge, dysmenorrhoea and menstrual irregularities is often obtained. Pain starts and continues in the lower abdomen and there is usually no preliminary central pain or discomfort. There is usually marked tenderness on vaginal examination.

In rupture of a right-sided tubal pregnancy the pain also starts in the lower abdomen and stays there. There is generally a history of a missed period, but on occasions this is absent. On vaginal examination the cervix is soft and there is intense pain when it is moved. The amount of bleeding into the peritoneal cavity varies, but may be large, leading to signs of severe blood loss, e.g. tachycardia, hypotension, pallor, sweating, shallow rapid respiration, and perhaps full-blown hypovolaemic shock. Since the condition occurs in young and generally otherwise fit women there may be considerable physiological adaptation to blood loss, especially an increase in the peripheral resistance by shut down of the splanchnic and other non-essential vascular beds. There may, therefore, be relatively little increase in heart rate or change in blood pressure etc. However, as soon as general anaesthesia is induced the peripheral resistance may fall abruptly and severe hypotension and other signs of hypovolaemic shock may suddenly present. It is wise, therefore, when a diagnosis of possible rupture of an ectopic pregnancy is entertained, to group the patient and cross-match several units of blood to be available before induction of anaesthesia.

Complications of ovarian cysts, notably torsion, rupture or haemorrhage into the cyst, can all come into the differential diagnosis of acute appendicitis. In all three instances the onset of pain is sudden, and usually located quite low in the iliac fossa. Marked tenderness is elicited on performing vaginal examination but if the tenderness is not excessive the fullness of the cyst mass may be palpable on the relevant side of the pouch of Douglas.

Pneumonia and right-sided pleurisy may occasionally give rise to referred abdominal pain. Chest signs may therefore be sought and X-ray of the chest may be helpful.

Perforated peptic ulcer may sometimes mimic acute appendicitis if the maximum tenderness appears to be concentrated in the right iliac fossa.

Acute cholecystitis can sometimes resemble acute appendicitis. Confusion is more likely to arise when the inflamed appendix lies in a high retrocaecal position. In some cases an urgent ultrasound examination may be helpful.

Ureteric colic should be diagnosed by the typical distribution of the pain in this disease. If stone colic is present microscopic examination of the urine will reveal haematuria, and this is a very useful means of confirming the diagnosis.

In acute pyelonephritis, frequency of micturition, tenderness confined to the right loin, pus in the urine and high temperature with rigors are the chief features which should help to distinguish it from acute appendicitis. This distinction may be more difficult in pregnancy.

Diabetes is another possibility which should always be kept in mind, as sometimes diabetic coma is preceded by attacks of abdominal pain. The urine should always be examined for sugar routinely on admitting a patient with abdominal pain.

Notwithstanding the above list of the more important diagnostic problems, surgical teaching remains that pain in the abdomen with nausea, anorexia, fever and tenderness in the right iliac fossa should be diagnosed and treated as appendicitis unless there are clear indicators to some alternative pathology.

Management

The treatment of acute appendicitis is appendicectomy. Operation is carried out as soon as possible, and the result should be complete cure.

If the patient presents with signs and symptoms of generalized peritonitis, rapid correction of any fluid or metabolic disturbance may be needed by intravenous therapy and gastric suction, and antibiotics may be started. As soon as the patient is judged fit to withstand surgery, appendicectomy is carried out.

The only exception to urgent operation is if, when the patient is first seen, a well defined appendicular mass has developed. It is then worth trying an expectant line of treatment in the hope that the inflammatory mass will subside, and appendicectomy can be performed more safely at a later date, usually in 6–8 weeks. The essentials of this expectant line of treatment are as follows:

1. Absolute bedrest.

2. Only water is allowed by mouth in the first few hours. If the condition appears to be settling down, other fluids are also then allowed. Solid food is not given as long as the mass persists.
3. A broad-spectrum antibiotic is exhibited.
4. An hourly record of pulse rate and a 4-hourly record of temperature is kept.
5. The mass in the abdomen is marked with a skin pencil and its size is judged in relation to this outline every day till the mass disappears or the line of treatment is changed.

The majority of the patients settle down on this regimen. When all signs and symptoms have disappeared, the patient is sent home with the advice to return for appendicectomy after 6–8 weeks.

If the patient does not show signs of improvement on this regimen in the next 24 h, this line of treatment is discontinued. Indicators of deterioration are a rise in the pulse rate, elevation of temperature, increase in the size of the abdominal mass, increase in pain or vomiting or the abdominal tenderness becoming more widespread. These symptoms and signs point to the fact that the inflammation is not being contained and overcome, and is no longer well localized. Laparotomy is indicated and the exact procedure depends on the operative findings. If an abscess is present this should be evacuated and a drain is left emerging from its depths through the wound. If, on the other hand, the mass comprises the swollen appendix plus adherent omentum and loops of intestine, a careful and taxing dissection may be required to dissect free and remove the appendix.

RECURRENT APPENDICITIS

Recurrent but mild attacks of acute appendicitis do occur in some patients and probably the majority eventually present with a severe enough attack to merit appendicectomy.

TUMOURS OF THE APPENDIX

The appendix is an infrequent site of tumour formation. Rarely a lipoma, adenoma or myoma are encountered as coincidental findings during laparotomy or appendicectomy.

Among the more active tumours, carcinoid tumour is the most likely to be met in clinical practice. Unlike similar tumours in the small intestine, it usually does not give rise to metastasis. The majority of the carcinoids are situated near the tip of the appendix and only a small number are found at the base. The tumour can usually be recognized on naked-eye examination because the cut surface is yellow.

Clinically, the commonest presentation is that of acute appendicitis. Any 5-hydroxytryptamine secreted by the tumour would be inactivated by the liver, so that there will be no hormonal effects of the carcinoid syndrome, e.g. facial flushing and diarrhoea. The latter arise only when metastatic deposits in the liver, which arise only from small intestinal carcinoid, secrete 5-hydroxytryptamine directly into the systemic circulation in the hepatic vein. If the removed appendix bears the tumour near the tip, nothing further needs to be done. If the tumour is situated near the base and excision appears to be incomplete, right hemicolectomy is recommended.

Adenocarcinoma is also rarely found in the appendix. The pathology, clinical features and treatment are similar to those of identical tumours of the caecum. The condition is described in Chapter 35.

35. The large intestine

The proximal part of the large intestine, from the caecum to the junction of the middle and lateral thirds of the transverse colon, is a part of the embryological midgut and the rest develops from the hind gut. The former, therefore, receives its blood supply from the branches of the superior mesenteric artery and the latter from the inferior mesenteric artery. Visceral pain arising from the proximal part, including the appendix, is felt round the umbilicus in the centre of the abdomen, whereas visceral pain from the descending and pelvic colon is felt in the lower abdomen below a line joining the anterior superior iliac spines.

The large intestine is smaller in length than the small intestine but is larger in circumference. In gross intestinal obstruction, however, there may be enormous distension of the small intestine, and the two may be distinguished from each other on X-ray by the presence of haustrations produced by taenia coli in the large intestine.

Neighbouring structures which are encountered in surgical mobilization of the colon and whose integrity should be maintained by careful dissection are the ureters, and on the right side the mid-parts of the duodenum.

The chief functions of the large intestine are absorption of water and some electrolytes and the forward transmission of the residue and its temporary storage till convenient for defecation. Normally, about 900 ml of water is absorbed daily from the large intestine. A greater part of the absorption occurs on the right side, as evidenced by the fact that more fluid faeces is passed through a caecostomy than through transverse or pelvic colostomy. However, absorption of water from the colon is not of critical importance in the sense that many individuals can lead a healthy life after complete removal of the colon for diseases like ulcerative colitis, regional enteritis or cancer.

Very small quantities of amino acids are absorbed in health from the colon. A small quantity of nitrogenous material, produced by the bacterial digestion of protein, is also absorbed and taken to the liver where it is detoxicated. In portal hypertension, there is enlargement of portasystemic communications which may be further increased by portacaval anastomosis produced surgically. In these conditions, nitrogenous products of bacterial action on protein may be directly absorbed into the systemic circulation and cause deleterious effects on the central nervous system, giving rise to portasystemic encephalopathy. This can be checked either by omitting protein from the diet or by reducing the bacterial population of thc colon by antibiotic therapy. Giving enemas may avoid the intestinal residue remaining long enough in the colon for significant absorption to occur.

Defecation is a reflex act which is initiated by distension of the rectum by bowel content. This is followed simultaneously by the development of a wave of mass contraction in the proximal bowel and relaxation of external and internal sphincters with consequently the expulsion of the faeces. In this reflex only the neural plexuses of the colon and the short sacral nerves are involved.

CONGENITAL DISORDERS

There are two congenital lesions of the large intestine which are of surgical interest. These are familial multiple polyposis and congenital megacolon (Hirschsprung's disease).

Familial polyposis of the colon is a rare disease of congenital origin, characterized by the development of multiple polyps in the large intestine. It is transmitted as a Mendelian dominant by both sexes to both sexes. The tumours are not normally present at birth and probably develop during adolescence and early adult life. Most cases become symptomatic at about 20 years of age. The rectum and sigmoid colon are the commonest sites affected but polyps may develop in any part of the large bowel from the ileocaecal region to the anus.

In the early stages, there are raised sessile areas of mucosa which are separated from each other by normal mucosa. Later, with further proliferation of the glandular tissue of the affected mucosa, the sessile patches become pedunculated. The number of sessile and pedunculated tumours varies greatly, sometimes amounting to hundreds scattered throughout the large intestine. The risk of one or more becoming frank adenocarcinoma is extremely high; the majority of patients develop cancer sooner or later if they live long enough. On average the age of developing this cancer of bowel is much younger than that not associated with familial polyposis, the condition being not uncommon even in the 30s.

Clinically, symptoms of familial multiple polyposis usually develop in the late teens or early 20s. There are attacks of lower abdominal pain, possibly diarrhoea and the passage of mucus and blood per rectum and sometimes tenesmus.

Rectal examination may reveal multiple sessile or pedunculated rounded masses in the rectum. This is confirmed by sigmoidoscopy. A contrast barium enema should be done to search for other proximal polyps which show as multiple filling defects. Colonoscopy will allow an even more accurate assessment of the number, size and distribution of the lesions, and also biopsy of any which may appear to be in any way irregular or otherwise suspicious of malignant change.

All patients in whom the disease has been diagnosed should be advised to have surgical removal of the colon.

Ideally the only way to provide a complete protection against malignant disease is to remove every bit of mucosa at risk, i.e. panproctocolectomy, leaving the patient with a permanent ileostomy. However, this is understandably difficult for many patients to accept, for many different reasons, and therefore the slightly lesser procedure of total colectomy, with preservation of the distal rectum and ileorectal anastomosis, may be preferred. With this operation, however, it will be strongly desirable to make regular, 6-monthly review proctoscopic examinations to detect, hopefully at an early stage, any malignant change in the residual rectal or anal canal mucosa. If this is detected then it becomes necessary to remove the rectum at a second operation and create an ileostomy.

All sibs of any patient presenting with familial polyposis should be strongly exhorted to have at least screening sigmoidoscopy and double-contrast barium enema. It is likely that several will be discovered to have multiple polyps, and these should be advised also to undergo total colectomy even if asymptomatic, so high is the risk of carcinoma of the colon developing in them. This is a difficult decision to accept, but it is a wise course of action to take, rather than wait till frank carcinoma develops, when it may well be too late to cure the patient. Should operation be refused, the patient should at least be kept under regular surveillance, at least 6-monthly, preferably with repeat barium enema or colonoscopy.

HIRSCHSPRUNG'S DISEASE

Primary megacolon or Hirschsprung's disease is an uncommon congenital condition in which there is an absence of parasympathetic ganglia in a segment of the terminal part of the large intestine, i.e. the anal canal, the rectum and a variable part of the more proximal colon. In the majority of cases, however, the absence of ganglia extends only to the pelvirectal junction. Rarely, the whole of the colon or even the whole gut is involved.

The affected part of the bowel is spastic and remains contracted but otherwise looks normal. Immediately above this contracted part there is a segment of the bowel in which the ganglion cells are present but only in small numbers. Usually, this transitional zone is about 2–5 cm long. Above this transitional zone the bowel contains the normal number of ganglia. Looking at the bowel, the aganglionic segment appears collapsed. The transitional zone above it is in the form of a cone with its apex directed downwards, and the bowel with the normal number of ganglia is grossly dilated. Histological examination of the aganglionic segment shows an absence of Meissner's plexus from the submucous plane, and of Auerbach's plexus from the intermuscular plane.

The physiological effect of the aganglionic segment is intestinal obstruction, as propulsive waves do not pass through it and therefore the contents of this part of the intestine do not move. There is dilatation of the proximal unaffected colon, all coats of which show compensatory hypertrophy.

Clinical features

The disease tends to run in families and boys are affected seven to eight times more often than girls.

In virtually all cases, symptoms of constipation appear soon after birth. The baby may fail to pass meconium. Rectal examination at this stage reveals an empty rectum and the examining finger appears to be gripped tightly by the anus and the rectum. Following rectal examination some meconium may be passed. There is increasing abdominal distension and loud borborygmi may be noticed.

In about 10% of cases, the disease manifests itself in the form of chronic constipation. The baby has a protruberant abdomen and fails to thrive. There is anaemia, and in contrast to the protuberant abdomen, the rest of the body looks emaciated.

Diagnosis is established on the basis of clinical examination, radiology and biopsy of the rectal wall. Barium enema is performed using a fine emulsion of barium in normal saline. Tap water is not used as the dilated hypertrophic proximal colon absorbs water rapidly and there is real danger of water intoxication and death. Barium enema X-ray shows a contracted rectum; a cone-shaped area of bowel above it and distended colon above the transitional zone.

Rectal biopsy will reveal the absence of Auerbach's and Meissner's plexuses if the biopsy has been taken sufficiently deeply. A superficial bite which includes only mucosa will not be adequate.

Management

The only curative treatment of the condition is the excision of the aganglionic segment and restoration of continuity of the intestine, usually by anastomosis of the unaffected colon to the anal canal. In cases of acute intestinal obstruction, it is best if a transverse colostomy is performed and the definitive operation is postponed to a later date.

DIVERTICULAR DISEASE

Diverticula are present in the large intestine in many individuals, one estimate suggesting in about 5% of white people of both sexes above the age of 40 years. The sigmoid colon is the part most commonly affected, and the caecum and ascending colon the least often. Rarely there is a solitary diverticulum in the caecum which, if it becomes inflamed, can mimic either acute appendicitis or carcinoma of the caecum. Chronic constipation may be a predisposing factor in the development of the diverticula, and there is much suspicion that the western-type diet, low in bran and vegetable roughage, is responsible, by reducing faecal bulk and encouraging localized segments of colon to be temporarily occluded; pressure rises and this may lead to 'blow-outs' of mucosa through points of weakness in the muscular layers of the bowel (Fig. 35.1). Most diverticula develop near the me-

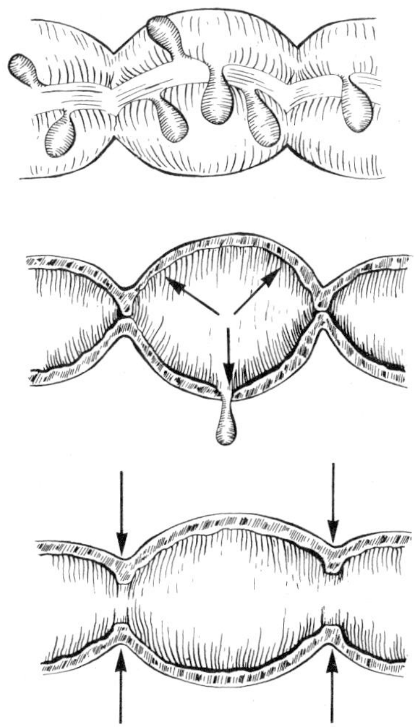

Fig. 35.1 Likely mechanism of production of diverticula. An isolated segment of colon is temporarily closed at either end by firm contraction waves completely occluding the lumen. As a result of the increased pressure a pouch of mucosa protrudes at the weakest point in the bowel wall, where the blood vessels penetrate it.

senteric border of the bowel at points of entry of the blood vessels, and these are natural points of weakness. The diverticula do not possess a muscular coat but comprise only mucosa and serosa. The opening into them may be wide or narrow.

In many individuals, the diverticula remain symptomless. However, it is easy to understand how inflammation and infection can arise because of stasis and obstruction of the neck of one or more diverticula, and when this occurs the disorder is termed diverticulitis. The mucosa becomes oedematous and congested and the overlying visceral peritoneum is also inflamed. In acute cases, an abscess may develop in the inflamed diverticulum or in the paracolic region. This may remain well localized or leak into the general peritoneal cavity, causing peritonitis.

In more chronic cases as a result of repeated inflammatory episodes, the involved segment may become adherent to the bladder or a loop of small intestine, and a fistula may develop into either structure.

Furthermore chronic inflammatory thickening and fibrosis of the involved colon result in narrowing of its lumen and shortening of its length, thus causing either acute or subacute obstruction. Rarely profuse haemorrhage can arise from erosion of the vessels passing through the weak points, which were the source of the diverticula in the first place.

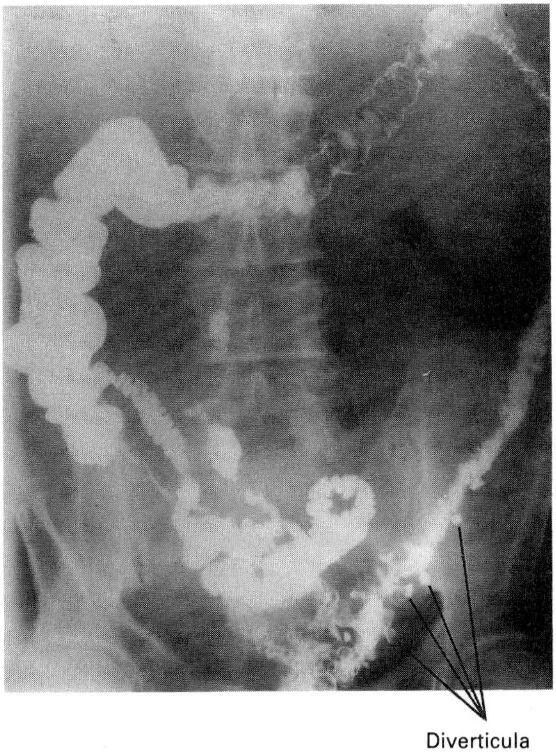

Fig. 35.2 Diverticular disease of the sigmoid colon. The multiple rounded diverticula are clearly shown filled by barium during a barium enema . The sigmoid colon is the commonest site for these, but a few are also seen in part of the descending colon.

Clinical features

As has already been mentioned, the disorder is often asymptomatic and may remain unnoticed unless a barium enema examination is performed for some other reason (Fig. 35.2).

When symptoms do arise, they may be relatively mild, with occasional lower abdominal discomfort, slight alteration in bowel habit towards either diarrhoea or constipation, feeling of distension, and passage of increased amounts of flatus. Most of these complaints are due to increased spasm and disordered bowel activity and perhaps minimal inflammatory changes.

When episodes of local infection with or without an associated paracolic abscess occur, there are the more acute symptoms of nausea, anorexia, fever, severe lower abdominal pain, perhaps vomiting and either marked constipation or profuse diarrhoea. On examination there is often a definite tender mass in the left iliac fossa representing the inflamed, swollen, thickened colon or abscess. Temperature, white cell count and erythrocyte sedimentation rate are all usually elevated. With appropriate treatment the symptoms and signs will usually gradually resolve over a few days to a week, but perhaps to be followed by recurrence at a later date.

The various complications which may arise will present their own clinical manifestations. Perforation gives the picture of peritonitis, with severe general abdominal pain aggravated by any movement, and severe toxicity; bleeding is usually the passage of fresh red blood per rectum with the accompanying signs of blood loss; fistula into the bladder will cause dirty urine with sediment or even gas bubbles passed along with the urine; and complete obstruction.

Management

Those with the mildest form of complaints from diverticular disease may require only to regulate their diet, paying particular attention to having a regular daily intake of bran, vegetable and fruit. If this is not sufficient one of the proprietary preparations which adsorb water and thereby increase faecal bulk may be helpful.

If the lower abdominal pain is troublesome an antispasmodic such as mebeverine, hyoscine butylbromide or dicyclomine hydrochloride can give relief.

More severe episodes of infection and abscess formation will require rest in bed, a broad-spectrum antibiotic, fluid–only diet, and close observation for possible complications.

For the patient who has disease localized to one segment of the colon, usually the sigmoid, and who has had several acute disabling attacks, the question of elective resection of the diseased bowel arises. As long as this is done in an interval between flare-ups, a straightforward end-to-end anastomosis can be made. This operation may free the patient of further symptoms, but it is wise to encourage adhering to a high-roughage type of diet to minimize the chances of further diverticula occurring in other parts of the colon.

Surgical treatment will also be required for the complications of peritonitis and obstruction, fistula, and on rare occasions when severe bleeding fails to stop spontaneously. Where there is leakage into the peritoneum, laparotomy, thorough saline lav-

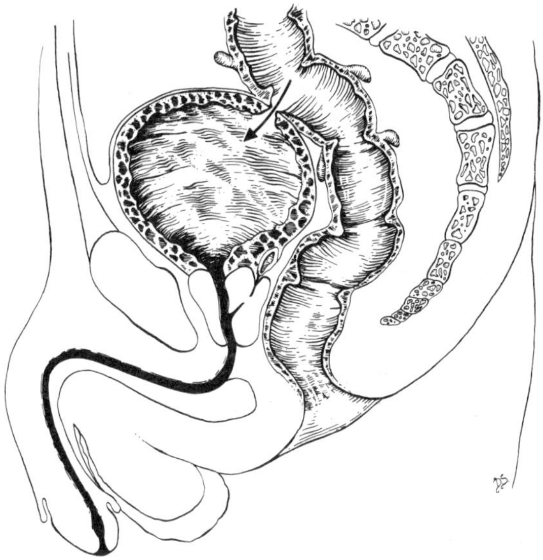

Fig. 35.3 Vesicocolic fistula: an infected diverticulum has become adherent to the wall of the urinary bladder and the inflammatory process has penetrated through the latter to produce direct communication—the fistula.

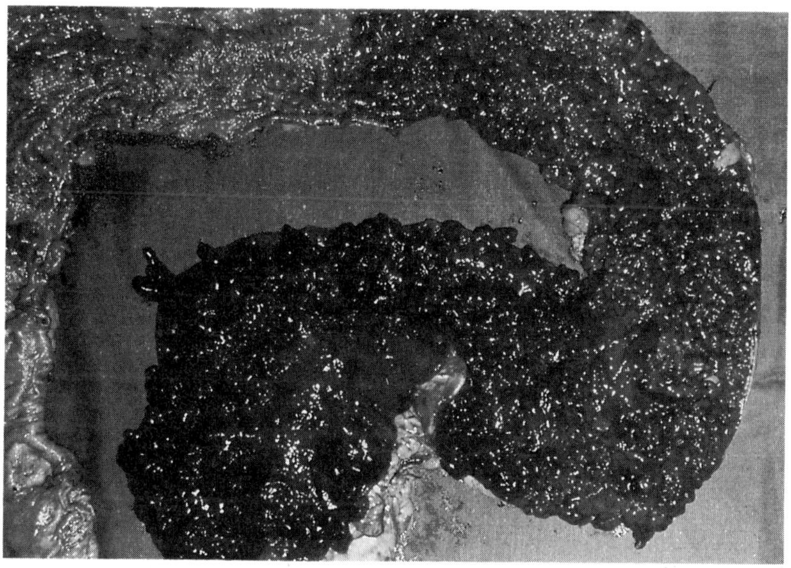

Fig. 35.4 Ulcerative colitis: resected colectomy specimen showing gross changes more in the distal segments. There is loss of the normal mucosal folds, and considerable pseudo-polyp formation-nodular attempts at repair of the denuded areas.

age, and either resection or some form of repair is necessary, and it is safest to add a proximal colostomy, usually in the transverse colon. Obstruction is again usually managed by colostomy and resection of the diseased segment either at the same time, or more likely as a second delayed procedure, so that the anastomosis does not involve distended, weakened bowel. A vesicocolic fistula (Fig. 35.3) is usually a small, well defined track which after appropriate bowel preparation and antibiotics to minimize the bladder infection can often be disconnected quite easily, with suture repair of the bladder defect and resection of the diseased colon with end-to-end anastomosis.

If all attempts to control bleeding from a segment of diverticular disease have failed resection of the segment may rarely be the only way of stopping exsanguination.

Surgical drainage may be required for large paracolic abscesses, if these are clearly outlined and seen to be 'pointing'. Any faecal fistula which may develop at the site following drainage can be expected to dry up spontaneously provided there is no distal obstruction.

Finally, it is worth stressing that the differential diagnosis between diverticular disease and carcinoma of the sigmoid or neighbouring areas of colon may on occasions be extremely difficult. Both are common in the same age group; both may cause lower abdominal discomfort, bowel irregularity, bleeding, and a palpable mass in the left iliac fossa. Although each has its own classical features on X-ray the picture may be atypical and confusing. Finally, both may be present together in the same patient. For all of these reasons it is understandable that great diagnostic uncertainty can arise. Where there is such doubt it is particularly important to get good endoscopic visualization and biopsy material from the diseased part of bowel.

ULCERATIVE COLITIS

Ulcerative colitis is a disease of unknown aetiology, almost always affecting the rectum and spreading back to a variable extent into the colon. Sometimes in its mildest forms it remains limited to the rectum, but when it is most severe it can involve the entire large bowel right back to the caecum. Pathologically it is characterized by patchy diffuse inflammation of the mucosa, granularity and eventual ulceration of the mucosa (Fig. 35.4). Although the exact cause of the disease is not known, a number of factors have been implicated from time to time. These include emotional stress, allergy to milk and its products, secondary infection and autoimmune phenomena.

It is usually a disease of the young, the highest incidence being in the 20s, and it may occasionally occur in children.

At first there is congestion of the mucosa which becomes oedematous and bleeds easily to the touch. Minute, discrete, superficial abscesses develop into ulcers which later may coalesce to form large ulcers. Microscopically, there is intense infiltration of the mucosa with leukocytes, plasma cells and eosinophils. In response to the inflammatory damage fibrous tissue laid down may produce shortening of the colon, and loss of the normal haustration pattern.

Mucosa adjoining ulcerated areas may become heaped up and oedematous and overhang the ulcers as pseudopolyps. Ulcerative colitis is a premalignant condition; the risk of carcinoma increases with the duration of the disease, the severity of attacks and the extent of colonic involvement.

In acute phases of the disease, segments of the colon may become extremely dilated—the so-called toxic dilatation. This complication carries a very real risk of perforation occurring, with the escape of highly dangerous bowel contents into the peritoneal cavity.

The profuse diarrhoea, with the discharge of mucus and blood in the acute stage of the disease, may lead to hypovolaemia, anaemia and vitamin deficiencies.

In addition to the gastrointestinal symptoms various systemic complications may arise, particularly after the disease has been present for some time. These include stomatitis, skin lesions, e.g. erythema nodosum or pyoderma gangrenosum, liver damage including cirrhosis, iritis, renal disease, polyarthritis and ankylosing spondylitis.

Clinical features

Typically there are attacks of diarrhoea with remissions. During an attack, there is classically watery diarrhoea with the rectal discharge of blood and mucus, and sometimes frank pus, and as many as 10–20 bowel actions per day may take place. The periods of remission which may occur spontaneously or be induced by treatment may be weeks, months, or in mild cases, even years.

In those severely affected by the disorder there may occasionally occur a fulminating pattern of relapse, with prostration, fever, malaise, and an almost incessant outpouring of bloody diarrhoea. The patient may well become obviously dehydrated, anaemic and hypoproteinaemic. The abdomen will often become distended with discomfort or pain and tenderness. In these severe attacks there is the real risk of segmental toxic dilatation and subsequent perforation, unless the attack is rapidly and effectively brought under control.

At the other end of the severity spectrum, and probably part of the same basic disorder, is the patient who may be troubled only by recurrent mild episodes of proctitis, with local discomfort and the passage of small stools mixed with blood and mucus, but in whom the pathological changes never extend above the rectum and the course is a relatively mild one.

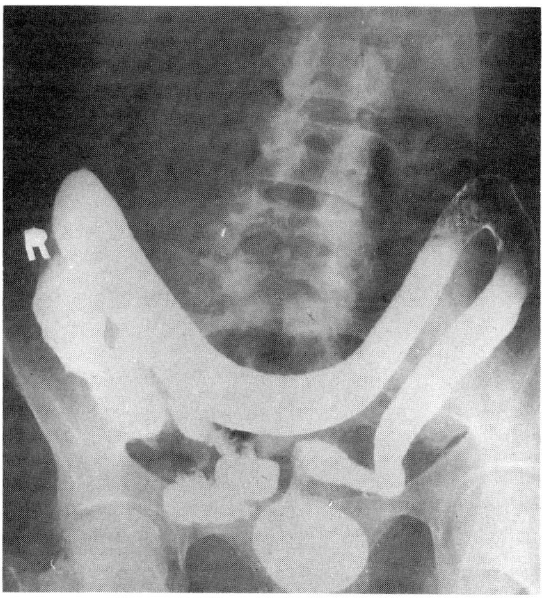

Fig. 35.5 Typical barium enema appearances in severe ulcerative colitis. The entire colon seems shortened, and there are no signs of normal haustral or contraction-wave patterns anywhere along the bowel, hence the oft-used term *hosepipe* to describe the picture. The small area at the splenic flexure showing the mucosal pattern reveals no normal folds, but rather a finely mottled appearance indicating areas of damage or destruction.

The diagnosis is usually established on the basis of the clinical history, physical examination, sigmoidoscopy and barium enema findings.

On sigmoidoscopic examination, in early cases, the mucosa appears to be oedematous and red and bleeds easily to the touch. At a later stage ulcers and pseudopolyps may be seen. A biopsy should be taken for histological examination.

A barium enema shows loss of haustrations in the early stages (Fig. 35.5). Later on, the colon may appear shortened as a narrow pipe. Pseudopolyps, if sizeable, may appear as filling defects on good-quality air contrast films.

Management

Patients having severe attacks should be admitted to hospital and will require intravenous fluid replacement, perhaps blood transfusion, and either prednisolone in a dose of 40-60 mg/day or adrenocorticotrophic hormone 80–120 mg parenterally. If there are no signs of distinct clinical improvement within 2–3 days, and particularly if there is evidence of toxic dilatation, urgent surgical resection—almost certainly total colectomy—may be required. Usually, however, these measures do bring the acute attack under control.

Less severe attacks may be helped by smaller doses of oral prednisolone, e.g. 20-40 mg/day, for 2–3 weeks, and then discontinued. For disease confined to the rectum or distal colon, prednisolone may be given either as retention enema or suppositories, or a foam rectal instillation.

Sulphasalazine (Salazopyrin) is also useful in many patients to induce remission, and furthermore if continued after the attack has subsided will decrease the chances of further relapse. It is often, therefore, used as maintenance therapy. Corticosteroids do not seem to act in this way and should not be continued long-term in a prophylactic manner.

In the follow-up of patients with ulcerative colitis attention should be paid to nutrition, vitamin and haematinic requirements.

Surgical treatment

As already mentioned, operation may be urgently required for those with severe fulminating disease or toxic dilatation who fail to respond quickly to steroid treatment and fluid replacement, or for severe blood loss.

Elective operation should be considered when the disease is progressive, disabling the patient, interfering with nutrition or associated with the systemic complications outlined above. In children the disease may interfere with normal growth and development and for this reason operation to rid the patient of the cause of retardation may be wise. Finally the risk or actual development of carcinoma of the colon in patients with extensive involvement of bowel and several years' history of the complaint may be the reason to advise operation.

The aim of surgery is to remove the diseased tissue, and for many years , this implied panproctocolectomy, with the formation of a permanent spout ileostomy (Fig. 35.6). More recently the less radical approach of total colectomy with preservation of the rectum and ileorectal anastomosis has been advocated by some surgeons. A further refinement has been the coring out of the rectal mucosa and anastomosis of the ileum to the lower part of the denuded rectum or anal canal. Direct end–to–end anastomosis of ileum to rectum is likely to lead to very liquid motions, urgency and incontinence, and much better bowel function and control may result if a pouch is created from the ileum and this is joined to the rectum. Various patterns of pouch have been advocated, from a simple J–shape to more elaborate W- and S–shaped ones (Fig. 35.7). Although these procedures clearly avoid the necessity of an ileostomy they may lead to difficulty with

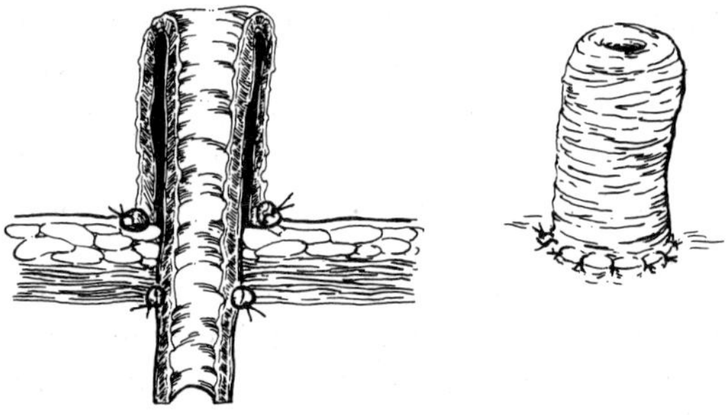

Fig. 35.6 Terminal ileostomy. After removal of the entire colon (and rectum) the divided end of the ileum is brought out through a neatly fitting circular wound, to project several centimetres beyond the skin. Then the wall is turned out on itself so that a spout is formed, and the edge of the mucosa is sutured exactly to the skin edge.

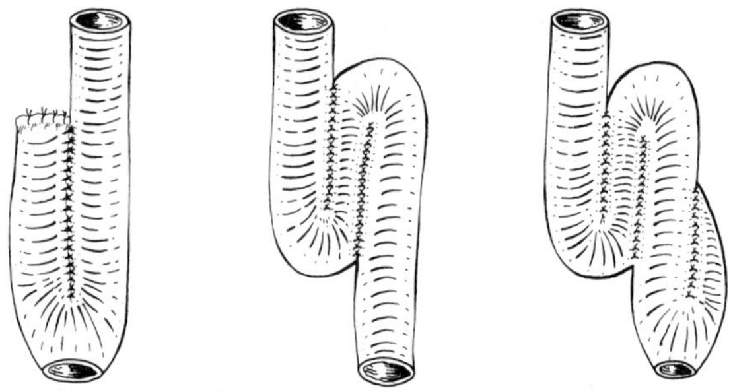

Fig. 35.7 Various patterns of ileal pouch, which can be formed to be brought down into the pelvis, and anastomosed to a residual stump of the rectum or anal canal. The simplest is a J-type, with a single segment folded back, but more elaborate and larger-volume pouches can be created by using a greater number of folded segments.

anal continence and will require careful and prolonged follow-up in case of complications in any small rectal stump which remains.

If a straightforward end ileostomy is fashioned it is important to have good mucosa-to-skin apposition and a spout of ileum projecting 3–4 cm out of the skin wound, so that the potentially erosive contents can be led clearly into a closely fitting adhesive connected plastic ileostomy bag. Once the patient is trained on its emptying, care and regular replacement, he or she should be able to resume a full range of normal activities. Several means of creating continent ileostomy pouches have been devised, but these require considerable skill and may pose various difficulties to both patient and surgeon.

REGIONAL ENTERITIS (CROHN'S DISEASE)

The aetiology and pathology of regional enteritis are dealt with in Chapter 33, but as mentioned there, the colon can also become involved by this disease. There is, in fact, evidence that colonic involvement is being increasingly recognized in many western countries. The course of this disease in the colon often simulates that of ulcerative colitis: both are characterized by attacks of diarrhoea and bleeding. Treatment is also more or less along the same lines. However, there are some differences in pathology, clinical features and details of treatment.

In regional enteritis there may be 'skip' areas of

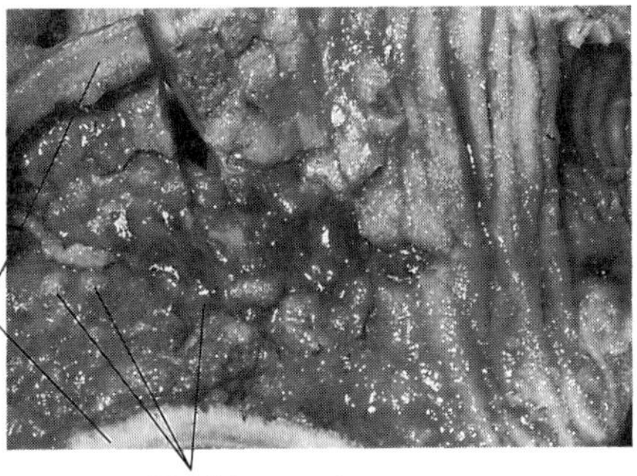

Fig. 35.8 Crohn's colitis: a resected portion of colon has been opened to demonstrate patch 'cobblestone' formation in affected mucosa to the left, and gross thickening of the wall, seen at the line of section. This latter is mostly in the submucous layer.

diseased bowel with intervening segments appearing normal, whereas in ulcerative colitis the inflammatory changes are continuous over the entire involved segment. Thickening of the bowel wall and of the mesentery is a marked feature of the former but is absent in the latter (Fig. 35.8). There are no pseudopolyps in regional enteritis and involvement of the rectum is less common in this disease, whereas it is almost 100% in ulcerative colitis. Because of this difference, rectal and anal-preserving operations for the removal of the colon are carried out more frequently in regional enteritis of the colon than in ulcerative colitis. However, excision of the rectum may be required for extensive involvement of the anal and perianal tissues with Crohn's disease.

TUMOURS OF THE LARGE INTESTINE

The large intestine is a much commoner site for tumours than the small intestine.

Among the benign tumours encountered are juvenile polyp, adenomatous polyp, villous adenoma, haemangioma and lipoma. Occasionally, the colon is also involved along with the small intestine in Peutz–Jeghers syndrome.

Bleeding per rectum and intestinal obstruction due to intussusception of the tumour are the two symptoms by which these benign tumours usually declare their presence.

Juvenile polyps

These tumours are encountered most frequently in children, who are brought with the complaints either of bleeding per rectum or a noticeable swelling prolapsing through the anus. The polyp can often be felt, and indeed brought out by the finger through the anus. It is excised after ligating the pedicle. Histologically it appears more like a hamartoma than a genuine tumour.

Adenomatous polyps

These are usually small sessile or pedunculated tumours, and when situated in the rectum may be felt by digital examination. They are common, and often detected during digital, endoscopic or barium enema X-ray examination as incidental findings. Many carcinomas appear to arise from or involve adenomatous polyps, and there has therefore arisen controversy as to a link between the two conditions. However, it remains uncertain whether only certain patterns of polyp have a premalignant nature, whether all do, or whether the finding of both together is coincidence. The current attitude is not to regard the single isolated adenomatous polyp of less than 1 cm diameter as of serious prognosis, but to be more suspicious of larger, and more multiple and sessile ones. Where any doubt arises, excision biopsy including the base is desirable for histological confirmation.

Villous adenoma

The villous adenoma is a tumour encountered in adults. It is sessile and has a velvety surface. The rectum is most often involved, but it may arise more proximally. Although it may be difficult to feel because of its soft slippery nature, on inspection through an appropriate endoscope it has a characteristic frond-like surface due to the abundant villous-like projections all over it. Histologically mucin-secreting cells are abundant in the epithelial linings of the villi.

Clinically the patient often presents with watery loose motions, the passing of visible mucus per rectum and/or some rectal bleeding. Sometimes the potassium lost in the mucus and other secretions is sufficient to cause frank hypokalaemia, with muscle weakness and cardiac irregularities.

Because of their known tendency to become malignant, villous adenomas should be excised completely along with the base. If this cannot be achieved by endoscopic means, then local resection and re-anastomosis may be required.

Other benign tumours

Rarely haemangiomas and lipomas arise in the large bowel and if symptomatic will require either local excision or resection of the segment from which it arises.

A haemangioma is a submucous tumour and may cause haemorrhage. In many cases it is not possible to visualize the tumour by barium studies, and it is only recognized at laparatomy, if performed during active haemorrhage. The part of the bowel containing blood is closely examined to discover the tumour. The portion of the colon bearing the tumour is excised.

A lipoma is more likely to produce intussusception than any other benign tumour of the colon. It should be removed.

Malignant tumours

Carcinoma of the large intestine is common and the majority of these tumours are adenocarcinomas. While the aetiology remains obscure in the vast majority of cancers of the colon, a minority develop as a complication of ulcerative colitis, of familial polyposis coli or villous adenoma.

Men are more commonly affected than women and the majority of the patients are middle-aged or elderly, though it may occur in younger people, especially as a complication of ulcerative colitis and polyposis coli. The rectum is the commonest site, the sigmoid next, followed in frequency by the caecum and ascending colon, the transverse colon, descending colon, and last the hepatic and splenic flexures. The gross appearance of the lesion in the rectum is commonly an ulcer with raised undermined edges; in the caecum is a large proliferating cauliflower–type mass, and in the left colon a small tight encircling stenotic mass. There are, however, exceptions to this generalization. Microscopically, the tumours are adenocarcinomas. A few other varieties of malignant tumours are occasionally encountered.

The cancer spreads by local infiltration and metastasizes both by lymphatics and by the blood stream. All carcinomas arise from the mucosa but the other coats of the bowel are infiltrated as time goes on. The tumour also spreads longitudinally in the wall of the colon. Retroperitoneal structures such as the ureters may become involved, and adjacent viscera like the bladder, the prostate or the vagina may be infiltrated by growths of the rectum. Proliferation of tumour cells in the wound or at the site of anastomosis after an operation may occur, and is another example of local infiltration.

Lymphatic spread is to the regional lymph nodes. These are first to the nodes close to the bowel and then to the nodes accompanying the branches of the mesenteric veins and, finally, to the para-aortic glands. In carcinoma of rectum metastatic deposits may also travel to the iliac group of nodes.

Blood-borne metastases are found mostly in the liver.

Clinical features

The presenting symptoms fall into three broad categories characteristic of carcinoma of the rectum, left or right side of the colon.

Carcinoma of the rectum

Carcinoma of the rectum presents with bleeding—usually small amounts of fresh blood streaking an otherwise normal stool; the passing of mucus—again usually small amounts of slimy material sometimes accompanying the blood, and tenesmus—a feeling that there is something present in the rectum even after the bowel has moved.

Carcinoma of the left side of the colon

Typical of left-sided colon carcinoma is some alteration to bowel habit, either towards constipation or looseness; dull pain or discomfort in the left iliac fossa or lumbar region; perhaps passage of blood per rectum, either fresh or slightly altered, and subacute or acute large bowel obstruction. There will then be increasing symptoms to absolute constipation, colicky abdominal pain, abdominal distension most noticeable first in the flank and, if the obstruction remains unrelieved, nausea and vomiting.

Carcinoma of the right side of the colon

Right-sided tumours are commonest in the caecum, and since this is a spacious part of the bowel and the tumour tends to be proliferative, it can grow to quite a size before causing symptoms. The clinical presentation may be the patient's own discovery of a mass in the right iliac fossa, or there may be progressive anaemia due to repeated small losses of blood from the ulcerating, necrosing tumour. Very rarely is this loss rapid and large enough to alter the colour of the motions.

Diarrhoea alternating with constipation is a typical symptom of colonic carcinoma, usually of the left side. Constipation is due to narrowing of the bowel. In diarrhoea two factors may be involved. First, mucus is produced in large amounts due to irritation of the mucosa by the impacted faeces and the tumour itself. Second, as a result of putrefaction of a part of the stool above an obstruction and impaired water absorption, some liquified faeces may pass the tumour and harder stools, giving the so-called spurious diarrhoea.

On examination, the patient may be anaemic due to loss of blood from an ulcerating growth, particularly of the caecum. A tumour mass may be felt along the line of the colon. In advanced cases an enlarged irregular and hard liver may be felt and ascites may be present.

Most carcinomas of the rectum come at least partly within reach of the examining finger per rectum and this important examination may also reveal masses in the pelvic pouch from more proximal lesions and there may be evidence of blood on the glove on completion of the examination. It is an important part of the initial assessment.

All patients in whom there is even a suspicion of carcinoma of the large intestine should be examined endoscopically, preferably with a fibreoptic instrument which can be passed at least into the sigmoid colon (Fig. 35.9), or at least with a conventional rigid sigmoidoscope(Fig. 35.10). In cancers of the rectum and lower part of the sigmoid colon, the growth is seen and biopsies are taken.

If the sigmoidoscopic examination is negative, a barium enema should be performed, ideally by a double contrast technique(Fig. 35.11). Most cancers are visualized by this method as a filling defect or stenosis. It can be argued that even when a distal carcinoma is confirmed visualization of the rest

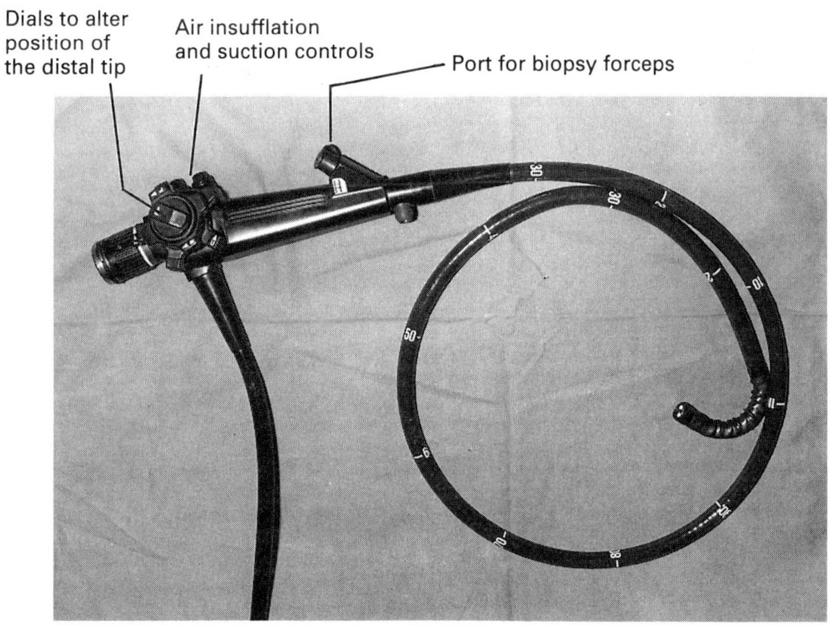

Fig. 35.9 Flexible sigmoidoscope: the flexibility is due to the fibreoptic cables which transmit the light to the distal end and also the image to the eyepiece. This instrument should allow examination of the proximal sigmoid colon. A full-length colonoscope is available which, with skill and care, can be negotiated right round to the caecum.

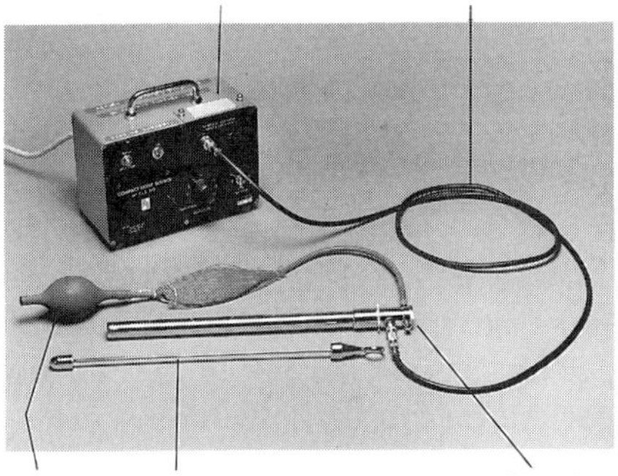

Fig. 35.10 Rigid sigmoidoscope. This is introduced with the obturator in place, and once the inner end reaches the rectum, the obturator is withdrawn, and the eyepiece, fibreoptic cable and hand-bellows are attached. Gentle air insufflation carries the mucosa away from the tip of the instrument to improve vision and ease further introduction. Biopsies of the mucosa can easily be taken by means of specially designed long-handled forceps.

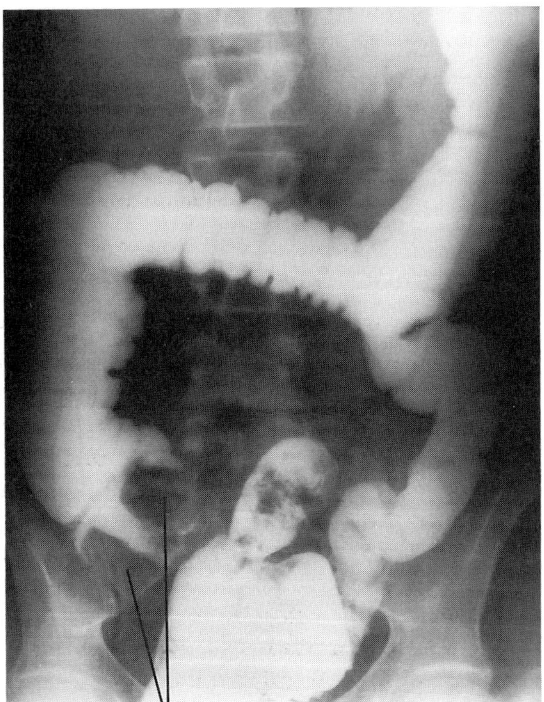

Fig. 35.11 Carcinoma of the caecum on barium enema. There is gross deformity of the shadow caused by the radiolucent tumour masses projecting into the lumen.

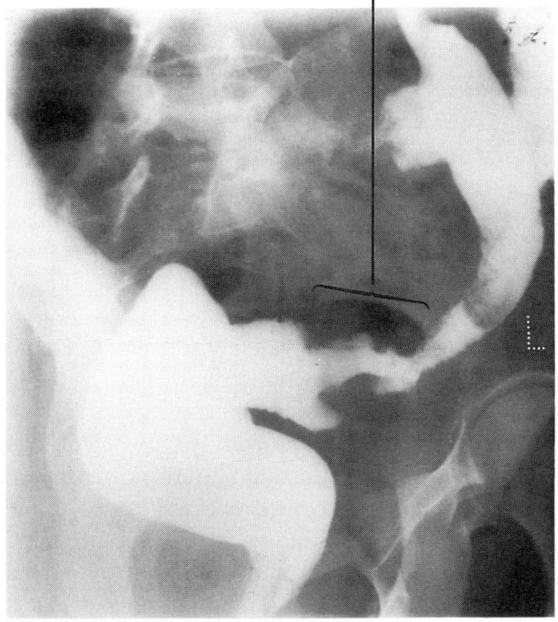

Fig. 35.12 Carcinoma of the sigmoid colon on barium enema. The encircling tumour, encroaching on the lumen, has an apple-core appearance.

of the colon should be sought to determine whether any further malignant or premalignant lesion is present at another level (Fig. 35.12). Colon cancer is one of the few which may at times be multifocal in origin.

If these investigations give uncertain results and colonoscopic expertise is available, this procedure should be undertaken. With skill the entire mucosa round to the caecum can be visualized and biopsy taken of any suspect area.

Management

The treatment of cancers of the large intestine is surgical. The objective is to remove en bloc the tumour-bearing part of the intestine with a wide margin of apparently normal bowel proximal and distal to the lesion, plus the regional lymph nodes (Fig. 35.13). On the right side of the colon this implies a right hemicolectomy with ligation of the ileocolic and right colic arteries at their origins and removal of terminal ileum, caecum, ascending colon, hepatic flexure and the right few centimetres of transverse colon and end-to-end anastomosis.

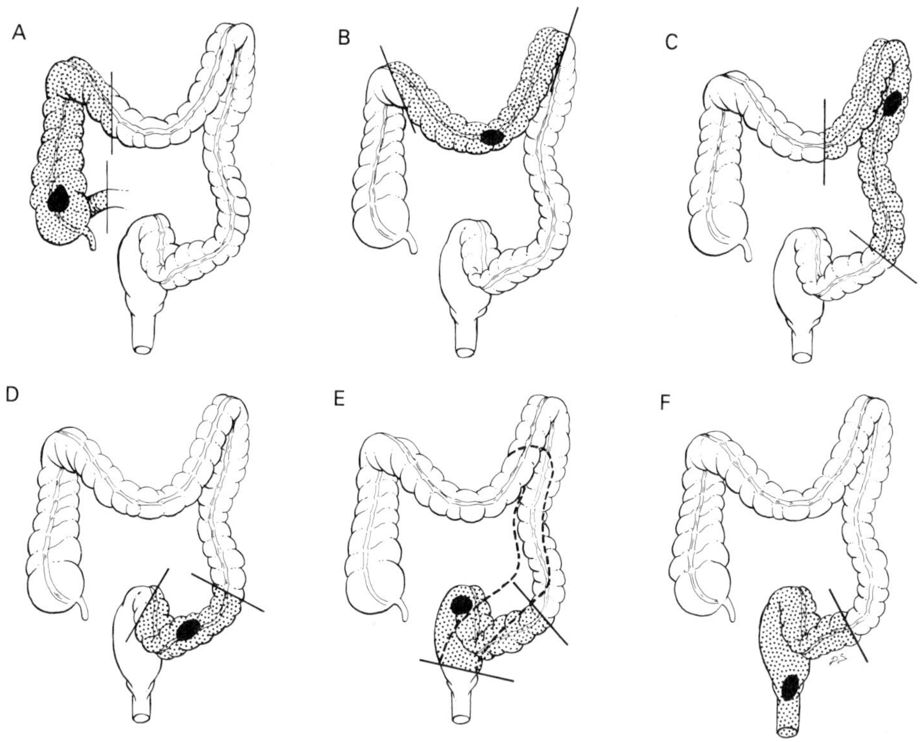

Fig. 35.13 Various types of resection performed for carcinoma of different sites within the colon. (**A**) Right hemicolectomy; (**B**) resection of transverse colon; (**C**) left hemicolectomy; (**D**) resection of sigmoid colon; (**E**) anterior resection of rectum; (**F**) adominoperineal resection of rectum. In (**A–E**), following resection, bowel continuity is restored by direct end-to-end anastomosis of the ends of the remaining bowel which, in the case of anterior resection of the rectum, may require mobilization of the splenic flexure and descending colon. In (**F**) abdominoperineal resection of the rectum, the proximal sigmoid colon end is brought out to the skin surface of the anterior abdominal wall, usually in the left iliac fossa, as a permanent colostomy.

Cancer of the transverse colon is treated by the removal of the involved colon together with the greater omentum and transverse mesocolon. The middle colic artery and the ascending branches of both the right colic and the inferior mesenteric arteries are ligated. Cancers in the segment from the splenic flexure to the proximal sigmoid are treated by left hemicolectomy, removing from the left part of transverse colon to upper sigmoid, and division of the main vessels from the inferior mesenteric root.

For lesions in the distal sigmoid colon and proximal rectum, where at least the distal 8–10 cm of rectum can be spared, the procedure of anterior resection of the rectum is appropriate. The pelvic peritoneum is opened, the upper rectum and whole sigmoid are mobilized, and after division of the main inferior mesenteric vessel close to its point of origin from the aorta, the divided proximal sigmoid is brought down into the pelvis (if necessary after further freeing of the splenic flexure and descending colon), and end-to-end anastomosis is performed. Ring stapling devices often facilitate this operation.

Finally, for carcinoma in the lower rectum the only satisfactory way of trying to rid the patient of the tumour is to remove the anal canal, rectum and distal sigmoid colon by a combined, usually simultaneous abdominoperineal approach, bringing the divided proximal end of the sigmoid colon out through the abdominal wall in the left iliac fossa as a permanent colostomy.

If the patient comes with signs and symptoms of acute intestinal obstruction, decompression of the obstructed bowel is carried out in the first instance either by a transverse colostomy if the growth is in the left side of the colon or by an ileotransverse anastomosis if the growth is in the right side of the colon. If the lesion is operable the resection is better postponed till the local and systemic effects of the obstruction have settled.

Even if distant metastases are present it is often good palliation to perform local excision of the tumour-bearing part of the colon, if this is technically feasible. If removal is not possible then some form of bypass of the tumour, e.g. ileotransverse colostomy for right-sided lesions, or proximal colostomy for more distal lesions if there appears to be an element of obstruction, may give temporary respite.

The prognosis for early cancer of the large bowel coming to operation is reasonably good. If the growth has remained confined to the bowel, the 5-year survival rate should be about 75%. If the growth has infiltrated pararectal tissue but there is no evidence of lymphatic spread, the 5-year survival rate is in the region of 60%. In advanced disease with penetration into surrounding tissues and lymphatic node involvement, the 5-year survival rate is only 5–10%. The overall 5-year survival rate is about 30–35%.

36. Intestinal obstruction

INTRODUCTION

Causes of intestinal obstruction may be congenital or acquired. Examples of the former are atresia, stenosis and malrotation of the gut, meconium ileus, Hirschsprung's disease of the colon and imperforate anus.

Acquired conditions are commoner, and include the following:

1. Inflammatory, e.g. tuberculosis, regional enteritis, and postoperative adhesions.
2. Mechanical, e.g. obstructed hernias, volvulus, intussusception and luminal obstruction by gallstones, foreign bodies and faecal masses.
3. Neoplastic—both benign and malignant tumours.
4. Neurogenic—paralytic ileus.
5. Vascular occlusion, e.g. thrombosis in mesenteric arteries or veins, and embolism of mesenteric arteries.

In adults the commonest causes in most countries are hernias and postoperative adhesions.

Whatever may be the cause, certain local and general changes occur in all forms of intestinal obstruction.

In non-neurogenic obstruction the intestine proximal to the site of obstruction displays vigorous peristaltic efforts to overcome the blockage. This may continue for several hours or even days. Later on, if the obstruction remains unrelieved, the peristalsis slows down and finally this part of the gut may become flaccid and distended. The bowel distal to the site of obstruction shows normal propulsive movements at first, and its contents are conveyed onwards. Evacuation may take place, after which this segment of the gut remains empty and motionless.

Distension of the proximal bowel is due to the collection of both gas and liquid. The gas mostly consists of swallowed air, but a small quantity is diffused from the blood vessels into the intestine and a still smaller proportion is produced by bacterial fermentation of the intestinal contents. The liquid consists of ingested material plus the secretions of the alimentary tract above the site of obstruction (Fig. 36.1). Normally, the distal ileum

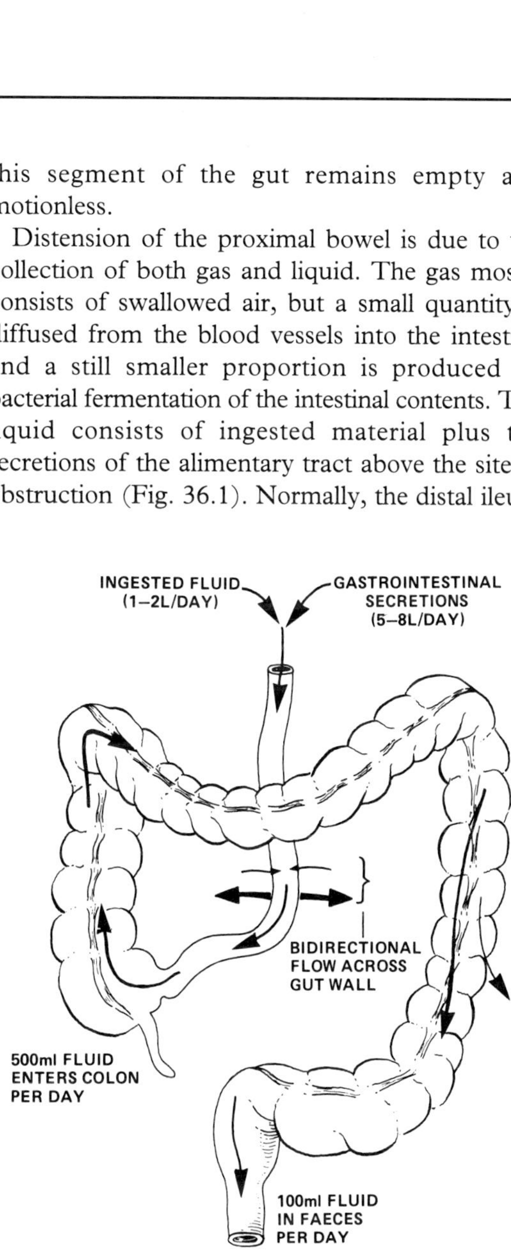

Fig. 36.1 Normal pattern of ingestion, secretion and absorption of fluids in the gastrointestinal tract.

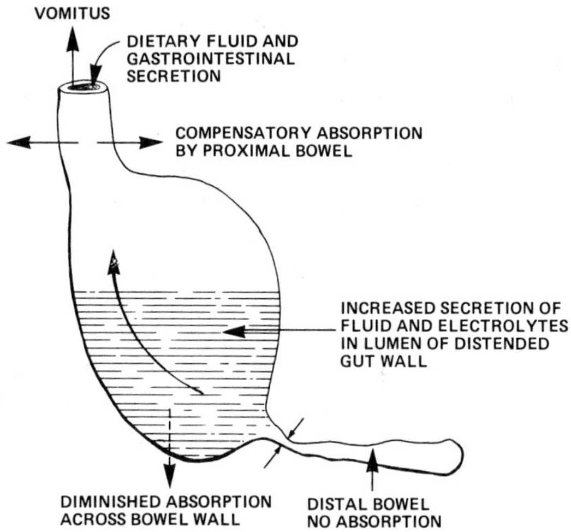

Fig. 36.2 Various effects of small bowel obstruction on the movements of fluids in and across the bowel.

and the colon are the chief sites for the absorption of fluids. If the site of obstruction is in the proximal bowel, absorption of fluid is hampered by two factors (Fig. 36.2). Firstly, the predominantly absorptive surface of the intestine distal to the site of obstruction is inaccessible to the fluid. Secondly, as a result of the distension, the venous plexus of the wall of the proximal intestine is stretched and compressed, so that its capacity to absorb fluid is markedly diminished.

Normally about 8 l of digestive juices is secreted in 24 h. This consists of:

Saliva	1.5 l
Gastric juice	2.5 l
Bile and pancreatic juice	1.0 l
Succus entericus	3.0 l

A very small proportion of this fluid is absorbed in high intestinal obstruction, i.e. that which is in the proximal part of the jejunum or in the duodenum. In large bowel obstruction, however, a relatively large part of this fluid may be absorbed from the bowel proximal to the site of obstruction, as long as gross distension does not compromise the viability of the bowel.

The fluid in the intestine consists of water, electrolytes and enzymes. Water and electrolytes come from the circulating blood, and the enzymes from the alimentary secretions. When a large quantity of fluid is trapped within the lumen of the intestine, hypovolaemia may develop, together with salt deficiency. If the situation is not reversed in time, hypovolaemia may lead to hypotension and hypoxia of the vital centres, with a fatal result.

In addition to the fluid loss, distension of the intestine with fluid and gases has other harmful effects. The abdominal distension, if gross, may cause respiratory difficulties. Increased pressure on the gut-wall venules may cause additional fluid loss through the numerous capillaries, thereby aggravating the total loss to the extracellular fluid volume. If the degree of increased local pressure causing the obstruction to the bowel lumen becomes even greater it may become sufficient to compress the venous flow completely or even cut off the arterial supply. In either event this will effectively stop the circulation to the affected segment of intestine and lead to gangrene. This process is termed strangulation. It is a serious, life-threatening complication, and its possible occurrence is the main reason for urgent correction of any intestinal obstruction.

Gangrene of the bowel may, of course, lead to its perforation and peritonitis. Even if perforation does not occur, the devitalized wall of the intestine may allow bacteria, bacterial toxins, and toxins produced by tissue autolysis to pass from the lumen into the peritoneal cavity. Absorption of these toxins further threatens the patient's life. The rate of toxin absorption depends upon the area of the peritoneum exposed to these products. It is rapid if strangulation has occurred inside the abdominal cavity, and comparatively slower from the sac of an external hernia. Absorption of the toxins may give rise to endotoxic shock, described in Chapter 11. Since some blood loss also results from back-pressure on the vessels in strangulation, escaping into the bowel wall and mesentery, this may be a significant loss if the damaged segment is long.

Chronic or subacute intestinal obstruction is the term used to designate the clinical situation in which the lumen of the bowel is not completely occluded but is so much narrowed that contents pass onward with difficulty. This is seen in some inflammatory conditions like tuberculosis and Crohn's disease and in some neoplastic conditions, when the lumen is gradually narrowed. When chronic obstruction becomes complete the condition is described as acute on chronic obstruction.

Clinical features

Pain is the predominant symptom in all forms of acute intestinal obstruction, except adynamic ileus. It is usually of sudden or rapid onset, cramping in character, severe in intensity and colicky in nature, i.e. rhythmically intermittent. It is not sharply localized but experienced across the abdomen, the level depending on the site of the obstruction. If this is located between the second part of the duodenum and the right part of the transverse colon the pain will be across the centre of the abdomen from lumbar and umbilical regions; if at a more distal level then it will be across the lower abdomen, iliac and hypogastric regions, and symmetrical as far as the distribution across the two sides (Fig. 36.3). Each spasm lasts for a few seconds or minutes and then slowly wanes. There is usually more or less complete relief between bouts of pain unless strangulation has occurred, in which case the pain becomes more continuous. The patient is often found to be grimacing in pain at the height of a paroxysm, and may hold the abdomen with the hands and roll about in the bed.

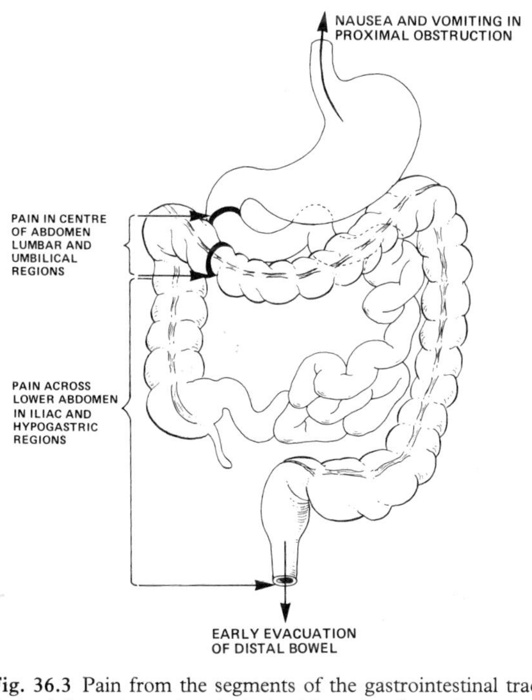

Fig. 36.3 Pain from the segments of the gastrointestinal tract derived from the embryological midgut, i.e. from the second part of the duodenum to the right side of the transverse colon, is felt in the central abdomen. Pain from the points distal to the right side of the transverse colon is felt across the lower abdomen.

Nausea and vomiting occur early and repeatedly in high small intestinal obstruction and later in large bowel obstruction. At first the vomited material is often of the most recently ingested substances, but as it progresses copious volumes of bile-stained dark liquid are brought up usually with little effort, and little or no relief of the pain follows. The vomitus in intestinal obstruction has in the past been described as faeculent because of its offensive taste and smell, and dark-brown colour. The fluid is, however, simply a mixture of retained secretions which are heavily bile-stained and undergoing some bacterial digestion.

Inability to pass faeces and flatus, called *absolute constipation*, occurs sooner or later in most varieties of obstruction. Shortly after the onset the bowel distal to the site of obstruction may be evacuated, after which absolute constipation becomes apparent. However, there are certain varieties of obstruction in which absolute constipation does not occur. These include mesenteric vascular occlusion, incarcerated Richter's hernia, pelvic peritonitis, intussusception and gallstone ileus.

Abdominal distension is a feature of distal obstruction and it is negligible in high jejunal or duodenal obstruction. When the greater part of the small intestine is distended, e.g. in ileal obstruction, the distension is mainly central, but when the site is in the distal colon then the distension is principally of the flanks where the ascending and descending colon are located.

On examination it may be possible, in a good light, to see waves of visible peristalsis taking place in distended bowel loops in any form of mechanical obstruction, but not in cases of adynamic ileus. Local tenderness, and especially rebound tenderness, is a grave omen, and signifies the presence of strangulation.

On auscultation in all varieties of obstruction exaggerated high-pitched bowel sounds are heard, but again with the exception of adynamic ileus, in which case the abdomen is silent.

On rectal examination, the rectum is usually found to be empty of faecal matter. If the obstruction has remained unrelieved for several hours the patient may develop general signs of dehydration, such as a dry tongue, shrunken eyes, an inelastic skin and rapid pulse, and these indicate a major loss of fluid and electrolytes from the blood volume and extracellular space.

A plain X-ray of the abdomen is taken if the signs and symptoms are equivocal. The characteristic findings in obstruction are distended loops of intestine and multiple fluid levels due to the accumulation of fluid and gas in the intestine. These horizontal lines are best demonstrated by X-ray films taken with the patient in the erect posture (Figs. 36.4 and 36.5).

Management

Most patients with intestinal obstruction will require prompt surgical relief, but operation is not indicated for adynamic ileus, and a small proportion of patients with obstruction due to postoperative adhesions will spontaneously settle without surgical intervention.

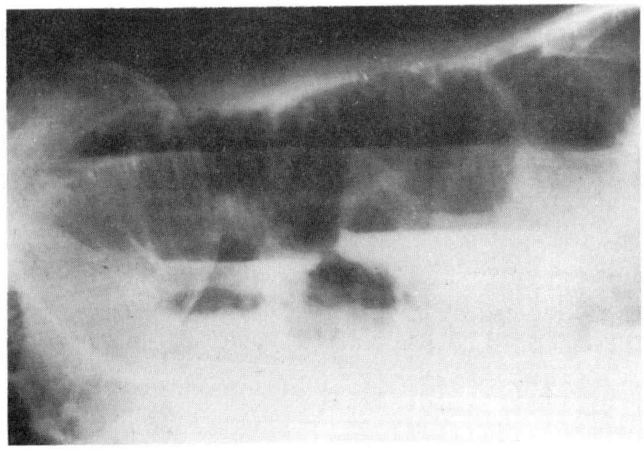

Fig. 36.5 This patient was too ill to be put in the erect position for the X-ray. Even when the films are taken with the patient lying down and turned to one side, fluid levels may be quite obvious, as in this case.

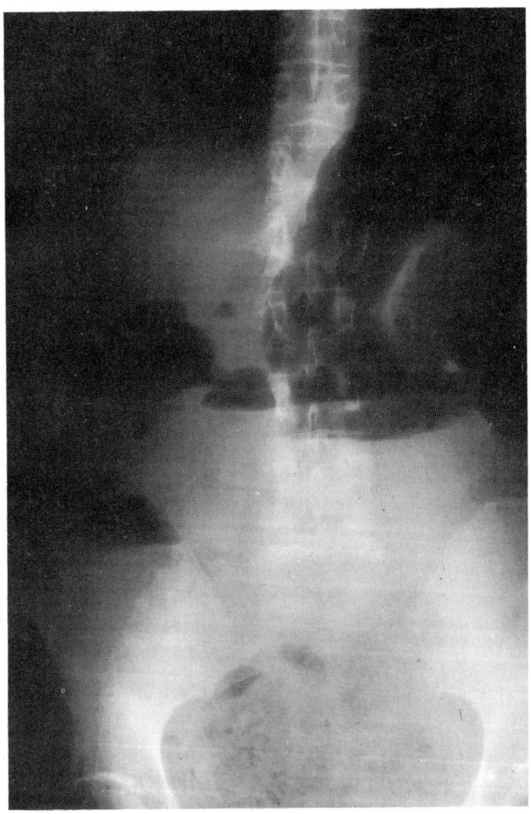

Fig. 36.4 Multiple fluid levels in the small intestine seen on a plain X-ray of the abdomen, with the patient erect. The horizontal straight lines represent the interfaces between liquid and overlying gas.

Whether operation is required or not the initial steps in management are the same—aspiration of the stomach contents and the establishment of a good intravenous infusion line and replacement of at least some of the fluid losses.

Gastric suction

A relatively wide-bore nasogastric tube should be passed and continuous low-pressure suction applied. This will prevent further vomiting, make the patient more comfortable and more importantly, will avoid the risk of aspiration of regurgitated gastric contents into the respiratory passages during induction of anaesthesia.

In the past the use of a much longer tube, with a balloon situated towards its end—the Miller–Abbott tube—was popular. The idea was to try to guide the inflated balloon into the small intestine so that propulsive waves would carry it distally and thereby allow emptying of a large part of the bowel proximal to the actual obstruction. However, this was often difficult or impossible to achieve, quite distressing for the patient, and has been largely abandoned.

Intravenous fluid infusion

Since in every patient with intestinal obstruction some fluid and electrolytes will be at least temporarily lost from the extracellular space, particularly from the circulating blood volume, and sometimes the amount is considerable, it should be routine to secure a freely running drip in a good-sized peripheral vein. Whenever it is anticipated that major problems in maintaining balance will arise or very large quantities of infusion will be required, then a central venous line should be inserted at the outset. This will permit a safer rate of infusion—a good general guide being for the central venous pressure not to exceed 5 cm of water.

Since the main objective is to make the patient fit for operation as quickly as possible and foremost of all to restore an adequate circulating blood volume, it is an unnecessary counsel of perfection to try to replace all losses completely and accurately. The most useful clinical guides are the vital signs of pulse, blood pressure, central venous pressure if available, and urine output. The latter is best measured hourly and this requires catheterization for accuracy. An hourly output of at least 50 ml/h and the presence of chloride in the urine should be achieved. In most instances, when the obstruction has been present for up to 24 or even 48 h, nutritional requirements can be ignored in calculating the initial fluid and electrolyte replacement. Rough guides as to the likely infusion requirements are as follows.

The first general principle is to give the daily fluid and electrolyte requirements to compensate for physiological losses, plus the amount estimated to be lost in vomit or aspirated content, and lying in the lumen of the dilated obstructed gut. This latter can, at best, only be a rough estimate.

If gross clinical signs of dehydration are present it can be assumed that the patient has lost about 6% of total weight. This means that in an average man of 60 kg weight, there is a deficit of about 3.6 1 of fluid. Approximately half of this quantity can be given in the form of 5% glucose and the rest in the form of normal, i.e. 0.9%, saline.

Another broadly acceptable policy is to replace all the fluid lost in vomiting and gastric suction by 0.9% saline solution. Over and above this, the fluid lost in urine plus 1.5 l—to allow for the loss in respiration and insensible perspiration—is replaced half by normal saline and half by 5% glucose. The rate of transfusion for meeting solely the daily requirements of fluid is about one 500 ml bottle in each 4 h.

The daily fluid requirements of children are about 35 ml per kg weight. In the newborn, the basic requirements may be calculated by the following formula:

$$\text{Fluid (ml)} = \frac{\text{age (days) x weight (kg) x 150}}{7}$$

Treatment by intravenous therapy and gastric suction brings great relief to the patient suffering from any form of intestinal obstruction. In adynamic ileus both of these measures will have to be continued, perhaps over many days, until gut activity returns, and in some cases of obstruction generally due to postoperative adhesions the obstruction may spontaneously become relieved during this management alone. In all other cases operative relief is necessary.

As soon as a treatment policy is decided the patient should be given a suitable strong analgesic such as omnopon or pethidine, and it is usual to give a large loading dose of a broad–spectrum antibiotic just before operation if there is any likelihood of strangulation or the need to resect and anastomose bowel.

SPECIFIC TYPES OF INTESTINAL OBSTRUCTION

Hernias

The diagnosis and management of obstructed hernias are discussed fully in Chapter 22. It is important to stress that these are common causes of obstruction and clinical examination of the potential sites for hernia should be routine in the assessment of all patients presenting with signs and symptoms suggesting intestinal obstruction.

Also considered elsewhere are obstruction due to congenital atresia (Ch. 33), neoplasia (Ch. 35) and inflammatory bowel disease (Ch. 33). Five further causes remain for separate discussion—volvulus, intussusception, postoperative adhesions, mesenteric vascular occlusion and adynamic ileus.

Volvulus

Volvulus is the twisting of a loop of intestine around a pedicle of its mesentery in such a way that its

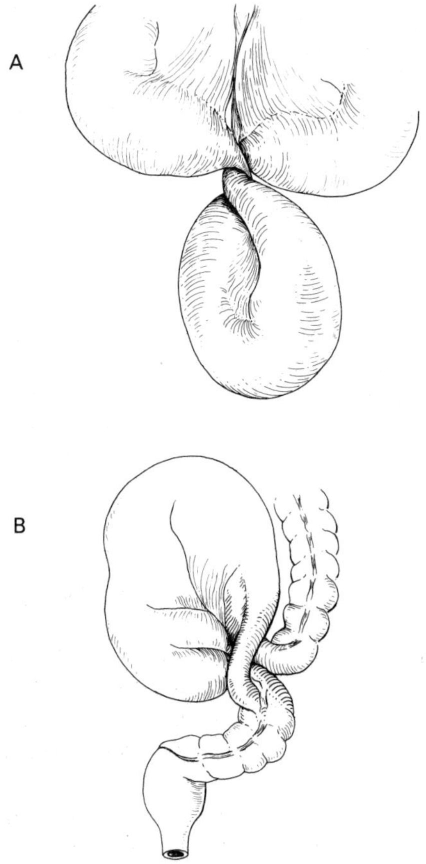

Fig. 36.6 Volvulus (**A**) of small intestine and (**B**) of sigmoid (pelvic) colon.

lumen is obstructed, as one loop overlies another, and its mesentery is so twisted that its blood supply may be obstructed. Potentially, therefore, every volvulus may, if unrelieved, lead to strangulation.

Volvulus neonatorum is described in Chapter 33. In India, the commonest portion of the gut to become twisted is the small intestine (Fig. 36.6A), whereas among African, European and American people, it is the pelvic colon which is more likely to undergo volvulus (Fig. 36.6B). A particularly mobile caecum and ascending colon are sometimes also the site of volvulus formation.

There is a belief that a bulky diet of grain and high vegetable content, which is the staple diet of many people both in India and Africa, may have some aetiological significance.

Volvulus of the pelvic colon occurs when the mesocolon is long and has a narrow base. Overloading of the colon with faeces probably acts as a predisposing factor. Sometimes a band of adhesion passes from the colon to the parietes, thus acting as an axis for torsion.

Clinical features

There are no specific pathognomonic signs and symptoms of volvulus of the small intestine. The picture is that of an acute intestinal obstruction and the diagnosis of volvulus is established at laparotomy. In the case of the volvulus of the pelvic colon, however, a significant feature is the rapid onset of abdominal distension, and in a thin patient the outline of an inverted U-loop of grossly distended pelvic colon may be seen on inspection of the abdomen. The gas-filled grossly dilated loop is often striking on plain X-ray of the abdomen. Probably in no other acute abdominal condition is the distension so rapid as in volvulus of the sigmoid colon.

At operation in the case of volvulus of the small intestine, untwisting is all that is usually necessary, provided there is no gangrene. In volvulus of the caecum and ascending colon the caecum should be fixed to the posterior wall of the right iliac fossa after undoing the rotation, so that the condition may not recur.

It is often possible to make a confident diagnosis of volvulus of the pelvic colon and in such cases it is worth trying to pass a wide-bore rectal tube through a sigmoidoscope. The main difficulty may be in guiding the tip of the tube around the acute angle of the rectosigmoid junction, past the distal point of obstruction, into the dilated loop. Various manoeuvres, e.g. placing the patient in the knee-elbow position, may help, by encouraging the bowel to fall forwards and upwards. If the tube can be passed there is an immediate explosive passage of flatus and liquid faeces, as the volvulus is undone, and the signs and symptoms subside. If this method does not succeed, laparotomy is undertaken, and the bowel is untwisted. If a part or whole of the involved colon has become gangrenous, it is excised, preferably by the Paul-Mikulicz method, exteriorizing temporarily both the proximal and distal divided ends of the bowel. If the volvulus is recurrent, then some surgical means of fixing the segment to the lateral pelvic wall or excision of the long central redundant segment is advisable.

Intussusception

Intussusception is the invagination of a part of the intestine into an immediately adjoining, usually more distal, portion.

In adults, the starting point of the invagination may be a tumour, benign or malignant, or the inflamed base of Meckel's diverticulum. In infants, there is an idiopathic variety, but certain features have been noted in association with its occurrence. The patient is usually a male child between 6 and 9 months of age. During this period, in European countries, most babies are weaned from milk and there may be a change in the intestinal flora. The new organisms may cause inflammation of the Peyer's patches in the ileum, which may become the starting point of the intussusception. If the condition is not relieved the apex of the intussuscepting bowel advances further and further into the more distal segment, drawing its mesentery and the contained blood vessels along with it (Fig. 36.7). The length of the intussuscepted mass may extend considerably, and in the case of one whose apex is at the ileocaecal valve, the commonest site in infants, this may travel up the ascending colon, into the transverse colon and even, in extreme instances, down to the rectum.

The compression of the inner by the outer layers of bowel causes obstruction to the lumen, giving rise to intestinal obstruction. At the same time, the mesenteric vessels between the inner and the middle tubes are compressed, and this threatens the viability of the bowel. There is therefore a risk of intestinal strangulation.

A

B

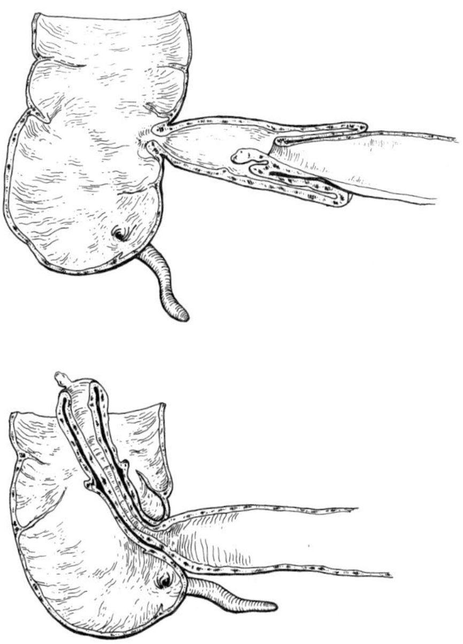

Fig. 36.7 Intussusception. (**A**) A portion of ileum has become invaginated into the immediately distal segment; the apex of this portion is represented here as a small pedunculated polyp. Attempts by muscular contraction of the bowel wall to propel the polyp distally may start this intussusception process. (**B**) The degree of invagination has increased, passed through the ileocaecal valve and is being further propelled up the ascending colon.

Clinical features

The onset is usually quite sudden. In the infantile variety, the baby suddenly cries and doubles up with pain, often drawing up the legs. The spasm passes off in a few seconds and the infant stops crying temporarily, but lies listless until the next spasm occurs a minute or two later. Repeated vomiting is usual.

At first there may be a normal bowel action, but later on, small quantities of blood-stained mucus, picturesquely described as redcurrant jelly stool, may be passed several times.

On examination a sausage-shaped lump may be felt in the abdomen anywhere along the course of the large intestine. By contrast, the right iliac fossa may feel empty. On rectal examination, the examining finger may be stained with blood and mucus, and very occasionally the apex of the intussusception may be felt, if it has extended as far as the rectum.

Usually the diagnosis is fairly obvious on clinical grounds and no special investigations are necessary.

Treatment

When the condition is diagnosed early in infants and there is no suspicion of strangulation, it is sometimes possible to achieve reduction by means of a barium enema. This should only be done by an experienced paediatric radiologist, under carefully controlled supervision and with a surgeon available in case of failure or any complication, such as leakage from the bowel. If such a reduction is successful the intussusception rarely recurs.

However, if there is any doubt at all about the safety of this approach, or clearly if it fails to give completely satisfactory evidence of reduction, laparotomy is required. At operation it is generally a relatively easy matter to reduce the intussusception by gentle but firm manipulation, more pressing the apex back proximally than pulling from above. Once again in infants it is rare for there to be any recurrence.

In adults there is usually a precipitating cause for the disorder, and this will need appropriate measures, e.g. excision of a tumour, or removal of a diverticulum.

Postoperative adhesions

Following any abdominal operation some usually fine fibrous adhesions form between neighbouring structures, e.g. coils of intestine, or intestine and parietal peritoneum. To a large extent these can be regarded as beneficial, strengthening the protection of damaged or diseased tissue, anastomoses, or raw surfaces. On occasions these adhesions are more numerous and substantial, particularly when there has been previous intra-abdominal sepsis or any degree of local ischaemia of tissue. These adhesions may lead to obstruction either by trapping a loop of intestine (Fig. 36.8) by compressing or angulating a segment, or by acting as an axis for a volvulus (Fig. 36.9). It must, however, be emphasized that if the obstruction is not relieved within 24 h, laparotomy should be undertaken to relieve it. If this is not done, there is real danger of strangulation, which may easily be overlooked because the patient remains relatively comfortable as a result of the treatment with drip and suction.

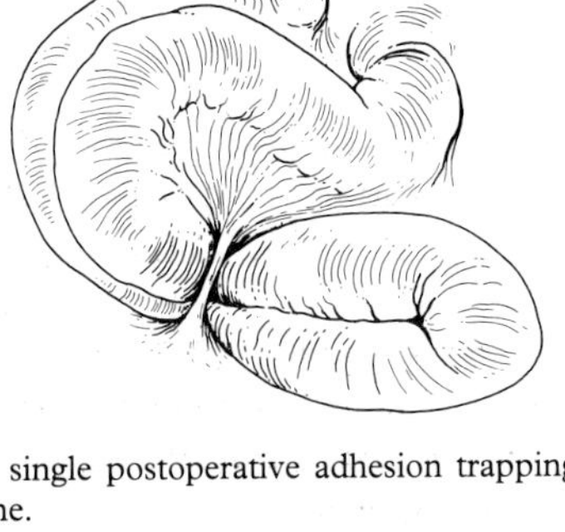

Fig. 36.8 A single postoperative adhesion trapping a loop of small intestine.

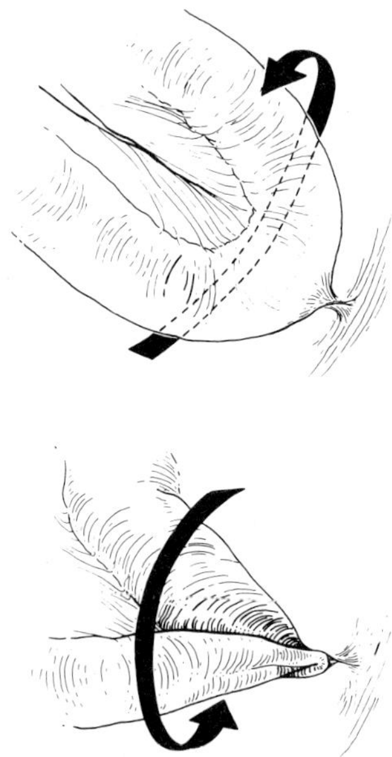

Fig. 36.9 An adhesion between the apex of a loop of intestine and the abdominal wall, acting as an axis for a volvulus.

Often all that is required at operation is the simple division of the obstructing band adhesion. More elaborate undoing of multiple sheets of adhesions, however, may be necessary. In patients presenting with repeated episodes of adhesion/obstruction, various techniques of fixation or plication of the intestinal loops have been advocated, but without universal enthusiasm.

Mesenteric vascular occlusion

Either the mesenteric veins or arteries may become occluded, the former by thrombosis and the latter by either thrombosis or embolism. The superior mesenteric artery is affected by embolism more often than the inferior mesenteric artery. The embolus may be released proximally from vegetations on the mitral valve, or from an atheromatous plaque in the aorta. Mesenteric venous thrombosis may occur in suppurative conditions such as pyelophlebitis or even acute appendicitis. It may also occur in portal hypertension.

No matter whether the occlusion is in the artery or in the vein, the end-result is ischaemic gangrene of the intestine. If the occlusion occurs in one of the branches of the artery, or in a tributary of the vein, the result is less disastrous, for in such cases only a segment of the intestine may become gangrenous.

When arterial occlusion occurs, the part of the intestine supplied by it becomes pale and then, as there is retrograde flow from the valveless veins, it becomes engorged and cyanosed. The venous engorgement gives rise to capillary haemorrhage into the lumen of the bowel, into its wall, and into the peritoneal cavity. The affected part of the intestine then becomes gangrenous. In venous occlusion, the overall effects are much the same.

Clinical features

The patients are usually middle-aged or old, but when this condition occurs in younger persons there is often a history of mitral valve disease.

Abdominal pain, vomiting and the passage of blood per rectum are the cardinal symptoms of the disease. The onset may be sudden or deceptively gradual, with severe abdominal pain, which is continuous and is felt mainly in the centre of the abdomen. The vomiting is usually repeated, and if blood is passed per rectum it may be either fresh or altered.

On examination, the patient usually appears to be in shock, with a rapid pulse rate and low blood pressure. Varying degrees of abdominal tenderness and muscle guarding are elicited. If only a localized segment of the bowel is involved, a tender mass may be felt in a thin patient. The diagnosis is usually established at laparotomy which should be performed as soon as the condition is suspected from the clinical features.

At operation, if the affected segment is localized and there is viable bowel both proximal and distal to it then resection, with either end-to-end anastomosis or exteriorization of the two divided ends, is performed. Where the entire small intestine is gangrenous, and the changes perhaps extend into the colon, clearly total resection is not compatible with survival without lifelong parenteral nutrition and in most instances is not a realistic option. Attempts can be made to perform embolectomy or thromboendarterectomy of the main occluded vessels, but results are generally bad and rarely is successful revascularization accomplished.

Following any successful procedure anticoagulation should be considered to discourage further vascular occlusive episodes.

Paralytic or adynamic ileus

In this condition there is no mechanical obstruction of the intestine but the neuromuscular mechanism responsible for the propulsion of the intestinal contents fails. The following are the more important causes of adynamic ileus:

1. Peritonitis, due to any cause.
2. Retroperitoneal haematoma, fractures of the ribs or spine or even the application of a plaster jacket.
3. Postoperatively after abdominal operations under general anaesthesia.
4. Uraemia.
5. Potassium depletion.

The exact mechanism by which adynamic ileus is produced remains obscure. It is thought that there are two levels at which dysfunction occurs—at the myenteric plexus, and in the muscle fibres of the intestine. Normal peristalsis ceases and the contents remain stagnant. The condition is further aggravated by the accumulation of gas, which is mostly swallowed air. This leads to the distension of the intestine, which in turn, by pressure on the veins, hampers the absorption of fluid. Alimentary juices, therefore, also accumulate in the intestine. Thus a vicious circle of abdominal distension, fluid loss and hypovolaemia sets in which, if not broken, may lead to a fatal outcome.

Clinical features

Adynamic ileus is characterized by abdominal distension, absolute constipation and vomiting. There is no pain in the abdomen, except that which is caused by the underlying condition, e.g. peritonitis, postoperative pain, etc. Normal bowel sounds are absent, but sometimes an occasional tinkling sound is heard due to passive shifting of the fluid in the intestine.

Treatment

The mainstays of treatment are continuous naso-gastric suction and intravenous therapy. Morphine may be given to allay anxiety. Any predisposing condition, e.g. peritonitis or uraemia, should be vigorously treated. If this fails, some surgeons advocate laparotomy to pass a Miller-Abbott type of tube through the nose and guide it through the duodenum and jejunum into the terminal ileum. With the tip of the tube in the terminal ileum, the abdomen is closed and low–power suction applied through the tube. This approach has not, however, found general favour.

More important is to make every endeavour to exclude or deal with any contributing factor; to maintain as accurate a fluid and electrolyte balance as possible; to continue the gastric aspiration, and wait patiently for the gradual return of intestinal activity as manifest by the reappearance of normal bowel sounds on auscultation over the abdomen, and finally evidence of the patient passing a small amount of flatus per rectum.

37. The anus and perianal region

INTRODUCTION

A short account of embryology and anatomy is followed by the description of the congenital and acquired disorders of the region under the following headings:

1. Congenital abnormalities.
2. Haemorrhoids.
3. Fissure-in-ano.
4. Fistula-in-ano.
5. Prolapse of the rectum.
6. Anorectal infections
   a. Perianal abscess.
   b. Ischiorectal abscess.
   c. Pilonidal sinus.
7. Malignant tumours of the anus
   a. Carcinoma.
   b. Melanoma.

DEVELOPMENT

At an early stage in development both the lower urinary tract and the distal bowel open as a single channel in the cloaca. A urorectal septum then forms to separate the anterior urethra from the posterior anorectum and the future anus forms and migrates posteriorly.

The three main groups of congenital abnormality affecting this region result from failure of a portion of the anorectum to develop and cannulize; failure of the canal opening to migrate posteriorly to the full extent, and an excess degree of fusion of the lateral genital folds covering over the anus in part or completely.

ANATOMY

The dentate line, which marks the site of fusion of the endodermal hindgut with the invaginated skin epithelium, is indicated by the anal valves, which are folds of mucosa joining the anal columns. It also marks a watershed between the portal venous drainage above the line, through the superior rectal vein, and the systemic drainage below the line, through the inferior rectal veins and hence into the internal iliac veins. The mucosa above the dentate line is not sensitive to pain but the lining below the line is very sensitive. Biopsy of the rectum and upper anal canal can therefore be taken without anaesthesia whereas biopsy from the lower part of the anal canal will require some form of anaesthesia.

The ischiorectal fossa is the fat-filled space on either side of the anal canal. It is pyramidal in shape bounded below by the skin, medially by the levator ani muscle above and the anal canal and sphincter muscles below, and laterally by the fascia covering the obturator internus muscle. The medial wall below the levator ani is weak and so an ischiorectal abscess is more likely to burst through it into the anal canal earlier than through the skin, thereby leading to the formation of a fistula-in-ano.

CONGENITAL ABNORMALITIES OF THE ANUS

It is estimated that 1 in every 4500 babies is born with an anal malformation. A completely imperforate anus is the commonest cause of intestinal obstruction in the newborn. The following are the

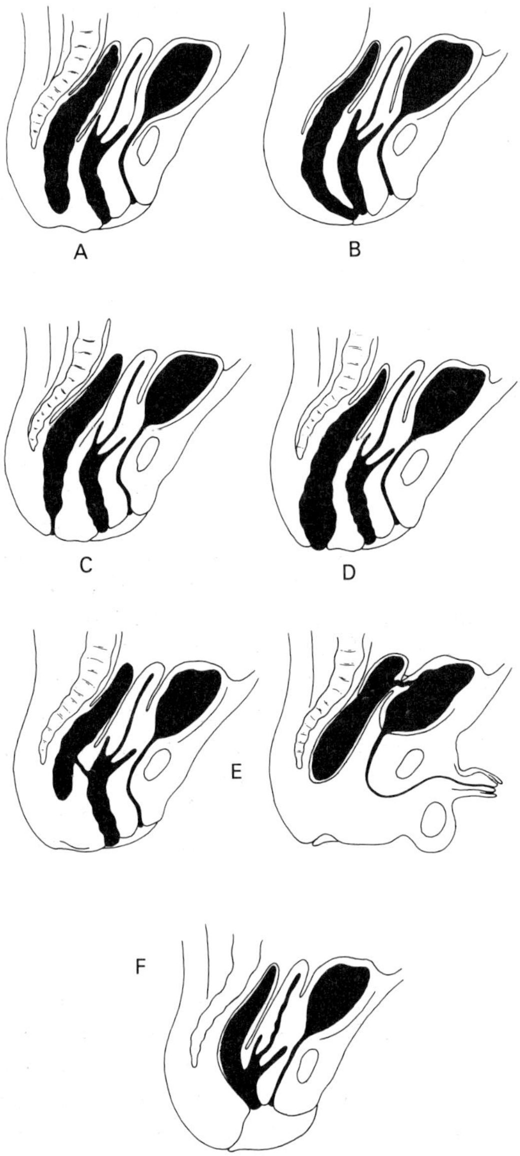

Fig. 37.1 Various patterns of congenital defects in the development of the anus and perianal region. The letters (**A–F**) correspond to the text descriptions

most common varieties of abnormality encountered (Fig. 37.1):

a. *Covered anus.* In this condition the anal canal and rectum are normal but the anal orifice is covered with a bar of skin which runs forward forming the inferior wall of a track which opens near the perineal body.

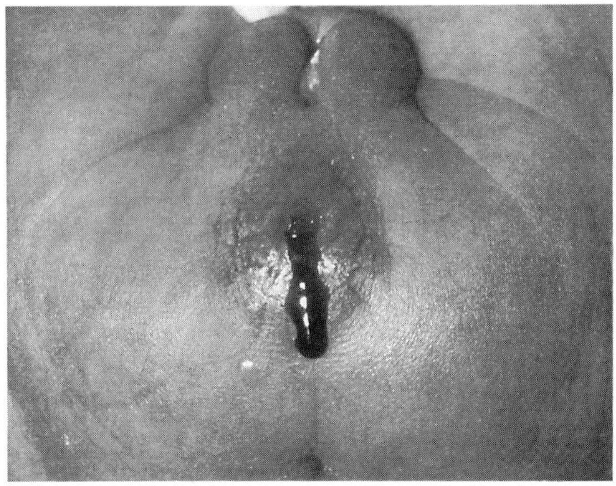

Fig. 37.2 Imperforate anus: only a pinhole opening permits the escape of a few drops of liquid meconium.

b. *Ectopic anus.* In this condition the anal canal is normally formed, but the opening of the canal is anterior to the normal position and in female babies, this may be in the vulva or even in the vagina.
c. *Stenosed anus.* In these cases the anal opening, in an essentially normal location, is of a size much smaller than the normal (Fig. 37.2).
d. *Membranous stenosis.* In this rare condition the anus is covered with a membrane through which meconium can be seen.
e. *Anorectal agenesis.* This is characterized by failure of a variable length of the anorectal canal to develop. In the most extreme cases of failure the distal end of the rectum ends blindly above the level of the pelvic floor. Usually there is also a rectovesical fistula in the male, and a rectovaginal fistula in the female. In less severe examples there may be only a short uncanalized segment separating distal rectum from the anal skin.
f. *Persistence of cloaca.* This is found only in female babies, and is the most severe form of congenital abnormality. In this condition there is a common opening for the urinary, genital and the alimentary tracts, and it is often associated with other abnormalities in the body.

Clinical features

Complete imperforate anus and agenesis will, of course, present as neonatal intestinal obstruction.

The absence of a normal anus is usually detected by the parents or medical attendants. In a stenosed anus, the opening may be found only on very careful inspection. Where a rectovesical fistula exists, the passage of air or faeces through the urethra may be noticed.

Management

If, on clinical examination, a firm diagnosis cannot be made as to whether an obstructing anomaly is of a low or high type, X-ray examination 8–10 h after birth may be helpful. The baby is held upside down and a radiopaque marker is placed at the site where the anus is normally situated and an X-ray picture is taken. Air in the distal bowel ascends as the baby is held bottom up, and the distance between the distal mass or shadow and the marker indicates the level of the lesion. If it is more than 2.5 cm, a high anomaly is diagnosed.

In low anomalies all that may be required is immediate excision of the skin bar or membrane in the covered anus. In cases of stenosed anus it is usually possible to define the opening and dilate it with a probe. A series of dilating instruments of increasing diameter are then used until the surgeon's little finger can be passed. The mother can be taught to dilate the anus of the baby every day with her gloved finger.

No immediate treatment is necessary for ectopic anus provided the opening is big enough.

In the high type of anorectal agenesis, if there is a rectovaginal fistula no further immediate treatment is necessary specifically for it. The patient is referred to a paediatric surgeon for definitive correction at a later date.

If rectal agenesis is associated with a rectovesical fistula or if there is no fistula, urgent surgical treatment is indicated. In rectovesical fistula, at least a defunctioning colostomy is performed. If the baby is in good condition and the surgeon is experienced in this type of work, the fistula may also be resected at the same sitting. Alternatively, the fistula can be resected later on and the colostomy closed when the surgeon is satisfied that the fistula has been effectively sealed.

In non-fistulous cases, colostomy is performed to relieve the intestinal obstruction. A definitive restorative procedure may be undertaken at the same sitting or later on, depending upon the condition of the baby and the surgical skill available.

There is no satisfactory treatment for cloaca.

HAEMORRHOIDS

The venous plexuses of the anorectal region are drained by the superior, middle and the inferior haemorrhoidal veins. The superior rectal vein is a tributary of the inferior mesenteric vein, which is part of the portal system of veins. In this system there are no valves. In the erect position, therefore, there is considerable pressure of a long column of blood in the veins of the internal plexus. Moreover, these veins lie in the submucosa which is lax and so the vessels are easily compressed by hard faeces. These factors could account at least in part for mechanical dilatation of the anal veins. Other theories include possible hyperplasia of the plexus, weakening of the anal 'cushions', and development of constricting fibrous bands within the anus.

Clinically haemorrhoids are quite often encountered where there is constipation, venous obstruction due to pressure by a gravid uterus, rectal and other neoplasms in the pelvis.

Theoretically haemorrhoids should be common in portal hypertension but this, however, is not the case.

Clinical features

Bleeding per rectum is the principal and often the only symptom. With the smallest of haemorrhoids this may be noticed as slight streaking on the stool or reddening of the toilet paper on wiping, but with larger piles there may be dripping or squirting of bright red blood on straining at stool. If they enlarge they may also prolapse.

By convention three degrees of haemorrhoids are described:

1. If there is no prolapse, and bleeding is the only symptom—first-degree.
2. If the prolapse occurs only at defecation and spontaneously returns to within the anal canal—second-degree.
3. If the piles remain prolapsed continuously, or promptly re-prolapse after manual replacement—third-degree.

Discharge of mucus is a further complaint, especially in the presence of second-or third-degree haemorrhoids. In these circumstances there is also often pruritus.

Clinical assessment

This should start with a careful abdominal examination to look for any underlying cause for haemorrhoids, e.g. colonic neoplasm, loaded bowel etc. Next the anal region should be inspected, with the patient lying in the left lateral position and the buttocks gently separated. If there is no obvious prolapse, the patient should be asked to strain down, when prolapse of second-or third-degree haemorrhoids may become obvious. First-degree piles, however, will not show any visible sign.

Uncomplicated haemorrhoids are not palpable to the examining finger, and digital examination will feel quite normal. However, it is important to feel for any tenderness, which may indicate a concomitant fissure, or local sepsis, or any anorectal tumour.

The principal method of confirming the presence of internal haemorrhoids is proctoscopy. With the patient remaining in the left lateral position, the instrument is inserted to its full length with the obturator in place. The latter is then removed and inspection carried out, while gradually withdrawing the instrument. As the level of the dentate line is reached the dark red to purple pile masses will be seen to bulge over the inner edge of the proctoscope (Fig. 37.3). If necessary the patient may be asked to strain down to make any doubtful masses distend. Because of the anatomical arrangement of the main draining veins, the piles are usually located one on the left lateral position and two on the right, one being anterior and the other posterior. Thus, one, two or three primary piles may be present, and in addition secondary smaller ones may arise between these. By the convention of regarding the patient in the lithotomy position and using the clockface, the classical locations of the three primary haemorrhoid sites are 3, 7 and 11 o'clock.

Even when haemorrhoids are clearly confirmed if there is any reason at all to harbour a suspicion of carcinoma of the bowel, particularly in middle-aged and elderly patients, it is wise to proceed with a barium enema examination and/or more proximal endoscopy.

Treatment

For early first-degree haemorrhoids, discovered either incidentally on examination, or causing only minimal occasional bleeding, dietary regulation, with perhaps the addition of one of the bulk-increasing and stool-softening preparations, may be all that is required.

More troublesome first-or second-degree piles may be dealt with by either injection of a sclerosant (Fig. 37.4), or the application of special rubber bands, as an outpatient procedure.

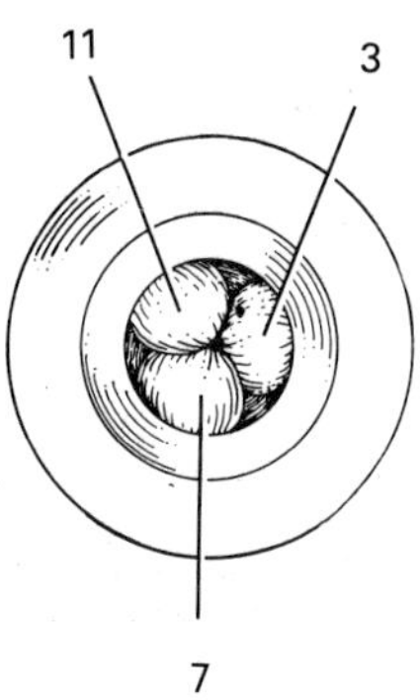

Fig. 37.3 View of three typical primary internal haemorrhoids through the proctoscope, with the patient examined in the lithotomy position. The numbers represent the numerals on a clock, i.e. the 3, 7 and 11 o'clock positions.

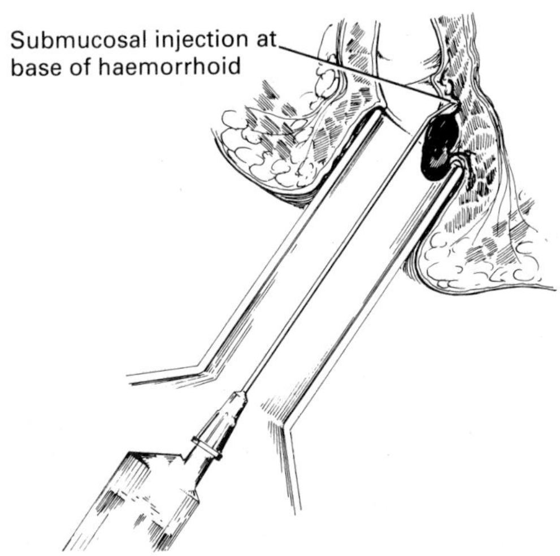

Fig. 37.4 Injection of sclerosant (conventionally 5% phenol in almond oil) in a long, angled, shouldered needle into the base of the pile.

The sclerosing agent traditionally used to stimulate fibrosis in the submucosa at the level of the haemorrhoid is 5% phenol in almond oil. Through a proctoscope about 3–5 ml is injected via a long shouldered needle introduced through the anal mucosa, clearly above the dentate line to avoid any pain. The mucosa over the injected site is seen to swell, and at most the patient should be aware of a slight aching as the injection is made. If pain is felt, the injection is being made too low.

In band ligation, again through a proctoscope, specially designed holding forceps are used to pull the pile down while an applicator slides the stretched-out rubber band down to the neck of the pile and releases it to cause tight constriction at this level (Fig. 37.5).

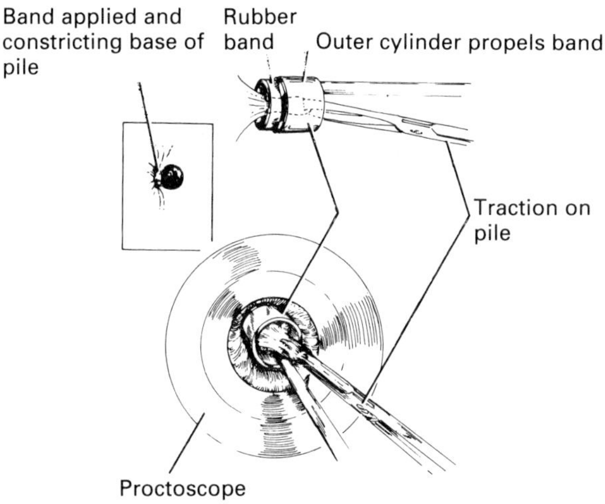

Fig. 37.5 Band ligation of pile. The proctoscope is first introduced and on being gently withdrawn demonstrates the pile projecting over the rim. The apex of the pile is then drawn gently down through the lumen of the cylindrical band applicator, the end of which is manoeuvred to the neck of the pile. Closing the handles of the applicator moves the outer cylinder over the inner one, thereby pushing the rubber band off the end, to ensnare the neck of the pile.

After either of these forms of treatment there may be mild discomfort, occasionally secondary or reactionary bleeding and still more rarely, local ulceration or necrosis.

Other methods of non-operative management of haemorrhoids advocated in recent years include cryotherapy, carbon dioxide laser application and forcible anal dilatation under general anaesthesia.

Formal haemorrhoidectomy

This is recommended when third-degree haemorrhoids are present, when lesser methods have failed to deal with the problem, or when other perianal lesions, e.g. external anal tags, also require removal. With the anaesthetized patient in the lithotomy position, each pile mass in turn is identified, dissected out from its pedicle separated from the lower fibres of the internal sphincter muscle, transfixed at the base of the pedicle by a stout absorbable stitch which is then doubly tied as a figure-of-eight around it, and the main pile mass is then cut away (Fig. 37.6). Usually a rounded portion of contiguous perianal skin is removed along with the pile. It is important to leave a good bridge of this skin intact between the excision area of each pair of piles, to prevent serious contracture of the anus developing.

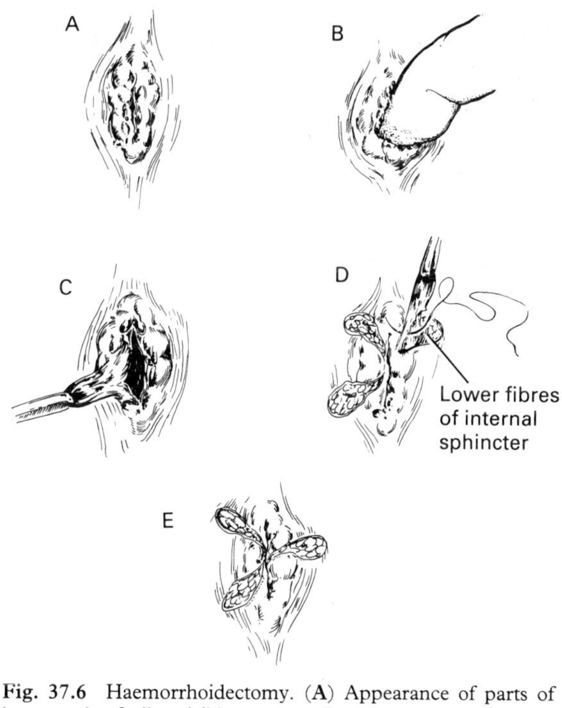

Fig. 37.6 Haemorrhoidectomy. (**A**) Appearance of parts of lower ends of piles visible at anus. (**B**) Pile mass being identified and made prominent by the examining finger. (**C**) Apex of pile at 7 o'clock position being grasped by forceps. (**D**) Pile mass at 3 o'clock position having been dissected down to its neck, where it is being transfixed with a stout absorbable stitch, at a point just below the exposed lower fibres of the internal anal sphincter muscle. (**E**) Final appearance: ligated pedicles have retracted into the anal canal: ellipses of perianal skin have been excised around each excised pile to discourage tag formation during healing.

Postoperative pain usually requires powerful analgesics in the first day or two, and it is wise to prescribe stool softeners, e.g. methylcellulose, at least for the time of the first few bowel movements to diminish local trauma and make defecation less uncomfortable. Complete healing of the raw areas can usually be expected in about 3–4 weeks. Again, reactionary or secondary haemorrhage may occur as an occasional complication and require active intervention, e.g. religation for the former and firm packing for the latter.

Thrombosed haemorrhoids

This painful complication is what is often referred to as an acute attack of piles. Probably the initiating factor is tight contraction of the sphincter muscles temporarily constricting the venous outflow from the haemorrhoids and the resultant stasis leading to clot formation. The prolapsed pile masses then become distended, tight, engorged, painful and tender. If the episode is encountered very early on it may be possible by gentle but firm manual pressure to reduce the mass into the anal canal, but usually this is not possible and the episode is treated by bed rest, potent analgesia, the local application of cool saline dressings and the prescription of stool-softening agents. Resolution generally takes 7–10 days, and if the piles remain, formal haemorrhoidectomy can be arranged at a later date. Sometimes, however, the piles may be obliterated as a result of the thrombosis and no further treatment may be needed.

Perianal haematoma

This disorder is characterized by the sudden appearance of a tense, painful, tender rounded swelling to one side of the anal ring immediately after straining at stool. Occasionally it may develop apparently spontaneously at other times. On inspection there is an obvious purple-blue, smooth, rounded swelling and the diagnosis is straightforward: One of the small perianal venules has ruptured and the leaked collection of blood thromboses in the subcutaneous space.

This condition used to be referred to as a thrombosed external pile. However, it is quite different from internal haemorrhoids, and to avoid unnecessary confusion it is better if the term external pile is abandoned, and the condition under present discussion is more properly termed perianal haematoma.

Immediate relief can be obtained by simple incision over the summit of the perianal haematoma, under general or local anaesthesia, evacuation of the clotted blood and leaving the wound to granulate and heal.

FISSURE-IN-ANO

This common condition is a longitudinal split in the sensitive skin of the lower part of the anal canal.

Most fissures are situated posteriorly, at the 6 o'clock position, but a small number—especially in women—are situated anteriorly. The long axis of the fissure is parallel to the long axis of the anus. Fibres of the internal anal sphincter may be seen in the floor of the fissure and in chronic cases a tag of skin may overhang the lower end of the fissure—the so-called sentinel pile. In acute fissures there is almost invariably intense spasm of the internal sphincter.

Clinical features

Intense anal pain usually starts suddenly during the act of defecation, and often the patient will admit to being somewhat constipated and having to strain. The pain persists for up to several hours and then may subside, only to return the next time the bowel moves.

There may also be a slight spot or streak of blood with the motions, and a slight mucus discharge.

On examination with the patient in the left lateral position, a sentinel pile may be seen in chronic cases and on gently separating the buttocks it may be possible to see at least the lower end of the fissure (Fig. 37.7). In the acute stage, however, there is such intense spasm of the internal sphincter muscle that it may not be possible to visualize the fissure at all. In such cases, further examination may be possible after applying local anaesthesia, e.g. 5% Xylocaine, on cotton wool. After about 5 min, sufficient anaesthesia may be achieved to enable the surgeon to examine the anal canal.

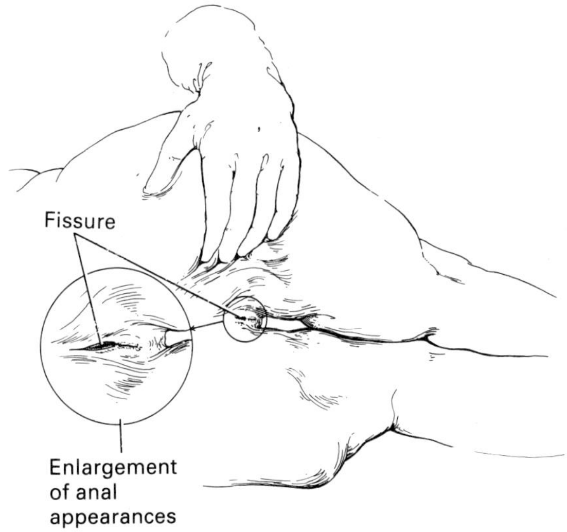

Fig. 37.7 Posterior anal fissure. With the patient in the left lateral position and as relaxed as possible, it may be possible to visualize the small linear fissure—almost always directly posterior—emerging from the anal margin. (However, often there is such severely painful spasm of the anal muscles that it is not possible to see it without some form of anaesthesia.)

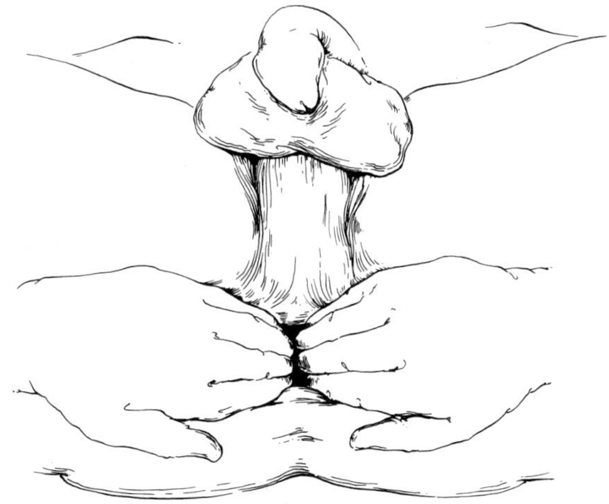

Fig. 37.8 Digital dilatation of the anus under general anaesthesia. Starting with the introduction of one and then two fingers and steady, firm separation to stretch the sphincter muscle gradually additional fingers may be inserted until six or even eight fingers can be accommodated.

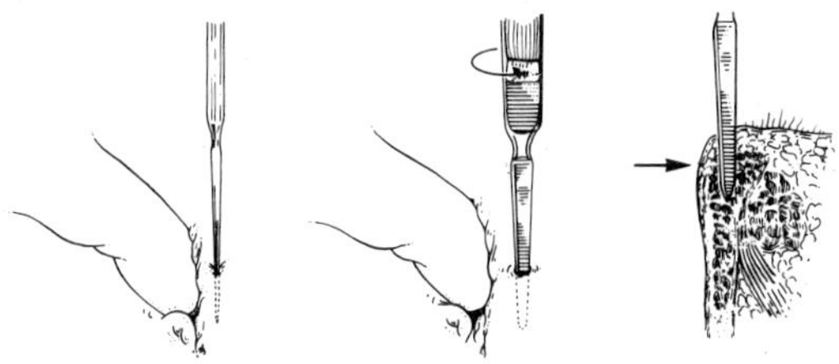

Fig. 37.9 Lateral sphincterotomy. A small tenotome is introduced through a stab wound, using a finger in the anal canal to guide the blade alongside the canal, to avoid puncturing it, and to bring the point to a level only part way up the sphincter. The blade is then rotated and the lowermost fibres of the sphincter muscle are divided. It is important not to divide too much of the sphincter, or continence will be impaired.

Treatment

Where the symptoms are minimal, dietary measures to ensure regular soft bowel motions and avoidance of straining at defecation plus the use of a local anaesthetic gel preparation prior to bowel action may suffice to permit healing within a few days.

For more painful lesions rapid relief can nearly always be obtained by manual dilatation of the anus under general anaesthesia. The purpose is to stretch the sphincter muscles and overcome the intense spasm for sufficient time for the fissure to heal over (Fig. 37.8).

If in spite of this the fissure recurs or a chronic one is established the operation of lateral sphincterotomy is advocated (Fig. 37.9). This involves cutting the lower fibres of the internal sphincter muscle by introducing a tenotomy knife through a small incision lateral to the anus, rotating the blade towards the lumen and dividing the sphincter fibres without damaging the mucosa.

FISTULA-IN-ANO

The fistula is an abnormal track communicating between the anal canal or rectum and the perianal skin.

Many arise as a result of either a perianal or an ischiorectal abscess, discharging both externally in the perianal region and internally into the anal canal or rectum. The track thus formed does not heal because of the persisting infection.

Crohn's disease (regional ileitis), ulcerative colitis, amoebic dysentery and tuberculosis are sometimes complicated by the development of fistula-in-ano, and occasionally one develops as a complication of colloid carcinoma of the rectum.

It is helpful to subdivide the different fistulas into high and low ones, depending on the point of

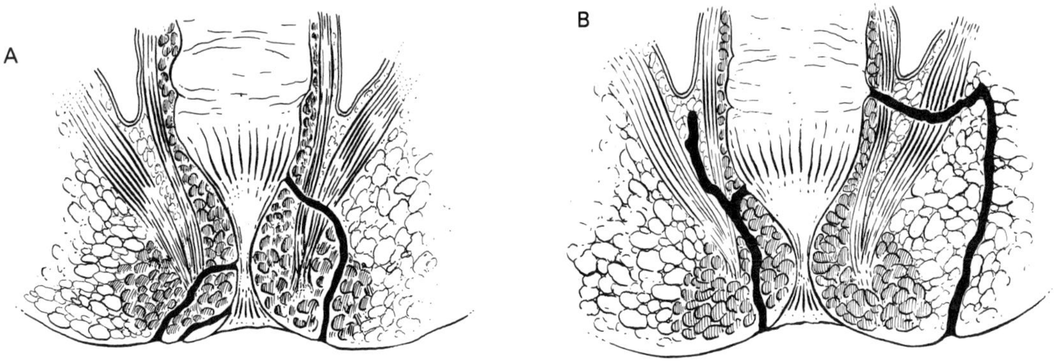

Fig. 37.10 Fistula-in-ano. Various patterns and levels of track. (A) Low: These fistulas enter the anal canal below the sphincter muscles or at most involving only the lower part of them; (B) high: these reach above the level of the sphincter muscles.

entry of the internal opening (Fig. 37.10). Fortunately low fistulas are much commoner and easier to cure, the internal opening lying below the pectinate line, and more importantly, below the anorectal muscle sling. In high-level fistulas the internal opening is above the muscle sling, and if the entire length of this sphincter muscle layer is divided the patient will be made incontinent.

Often the track is short and fairly direct, but sometimes, particularly with high-level fistulas and ones situated posteriorly the track may be long, tortuous and have several sidetracks. Successful treatment depends on knowing the full extent of the track.

Goodsall's rule is a generally reliable guide: namely, that if the external opening lies anterior to a transverse line across the centre of the anus, with

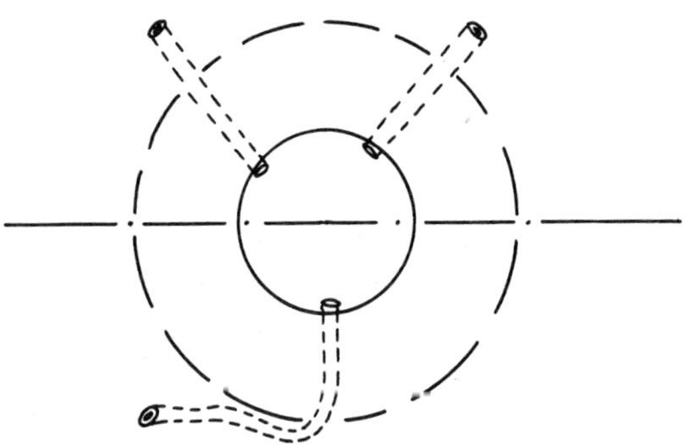

Fig. 37.11 Goodsall's rule: with the patient in the lithotomy position fistulas anterior to the midline pass directly into the anal canal, whereas those behind the midline usually follow a more tortuous path and enter the anal canal posteriorly.

the patient in the lithotomy position, then the track is direct to the nearest point in the anal canal, whereas if the external opening is behind this transverse line the internal anal opening is in the midline posteriorly (Fig. 37.11). Furthermore, the track in the latter may extend behind the anal canal on one or both sides before entering at the midline making a so-called horseshoe track.

Clinical features

The discharge of pus and mucus from a spot near the anus is the commonest symptom. Often there is a history of an abscess in that region which either had burst spontaneously, or was treated by incision and the discharge started shortly after that. Sometimes the discharge may stop for a few days, and a further abscess develops, again discharges and this cycle may be repeated.

Inspection shows an opening near the anus with discharging pus. On rectal examination the thickened track leading to the internal opening may be palpable, and pressure on this area may express the discharge of further pus from the external opening. In a high fistula, the internal opening may be felt to lie above the rectal sling. It may be possible to visualize the internal opening through a proctoscope, but often all that can be seen is an area of reddened and slightly swollen mucosa. Passage of a malleable probe along the track from the external opening may help to locate the inner opening. It is advisable also to perform full sigmoidoscopy to look for the presence of any associated disease, and biopsy of any unhealthy areas of mucosa.

Treatment

The treatment of a low-level anal fistula is complete surgical excision of the track. This is done under general anaesthesia by laying the track open from the outer to the internal opening and by excising all the granulation tissue lining the track, including any side-branches.

In high fistulas, this approach cannot be used as it will cause incontinence due to division of the rectal sling. It may still be possible to lay open the lower parts of the track, and any side-branches, but caution has to be exercised not to divide the sphincter muscles too deeply. One alternative is to pass a stout non-absorbable suture through the remainder of the track, out through the internal opening, tying it loosely. This can then be used postoperatively as a guide to the amount of remaining functioning sphincter muscle. Various methods of further excision of the residual track can then be considered, but are probably best referred to centres with particular expertise in this type of surgery.

For those fistulas which are associated with tuberculosis and inflammatory disease of the bowel treatment of the underlying disorder is, of course, indicated, but this in itself may not be enough to secure healing of the fistula and an appropriate operation may still be necessary (Fig. 37.12).

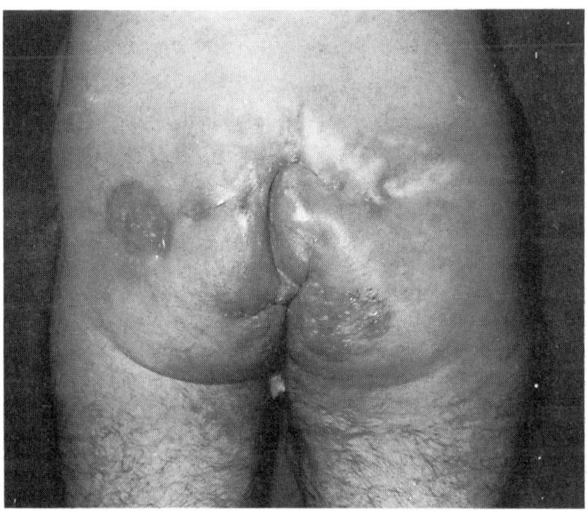

Fig. 37.12 Tracks and scars of multiple perianal abscesses, sinuses and fistulas in a patient with Crohn's disease.

PROLAPSE OF THE RECTUM

Protrusion of the rectum through the anus may be partial, when only the mucosa prolapses, or complete, when the whole thickness of the rectal wall protrudes through the anus (Fig. 37.13).

There are a number of factors which predispose to prolapse. In infants, the relative lack of the curve in the sacrum tends to make the direction of the rectum straight downwards and this is considered to be a factor facilitating prolapse of the mucosa. In children, there is often a history of repeated straining, as in whooping cough or on account of diarrhoea. Furthermore, a diminution in the amount of ischiorectal fat following any debilitating disease may reduce the support of the rectum (Fig. 37.14). In adults third-degree haemorrhoids sometimes initiate the process, and in women prolapse of rectum may be a part of a general pelvic floor weakness, associated with uterine prolapse. In elderly men straining during micturition due to an enlarged prostate may be a predisposing factor.

In complete prolapse, the protruding bowel may be as long as 15 cm and the mucosa is deep pink with circular folds. It consists of two complete layers of rectal wall. In the anterior part of a long prolapse, there may be a downward extension of the peritoneal pouch, which may contain a loop of intestine. The condition, therefore, is in effect a type of sliding hernia.

Clinical features

The complaint is of 'something coming down', initially only at defecation, but as it increases in size the prolapsed rectum may remain continuously out. In addition, there is often small amounts of contact bleeding and secretion of noticeable quantities of mucus. Local skin irritation follows.

Examination is best conducted after a bowel action when the prolapse may be obvious. It can be readily distinguished from an intussusception because in prolapse, a finger cannot be passed between the anal margin and the protruding mucosa, whereas it can in an intussusception.

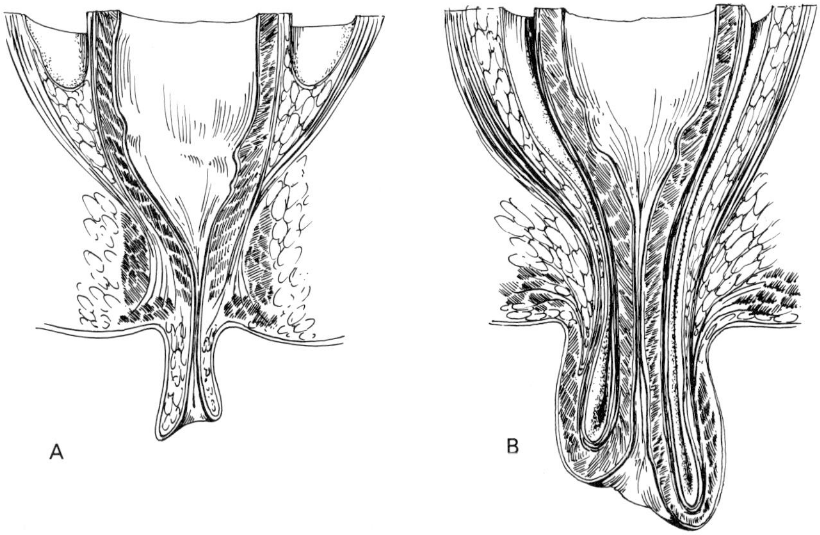

Fig. 37.13 Prolapse of the rectum. (**A**) Partial prolapse, with only mucosal layers being displaced downwards. (**B**) In the complete prolapse the entire thickness of the bowel has fallen through the anus, carrying even a protrusion of the pelvic peritoneum within the prolapsed mass.

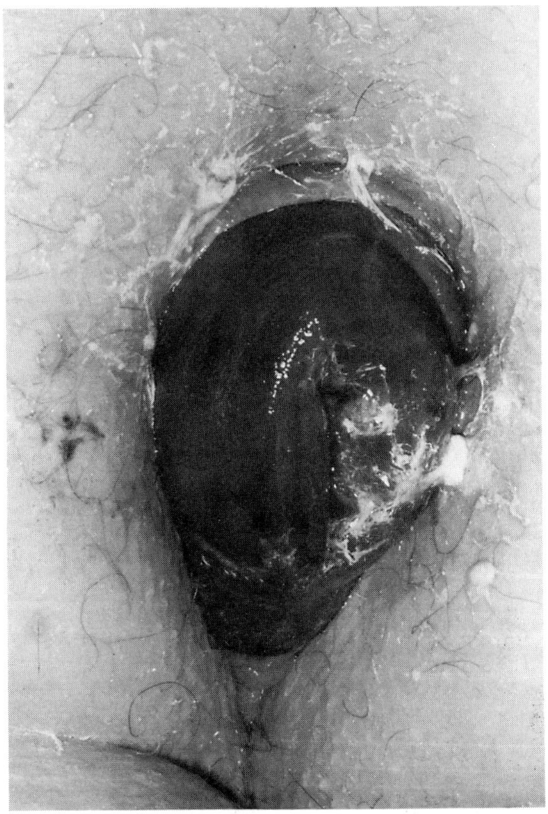

Fig. 37.14 Complete rectal prolapse in an elderly patient. While the bowel can be returned to above the anal ring by gentle manual pressure, it becomes extruded again as soon as the pressure is released.

Management

Predisposing factors such as weight loss, third-degree haemorrhoids, or prostatic obstruction should be corrected, but if the prolapse continues or there are no obvious precipitating factors, specific treatment is usually required.

In small degrees of partial prolapse, particularly in children, 5% phenol in almond oil may be injected into the submucosa after reducing the prolapse. If this fails or in adults simple excision of the cuff of redundant mucosa may be adequate.

For complete prolapse there are broadly two alternative types of procedure. First, in the frail and elderly judged to be unfit for any formal abdominal operation, the insertion of an encircling steel or stout nylon suture subcutaneously to narrow the anal ring (Thiersch operation) may prevent extrusion of the lax bowel (Fig. 37.15). However, there is a real danger of inducing faecal impaction unless bowel action is kept soft and regular, and the sutures also have a tendency to break or to work to the surface causing painful infected ulceration, and have to be removed.

The second approach, and usually more satisfactory, is to repair or reinforce the pelvic floor and/or use some method of fixing the rectum within the hollow of the sacrum. Various techniques have been developed. One which has become popular

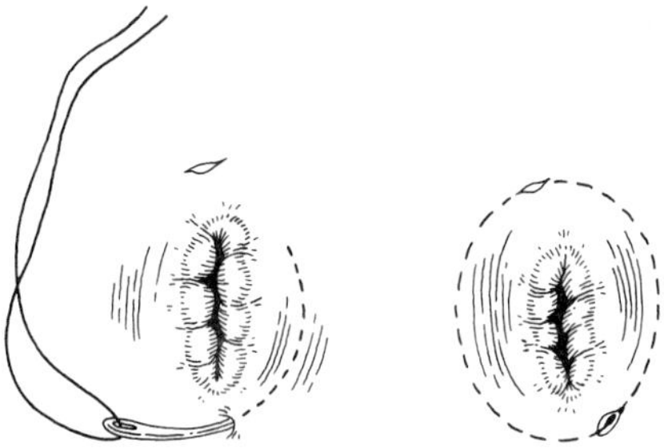

Fig. 37.15 Insertion of a Thiersch wire. Through a small posterior stab wound a half-circle needle carrying a braided metal wire is passed subcutaneously around one side of the anus. Having been brought out through a similar small anterior wound, it is then continued round to the original posterior wound and firmly knotted, using a finger inserted anally to judge the lumen size. The knot is buried, and the two small wounds are sutured.

and is relatively straightforward is fully to mobilize the rectum and proximal anal canal; these are then pulled well up into the pelvis and anchored to a partially encircling sheet of Ivalon sponge or other non-absorbable material by sutures (Fig. 37.16).

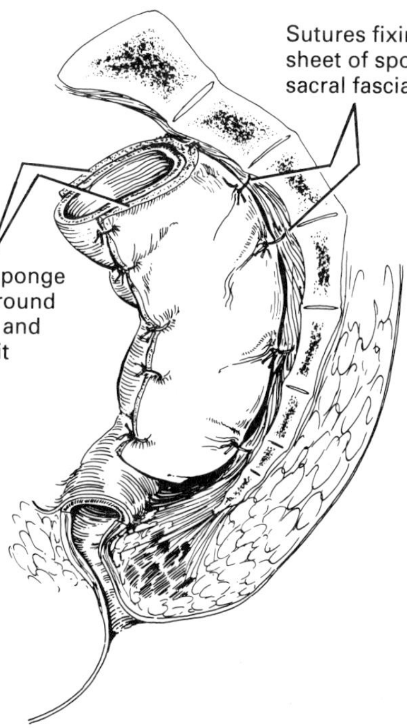

Fig. 37.16 Ivalon sponge fixation of rectum. The wrap-round is not complete, but leaves an anterior segment of the bowel wall uncovered, to diminish the chances of an obstructing stricture developing.

The induced fibrotic reaction further secures the anorectum in this restored position. The immediate and long-term results are generally much better than for the lesser procedures.

ANORECTAL INFECTIONS

The perianal region and the ischiorectal fossa are common sites for abscess formation (Fig. 37.17). Infection may spread to these spaces from suppuration in one or more of the anal glands. These glands, which lie in spaces between the muscle fibres of the external sphincter just deep to the perianal skin, are drained by ducts which open into the anal crypts.

In some cases the infection may be haematogenous, or may arise secondarily to a fissure, haematoma or thrombosed pile. In the majority of cases the infecting organism is one of the coliforms.

The clinical presentation is that of a steadily progressive painful swelling to the side of the anus over a few days. The swelling is acutely tender and may throb and defecation is painful. There may be mild systemic symptoms such as anorexia, sweating, fever and nausea. On inspection the area is reddened, tense, swollen and if pus has already formed and is starting to 'point' this may be seen as a yellow-grey circle in the middle of the swelling.

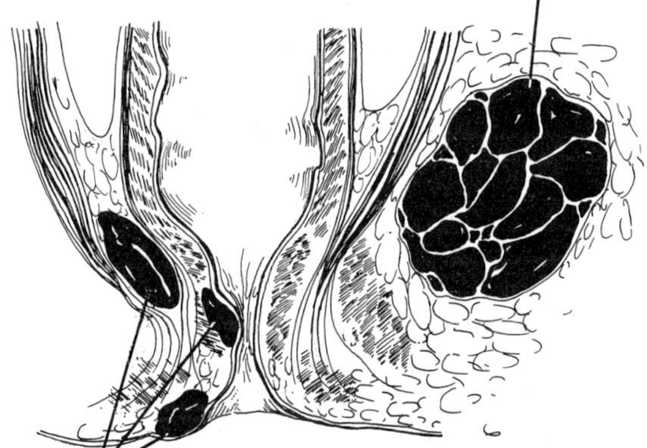

Fig. 37.17 Sagittal section through the lower rectum and anal canal showing different planes in which perianal and ischiorectal abscesses may develop.

Palpation should be extremely gentle and usually the degree of tenderness is so great that true fluctuation is impossible to demonstrate. The patient's temperature may be raised and there will be a leukocytosis.

Treatment

Both perianal and ischiorectal abscesses should be incised and drained under good general anaesthesia as soon as the diagnosis is made. It is important to evacuate all pockets of pus which may be present in loculi and recesses of the main abscess cavity. It is usual to make a liberal cruciate incision over the summit of the abscess, to break down any septa within the cavity by the finger, and then leave one or more drains leading from the depths of the abscess secured firmly in place (Fig. 37.18). The skin wound is left wide open after excising the four triangles of skin defined by the cruciate incision. During convalescence a periodic check should be made to ensure that no further pocketing of pus occurs and that progressive healing from the depths towards the surface ensues within the next 1–2 weeks.

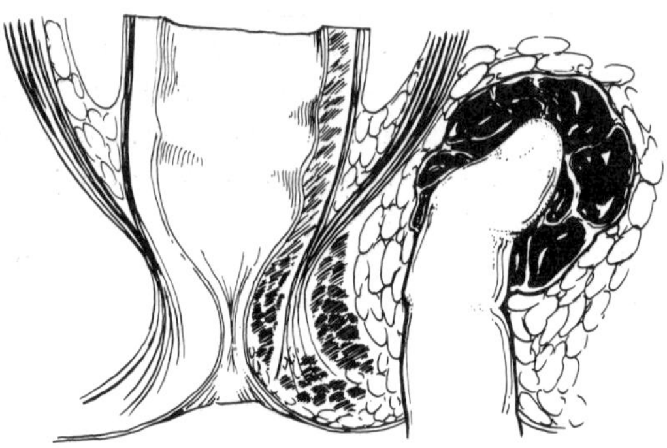

Fig. 37.18 Evacuation and drainage of an ischiorectal abscess. Under general anaesthesia and through a wide, usually cruciate incision, the abscess cavity is entered and a finger introduced to break down all septa containing loculi of the abscess. A drain is then left protruding from the emptied cavity.

Pilonidal sinus

This troublesome condition is commonest in young males, especially those well endowed with body hair. The almost invariable location of the opening or multiple openings is in the natal cleft about 2–3 cm posterior to the anus. The main direction of the track is towards the head, and although on following the track from the orifice it is at first single, there are often branches as it passes more deeply, and these side-branches may extend several centimetres laterally. The track is mainly granulation tissue, with a lining of some squamous epithelium, and nearly always contains one or more hairs within the lumen. These hairs point in towards the depths of the sinus, and have thus clearly been driven or

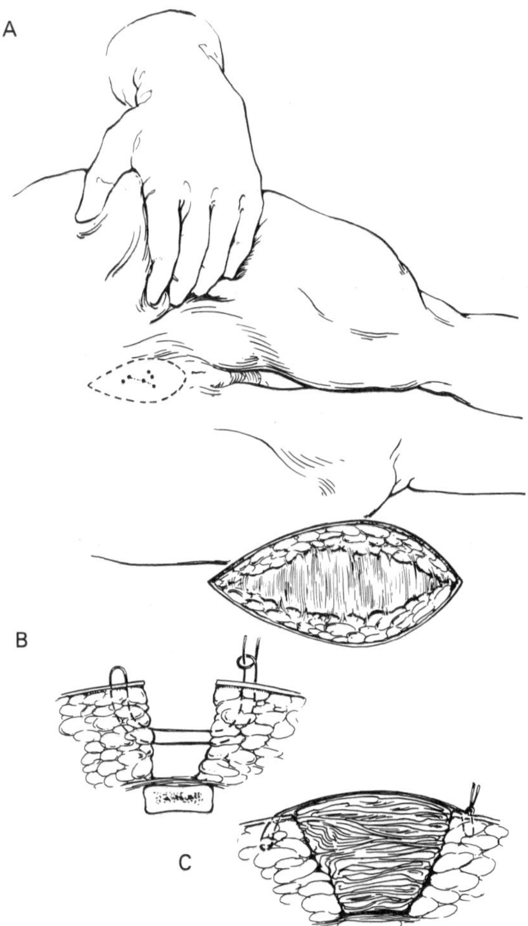

Fig. 37.19 Pilonidal sinus: the upper view shows the several black small pits at or near the midline of the natal cleft. The operation to excise the entire track usually involves an elliptical excision down to the sacral fascia (**A**). It may be possible to appose the wound edges by deeply placed sutures (**B**) or the wound may be left open (**C**), and packed with gauze or a mouldable silicone foam elastomer dressing.

sucked into the track rather than having grown out from its wall.

Some patients present with pilonidal sinus with a clear history of a localized abscess in the area and this may have discharged spontaneously or been incised. Recurrence of abscess formation or persistence of purulent discharge may have followed. Others present with the sinus already formed and complain only of a small amount of discharge and slight local discomfort or irritation.

The diagnosis is usually easy; characteristic black pinhead pits are seen in the upper part of the natal cleft on gently separating the buttocks (Fig. 37.19).

Treatment

The entire track should be either excised or laid open and allowed to granulate up from the depths. It is important to remove or lay open the entire extent of whatever branches may be present, otherwise recurrence of a sinus is inevitable. Excision and primary suture will, of course, lead to faster healing, but should be performed only when the full depth of the wound edges can be properly brought together by sutures without tension. If there is tension, or a subcutaneous space to fill with haematoma, the wound is very likely to become infected, break down and the sinus recur.

Various other less aggressive methods of treatment have been suggested, e.g. clearing the track by abrasive brushing, application of phenol, simple de-roofing, etc.

When in doubt about the advisability of any of these lesser methods, or excision plus primary suture, the time-honoured operation of laying the whole track open to leave a boat-shaped wound and packing this, e.g. with a silicone foam mould, usually gives a satisfactory resolution of the problem, although it requires several weeks of supervision of the change of dressings.

TUMOURS OF THE ANUS

Perhaps the most common benign tumour is simple papilloma, either single, or more frequently multiple. They are thought to be viral in origin and are to be distinguished from the lower, flatter and more rounded lesions of condylomata lata, a feature of secondary syphilis.

Benign papillomata may be removed either by diathermy or excision under anaesthesia.

Squamous carcinoma is very much rarer than adenocarcinoma arising from the true rectal or anal mucosa, but may present with symptoms similar to rectal carcinoma. An ulcerated swelling develops, causing bleeding and discharge of mucoid material and it often becomes infected. There is usually a tendency for it to grow around the anus, producing stenosis and interference with normal bowel action. Lymphatic spread may travel to the inguinal nodes, which should be palpated.

Since the tumour, arising basically from skin, is squamous it should be radiosensitive and radiotherapy is therefore an option. However, it is usually preferable to advise surgical excision, which implies an abdominoperineal resection of the anus, anal canal and rectum, and creation of a permanent colostomy.

38. Genitourinary system: general disorders

The genital and urinary tracts share much in common and it is helpful to think of them as a whole rather than as their individual components. An understanding of their common embryology is a great help in understanding congenital abnormalities affecting the urinary and the genital systems.

DEVELOPMENT OF THE GENITOURINARY TRACT AND ITS ANOMALIES

Urinary system

There are three separate stages in the embryological development of the kidneys (Fig. 38.1). Pronephros is a vestigial structure that disappears completely by the fourth week except for its primary duct. This primary duct gains connection to the mesonephros, the second stage of development. Whilst most of the mesonephric tubules also degenerate the mesonephric duct persists and opens into the cloaca. The ureteric bud develops at this latter point and starts to grow cranially to meet the metanephric blastema, which is the final phase of development. During the cranial migration and rotation the metanephric tissue progressively enlarges with rapid internal differentiation into the urinary tubules. The cephalad end of the ureteric bud expands within the metanephros to form the renal pelvis.

Consequences of failed development

Failure of the metanephros to ascend leads to an ectopic kidney. Failure to rotate during ascent causes a malrotated kidney. Horseshoe kidney results from fusion of the two metanephric masses. Bifurcation of the ureteric bud results in a bifid ureter. Development of an accessory bud leads to a duplicated ureter commonly meeting the same

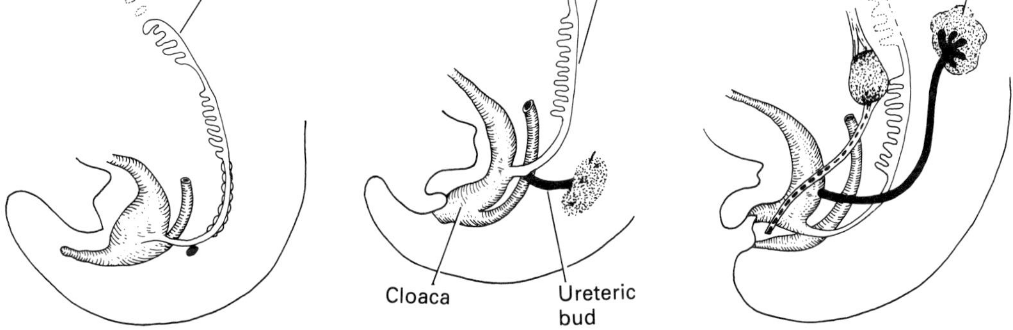

Fig. 38.1 Three stages in the embryological development of the urinary system.

nephric mass; rarely, each bud has a separate metanephric mass resulting in supernumerary kidneys. Failure of a ureteric bud to develop results in a solitary kidney and a half trigone.

Bladder and urethra

Division of the cloaca (the blind end of the hindgut) into a ventral (urogenital sinus) and a dorsal (rectum) segment is completed during the seventh week and initiates the early differentiation of the urinary bladder and urethra. The urogenital sinus receives the mesonephric duct and gradually absorbs its caudal end so that by the end of the seventh week the ureteric bud and the mesonephric duct have independent openings.

Congenital anomalies of the bladder and urethra

Failure of cloacal division results in persistent cloaca. Incomplete division is more frequent and results in rectovesical, rectourethral or rectovestibular fistulas, usually with imperforate anus or anal atresia. Development of genital primordia in an area more caudal than normal results in incomplete or complete epispadias. A more extensive defect results in vesical exstrophy. Failure of the urethral folds to fuse leads to various grades of hypospadias.

Prostate

The prostate develops at the end of the 11th week as five groups of outgrowths of urethral epithelium both above and below the entrance of the mesonephric duct. These form the five lobes of the prostate.

Gonads

Each embryo is at first morphologically bisexual; the development of one set of sex primordia and the gradual involution of the other are determined by the sex type of the gonad which starts to be differentiated during the seventh week. If the gonad develops into a testis the germinal epithelium grows into radially arranged cordlike masses that differentiate later into seminiferous tubules. If it develops into an ovary it becomes differentiated into a cortex and medulla; the cortex later differentiates into ovarian follicles containing ova.

The testis remains at the abdominal end of the inguinal canal until the seventh month, and then passes through the inguinal canal to the scrotum guided by the primary attachment of the gubernaculum. The ovary undergoes internal descent to enter the pelvis.

Anomalies arising from failed development of the gonads

Lack of complete testicular descent is known as crypto-orchidism. The descent to an abnormal site is known as testicular ectopia (ectopic testis).

In the male the genital duct system develops from the wolffian duct, which differentiates into epididymis, vas deferens, seminal vesicles and ejaculatory ducts. In the female the genital duct system develops from the müllerian ducts which fuse at their caudal ends and differentiate into the uterine tubes, uterus, and most of the vagina.

The external genitalia start to differentiate by the eighth week. The genital tubercle and the genital swellings develop into the penis and scrotum in the male and the clitoris and labia majora in the female.

With breakdown of the urogenital membrane in the seventh week the urogenital sinus achieves a separate opening on the undersurface of the genital tubercle. The expansion of the intratubercular part of the urogenital sinus will form the vaginal vestibule and the distal part of the vagina. The two folds on the undersurface of the genital tubercle unite in the male to form the penile urethra; in the female they remain separate, to form the labia minora.

Consequences of anomalous development

Failure of fusion in the male leads to hypospadias which is usually associated with incomplete formation of the prepuce with a dorsal hood and a ventral penile curvature. It is never proximal to the bulbus urethra, and continence is always preserved. Epispadias is a milder form of bladder exstrophy. If extensive, epispadias can extend to the bladder neck and is frequently associated with incontinence. A rudimentary penis or a hypertrophied clitoris is seen with pseudohermaphroditism.

APPLIED ANATOMY OF THE GENITOURINARY TRACT

The kidneys

The kidneys are paired organs lying behind the peritoneum on the posterior abdominal wall and separated from the surrounding fascia by perinephric fat. The renal vascular pedicle enters the renal sinus; the renal vein is anterior to the artery, and both are anterior to the renal pelvis. The renal artery divides in the renal sinus into anterior and posterior branches that undergo subdivisions with variable extents of distribution. They are end-arteries. The venous tributaries anastomose freely and usually drain into one common renal vein. Accessory vessels are common.

The renal parenchyma

The renal parenchyma consists of over 1 million functioning units (the nephrons) and is divided into a peripheral cortex containing the secretory elements and a central medulla containing the excretory elements. The nephron starts in the cortex as Bowman's capsule which surrounds the glomerulus and leads to a long tubular structure consisting of proximal and distal convoluted tubules with the loop of Henle in between them; it ends in a collecting duct that opens at the tip of a papilla into a minor calix.

The renal pelvis and calices

The renal pelvis and calices are within the renal sinus and function as the main collecting reservoir. The pelvis, which is partly extrarenal and partly intrarenal, branches into three major calices that in turn branch into several minor calices. These minor calices are directly related to the renal parenchyma and they receive the tips of the medullary pyramids (the papillae) and act as a receiving cup to the collecting tubules. The pelvicaliceal system is a highly muscular structure; the musculature runs in every direction and is directly continuous between the pelvis and the various calices, helping to synchronize their contractile activity.

The ureter

The ureter connects the renal pelvis to the urinary bladder. It is a small muscularized tube; its muscle fibres lie in an irregular helical arrangement and are meant primarily for peristaltic activity. The ureteral musculature is directly continuous with the renal pelvis cranially and with the vesical trigone distally. The pelvic and ureteric blood supply is segmental, arising from the renal, spermatic or ovarian and vesical arteries with rich, subadventitial anastomosis.

The bladder

The bladder is primarily a reservoir with a meshwork of muscle fibres that not only change from one plane to another but also branch and join each other to constitute a synchronized organ. Its musculature is directly continuous with the urethral musculature and this functions as a urethral sphincteric mechanism in spite of the lack of a true circular sphincter. The ureters enter the bladder postero-inferiorly through the ureteral hiatus; after a short intravesical submucosal course they lose their lumen and become continuous with the trigone which is superimposed on the bladder base, though deeply connected to it.

The urethra

The adult female urethra is about 4 cm long and is muscular in its proximal four-fifths. This musculature is arranged in an inner longitudinal coat which is continuous with the inner longitudinal fibres of the bladder, and an outer circular coat which is continuous with the outer longitudinal coat of the bladder. The outer circular fibres comprise the sphincteric mechanism. The striated external sphincter surrounds the middle third of the urethra. In the male the prostatic urethra is heavily muscular and sphincteric. The membranous urethra is within the urogenital diaphragm and is surrounded by the striated external sphincter. The penile urethra is poorly muscularized and traverses the corpus spongiosum to open on the tip of the glans penis.

The prostate

The prostate surrounds the proximal portion of the male urethra; it is a fibromuscular glandular cone-shaped structure about 2.5 cm long and weighing about 20 g. It is traversed from base to apex by the urethra and is pierced posterolaterally by the ejaculatory ducts that converge to open at the verumontanum on the floor of the urethra. The prostatic glandular elements drain through about 12 paired excretory ducts that open into the floor of the urethra above the verumontanum. The prostate is surrounded by a thin capsule derived from its stroma which is ridged in musculature, and part of the urethral musculature and the sphincteric mechanism. A rich venous plexus surrounds the prostate especially anteriorly and laterally. Its lymphatic drainage is into the hypogastric, sacral, vesical and external iliac lymph nodes.

The testis

The testis is a paired organ surrounded by the tunica albuginea and subdivided into numerous lobules by fibrous septa. Extremely convoluted seminiferous tubules gather to open into the rete testis, where they join the efferent duct to drain into the epididymis. Arterial supply is via the internal spermatic artery; venous drainage is through the pampiniform plexus which drains into the spermatic veins. The right spermatic vein joins the vena cava and the left joins the renal vein. The lymphatics drain into the lumbar lymph nodes.

SURGICAL PHYSIOLOGY OF THE URINARY SYSTEM

The function of the kidneys is to maintain and regulate homeostasis of body fluids and electrolytes and to excrete toxic byproducts of metabolism. In addition they have a regulatory role in blood pressure control and in haemoglobin production. The kidney regulates body fluids and electrolytes by three main mechanisms:

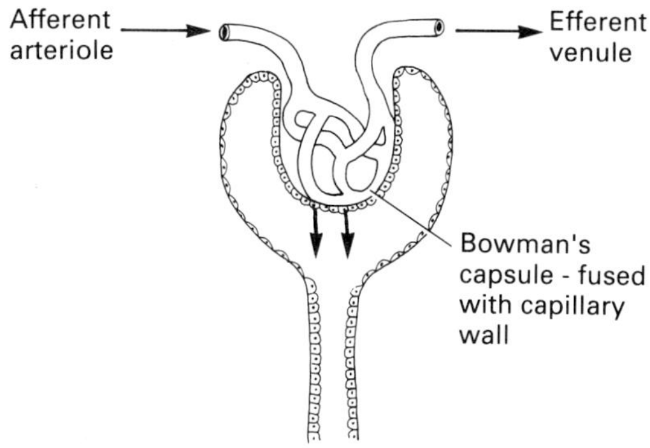

Fig. 38.2 Schematic representation of a glomerulus, in which the process of filtration across the combined membrane of the capillary wall and the single-cell-thick inner layer of the glomerulus takes place. Water, electrolytes and various larger molecules are filtered from the plasma in this process.

1. Firstly by glomerular filtration (Fig. 38.2): this is dependent on glomerular capillary arterial pressure minus plasma colloid osmotic pressure plus Bowman's capsular resistance. Creatinine clearance is a measurement of the volume of plasma cleared of creatinine per minute and it is calculated by measuring the amount of creatinine excreted in the urine per hour (urinary creatinine concentration × urinary volume per hour) divided by the plasma concentration of creatinine. The normal range is from 80 to 140 ml/min. Both simple plasma creatinine and blood urea levels reflect the glomerular filtration rate, rising as filtration rate diminishes and falling as filtration rate increases, but by themselves they are only very rough guides.
2. Clearly with such a large volume of plasma being filtered every minute through the glomerular basement membrane it is essential that effective reabsorption takes place through the tubular wall (Fig. 38.3), and under normal circumstances about 99% of the filtered volume will be reabsorbed through the tubules, together with all the valuable constituents of the filtrate (chlorides, glucose, sodium, potassium, calcium and amino acids). Urea, uric acid, phosphates and sulphates are also reabsorbed to varying degrees. The process of reabsorption is partly passive by diffusion and partly active. Reabsorption of water and electrolytes is under control of the adrenal, pituitary and parathyroid glands.
3. Tubular secretion is the third main function of the nephron. This helps to eliminate and thus

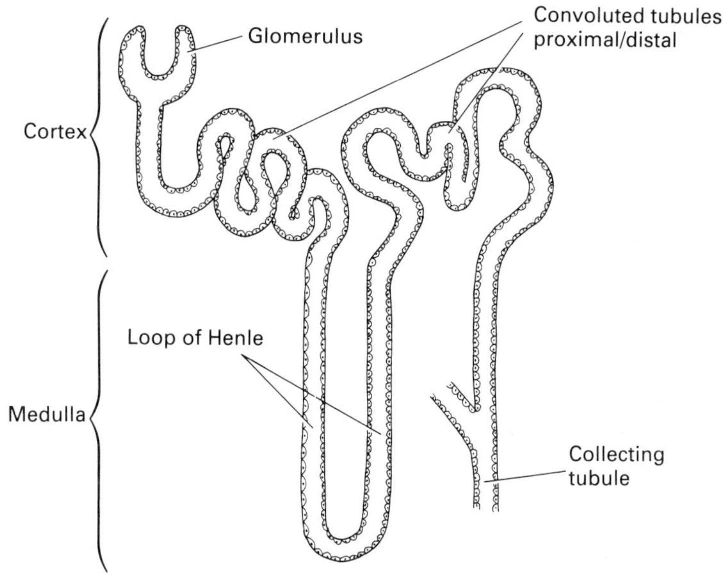

Fig. 38.3 Diagram of disposition of different parts of the nephron. The main roles of the proximal and distal tubules and the loop of Henle are concerned with the reabsorption of most of the glomerular filtrate, the regulation of electrolyte losses, and some secretion of substances to maintain acid–base balance.

maintain plasma levels of certain substances or to exchange valuable ions from the filtrate for less desirable ions in the plasma, e.g. sodium ion from the urine for a hydrogen ion in the plasma. Failure of adequate secretory function leads to acidosis, commonly encountered in chronic renal disease. The renal plasma flow can be calculated from the phenolsulphonphthalein clearance and this serves as a clinical measurement of renal blood flow.

The ureteropelvicaliceal system

This system is one continuous tubular structure with adequate musculature which is imperceptibly moving from one segment to the other to maintain autonomic continuity and physiological synchrony at various levels. Cinepyelography indicates that there are sphincters at the junction of the minor and major calices and at the pelviureteric junction. Each segment of the caliceal system fills before its contents are passed into the next chamber. Ureteral filling is primarily passive; ureteral emptying is primarily active. Ureteral peristaltic activity is essential in order to transport urine across points of resistance, e.g. the ureterovesical junction (and to prevent retrograde flow).

The ureterovesical junction

The ureterovesical junction allows free flow of urine from the ureter to the bladder and at the same time prevents retrograde flow. The continuity and specific muscular arrangement of the intravesical ureter and the trigone provide a muscularly active valvular mechanism that can efficiently adapt itself to the variable phases of bladder activity during filling and voiding. Progressive bladder-filling leads to firm occlusion of the intravesical ureter against retrograde flow and increased resistance to antegrade urine flow due to trigonal stretching. During voiding trigonal contraction completely seals the intravesical ureter against any antegrade or retrograde flow.

The urinary bladder

The urinary bladder functions primarily as a reservoir that can accommodate variable volumes without increasing its intraluminal pressure. Emptying of the full bladder involves voluntary activation of the detrusor muscle, which contracts uniformly and maintains its contraction until the bladder is completely empty. Funnelling of the bladder outlet with progressive downward movement of the dome ensures complete emptying.

The vesical sphincteric mechanism is primarily a smooth-muscle sphincter in the male prostatic urethra and in the proximal four-fifths of the female urethra. There is no purely circular sphincteric entity but there are abundant circularly oriented muscle fibres which are directly continuous with the outer coat of the detrusor muscle. The sphincter has the same nerve supply as, and reacts simultaneously with, the detrusor.

DISORDERS OF THE URINARY SYSTEM

There are three general disturbances which affect the urinary system as a whole rather than its individual parts. These are obstructive uropathy, urinary infection and urinary stone formation. As a group of disturbances they are intimately related, and are generally regarded as the urological triangle, each leading on to the other as a complication, and as a final consequence of any one of them or indeed of all three of them, renal failure may result.

OBSTRUCTIVE UROPATHY

Obstruction is one of the most important pathological entities affecting the urinary tract since it eventually leads to decompensation of the muscular conduits and reservoirs, back-pressure and atrophy of the renal parenchyma; it also invites infection and stone formation which cause additional damage to the organ involved. Both the level at which the obstruction occurs and the degree of obstruction are important to an understanding of the pathological consequences of this group of disorders.

Level of obstruction

Any obstruction at or distal to the internal urethral meatus leads to back-pressure effects on both kidneys. Obstruction at or proximal to the ureteral orifice leads to unilateral damage unless the lesion involves both ureters simultaneously.

Degree of obstruction

Complete obstruction leads to rapid decompensation of the system proximal to the site of obstruction with immediate muscular failure. For example, acute retention occurs if the obstruction is distal to the bladder, and anuria occurs if obstruction involves both ureters. Partial obstruction leads to gradual progressive muscular hypertrophy, followed by gradual dilatation, decompensation and hydronephrosis.

Aetiology

Urinary tract obstruction may be congenital or acquired.

Congenital

1. Meatal stenosis, urethral stricture, postero-urethral valves, ureterovesical, and ureteropelvic junction obstruction.
2. Neurological deficiency, e.g. spina bifida.

Acquired

1. Urethral stricture, inflammatory or traumatic.
2. Bladder outlet obstruction (benign prostatic hypertrophy or cancer of the prostate).
3. Vesical tumour.
4. Urogenic bladder (paraplegia).
5. Extrinsic ureteral compression (retroperitoneal fibrosis, tumour, enlarged lymph nodes).
6. Ureteral or pelvic stones.
7. Ureteral strictures.
8. Ureteral or pelvic tumours.

Pathogenesis

Regardless of its cause, acquired obstruction leads to the same changes in the various segments in the urinary tract, depending on its severity and duration.

Urethral changes

Proximal to the obstruction the urethra dilates and balloons. A urethral diverticulum may develop, and dilatation and gaping of the prostatic and ejaculatory ducts may occur.

Bladder changes

Early, detrusor and trigonal thickening and hypertrophy compensate for the outlet obstruction and lead to complete bladder-emptying (Fig. 38.4). This change leads to progressive development of bladder trabeculation, cellules, saccules and then diverticula. Beyond a certain phase bladder decompensation occurs, and is characterized by the above changes, plus variable amounts of residual urine. A very late change with persistent obstruction (more frequently encountered with neurogenic dysfunction) is decompensation of the uretero-vesical junction, leading to reflux which aggravates the back-pressure effect on the upper tract by exposing it to abnormally high intravesical pressures, in addition to favouring the onset or persistence of urinary tract infection. If ureteral obstruction is unilateral, compensatory hypertrophy of the contralateral kidney will develop. Total renal function, therefore, may remain normal.

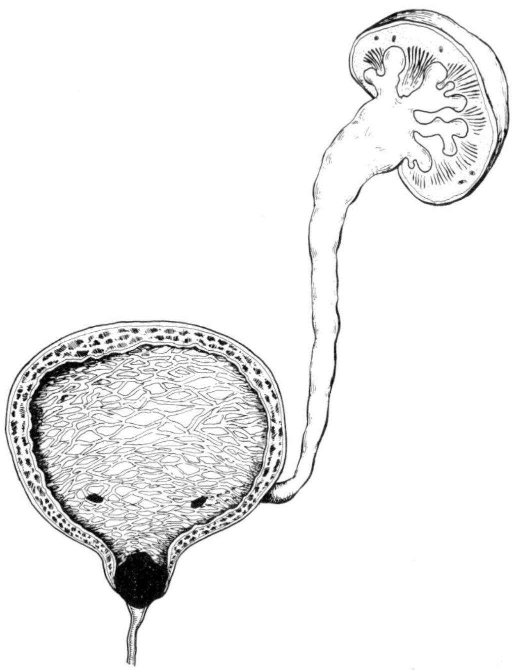

Fig. 38.4 Various effects of obstruction to the bladder outflow. The bladder wall is thickened and the mucosa trabeculated: the ureteric orifices are widened, the ureters and pelvis dilated, and the calices expanded and rounded. The next change, if unrelieved, would be thinning of the renal substance, leading to renal failure.

Ureteral changes

The first noted change is gradual progressive increase in ureteral distension. This increases ureteral wall stretch, which in turn increases contractile power and ureteral hyperactivity and hypertrophy develop. Because the ureteral musculature runs in an irregular helical pattern, stretching of its muscular elements leads to lengthening as well as widening. This is the start of decompensation when tortuosity and dilatation become obvious. These changes can progress, leading to marked ureteral dilatation and lengthening, and the ureter becomes atonic with infrequent or completely absent peristalsis.

Pelvicaliceal changes

When subjected to progressively increasing volumes of retained urine, the renal pelvis and calices progressively distend. The pelvis first shows evidence of hyperactivity, hypertrophy and then progressive dilatation and atony. The calices show the same changes to a variable degree, depending on whether the renal pelvis is intrarenal or extrarenal. In the extrarenal pelvis the caliceal dilatation may be minimal in spite of marked pelvic dilatation. In the intrarenal pelvis caliceal dilatation and renal parenchymal damage are maximal. The successive phases seen with obstruction are rounding of the fornices, followed by flattening of the papillae and finally clubbing of the minor calices.

Renal parenchymal changes

With progressive pelvic caliceal distension, there is parenchymal compression against the renal capsule. This, plus the more important factor of compression of the vessels by the distending calices, results in a marked drop in renal blood flow. This phenomenon leads to progressive parenchymal compression and ischaemic atrophy.

Clinical findings

Symptoms and signs

These vary according to the site of obstruction.

Intravesical obstruction. Intravesical obstruction leads to difficulty in initiation of voiding, a weak stream, and a diminished flow rate with terminal dribbling. Burning and frequency are commonly associated symptoms. A distended or thickened bladder wall may be palpable. Urethral induration of a stricture, benign prostatic hypertrophy or cancer of the prostate may be noted on rectal examination. Meatal stenosis and impacted urethral stones are readily diagnosed.

Supravesical obstruction. Renal pain or renal colic and gastrointestinal symptoms are commonly associated with acute obstruction. Supravesical obstruction may be completely asymptomatic when it develops very gradually over a period of several weeks or months. An enlarged kidney may be palpable. Costovertebral angle tenderness may be present.

Laboratory findings

Evidence of urinary infection, haematuria or crystalluria may be seen. Impaired kidney function is noted by elevation of the blood urea or the serum creatinine, with the ratio well above the normal 10 : 1 because of significant urea reabsorption.

X-ray findings

Radiological examination is usually diagnostic in cases of stasis, tumours and strictures. Dilatation and anatomical changes occur above the level of obstruction, whereas distal to the obstruction the configuration is usually normal. An intravenous pyelogram will usually demonstrate the level and the extent of obstruction, except when the obstruction has been long-standing and renal function is poor, in which event a triple dose of contrast medium is given as an intravenous infusion and delayed pictures taken at 12, 24 and 48 h. Cystoscopy and retrograde pyelography are often helpful in identifying the level of obstruction in a ureter where the kidney is not functioning sufficiently to show up on intravenous urogram.

Ultrasonography

Ultrasonography provides an ideal non-invasive method for screening the kidney to exclude the presence of obstruction. At the same time it offers a precise method for cannulating the kidney in order to perform an antegrade pyelogram. Ultrasonic examination of the kidney has largely replaced the intravenous urogram as a screening test for renal obstruction.

Isotope renogram

The isotope renogram is another relatively non-invasive way of examining the poorly functioning kidney in order to determine the degree of obstruction. It has the singular advantage of being a functional test and when combined with an intravenous injection of frusemide can distinguish flaccidity from mechanical obstruction. An intravenous injection of frusemide will induce an immediate emptying of a flaccid, dilated pelvicaliceal system.

Complications

The most important complications of urinary tract obstruction are renal parenchymal atrophy, infection and stone formation. A combination of infection and obstruction leads to rapid kidney destruction.

Treatment

The aim of therapy is relief of the obstruction. For example, in acute urinary retention, treatment consists of bladder drainage by a catheter. Surgery is often necessary. Simple urethral stricture may be managed conservatively by dilatation. Urethrotomy or urethroplasty may be required. Urethral valves must be ruptured. Benign prostatic hypertrophy and obstructing bladder tumours require surgical removal. Impacted stones must be either removed or bypassed by a catheter in order to be surgically removed later, or to be given a chance to pass spontaneously. Ureteropelvic obstruction requires surgical revision and plastic repair. Preliminary drainage above the obstruction is sometimes needed to improve kidney function. Occasionally permanent drainage and diversion by cutaneous ureterostomy, ileal or colonic loop diversion or permanent nephrostomy are required.

Prognosis

The prognosis depends on the cause, site, duration and degree of kidney damage. In general, relief of obstruction leads to improvement in kidney function except in seriously damaged kidneys, especially those destroyed by inflammatory scarring.

INFECTIONS OF THE URINARY TRACT

Urinary tract infections are so common and so serious in long-term effects that meticulous attention must be paid to the details of diagnosis and treatment. Urinary tract infection is undoubtedly the commonest cause of 'renal hypertension' in women, and a frequent cause in men. Because the chronic form of the disease is associated with few symptoms the diagnosis is often not established until signs of renal insufficiency or hypertension appear. Resistance to treatment is remarkable, and relapses are frequent and often associated with anatomical abnormalities. The following clinical classification provides a useful approach to the patient:

1. Acute infection, uncomplicated.
2. Acute infection, complicated
   a. with anatomical defect not demonstrable.
   b. with anatomical defect demonstrable.
3. Asymptomatic bacteriuria.
4. Chronic infection.

Acute infection of the upper urinary tract

Essentials of diagnosis

The common symptoms and signs are the sudden onset of chills and fever, with urinary frequency, urgency and burning on micturition; pain and tenderness in the costovertebral angle over the kidneys, headache, prostration, nausea and vomiting; urine containing pus (pyuria), few or many red cells, granular and white cell casts, small-to-moderate amounts of protein, and bacteria; leukocytosis, rapid sedimentation rate and occasionally bacteraemia. Acute urinary tract infection may be confined to the bladder, but more often the infection involves the ureters and kidneys as well. In many cases anatomical defects of the genitourinary tract produce obstruction or stasis which favours invasion and persistence of pathogenic organisms

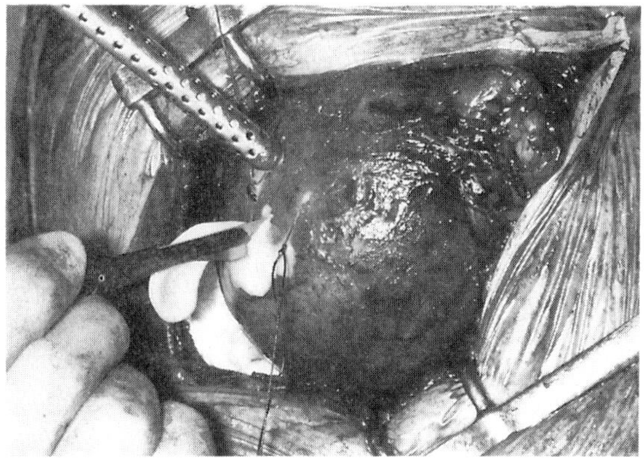

Fig. 38.5 Pyogenic infection in a grossly hydronephrotic kidney led to a large collection of pus in the distended kidney—pyonephrosis. The pus can be seen pouring from the incision.

(Fig. 38.5). The organisms most frequently found are Gram-negative bacilli, i.e. *Escherichia coli, Enterobacter (Aerobacter) aerogenase,* paracolon species, *Pseudomonas aeruginosa, Proteus vulgaris* and *Salmonella*; and the Gram-positive cocci, i.e. streptococci (enterococci and staphylococci). In acute urinary tract infections the causative organism is present in great numbers, ranging from 10 000 to hundreds of millions of bacteria per millilitre of urine.

Predisposing factors are of importance. In young people infection is much more frequently encountered in the female; in the older age groups infection is more common in the male since urinary tract obstruction is more frequent. Pregnancy, diabetes mellitus, papillary necrosis, metabolic disorders with nephrolithiasis, obstructive uropathy, neurogenic bladder and genitourinary instrumentation are all associated with a high incidence of acute urinary tract infection.

Differential diagnosis

Acute infection involving the upper urinary tract must be differentiated from other acute causes of abdominal pain. The presence of pus and bacteria in the urine will usually confirm the diagnosis.

Laboratory findings

The white blood count is usually 14 000–20 000 mm^3, with an increased polymorphonuclear neutrophil count. The sedimentation rate is very rapid. The urine contains large numbers of polymorphonuclear leukocytes, granular and leukocyte casts, some red cells and epithelial cells, shreds of mucus, protein and at times visible organisms. Cultures of the urine reveal multitudes of bacteria, and blood cultures are occasionally positive as well. Examination of the urine is extremely important, for only if the organism is identified can therapy be properly directed. A Gram-stain smear of the sediment obtained from 5–10 ml of urine will show identifiable bacteria when these are present in concentrations of 10 000 or more per ml of urine. Urine cultures should be performed either on fresh catheterized specimens or on fresh midstream specimens after proper cleansing of the urethral meatus and, in the female, exclusion of the labial and vaginal contaminants. Percutaneous aspiration of urine from the bladder using a sterile needle and syringe and strictly aseptic technique have the advantage of avoiding the hazards of catheterization, but involve the more serious risk of puncturing the peritoneum or gut unless the procedure is performed carefully.

Treatment

Specific measures

Give specific antimicrobial drugs chosen on the basis of cultures and sensitivity tests. The sulphonamides, penicillins, nitrofurantoin and the tetracyclines should be employed in doses sufficient to produce adequate levels in the renal tissues and urine. Chloramphenicol, the colistins, neomycin, and polymyxin should be reserved for cases which are refractory to other agents. The newer cephalosporins should be held in reserve for their own particular indications. In the uncomplicated case of the initial attack of urinary tract infection in the female, treatment with the appropriate antibiotic for 10 days will usually produce a cure.

Cultures should be repeated at 2 weeks and 3 months after therapy has ceased to confirm the absence of infection. In cases of recurrence or reinfection in females and in all cases of infection in males, complicating or predisposing anatomical defects or obstruction must be ruled out. When the acute phase has passed diagnostic studies should be undertaken to demonstrate any anatomical or metabolic defect: X-ray of the abdomen, intravenous urogram, cystoscopy, cystogram and cysto-urethrogram to determine reflux of urine into the ureters, and appropriate tests for coexisting metabolic diseases such as diabetes mellitus. Anatomical abnormalities which cause obstruction, stasis or reflux should be corrected if possible, for their persistence precludes permanent cure.

General measures

The patient should rest in bed and take a regular diet as tolerated, and keep up a high intake of fluids to maintain a high urine output. The intravenous administration of fluids may be required. Give antipyretics and analgesics as indicated.

Prognosis

In the absence of anatomical abnormality of the urinary tract appropriate antimicrobial therapy will usually result in cure. Recurrent or continued infection produces renal damage, and the ultimate development of renal insufficiency or hypertension.

Chronic urinary tract infection

Essentials of diagnosis

1. The condition may be asymptomatic except for exacerbations of symptoms of acute urinary tract infection.
2. End-stages of chronic infection are characterized by symptoms and signs of renal insufficiency, uraemia and hypertension.
3. The urine may be unremarkable, or may contain leukocytes, bacteria and protein.

General considerations

Chronic infection is often unsuspected unless a history of urinary tract infection or of unexplained and peculiar gastrointestinal symptoms is elicited. When hypertension is present the possibility of long-standing asymptomatic infection must always be entertained, since the disease is often unilateral and nephrectomy may be curative if the function of the other kidney is normal. Before renal insufficiency develops proper treatment may delay or prevent serious sequelae of continuing infection.

Clinical findings

There are none unless clear-cut exacerbations of more acute urinary tract infection occur. The late manifestations are those of renal insufficiency or of hypertension.

Treatment

Treatment of patients with chronic bacteriuria who have had bacteriological relapses with upper urinary tract involvement must be vigorous and of extended duration. Often 10–14-day courses of therapy are inadequate. The drug used must be selected on the basis of culture and sensitivity tests, with preference for oral agents. Treatment should continue for 2–6 weeks. All agents must be employed with caution in the presence of renal insufficiency. A thorough investigation is required to rule out obstruction, stone, anatomical defects and neuromuscular defects. Intravenous urograms, cystoscopy, ureteral catheterization, cystography and voiding cystourethrography may be necessary to delineate defects responsible for intractable infection. Surgical correction of anatomical abnormalities or relief of obstruction may improve the chances for cure.

Prognosis

Unless the infection is eradicated one or both kidneys will be damaged so severely that irremedial hypertension or renal insufficiency will result. However, the course of the disease may be protracted over many years, and with careful management these patients may lead reasonably comfortable lives even when the renal reserve is limited.

Lower urinary tract infection

Because the urinary tract is a continuous duct with relatively ineffective separation of the ureterocaliceal system from the urinary bladder, it is hazardous to assume that an isolated infection of the bladder exists. The principles of diagnosis and management of urinary tract infection as stated above apply to the so-called lower urinary tract infections or cystitis. Anatomical and neurogenic defects and metabolic diseases such as diabetes mellitus and those conducive to stone formation must be searched for and corrected. Cystitis with overt haematuria (haemorrhagic cystitis) requires hospital care, for bleeding may be severe. Cultures must be made and suitable antimicrobial agents employed. It is important to remember that a urinary tract infection is not an infection in the urine alone but in the tissues of the urinary tract as well.

Tuberculosis of the urinary tract

Essentials of diagnosis

1. Early symptoms usually include burning on micturition, frequency and nocturia.
2. Malaise, fatigue, fever and night sweats are common symptoms.
3. The urine classically contains pus without organisms.
4. Culture or guinea pig inoculation confirms the presence of *Mycobacterium tuberculosis.*
5. Urograms show a 'moth-eaten' appearance of calices, abscess cavities and varying degrees of kidney destruction.
6. Cystoscopy may reveal ulcers and granulomas on the bladder wall. Biopsy may aid in the diagnosis.

General considerations

Haematogenous dissemination of tubercle bacilli from foci in the lung or lymph nodes is the usual source of tuberculosis of the kidney; rarely does the infection originate in the genital tract. The genital organs may become infected by haematogenous spread or secondary to kidney infection. The prostate, seminal vesicles, epididymis and, rarely, the testes may be infected (Fig. 38.6). The fallopian tubes are more frequently involved than the ovaries and uterus. The kidney and ureter may show little gross change. Caseous nodules in the renal parenchyma and abscess formation with destruction of tissue and fibrosis often produce extensive damage. Calcification in the lesions is common. The ureter and calices are thickened, and stenosis may occur, with total destruction of functioning renal tissue above. The bladder shows mucosal inflammation and submucosal tubercles which become necrotic and form ulcers. Fibrosis of the bladder wall occurs late or upon healing. Tubercles with caseous necrosis and calcification are found in the genital organs. Microscopically, typical tubercles are found,

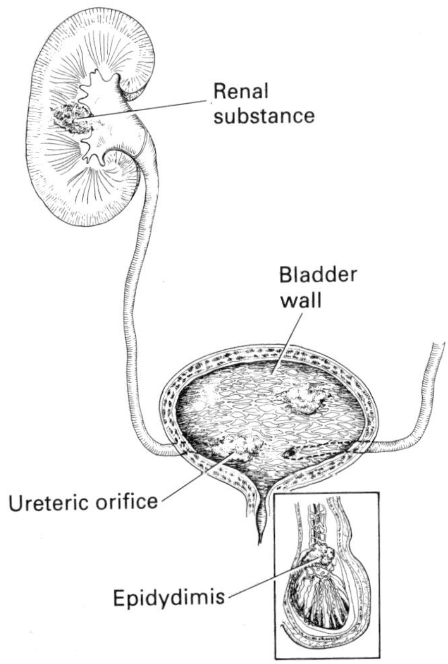

Fig. 38.6 Four sites in the genitourinary tract at which tuberculosis tends to arise.

and demonstration of tubercle bacilli in the lesions is usually easily accomplished. The search for tuberculosis elsewhere in the body must be complete whenever urinary tract tuberculosis is found.

Clinical findings

Symptoms and signs

Symptoms are not characteristic, but specific manifestations of chronic infection with malaise, fever, tiredness and night sweats may be present. Kidney and ureteric infection is usually silent. Bladder infection produces frequency, burning on urination, nocturia and occasionally strangury. If bleeding occurs with clot formation, ureteral or vesical colic may occur. Gross haematuria, which is painless, is a fairly common symptom. Genital involvement becomes apparent as enlargement of the epididymis, or as a sinus tract. Induration or nodularity of the prostate and thickening of the seminal vesicles indicate infection. Examination may reveal only costovertebral angle tenderness and the alterations of the genital tract organs available to palpation.

Laboratory findings

The urine contains pus without bacteria, red cells, and usually protein. Culture for tubercle and guinea pig inoculation confirm the diagnosis. If renal damage is extensive signs of renal insufficiency will be demonstrated.

X-ray and cystoscopic findings

Excretory urograms will reveal the 'moth-eaten' appearance of involved calices or the obliteration or stenosis of calices, abscess cavities, ureteral thickening and stenosis, or the kidney may be totally destroyed and therefore not show. Calcification of involved tissues is common. Thorough cystoscopic examination is required to determine the extent of any bladder wall infection, and to provide biopsy material if needed. Culture of urine obtained from ureteral catheters will help establish whether one or both kidneys are affected.

Differential diagnosis

The differential diagnosis is essentially that of sterile pyuria, which may also occur in chronic pyelonephritis and in chronic non-specific urethritis and cystitis. Culture should serve to distinguish tuberculosis from these.

Medical treatment

If renal infection is unilateral but gross necrosis is not evident or if renal infection is bilateral, the patient should rest in bed and be given antitubercular therapy. In the initial phase, the concurrent use of at least three drugs is designed to reduce the population of viable bacteria as rapidly as possible, and to minimize the risk of ineffective treatment in those patients infected by drug-resistant bacteria. Treatment of choice for the initial phase is the daily use of isoniazid and rifampicin supplemented by ethambutol. These drugs should be continued for at least 8 weeks, and preferably until the results of drug sensitivity testing is known. After the initial phase, treatment is continued with only two drugs, one of which, in the absence of contraindication, should always be isoniazid. The second drug may be rifampicin, ethambutol or streptomycin, and the duration of treatment depends on the combination of drugs used. When isoniazid with rifampicin is given daily throughout the treatment a 9-month course is sufficient for most patients.

Surgical treatment

If renal infection is unilateral and the involved kidney is severely damaged, combined medical treatment as above plus nephrectomy is indicated. If one kidney is severely involved by a caseous hydronephrosis or is bleeding severely, nephrectomy and medical therapy may be necessary even though the other kidney is infected. Combined therapy may be required also for advanced genital organ or vesical tuberculosis.

Prognosis

The prognosis varies with the extent of renal involvement and damage to renal function. Antimicrobial therapy has improved the outlook remarkably. Anatomical defects resulting from scar and healing or from stenosis of the ureter with hydronephrosis may delay or preclude cure. Vesical or genital tuberculosis responds less well than does uncomplicated renal infection. There is often chronic progressive contraction of the bladder until its capacity is so small that it causes great distress to the patient.

URINARY STONES

Urinary stone is one of the most common diseases of the urinary tract. It occurs more frequently in men than in women, but is rare in children; a familial predisposition is often encountered. If a stone is not obstructive it is not apt to cause injury or symptoms. If it blocks the urinary passage (for example, the pelviureteric junction), it leads to severe symptoms and renal damage. Since stones tend to recur, a patient with non-obstructive stone may later form a stone which will cause obstruction; for this reason, investigation of the cause of the first stone is of importance in the prevention of later renal injury.

Renal stone

Aetiology

All the causes of renal stone formation are not known, but in most cases multiple factors are involved. At least 90% of stones contain calcium or magnesium in combination with phosphate or oxalate. The remainder are of organic composition (cystine, uric acid). The following factors are known to influence the formation of stones:

1. Hyperexcretion of relatively insoluble urinary contents.
   a. Calcium. The major calcium foods are milk and cheese. Marked hypercalciuria may be seen in the adult who drinks 1 litre or more of milk each day. It has been shown that the lactose in milk causes increased absorption of calcium from the gut. The amount of calcium contained in hard water has also been said to cause hypercalciuria. Prolonged immobilization (such as spinal cord injuries, fractures, poliomyelitis) and certain bone diseases (for example, metastatic cancer, myeloma, Paget's disease) cause hypercalciuria. Under these circumstances calcium excretion may reach 450 mg/day. Primary hyperparathyroidism causes hypercalciuria and hyperphosphaturia as well as hypercalcaemia and hypophosphataemia, and two-thirds of these patients have renal stones. Idiopathic hypercalciuria is almost exclusively seen in males, and in this condition the serum calcium is normal, serum phosphate is low, and even on a low calcium intake these patients may excrete as much as 500 mg of calcium in 24 h.
   b. Oxalate. At least 50% of renal stones are composed of calcium oxalate. Cabbage, rhubarb, spinach, tomatoes, celery and cocoa contain considerable quantities of oxalate, but limitation of these foods has little effect in prophylaxis because the major source of oxalate is endogenous. Hyperoxaluria is a genetic disorder affecting the metabolism of glyoxylic acid, which forms oxalate rather than glycine. It is a rare phenomenon, but it is one of the common causes of nephrolithiasis and neprocalcinosis in children, and it is often fatal.

c. Cystine. Cystinuria is a hereditary disease. It is uncommon and only a small percentage of these patients form stones.
d. Uric acid. Uric acid stones may form when there is a rapid tissue breakdown, i.e. in chemotherapeutic treatment of leukaemia, polycythaemia and carcinoma; for this reason it is important to maintain an alkaline urine when treating these diseases. Uric acid-formers have a consistently low urinary pH, which may be caused by a decreased tubular formation of ammonia. Elevated serum uric acid concentration is often observed secondary to thiazide diuretic therapy, but this can be controlled by giving probenecid. Many patients with gout form uric acid calculi, although gout is not a necessary condition for the formation of uric acid stones.
e. Silicon dioxide. Long-term use of magnesium trisilicate in the treatment of peptic ulcer may rarely lead to the formation of radiopaque silicon stones.

2. Physical changes which occur in the urine.
   a. Increased concentration of salts and organic compounds. This may be due to low fluid intake or excessive water loss. The latter may occur in febrile disease, in hot climates or in occupations causing excessive perspiration, or may be due to vomiting and diarrhoea.
   b. Urinary pH. A mean urinary pH is 5.85. It is influenced by diet and is altered by the ingestion of acid or alkaline medications, for example in the treatment of peptic ulcer, and carbonic anhydrase inhibitors, i.e. acetazolamide used in the treatment of glaucoma which causes an increase in urinary pH. Urea-splitting bacteria, by liberating ammonia, make the urine strongly alkaline—pH>7.5. The inorganic salts are less soluble in alkaline medium—calcium phosphate forms at pH 6.6 and magnesium ammonium phosphate precipitates at pH 7.2. Organic substances, for example cystine and uric acid, are least soluble at pH below 7.
3. Nidus formation. Randall observed that calcific plaques are commonly seen in the renal papillae. He believed that they develop as a result of injury to the cells of the collecting tubules secondary to infection elsewhere. Randall postulated that when the overlying mucosa finally ulcerates, the calcification acts as a nidus to which the insoluble substances in the urine can adhere. It has also been shown that most stones develop by precipitation of crystals, e.g. calcium oxalate, on an organic matrix formed of amino acids and carbohydrates. Other masses that can act as nidi include blood clots, clumps of epithelial or pus cells, or even bacteria. Necrotic ischaemic tissue and foreign bodies may encourage the precipitation of relatively insoluble substances.

Pathology

The size and position of the stone govern the development of secondary pathological changes in the urinary tract. The obstruction caused by a small stone lodged in the pelviureteric junction or in the ureter may slowly destroy a kidney whereas a relatively large stone may be so placed as to cause little renal damage. Infection is a common complication of an obstructing renal stone, because of the stasis which it causes. The presence of such a foreign body seems to decrease the local resistance to haematogenous infection. The parenchymal ischaemia caused by local pressure from an enlarging 'staghorn' stone may progressively damage a kidney.

Types of urinary calculus

1. Calcium phosphate stones (often mixed with magnesium ammonium phosphate) may be soft or hard. They are usually yellow or brown and often form staghorn masses (Fig. 38.7).
2. Magnesium ammonium phosphate stones are usually yellow and friable. Staghorn formation is common.
3. Calcium oxalate stones (jack stones, mulberry stones) are usually small, rough and hard. Spicules radiating from the central core can often be seen on X-rays.
4. Cystine stones are smooth and light yellow or yellow-brown in colour. They have a waxy appearance, and are usually multiple and bilateral. They may enlarge quite rapidly sometimes, coalescing to form staghorn calculi (Fig. 38.8). Although their density is relatively low they can be identified on X-ray as homogeneous, slightly opaque, smooth rounded bodies.

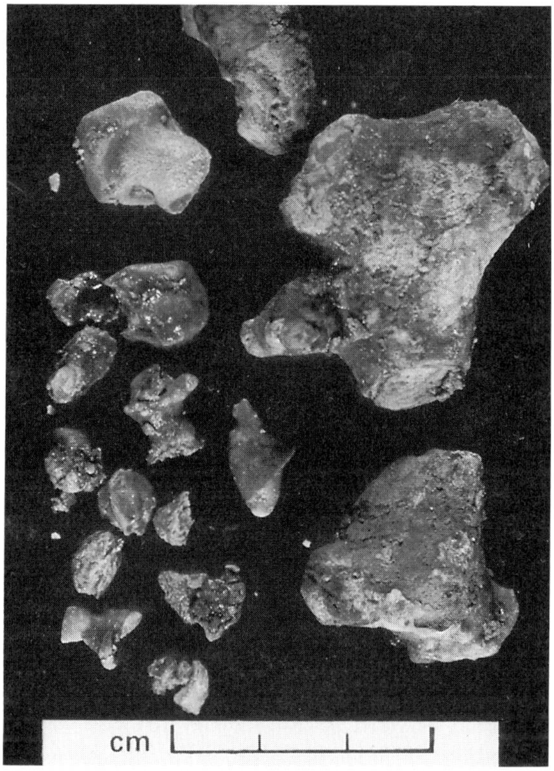

Fig. 38.7 Fragments of a staghorn calculus, which had to be broken down at operation into pieces small enough to be removed through the incision in the renal pelvis.

5. Uric acid stones: uric acid crystals can precipitate in the renal parenchyma; the stones so formed from these crystals are usually small and hard, varying in colour from yellow to reddish-brown. They may be multiple, and if they are composed of pure uric acid crystals they cannot be seen on X-ray. On intravenous pyelogram they are seen as negative shadows.

Radiopacity

Radiopacity is directly related to the density of the stone compared to that of water. Calcium phosphate is very dense. Uric acid is at the other end of the scale and non-opaque.

Clinical findings in urinary stones

Symptoms

Diet, the amount of milk and cheese, drugs, alkalis, analgesics, acetazolamide, vitamin D, periods

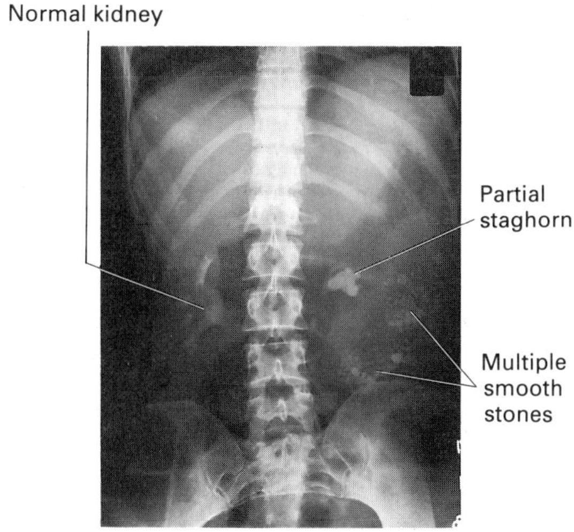

Fig. 38.8 Multiple radio-paque stones in the left kidney and pelvis. The numerous rounded, smooth shadows are typical of the appearance of cystine stones. Furthermore these also tend to coalesce to form staghorn masses, as seen in the upper part of the pelvis. There is no significant excretion of the contrast medium from the left kidney but fortunately there is good excretion from the normally outlined right one.

of immobilization, previous passage of stones, and the presence of gout may all be relevant. There may be a family history of stone formation due to hereditary hyperoxaluria, cystinuria, hyperuricaemia or renal acidosis. If the stone is still submucosal (Randall's plaque) or adherent to the parenchyma there are no symptoms. The same is usually true of a small stone trapped in a minor calix. If the stone is free and obstructs a calix or the uretero-pelvic junction there will be dull flank pain from parenchymal and capsular distension, colic from hyperperistalsis, and smooth-muscle spasm of the calices and pelvis, haematuria, nausea, vomiting and abdominal distension. Chills, high fever and bladder irritability are only present in association with infection. Staghorn calculus may be asymptomatic even when infection is present.

Signs

Tenderness in the costovertebral angle or over the kidney may or may not be present. Acute renal infection may cause more definite findings. If marked hydronephrotic atrophy has occurred as a result of prolonged ureteral obstruction, a mass in the flank may be seen, felt, or percussed. Some muscle rigidity over the kidney may be found, and rebound tenderness may be elicited, particularly if acute infection is present. Abdominal distension and diminished peristalsis usually accompany acute renal colic.

Laboratory findings

1. Haematological indices. The white cell count may be increased as a result of complicating infection, and if renal function has declined then anaemia may be present.
2. Urinalysis. Protein may be noted, because of the presence of red blood cells. Pus cells and bacteria may be seen. Oxalate bodies are often observed in hyperparathyroidism, in renal tubular acidosis, and in hyperoxaluria. Calcium phosphate casts suggest hypercalciuria. If the pH of the urine is higher than 7.6, urea-splitting organisms must be present, because the kidneys cannot produce urine in this range of alkalinity. Such a finding strongly suggests that the stones are composed of magnesium ammonium phosphate. Fixation of the pH at 6.5 is compatible with renal tubular acidosis. Consistently low pH is a common cause of the formation of uric acid calculi.
3. Renal function tests. Renal function can be assessed by measuring the 24-h urea and creatinine clearance and performing a dilution concentration study.
4. Blood chemistry studies. Fasting serum calcium and phosohorus concentrations should be determined on at least three occasions. The serum protein level should also be estimated, since almost half of the calcium is normally un-ionized and bound to protein. If serum proteins are low but total calcium is normal an increase in ionized calcium is indicated. Hypercalcaemia with hypophosphataemia strongly suggests a primary hyperparathyroidism, but normal serum phosphate is found in 60% of these patients. Elevated serum uric acid is found in 50% of uric acid stone formers.

X-ray findings

At least 90% of renal stones are radiopaque and are readily visible on a plain film of the abdomen, unless they are small or overlie bone. It is necessary to differentiate renal stone from calcified mesenteric lymph nodes, calcium in rib cartilage, gallstones and solid medication such as tablets present in the intestinal tract. Because the plain film is two-dimensional, it has only presumptive value, except in the case of a staghorn stone which is never confused with any other finding. The morphology of the stone may give a clue to its chemical nature. Bone disease may also be seen in the ribs, spine, pelvis or femoral heads. This may afford a clue to the aetiology of hypercalciuria, for example, hyperparathyroidism, metastatic carcinoma or Paget's disease. Excretory urograms are necessary because they accurately localize the calcific shadow unless the kidney is without function or unless it is acutely blocked by stone. Oblique views may also be helpful. If a urogram is not obtained by the kidney but the kidney shadow becomes dense (nephrogram), acute obstruction of a good kidney has probably occurred. If the stone is non-opaque the films will demonstrate obstruction by dilatation and the stone may appear as a darker area, a negative shadow in the renal pelvis. Excretory urograms also give an indication of renal function. If renal function is poor, retrograde urograms may be needed.

Renal scan

If renal function is poor isotope studies may prove helpful in further assessing this factor. If the damage is irreversible, the ^{131}I hippuran scan will show little uptake by the tubules: technetium ^{99m}scan will reveal poor vascularity. Such findings may indicate the need for nephrectomy rather than nephrolithotomy.

Ultrasound examination of the kidney

Ultrasonography is a very good non-invasive method for assessing obstruction of the kidney and locating a stone. It also provides a medium for accurately placing a probe into the renal pelvis in order to carry out an antegrade pyelogram or indeed to clasp and destroy the stone by ultrasonic resonance.

Instrumental examination

Cystoscopy for diagnostic purposes is seldom necessary if the excretory urograms are satisfactory.

Ureteral catheterization may prove helpful in localizing obstruction and measuring renal function.

Such studies in conjunction with retrograde urograms may be the deciding factor in the choice of treatment (pyelolithotomy versus nephrectomy).

Examination of the stone

It is important that every stone removed from the urinary tract is examined biochemically in order to attempt to establish an aetiology of stone formation. It is particularly helpful in differentiating primary metabolic stones from secondary stones caused by infection, etc.

Differential diagnosis

This may be difficult particularly in the presence of infection. The differential diagnosis includes pyelonephritis, renal tumour, tumour of the renal pelvis or calix, renal tuberculosis, and finally, papillary necrosis.

Complications

The presence of a stone lowers resistance to bacterial invasion, and this is particularly true if the stone is obstructive. Calculi complicated by infection may cause pyonephrosis, and ultimately complete destruction of the kidney, which becomes a cavity containing stones and purulent material only. Obstruction of the ureter at the ureteropelvic junction leads to hydronephrosis. If this progresses the parenchyma of the kidney is ultimately destroyed.

Treatment

1. Conservative measures.
   a. No surgery is necessary in the following instances:
      i. Randall's plaque requires no treatment as long as it remains submucosal. Later, however, it may become free and pass down the ureter and cause obstruction.
      ii. A small stone trapped in a minor calix and causing few if any symptoms and no renal damage is best ignored.
      iii. A conservative approach is usually indicated for coralliform stones, particularly in the elderly, as long as the symptoms remain minimal or absent, since extensive incisions into the renal parenchyma are necessary for their removal.
      iv. Stones due to renal tubular acidosis should be treated conservatively, even if multiple, since they may pass spontaneously with adequate medical treatment using alkalis.
   b. Combat infection. This is of particular importance if the bacteria are urea-splitting, for they encourage the progression of calcium phosphate or magnesium stones. Unfortunately, in the presence of stones it is often impossible to eradicate infection.
   c. Attempts at dissolution. Chemical dissolution of renal stones requires indwelling ureteral catheters for constant through and through irrigation with G (or M) solution, and is usually mechanically impracticable. Sand and stone fragments occlude the catheters and cause acute obstruction. This may lead to exacerbations of pyelonephritis, and bacteraemia and renal cortical abscesses may result. Some uric acid stones may dissolve with allopurinol therapy. Cystine stones may likewise disappear when penicillamine D is administered.
2. Invasive measures. Surgical removal of the stone is indicated if the stone is obstructive and causes undue pain or progressive renal damage, or if the infection complicating a stone cannot be eradicated. Nephrectomy may be necessary if obstruction and infection have markedly impaired renal function. Ultrasonic dissolution of stones has added a new dimension to surgical

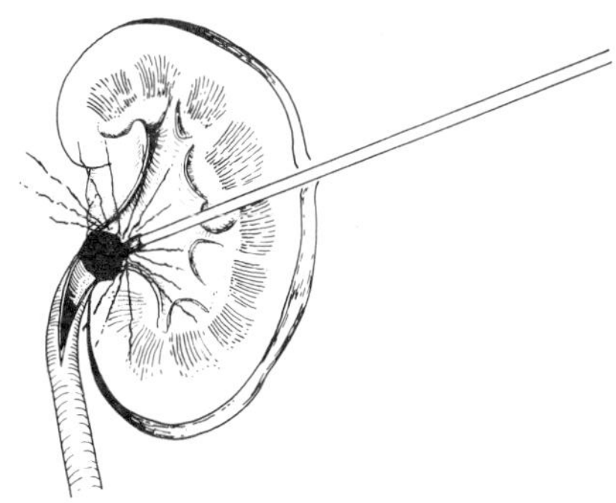

Fig. 38.9 Ultrasound disintegration of a stone in the renal pelvis, by means of a probe passed directly through the kidney into the pelvis to make direct contact with the stone. This is an endoscopic procedure.

measures of treatment of stones. This can be carried out either by passing a probe into the kidney and localizing the stone precisely using ultrasound (Fig. 38.9), and then disintegrating it by ultrasound resonance and washing it out through a nephrostomy, or alternatively by placing the patient in a water bath and focusing ultrasound on the stone through the water (Fig. 38.10).

3. Prevention. Patients who have formed stones should be managed prophylactically in an attempt to prevent recurrences. Effectiveness of preventive measures depends on the diagnosis of stone-forming.
   a. General measures. Stone-formers must maintain a high urine volume to keep solutes well diluted. Combat infection by use of appropriate antibiotic. Eliminate obstruction and stasis by any surgical means. Avoid recumbency. Calcium stone-formers should be persuaded to maintain an acid urine.
   b. Specific measures. Prophylactic treatment specific for various types of stone is as follows:
      i. Calcium and magnesium ammonium phosphate stones if caused by primary hyperparathyroidism—the parathyroid glands should be explored.
         Diet—eliminate milk and cheese if hypercalciuria is discovered.
         Urinary pH—calcium phosphate and magnesium ammonium phosphate stones form most readily in neutral or alkaline urine. The pH of the urine should be kept below 6. It can be tested by the patient with litmus paper. Alkaline urine can be effectively acidified by prescribing cranberry juice, 200 ml four times a day, or ascorbic acid 1 g four times a day, or sodium or potassium acid phosphate.
         In renal tubular acidosis *alkali* should be given in the form of sodium or potassium citrate; this will dramatically reduce the output of urinary calcium.
         Diuretics. Thiazide diuretics decrease the calcium output in the urine.
      ii. Oxalate stones. There is no effective method of decreasing the amount of oxalate in the urine, even in hyperoxaluria. Foods high in oxalate should be deleted from the diet, though the effect of this is questionable. The administration of magnesium oxide 150 mg three times a day may control recurrence of oxalate stones, but it does not diminish the level of urinary excretion.
      iii. Metabolic stones (uric acid, cystine). The pH of the urine should be maintained at 7 or higher, thereby increasing the solubility of these substances. This can be done with an alkaline ash diet (high in vegetable and fruit content, low in protein) but added alkalis are usually needed, such as 50% sodium citrate solution, 5 ml four times a day. Allopurinol, a xanthine oxidase inhibitor, by decreasing the endogenous production of uric acid, has proved very effective in preventing the recurrence of uric acid calculi. The dose is 300 mg

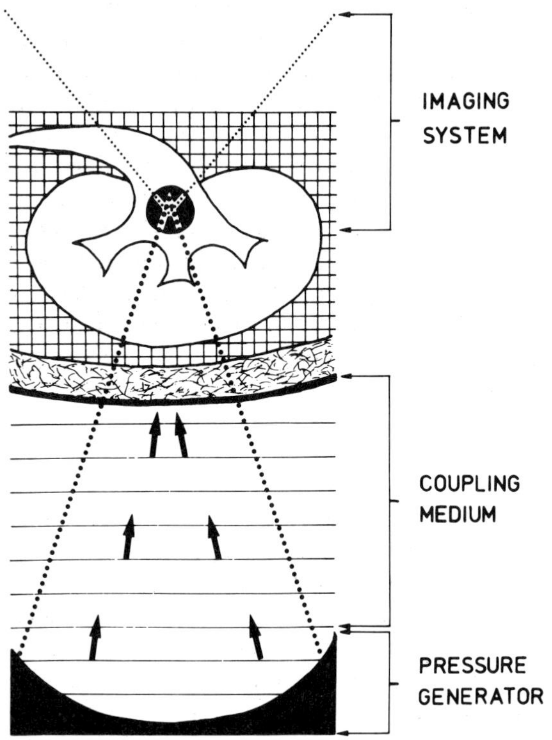

Fig. 38.10 Extracorporeal lithotripsy. Accurately focused beams of externally generated shock waves are directed, under ultrasound or X-ray control, on to the stone. Since the shock waves pass easily through fluid, the technique involves either placing the patient's trunk in a water bath, or directly applying a fluid-containing bag to the skin and transmitting the waves via this.

every 12 h. In severe cystinurics a low methionine diet may be necessary in order to decrease the amount of endogenous cystine, but this diet is not very palatable. If the above measures fail to decrease the urinary cystine to safe levels, penicillamine should be added to the regimen. This preparation, 30 mg/kg/day in divided doses, usually reduces the amount of cystine in the urine to 100 mg or less per day.

Prognosis

The recurrence rate of renal stone is significant, and the prognosis must therefore be guarded. The patient must be carefully followed for months or even years. The real danger is the possible progressive destruction of the kidney caused by obstruction and infection.

Ureteric stone

Ureteric stones originate in the kidney. Gravity and peristalsis both contribute to spontaneous passage into and down the ureter. Ureteric stones are seldom completely obstructive; they are usually spiculated so that urine can flow around them. Occasionally a stone will remain lodged in a ureter for many months without harming the kidney. If the stone passes within a few days no evidence of renal injury can be shown. However, if the stone is definitely obstructive and is allowed to remain for weeks or months, irreparable damage to the renal parenchyma can occur. A stone is apt to be arrested in the narrowest points of the ureter. If infection should complicate the urinary stasis, further renal damage results.

Clinical findings

Symptoms

Pain is usually abrupt in onset, and becomes severe within a matter of minutes. There are two types of pain:

1. The radiating, colicky, agonizing pain from hyperperistalsis of the smooth muscle of the calices, pelvis and ureter.
2. The rather constant ache in the costovertebral area and flank from obstruction and capsular distension.

The radiation of the pain at times suggests the position of the stone. If high in the ureter, the colic may radiate to the testicle. As the stone nears the bladder the pain may spread to the scrotum or appear in the vulva. This is due to the common innervation of these organs and the lower ureter. At times the pain comes on more slowly and may be felt more anteriorly, and occasionally may be quite mild. In these instances the diagnosis may not at first be obvious. Gastrointestinal symptoms are commonly associated with stone in the ureter. Nausea and vomiting almost always occur, and abdominal distension due to paralytic ileus is often present. These symptoms may be so severe that renal and ureteric pain may be overshadowed and an intraperitoneal lesion sought. Gross haematuria is observed in about one-third of cases; small clots may be passed. Even in the absence of infection, symptoms of urgency and frequency may develop when the stone approaches the bladder. Existing chronic renal infection may be exacerbated by ureteric obstruction. Chills and fever with increased back pain may be noted. It is not common for a stone to be complicated by acute new infection unless it is introduced by instrumentation. If this does occur, chills, fever and sepsis are to be expected.

Signs

The patient is usually in agony, pacing the floor rather than lying quietly in bed, as a patient with peritonitis would normally do. Nothing he or she does affords relief. The skin may be cold and clammy, and the patient may exhibit other signs of mild shock. There is marked tenderness in the costovertebral angle and the flank. Percussion posteriorly causes severe pain. Spasm of the abdominal muscles on the affected side is to be expected. Fever indicates that infection is complicating the picture. The ipsilateral testis may be hypersensitive if the stone is in the upper ureter. The scrotal skin may be hyperaesthetic if the stone lies low.

X-ray findings

A plain film of the abdomen may show a calcific body in the region of the ureter. This constitutes merely presumptive grounds for the diagnosis, however, for the observed shadow may be a phlebolith or other intra-abdominal calcification. An excretory urogram is invaluable. The uretero-gram places the calcification in the ureter and usually demonstrates dilatation of the ureter above the stone. It also reveals what is happening to the kidney, i.e. the degree of obstruction. On occasion no dye may enter the renal pelvis or ureter because of the obstruction, but a marked denseness of the renal shadow occurs. This is evidence of good kidney function and acute ureteric obstruction. In the case of a non-opaque stone a negative grey or black shadow is seen within the white area of the outlined ureter. This may be difficult to differentiate from a ureteric tumour or blood clot. The diagnosis of ureteric stone may be established by demonstrating that the suspicious shadow hugs the cystoscopically placed ureter catheter in both the anteroposterior and oblique views.

Differential diagnosis

Passage of crystals down the ureter may occur during treatment or an exacerbation of gout or in oxaluria after excessive ingestion of high oxalate foods. Symptoms and signs are the same as those seen in stone, and haematuria is just as common. X-ray examination, however, is usually normal. Tumour of the kidney or the renal pelvis may bleed and a clot or piece of necrotic tumour may pass down the ureter. This will simulate ureteric stone perfectly. Ureteric tumour is often obstructive and may cause colic. Haematuria is common. Obstructive chronic lesions of the ureter may cause severe recurrent pain. These include congenital ureteric stenosis and extraureteric obstructions such as may be caused by lymph nodes containing cancer. Acute pyelonephritis may start so abruptly and the pain may be so acute as to suggest stone. The finding of pyuria and bacteriuria with normal urograms should establish the diagnosis. Acute gallbladder disease and acute appendicitis may occasionally mimic ureteric stone, particularly if the pain is referred. An aneurysm of the abdominal aorta may cause pain suggestive of left renal colic. Palpation of the aneurysm, absence of haematuria and normal intravenous pyelogram will differentiate the two.

Complications

The major complication of ureteric stone is obstruction—usually only partial. Permanent renal damage is rare, except in cases which remain undiagnosed or are inadequately treated. Bilateral ureteric calculi may cause anuria, in which case drainage of the kidney by ureteric catheters or removal of stones must be accomplished immediately. Infection may gain a foothold in the presence of obstruction, but it is usually introduced by the cystoscopist during attempts to remove the stone.

Treatment

Specific measures

About 80% of stones which reach the ureter can pass spontaneously and should always be allowed to do so, as long as complications do not develop. Antispasmodics may be helpful. Physical activity should be encouraged and adequate fluid intake

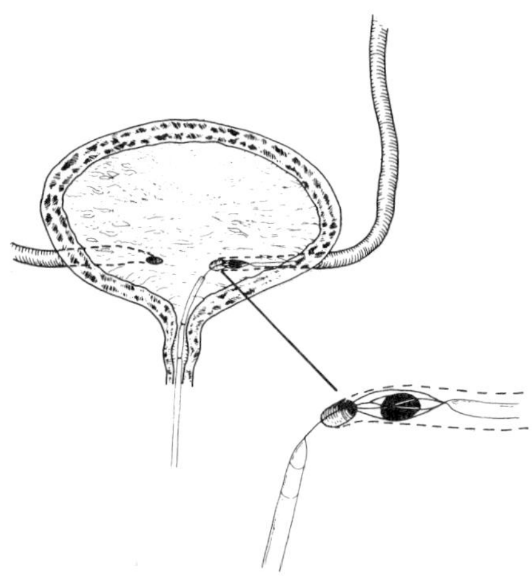

Fig. 38.11 Cystoscopic removal of a stone impacted at the lower end of the ureter. If necessary the ureteric orifice can be enlarged by a cutting diathermy point, and then the stone caught up in the web of a basket, also introduced along a channel of the cystoscope.

maintained to increase ureteric peristalsis. A stone small enough to pass down the ureter will have no difficulty in traversing the urethra. Cystoscopic manipulation (Fig. 38.11) or surgical intervention (ureterolithotomy) is necessary if the stone is too large to pass through the ureteric lumen spontaneously. Stones up to 0.5 cm in diameter and even a few up to 1 cm in diameter may pass without surgical or cystoscopic assistance. The onset of infection may require removal of the obstructing agent before sepsis can be controlled. If periodic excretory urograms show progressive hydronephrosis or if pain remains intense and incapacitating, removal of the stone is indicated.

General measures

Morphine or a similar opiate is necessary to control pain and should be given intravenously. Morphine sulphate 8 mg or a comparable drug in the same relative strength should be given immediately and repeated in 5 min. if relief has not been obtained. Pain can usually be controlled thereafter by subcutaneous injection. Initial subcutaneous morphine even in doses of 30 mg is disappointing for relief of pain of this degree. Atropine 0.8 mg subcutaneously is the antispasmodic of choice. Probanthine 0.1 g intravenously will usually relieve the pain; unfortunately it may paralyse bladder action for some hours as well. Other antispasmodics may be given by mouth but their efficacy is questionable. Heat to the flank or a hot bath is often helpful as an adjunct to drug analgesia.

Bladder stone

Primary bladder stones are rare in the UK but occur commonly in north-west India, the Middle East and parts of China. The cause is not known, but it appears to be dietary. The calculi may be secondary to vitamin B_6 deficiency. Once removed, these vesical stones rarely recur. A secondary vesical stone develops as a complication of other urological disease; 95% occur in men, the most common cause of secondary vesical stone being infection of residual urine with urea-splitting organisms, for example *Proteus*. This partial urinary retention may be due to prostatic or bladder neck obstruction, cystocele or neurogenic bladder. Stagnation is particularly marked in vesical diverticula, and stones are often found when diverticula are present. A stone passed through the ureter usually passes on through the urethra. In obstruction or stasis it may remain in the bladder and act as a nucleus for precipitation of more urinary salts. A markedly inflamed or ulcerated bladder may also predispose to stone formation, as is seen in vesical schistosomiasis, and following irradiation of the bladder. Foreign bodies occasionally are introduced into the bladder, particularly in women, and these may act as nidi for precipitation of calcific deposits. Infection complicates the picture, and quickens stone formation, particularly if the bacteria are urea-splitters.

Pathology

Vesical stones may be single or multiple. If single they are ovoid, and if multiple they are often faceted (Fig. 38.12). In addition to the infection which is uniformly present with secondary stones, their presence further increases the inflammation of the bladder. Most vesical stones are radiopaque (calcium phosphate, calcium oxalate, or ammonium magnesium phosphate) but a few are radiolucent (uric acid).

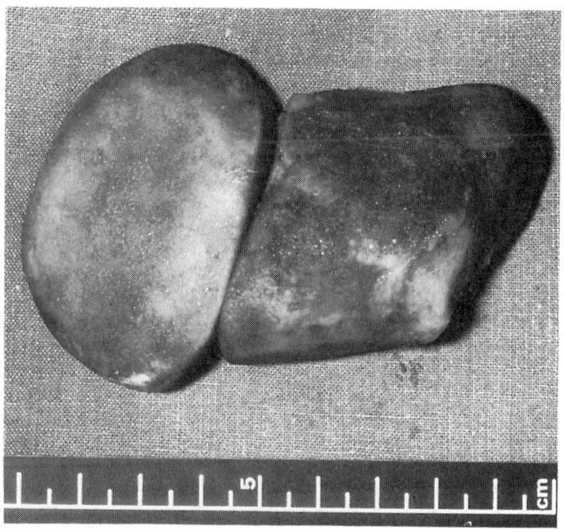

Fig. 38.12 Two large stones which had been present in the bladder for several years, and had become faceted by constant rubbing one against the other.

Clinical findings

Symptoms

Symptoms of chronic urinary obstruction or stasis and infection occur in most cases, for these are the common causes of vesical stone. There may be a history of the introduction of a foreign body into the bladder. The patient may complain of sudden interruption of the urinary stream associated with pain radiating down the penis when the stone rolls over the bladder neck. There may be inability to void, except in certain positions which cause the stone to move off the bladder neck. Considerable haematuria may be noted, although this can occur also with pure obstruction or infection.

Signs

Only giant calculi can be felt suprapubically. The bladder may be visible, palpable or percussible if there is a great deal of residual urine. Palpation of the urethra may reveal a thickening compatible with stricture. Rectal examination may demonstrate a relaxed anal sphincter (neurogenic bladder) or an enlarged or hard cancerous prostate.

Laboratory findings

The urine is always infected, and blood cells are commonly found in it.

X-ray findings

Vesical stones are usually visible on a plain film (Fig. 38.13). They must be differentiated from calcified ovaries and fibroids. Oblique films are usually helpful. Excretory urograms often show back-pressure changes in the kidney, and a film taken after voiding may reveal residual urine. Diverticula should be noted. Stones will be localized in the excretory or retrograde cystograms.

Instrumental examination

The attempt to pass a catheter or sound may lead to the diagnosis of a urethral stricture. Successful passage of a catheter after urination allows estimation of the degree of obstruction and stasis by recovering residual urine. The positive diagnostic step

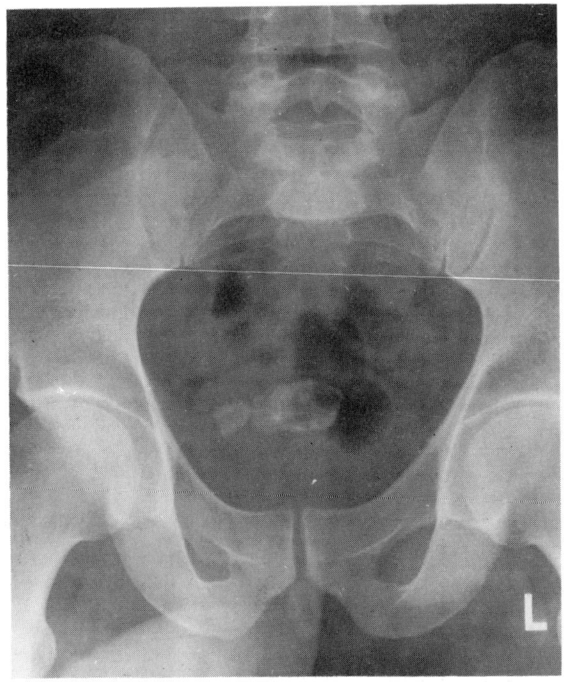

Fig. 38.13 Straight X-ray, showing clearly three radiopaque stones in the urinary bladder.

of sounding for stone may be accomplished by passing a sound into the bladder. The definite click of the instrument on the stone can readily be heard or felt. Cystoscopy usually visualizes the stone or stones and the obstructive lesion with its secondary vesical changes.

Differential diagnosis

A pedunculated tumour of the bladder may suddenly occlude the vesical orifice, thereby simulating vesical stone. Cystoscopy will make the differentiation. Extravesical calcification on X-ray of the vesical region may appear to be in the bladder, although it is actually in the veins, omental pads, ovaries or fibroids of the uterus.

Complications

A primary stone will lead eventually to infection. If infection is present it will be worsened by the presence of a stone, which in turn will defeat attempts to sterilize the urine. Vesicoureteric reflux is commonly associated with bladder calculi. Removal of calculi may cause spontaneous cessation of reflux.

Prevention

Stasis and infection, whether primary or secondary, must be eradicated.

Treatment

Specific measures — cystoscopy and surgical removal

1. transurethrally—small stones can be removed by cystoscopy manipulation, large ones can be crushed with a lithotrite (Fig. 38.14) and the fragments washed out. If the patient has an obstructing prostate, which can be removed by transurethral resection, both procedures may be undertaken at the same time.
2. suprapubic route—this route must be used for the removal of stones which are too large for transurethral removal or crushing. Suprapubic prostatectomy may also be indicated.

Chemical dissolution. This is usually successful, but fails to treat the cause of stone formation. It may be indicated if the patient is considered to be an unwarranted surgical risk or if he refuses surgery, or cystoscopic removal. In the dissolution of calcium and magnesium ammonium phosphate calculi excellent results can be obtained with hemiacidrim (remacidin): 30 ml of 10% solution is instilled, the catheter is clamped for 30–60 min, and this is repeated 4–6 times a day. A continuous drip used through a three-way Foley catheter may also be successful. Calcium salts and magnesium ammonium phosphate are highly soluble in citric acid (solution J). If this solution proves irritating the amount of sodium carbonate can be increased.

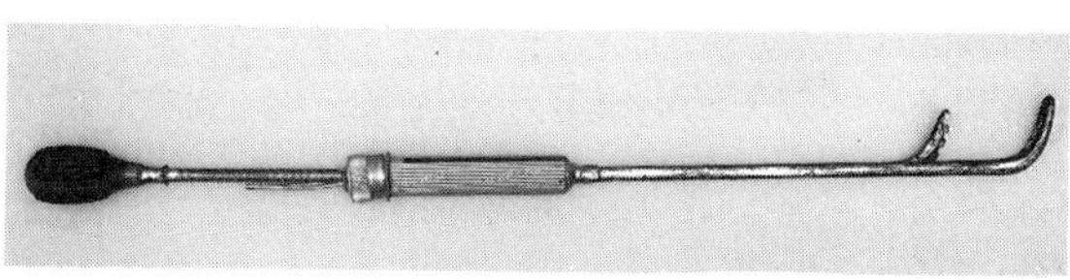

Fig. 38.14 Lithotrite. By turning the handle shown on the left the jaws are closed. This allows introduction per urethram into the bladder, when the jaws are opened. By manoeuvring the opened jaws to the lowermost part of the bladder the stone is allowed to fall into the open jaws and then crushed by closing them by rotation of the handle. The resulting small fragments can then be washed out of the bladder.

General measures

Analgesics for pain and antibiotics for control of infection are used for the relief of distressing symptoms until the stone can be removed.

Prognosis

The rate of recurrence of vesical stone is very low if the primary cause—obstruction—is successfully treated.

Prostatic calculi

Prostatic calculi are seldom of clinical importance. They are commonly seen in association with benign prostatic hyperplasia, although in rare cases in younger persons they may be secondary to an advanced but healing tuberculous prostatitis. Prostatic calculi are formed from desquamated epithelial cells which finally acquire a shell of calcium. They average about 1–2 mm in diameter and are brown or black in colour. They are situated between the hypertrophied adenoma and the surgical capsule. Therefore, on enucleation of the enlarged prostate or complete transurethral prostatectomy they tend to be extruded. On plain film they are situated in the region of the symphysis pubis. The importance of prostatic calculi lies in the fact that they cause indurated areas in the prostate which may be mistaken for carcinoma.

RENAL FAILURE AND RENAL TRANSPLANTATION

Acute renal failure occurs as a consequence of a profound underperfusion of the kidneys during peripheral circulatory collapse, septic or endotoxic shock. Provided the patient is resuscitated promptly and the cause treated, the period of renal impairment may be quite short and clinically non-significant. However, when the episode is of longer duration the patient becomes oligo- or anuric, retains fluid, becomes profoundly uraemic and hypercatabolic, with an increasing acidosis and tendency to hyperkalaemia. Survival depends upon the urgent application of haemodialysis which may be required continuously for the first 24–48 h and thereafter intermittently until a diuresis occurs. Recovery from acute renal failure is the general rule. The pathological basis is acute tubular necrosis; in rare instances, however, the whole cortex undergoes necrosis and recovery is impossible. Given prompt resuscitation and reversal of the original precipitating cause, usually haemorrhage, the period of recovery from acute tubular necrosis varies from a few days to 3 weeks. Some idea of the probability of recovery can be gained from sequential gamma-camera renograms using ^{123}I hippuran.

Chronic renal failure is most often the consequence of a progressive primary disease of the kidneys. Glomerulonephritis accounts for more than 56% of all patients presenting with end-stage renal failure, and pyelonephritis accounts for a further 35%. Renal damage secondary to diabetes mellitus is also a potent cause of chronic progressive destruction of the kidneys. Chronic renal failure—whatever its cause—is a slowly progressive disease, often taking many years to reach end-stage. Progressive failure can be slowed by protein-restricting diets, in which the protein content of the diet is reduced progressively from 60 g/day down to as little as 20 g/day. In addition fluid intake has to be restricted to equal the output, plus the extrasensory loss. Patients are required to weigh themselves each day, and if they are gaining weight or becoming oedematous, further fluid restriction needs to be implemented. When the patient's ability to clear creatinine falls below 10 ml/min there is usually need for dialysis support. At this stage attention to diet becomes critical, and at all costs patients must exclude potassium-containing fruits and chocolate from their diet, as the risks of sudden death from hyperkalaemia become very real. By now the patient is usually profoundly oliguric, and fluid restriction has to be severely imposed.

Haemodialysis is the commonest form of dialysis treatment in chronic renal failure, although it is slowly being overtaken by chronic ambulatory peritoneal dialysis (Fig. 38.15) as the most useful form of dialysis preparation for transplantation. Both forms of dialysis, when carried out expertly, will keep the patient in good health for many years, and allow many of them to return to work. The restrictions of dialysis, however, require strict self-discipline and continuous clinical monitoring.

Renal transplantation offers the prospect of a return to a normal life free from dialysis. Renal transplantation is severely restricted by the availability of kidney donors. Donors can either come from the family as live related donors or, more commonly in the UK, from cadavers after consent has been obtained from the relatives, and a diagnosis of brainstem infarction made by a responsible independent medical practitioner of more than 5 years' registration. Cadaver donors are most often the victims of head injuries as a consequence of road traffic accidents. A proportion are the victims of sudden catastrophic cerebrovascular haemorrhage. A diagnosis of brainstem infarction is made when the patient is unable to ventilate independently and when the craniofacial reflexes are no longer intact.

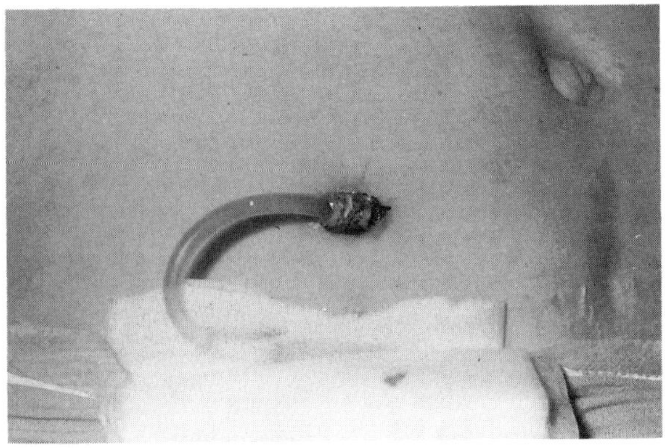

Fig. 38.15 Chronic ambulatory peritoneal dialysis. An in-dwelling (Tenchkoff) cannula is inserted through the anterior abdominal wall, and through this the dialysing fluid can be run into the peritoneal cavity as required. Time is allowed for filtration of the accumulated fluid and other materials which have not been excreted by the failed kidneys to occur, and then the dialysing fluid is returned to a collecting bag outside the abdomen.

Organs for donation are usually cooled in situ using a double–balloon catheter in the aorta and flushing the kidneys through with a hypertonic balanced electrolyte solution. The tonicity is usually increased by the addition of mannitol to the solution. In situ cooling, using this method, allows the kidneys to be removed at leisure, as they will be protected from damage in the cold for up to

48 h. The recipient is chosen on grounds of blood group compatibility and the least number of human leukocyte antigen mismatches.

Most often the cadaver kidney is implanted in the pelvis extraperitoneally, anastomosing the renal artery to the iliac artery, and the renal vein to the iliac vein. The ureter can then be attached to the bladder which is in the immediate proximity of the operation field. Following transplantation the recipient is immunosuppressed with cyclosporin, either by itself, or in combination with azathioprine and steroids. Acute episodes of rejection are determined by transient impairment of renal function, and these are treated usually with large doses of intravenous prednisolone. Steroid-resistant rejection can be treated with one of the mono- or polyclonal antibodies against lymphocytes.

Patient survival following renal transplantation reported to the UK Transplant Registry is around 98% at 1 year and 95% at 5 years. Graft survival for well matched kidneys is 85% at 1 year and 75% at 5 years.

Clearly renal transplantation has brought a new perspective to what was formerly a highly fatal disease. Following successful renal transplantation young children can be expected to grow with straight limbs, and in the absence of bone disease young women can expect to become fertile and have families, and young men can expect to return to a normal working life.

39. Kidneys and ureters

CONGENITAL ABNORMALITIES OF THE KIDNEY

The embryology of the kidney has been briefly discussed in Chapter 38. Congenital abnormalities of the kidneys are clearly a consequence of disorders in the embryological process.

Absence of one kidney

An absent or congenitally atrophic kidney is present in about 1 in 1500 individuals. No symptoms can be attributed to the absence of the kidney and its discovery is usually coincidental on investigation for some other reason, either by ultrasound of the upper abdomen or on pyelographic examination in which only one functioning kidney is seen.

Renal ectopia

This situation occurs once in approximately 1000 cases, the kidney being arrested in some part of its normal ascent, usually at the brim of the pelvis. Commonly the contralateral kidney is present in its normal position. Inflammation of the ectopic kidney may give rise to a tender mass which may be mistaken for an intra-abdominal abscess such as an appendix abscess or a pericolic collection.

Horseshoe kidney

Horseshoe kidney results from the fusion of the two metanephric masses. The kidneys fail to ascend completely. The adrenal glands, however, being developed separately, are found in their normal position. This abnormality, found approximately once in every 1000 cases, is more common in the male. Usually the bridge joining the lower poles lies in front of the fourth lumbar vertebra (Fig. 39.1). Fusion occurs very early, when the embryo is around 30 days old, at which time the two masses of mesoblast destined to form the kidneys lie very close together. Exceptionally it is the upper poles that are fused. Horseshoe kidneys are notoriously prone to become diseased, largely because the ureters are angulated as they pass over the fused isthmus (Fig. 39.2). This produces urinary stasis. Consequently, simple infection, tuberculosis and calculus formation are common complications. Although a fixed mass below the umbilicus may suggest horseshoe kidney, the final diagnosis is established by intravenous urography. While horseshoe kidney is not a contraindication to pregnancy, urinary complications are more frequent in pregnancy.

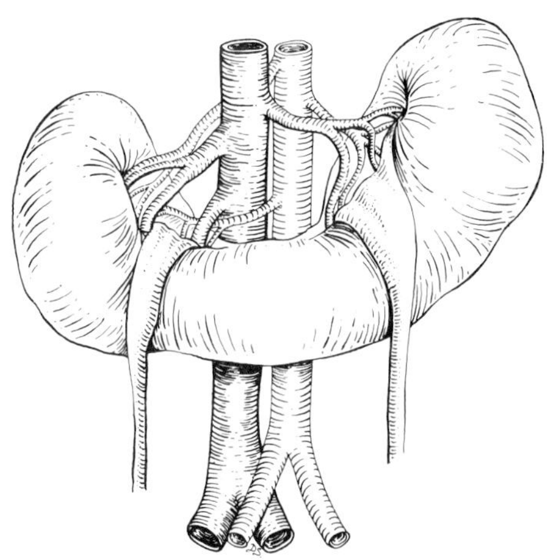

Fig. 39.1 Horseshoe kidney. The two lower poles are fused and continuous as a bridge across the aorta and inferior vena cava. The ureters are forced to lie more anterior-facing than normal.

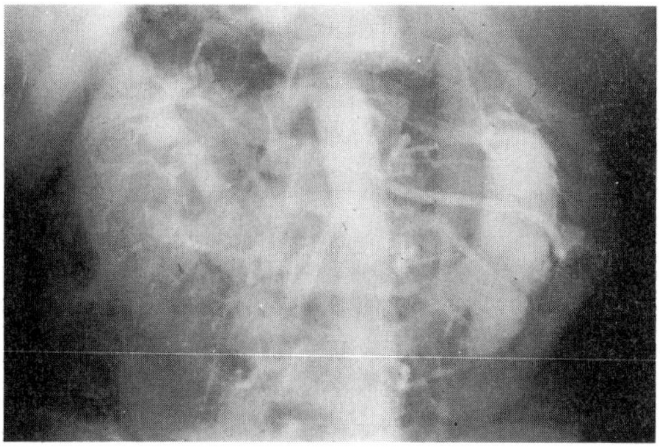

Fig. 39.2 Horseshoe kidney demonstrated by aortogram. The outline of the fused lower poles can be seen crossing the midline. The pelvis of the left renal mass is dilated and there are several arteries supplying each side.

Treatment

Treatment is only indicated in the presence of pain or non-specific infection. In these situations division of the isthmus is usually curative. If one-half of the horseshoe kidney is irreparably diseased, e.g. by stone or neoplasm, heminephrectomy should be performed.

Unilateral fusion (crossed dystrophia)

This condition is very rare. Both kidneys are situated in one loin. One kidney, carrying its own blood vessels and with the ureter opening into the bladder in the normal position, crosses the middle line and its upper pole fuses with the lower pole of the normally placed kidney. In this instance both kidney pelves are situated, one above the other, medial to the renal parenchyma.

Congenital cystic kidneys (polycystic kidneys)

Polycystic kidney disease is a familial disorder and it involves not only the kidneys but sometimes the liver and pancreas as well. A few cases are seen in infancy and early childhood. Renal cysts are thought to be due to a failure of union of the collecting and convoluted tubules. As the cysts enlarge, pressure is exerted on normal surrounding tissue, leading to its gradual destruction. The diagnosis is usually made during investigation for the cause of hypertension, or of uraemia discovered in the third or fourth decade of life. The sex incidence is about equal. Flank pain may be noticed if bleeding occurs into a cyst, and haematuria may then occur.

Examination reveals bilateral enlargement of the kidneys. The urine often shows red blood cells and evidence of infection. Serum creatinine or blood urea nitrogen measures the degree of renal insufficiency. Urograms reveal the enlarged kidneys, with marked bending and prolongation of the calices around the large cysts. Ultrasonography and computerized tomography scans make the correct diagnosis in a high percentage of cases. Surgery is not warranted unless a large extrarenal cyst obstructs the upper ureter.

When the condition is manifested in infancy the prognosis is poor. In the adult-type, death usually occurs 5–10 years after the onset of clinical symptoms, unless the patient is transferred to dialysis and subsequently transplanted.

Simple renal cyst

Simple cyst of the kidney is usually unilateral and single, but it may be multiple and bilateral (Fig. 39.3). Whether this disorder is congenital or acquired is not clear. By compression the cysts can destroy adjacent parenchyma. They contain fluid that resembles but is not urine. Most cysts are diagnosed after the age of 40 years. Flank pain may be the presenting symptom, though most renal cysts

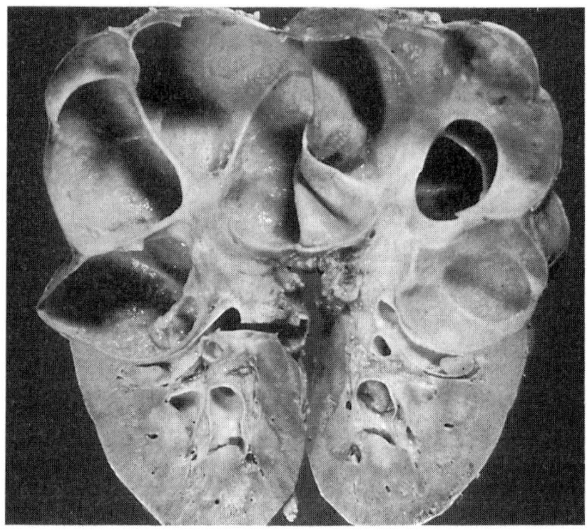

Fig. 39.3 Multiple congenital cysts occupying the upper half of a kidney, the lower half of which appears normal.

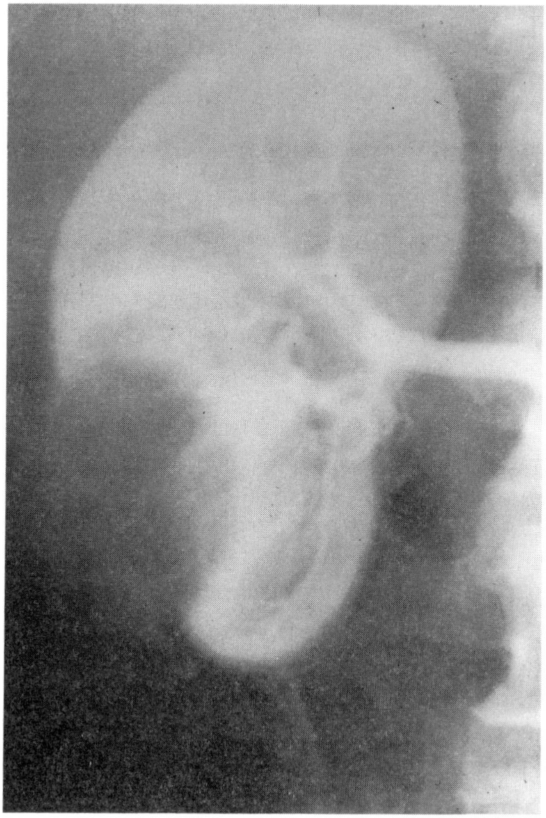

Fig. 39.4 Solitary benign cyst of the lower pole of an otherwise normally functioning kidney, outlined by selective renal artery arteriography. Since there is, of course, no blood supply to the cyst it shows up as a rounded translucent area, in contrast to the dye-filled normal renal substance.

are found coincidentally on urography done for other purposes. A mass may be felt in the renal area, and must be differentiated from tumour. Urinalysis and tests of renal function are usually normal. An excretory urogram reveals a mass in the kidney that distorts the adjacent calices (Fig. 39.4).

A simple cyst must be differentiated from adenocarcinoma of the kidney. If renal ultrasonography or computerized tomography scan confirms a cyst, a needle can be passed into the lesion, and if clear fluid is aspirated this implies a benign cyst. It should always be subjected, however, to cytological examination. A technetium gamma-camera scan will also demonstrate the absence of blood vessels in the cyst. Complications of unilateral cyst are rare, but bleeding into the cyst or infection of the cyst may occur.

Medullary sponge kidney

Cystic dilatation of the renal collecting tubules is occasionally seen. It represents a congenital ectasia of these tubules which may be complicated by the development of microcalculi. The lesion is often bilateral and may involve all calices. There is an increased incidence of infection in such kidneys, and the symptoms are usually those of pyelonephritis or stone, or haematuria. Excretory urograms reveal dilated tubules which show up as a 'blush' pattern. There is no specific treatment. Infection must be combated, and in the presence of calculi a prophylactic regimen of antibiotics should be prescribed.

Aberrant renal vessels (Fig. 39.5)

These are found more often on the left side than on the right, and in females more commonly than males. Most often they are unilateral. There is a view that aberrant renal vessels may cause hydronephrosis. However, it is unlikely that aberrant vessels by themselves cause the condition. It is more likely that their presence accentuates a hydronephrosis already present.

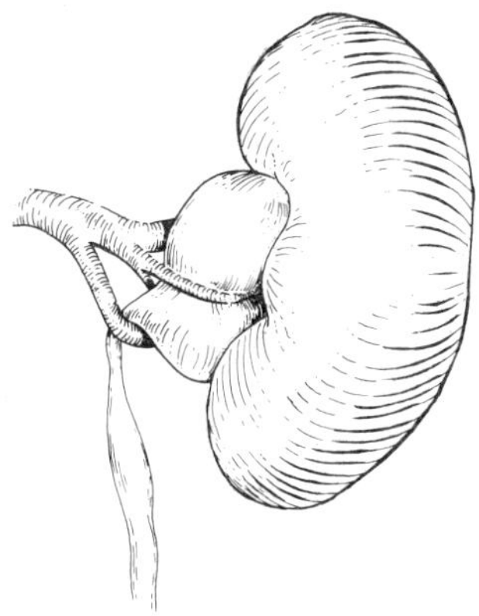

Fig. 39.5 Aberrant renal arteries. Several branches are shown, the lowermost of which crosses at the pelviureteral junction.

CONGENITAL ABNORMALITIES OF THE RENAL PELVIS AND URETER

Duplication of the renal pelvis

This is the most common congenital anomaly of the upper renal tract, and is found in about 4% of patients. It is usually unilateral and is somewhat more common on the left side than on the right. The upper renal pelvis is comparatively small and drains the upper group of calices. The larger lower renal pelvis drains the middle and lower group of calices.

Duplication of the ureter

Double ureters are present, in addition to double renal pelves, in about 3% of cases submitted to intravenous urography. The ureters often join, usually in the lower third of their course, and have a common orifice into the bladder. Less frequently, the ureters open independently into the bladder, in which case the ureter draining the upper pelvis crosses its fellow and opens below and medial to it.

Ectopic ureteric orifice

Should a second ureteric bud arise from the mesonephric duct later than usual, the orifice of the accessory ureter is prone to occupy a grossly abnormal position. This is a rare anomaly. In both sexes the existence of double ureter is determined by excretory urography. In the female an ectopic ureter opens either into the urethra, below the sphincter urethrae, or into the vagina and causes intractable incontinence of urine. The diagnosis can nearly always be made from the history alone. A girl or woman who has dribbled for as long as she can remember, despite the fact that she has a desire to void and does urinate, has an ectopic ureteric orifice.

Demonstration of this orifice is often extremely difficult because it is guarded by a valve. The diagnosis can be established by giving an intravenous injection of indigo carmine and placing one swab into the vestibule and another into the vagina. The one coloured blue signifies the position of the ectopic orifice. Sometimes laparotomy is the only way of finding or excluding the additional ureter.

In the male the aberrant opening may be situated at the apex of the trigone in the posterior urethra, in a seminal vesicle or in an ejaculatory duct. As in all these diverse situations, the ectopic ureteric orifice is situated above the sphincter urethrae, and therefore the male patient remains continent. A recurrent acute or chronic pyelonephritis is prone to supervene in the renal tissue served by the ectopic ureter.

Congenital megaloureter

This may be unilateral or bilateral, and in late stages is accompanied by hydronephrosis. Often the condition is symptomless until infection has occurred. If, however, the patient experiences pain the diagnosis can be made before the onset of infection. The ureteric orifice on the affected side is normal in size and shape but it is immotile, the efflux being a continuous trickle instead of intermittent ejections. A ureteric catheter passes easily. Excretory pyelography shows the ureter to be greatly dilated. In infected cases a cystoscopic meatotomy and drainage of the dilated ureter with a ureteric catheter for about 6 weeks may be effective in clearing up the infection. Reflux afterwards is likely, and so the condition is better treated by open excision of the lower 1–2 cm of ureter followed by reimplantation into the bladder using a nipple ureterostomy with a long intramural course for the ureter.

Ureterocele

Ureterocele is due to congenital atresia of the ureteric orifice which causes a cystic enlargement of the intramural portion of the ureter (Fig. 39.6). Usually the wall of the cyst is composed of mu-

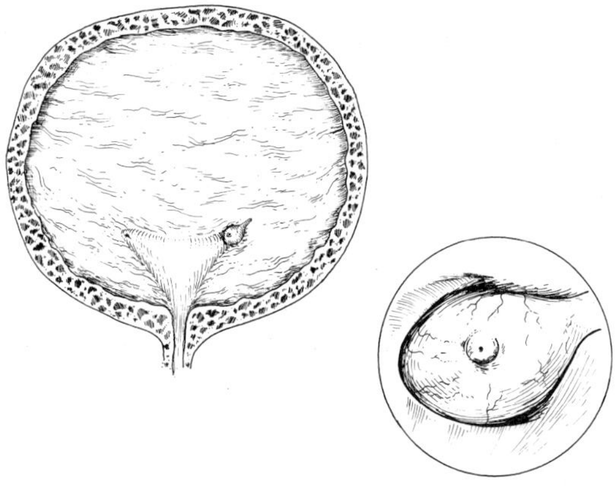

Fig. 39.6 Ureterocele. On account of stenosis of the ureteral orifice the distal segment has become dilated and has stretched the overlying mucosa around and proximal to the orifice.

cous membrane only, but infrequently the muscle coat is also included. This condition may be discovered in childhood, but often it is not recognized until adult life. Women are more often affected than men, and in 10% of cases the condition is bilateral. The condition, producing some obstruction, does render the patient more liable to stone formation and recurrent infection. Cystoscopic findings are characteristic; when the wall consists of mucous membrane, there is a translucent cyst over which blood vessels radiate. In the rare variety containing muscle in the wall the cyst is opaque. In either case the sac is seen to enlarge as it fills with urine. The pyelographic findings are characteristic.

Treatment

Most cases are symptomless and no treatment is required. Hydronephrosis, stone or recurrent infection may necessitate treatment. Cauterizing a hole through the wall of the cyst with a diathermy electrode is a simple and satisfactory procedure. A micturating cystogram should be performed 3 months later to exclude urinary reflux.

INJURIES TO THE KIDNEY

In civil life blows or falls upon the loin are the most usual causes of renal injury. Haematuria following minor injuries should suggest the possibility of pre-existing renal abnormality, viz. stone, hydronephrosis or tuberculosis. The degree of injury varies considerably from a small subcapsular haematoma to a complete tear involving the whole thickness of the kidney. In addition the kidney may be partially or wholly avulsed from its pedicle. Tears of the renal parenchyma follow the lines of the uriniferous tubules. The whole of one pole may be detached. The injury is extraperitoneal except very rarely in children, in whom there is little perinephric fat. In this situation the peritoneum may be intimately related to the kidney and is liable to be torn in addition to the renal capsule, allowing blood and perhaps urine to escape into the peritoneal cavity.

Clinical features

Rarely there is superficial bruising but there are likely to be local pain and tenderness. Haematuria is the cardinal sign of a damaged kidney, but it may not make its appearance until some hours after the accident. If the haemorrhage is profuse it may be followed by clot colic.

Severe delayed haematuria

Sudden profuse haematuria can occur between the third day and the third week after the accident in a patient who appears to be progressing favourably. It is due to a clot becoming dislodged.

Meteorism

In many cases of renal injury abdominal distension comes on about 24–48 h after the accident. In all probability it is caused by retroperitoneal haematoma implicating the splanchnic nerves. A perinephric haematoma should be suspected if there is even a slight flattening of the normal contour of the loin.

Management and treatment

Conservative treatment is usually successful. However, it must be remembered that injury to other organs may be associated with injury to the kidney. The patient must rest flat in bed until macroscopic haematuria has been absent for 2–3 days; morphine should be given for pain; an hourly pulse and blood pressure chart should be kept; a prophylactic antibiotic should be given, and the patient should be grouped and cross-matched in case a transfusion is required. An intravenous urogram should be obtained urgently to show—hopefully—that the other kidney is normal. Exploration is necessary only if there are signs of progressive blood loss or a swelling develops in the loin, or if there are signs of perirenal infection. The aim should be to conserve as much of the kidney as possible. In all cases at exploration the peritoneum should be opened to exclude damage to other organs.

Complications

Clot retention in the bladder can be cleared by bladder irrigation. Pararenal pseudohydronephrosis may occur in the course of a few weeks due to a combination of a complete tear of the renal cortex and ureteric obstruction. Hypertension may follow fibrosis of the kidney, usually after 3 months or more. Nephrectomy may then be necessary. Aneurysm of the renal artery is a rare complication of injury to the kidney.

INJURIES TO THE URETER

Rupture of the ureter can occur as a result of an accident causing hyperextension of the spine. The clinical diagnosis is impossible until a diminished quantity of urine is passed, followed by a swelling in the loin or iliac fossa. An intravenous urogram shows a diffuse shadow below the kidney on the injured side.

Injury to one or both ureters during pelvic surgery is considerably more common than the foregoing, and occurs most often during the course of a difficult hysterectomy. Preliminary catheterization of the ureters prevents such accidents for with catheters within them the ureters can be felt and seen unmistakably. The accidents include division of the ureter, ligating it, crushing it in a clamp, or removing a portion of its wall.

Injury recognized at the time of the operation

The ureterovesical continuity should be restored, usually by introducing a pigtail stent into the ureter and oversewing the defect or re-anastomosing the mobilized ureter.

Injury not recognized at the time of the operation

There are three possibilities in unilateral injury:

1. No symptoms. If one ureter is ligated securely and the contralateral kidney and ureter are normal the affected kidney most often undergoes silent atrophy, thus the accident remains unsuspected for many years.
2. Lumbar pain, hydronephrosis and pyenephrosis occur in less than half of the remainder. Excretory pyelography reveals no excretion on the side of the lesion. To avoid infection of the developing hydronephrosis nephrostomy should be undertaken early. A reparative operation may then be undertaken.
3. A urinary fistula develops through the abdominal incision or following panhysterectomy through the vagina. Again, a temporary nephrostomy should be performed and a reparative operation postponed until oedema and infection have abated, usually after about 6 weeks.
   In cases of anuria following ligation of both ureters during hysterectomy an attempt is made to pass ureteric catheters when both ureters will be found to be occluded. The wound should be explored and the ligatures removed.

Repair of the injured ureter

If the ends are clean-cut and no length has been lost, each end should be split for approximately 1 cm and the edges united over a pigtail stent (Fig. 39.7). If the division is low down it may be possible to re-implant the ureter directly into the bladder. Alternatively, a flap of bladder may be turned up

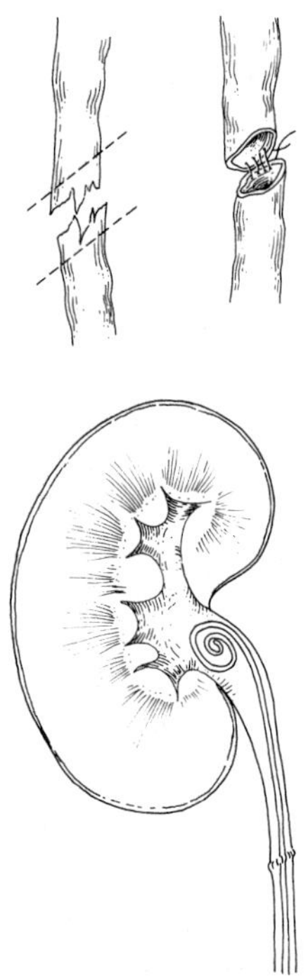

Fig. 39.7 Repair of damaged ureter. Making the anastomosis oblique gives a longer suture line and is less likely to result in stenosis than a directly transverse join. The lower illustration shows a pigtail stent in place after the repair. When signs of healing are adequate the stent can be removed simply by traction, when the coil at the inner end unfolds.

to replace the lower ureter. Occasionally it may be necessary to autotransplant the kidney into the pelvis in order to establish a connection between the shortened ureter and the bladder. Finally, as a last resort, a segment of ileum may be inserted to bridge the gap between the upper end of the ureter and the bladder.

HYDRONEPHROSIS

Hydronephrosis is an aseptic dilatation of the whole or part of the kidney due to partial or intermittent obstruction of the outflow of urine. Hydronephrosis may be unilateral or bilateral. The causes are described below.

Unilateral

Extramural

1. In a large number of cases of pelvic hydronephrosis an artery or a vein of the lower pole is found apparently obstructing the upper ureter. In many instances this is not an aberrant vessel but a normal inferior renal artery or vein that has been displaced downwards by the enlarging renal pelvis. This displaced vessel, while adding considerably to the rapid increase in size of the hydronephrosis, is not necessarily the primary cause (see Fig. 39.5).
2. Involvement of the ureter by growth outside it, e.g. carcinoma of the cervix, prostate, rectum, colon or caecum.
3. Idiopathic retroperitoneal fibrosis.

Mural

1. Congenital stenosis, physiological narrowing or achalasia at the pelviureteric junction.
2. Congenital atresia of the ureteric orifice.
3. Inflammatory stricture of the ureter following removal of a stone that was lodged in one portion of the ureter for a long time, or tuberculosis of the ureter. Stricture of the ureter also follows ureteroureteric anastomosis or trauma to the ureter during pelvic operations.
4. Neoplasm of the ureter or the bladder involving the ureteric orifice.

Intramural

A stone in the ureter or a small calculus in the renal pelvis; the latter often gives rise to intermittent hydronephrosis.

Bilateral hydronephrosis

This is generally the result of some form of urethral obstruction, but it can also be caused by one of the lesions described above occurring bilaterally. When due to lower urinary obstruction the cause may be:

1. Congenital
   a. Atresia of the urethral meatus.
   b. Phimosis (very rare).
   c. Congenital valves of the posterior urethra.
   d. Congenital contracture of the bladder neck.
2. Acquired
   a. A neoplasm of the bladder which involves both ureteric orifices.
   b. Prostatic enlargement or carcinoma.
   c. Acquired contracture of the bladder neck.
   d. Carcinoma of the cervix.
   e. Carcinoma of the rectum, involving both ureters.
   f. Inflammatory or traumatic urethral stricture.

When the obstruction lies in the urethra, muscular hypertrophy of the bladder occurs, and the ureters by reason of this hypertrophy become partially obstructed in the intramural portion of their course.

Pathology

The pathological changes differ in some respects according to whether the kidney has an extrarenal or an intrarenal pelvis, the former being more common. In a kidney with an extrarenal pelvis at first the pelvis alone becomes dilated. As time goes on if the obstruction is not relieved, the calices become increasingly dilated and the renal parenchyma is progressively destroyed by pressure atrophy. In a kidney with an intrarenal pelvis the destruction of the parenchyma occurs more rapidly. In either case it may be a matter of years before the diagnosis is made, by which time the kidney may be merely a lobulated sac containing pale uriniferous fluid of low specific gravity. On bisecting the specimen longitudinally a series of compartments representing the dilated calices will be found.

Unilateral hydronephrosis

Clinical features

The female: male ratio is 2 : 1, the right side being more commonly affected. Presenting features include:

1. Insidious pain, usually slight, which often amounts to only a dull ache or a sense of weight in the loin, may be brought on by alcohol or excessive fluid intake. On examination an enlarged—sometimes greatly enlarged—kidney is found. In these cases the obstruction is usually at the pelviureteric junction.
2. Attacks of renal colic may occur, and no palpable swelling may be found.
3. Intermittent hydronephrosis—after an attack of renal colic with its accompanying abdominal rigidity, the pain passes off and a swelling in the loin is detected. Some hours later, or on the next day following the passage of a large quantity of urine due to some reflex polyuria, the pain is relieved and the swelling disappears (Dietl's crisis).

Urography

Except during pregnancy, when X-rays are contraindicated for fear of causing a congenital malformation, the diagnosis is made by excretory urography (Fig. 39.8). Alternatively, ultrasonography or a computerized tomography scan will confirm the diagnosis. When hydronephrosis is advanced, films taken 6–24 h after the injection of medium may show a hydronephrotic kidney which was imperceptible on films taken at the routine times (Figs 39.9 and 39.10). As a rule the earliest pyelographic manifestation of a hydronephrosis is dilatation of the renal pelvis, for in the majority of cases the pelvis is extrarenal. The next change is decreasing concavity and then flattening of the minor calices and dilatation of the major calices, which are the first changes when the pelvis is intrarenal. In moderately sized hydronephroses the minor calices become convex and finally club-shaped and the major calices considerably broadened. In advanced cases there is extreme dilatation of the renal pelvis and the calices, or no excretion of opaque media. Localization of the site of obstruction can be obtained by passing a needle into the renal pelvis under ultrasound control and injecting a radiopaque dye (antegrade pyelogram). A pigtail stent passed

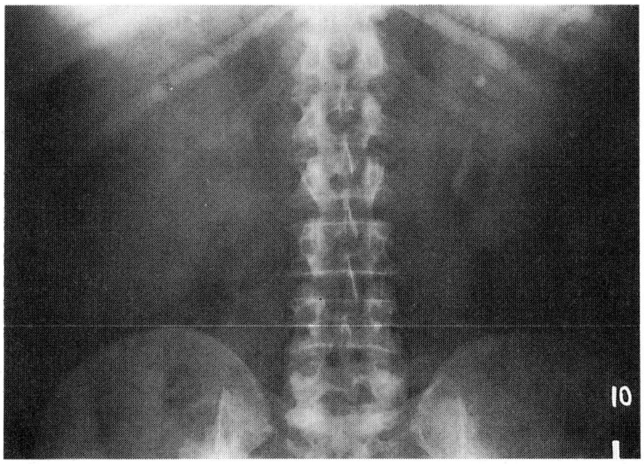

Fig. 39.8 Intravenous urogram showing a normal renal outline on the left, along with a normal-size and shaped pelvicaliceal system. By contrast, on the right there is an enlarged renal outline and no evidence of the pelvicaliceal system, on account of right-sided hydronephrosis.

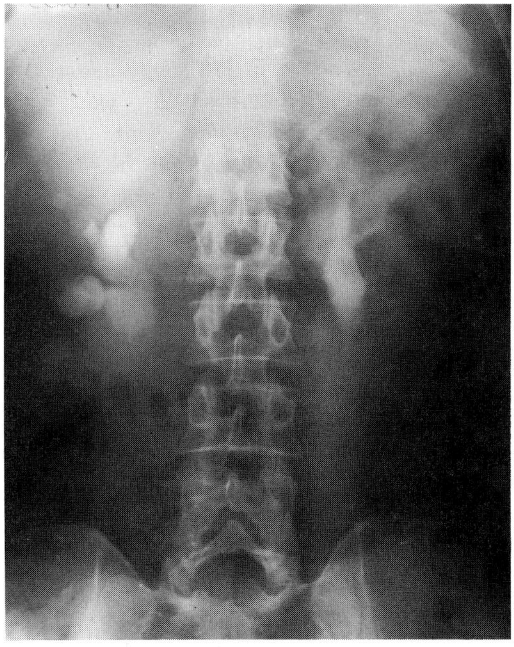

Fig. 39.9 Intravenous urogram taken at a longer interval after injection of the contrast medium. The dilated pelvis and rounded calices, particularly the lower ones, are evident on the right side, by contrast with a normal outline on the left.

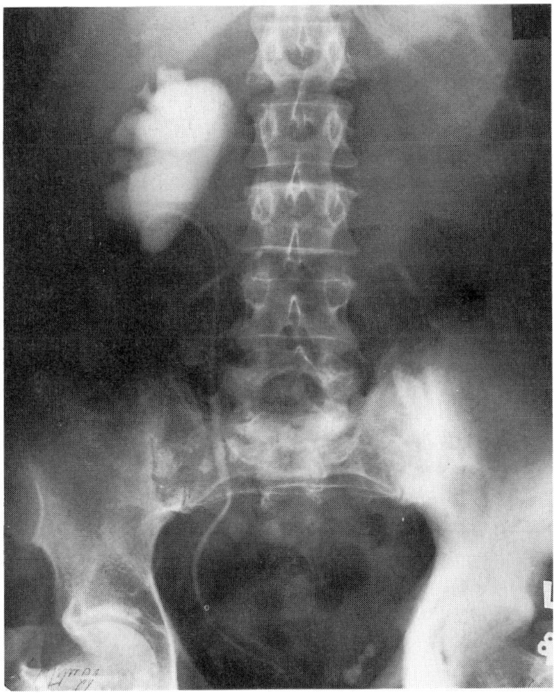

Fig. 39.10 Right-sided hydronephrosis demonstrated by retrograde catheterization via a cystoscope.

through the needle can then be used to drain the hydronephrosis until a correction is undertaken.

Treatment

Nephrectomy is indicated when the total parenchyma has been destroyed and the kidney is nonfunctioning. Most often the hydronephrosis can be reconstructed by excising the stricture or the site of obstruction and creating a plastic repair. For pelviureteric obstruction the Anderson-Hines pyeloplasty is the usual plastic repair (Fig. 39.11). In this operation the redundant renal pelvis is excised and the ureter re-anastomosed to the pelvis after excising the diseased segment.

NEOPLASMS OF THE KIDNEY AND URETER

Benign neoplasms

Adenoma

Pea-like cortical adenomas are sometimes found at necropsy. They give rise to no symptoms and are only of academic interest.

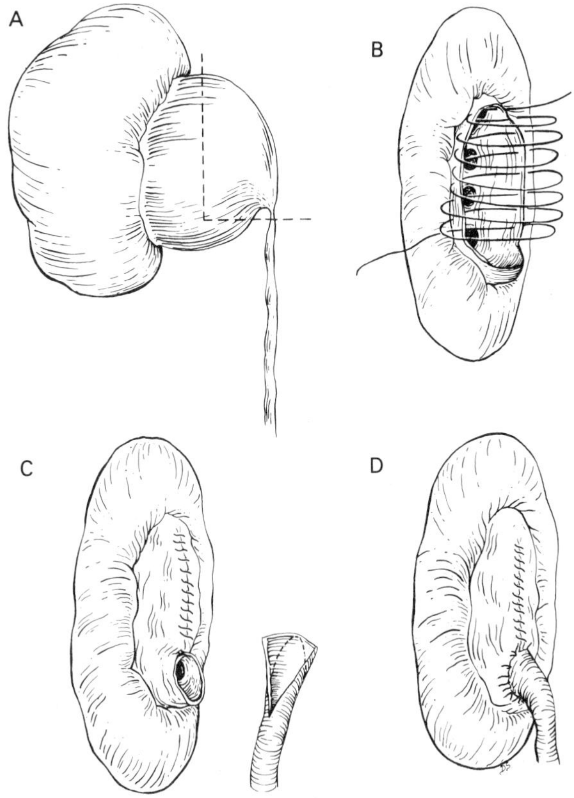

Fig. 39.11 Anderson–Hines repair of hydronephrosis due to congenital pelviureteral stricture. (**A**) The segment of dilated pelvis and proximal ureter excised; (**B**) closure of upper part of pelvis (**C**) fashioning a flap of the upper end of the ureter; (**D**) anastomosis of this flap to the lower part of the pelvis.

Angioma may give rise to profuse haematuria.

Truly benign tumours of the kidney are so rare that a good rule is that all neoplasms of the kidney which can be recognized correctly should be considered malignant and treated as such.

Malignant neoplasms of the kidney

Clinically neoplasms of the kidney are divided into two classes: children between the ages of 1 and 7 years and adults after the age of 40. Between the ages of 7 and 40 malignant neoplasms are unusual in the kidney.

Renal neoplasms in children

Wilms tumour (nephroblastoma)

This is a mixed tumour containing epithelial and connective tissue elements arising from embryonic nephrogenic tissue situated originally in one or other pole of the kidney. In infancy such tumours are very occasionally bilateral, but unilateral tumours are far more common. They usually occur during the first 4 years of life.

Pathology

Macroscopically on section the neoplasm is greyish-white or pinkish-white in colour. Its consistency varies with the rapidity of growth, i.e. the more rapid the growth, the softer the tumour.

Microscopically it is composed mainly of two types of cells—epithelial and connective tissue. Cartilage, bone and smooth or striped muscle fibres are occasionally found. The epithelial and connective tissue cells exist side by side, but one type is usually predominant. Thus the tumour is composed of mixed cellular elements, some of which are radiosensitive and some radioresistant. Consequently, the radioresistant elements show a continuance of activity despite radiotherapy. Metastases occur most commonly in the liver and lungs, rarely in the brain and bones. Nephroblastoma accounts for 8% of childhood malignancies.

Clinical features

Abdominal enlargement is the predominant feature in 60% of cases. Pain is present in 20%, haematuria in 15%, malaise, weakness, anorexia and weight loss in 10% and fever in 3% of patients. An abdominal mass is palpable in almost all cases. The mass is usually very large, firm and smooth and does not ordinarily extend across the midline. Hypertension is noted in more than 50% of patients and may be sufficient to produce congestive heart failure. Aniridia, hemihypertrophy, hypospadias, cryptorchidism and urinary anomalies are frequently associated. An intravenous urogram shows distortion of the calices and kidney. Non-visualization on urography indicates tumour extension into the ureter or renal vessels. Cystoscopy and retrograde urography are unnecessary. Renal arteriograms are helpful in differentiating retroperitoneal tumours and in detecting small or bilateral nephroblastomas. An inferior vena cavagram may show obstruction in the vena cava, but it does not differentiate compression from tumour invasion. Renal ultrasonography and computerized tomography scan may distinguish hydronephrosis from a solid tumour. Liver scan and chest X-rays will identify metastases.

Differential diagnosis is from abdominal masses such as hydronephrosis, multicystic or duplicated kidneys, neuroblastoma, teratoma, hepatoma and rhabdomyosarcoma. An intravenous urogram distinguishes nephroblastoma from the other tumours because caliceal distortion indicates intrarenal origin. Calcification occurs in 10% of cases of nephroblastoma and tends to be more crescent-shaped, discrete and peripherally located, whereas the calcification in neuroblastoma is finely stippled.

Complications

A tumour can extend into the renal vein and the inferior vena cava. These vessels should be carefully palpated during abdominal exploration and the tumour should be removed in such a way that tumour embolus will not occur.

Treatment

The preferred treatment is immediate nephrectomy and excision of all surrounding tissues within Gerota's fascia. Irradiation of the tumour bed is indicated if the tumour has extended beyond the capsule of the kidney. Large necrotic haemorrhagic tumours may require preoperative angiographic embolization to facilitate extirpation. Very large tumours may be treated with radiation therapy preoperatively to reduce the size of the tumour. A significant reduction in size usually occurs in 7–10 days, after which nephrectomy is more easily performed, usually through a long transverse or thoracoabdominal incision. Prognostic factors that influence survival include age, size of tumour, extension of tumour beyond the capsule, lymph node metastases and the histology of the tumour. Children under the age of 2 have better survival rates than older children. Tumours weighing over 375 g are associated with a poorer prognosis than smaller ones. Invasion of the renal capsule or renal sinus results in a survival rate of 60% compared to 80% when there is no capsular involvement. When regional lymph nodes are uninvolved the survival rate is 72%. Following surgical removal of the primary tumour, radiation therapy to the tumour bed and across the midline to include both sides of the spine is indicated when there is capsular invasion, residual non-haematogenous tumour, lymph node metastases or unfavourable histological features.

All patients should receive combination chemotherapy postoperatively consisting of dactinomycin 15 mg/kg/day for 5 days postoperatively, at 6 weeks and every 3–15 months, and vincristine 1.5 mg/m^2/day on the first and last day of the dactinomycin course. Doxorubicin 60 mg/m^2 to a total dose of 300 mg/m^2 should be given at 6 weeks and every 3 months. The cardiotoxicity of doxorubicin is significant, and the drug may be reserved for children with unfavourable prognostic factors. The addition of cyclophosphamide may be indicated for patients with unfavourable histological reports. Solitary metastases in the lung should be resected. Hepatic metastases and pulmonary metastases should be irradiated. Any residual tumour following radiation therapy, including multiple lesions, should be resected.

Bilateral nephroblastoma occurs in 5–10% of cases. X-ray therapy followed by bilateral nephrectomy and dialysis treatment for 4 or 5 years prior to a renal transplant is the favoured treatment.

Prognosis

Of those patients who die of nephroblastoma, 98% die within 2 years following treatment. Nephrectomy and X-ray therapy alone or with one course of dactinomycin provides a cure rate of 50% at best. A combination of dactinomycin and vincristine achieves 90% long-term survival. When pulmonary or hepatic metastases are present at diagnosis the survival rate following combined treatment with surgery, X-ray therapy and chemotherapy is 50%.

Renal neoplasms in adults

Renal adenocarcinoma (hypernephroma)

This is the commonest neoplasm of the kidney (75%). It arises in the cortex, probably from a pre-existing adenoma, or de novo in the cells of the uriniferous tubules.

Pathology

By the time of clinical presentation the tumour is usually of moderate size, spherical in shape, and it often occupies one or other pole, more commonly the upper one. On section it is characteristically yellow due to lipid, and less often it is dull white or semi-transparent. Haemorrhagic areas are often seen. The tumour is divided into numerous lobules by fibrous septa. The larger the tumour, the more extensive is its central haemorrhage and necrosis. Microscopically the most common appearance is of solid alveoli of cubical or polyhedral clear cells with deeply stained small rounded nuclei and abundant cytoplasm containing lipoid, cholesterol and glycogen. The cells may also be arranged in the form of papillary cysts or tubules. In a much smaller percentage the cells are granular and dark. Clear and dark cells can coexist in different parts of the same tumour. In all cases the stroma is scanty but rich in large blood vessels, the walls of which often appear in places to consist of tumour cells.

Spread

As the tumour enlarges it encroaches upon a group of calices and is prone to grow into the renal veins. Pieces of growth becoming detached are swept into the circulation to become arrested, particularly in the lungs ('cannon-ball' metastases) and bones. Occasionally when a secondary growth appears in a long bone it remains the only metastasis for perhaps a year or more. While spread in the blood stream predominates, spread by lymphatics also occurs. If the tumour bursts through the renal capsule into the perirenal tissues it then metastasizes to the lymph nodes in relation to the hilum of the kidney and from there to the para-aortic and other lymph nodes.

Clinical features

The tumour is twice as common in men as in women. Typically the first sign is intermittent painless haematuria. Clot colic may follow, and may be associated with a dragging pain in the loin. Occasionally, the first manifestation is a palpable renal swelling. In the adult male the rapid appearance of a varicocele is a rare but impressive sign associated with invasion of the renal vein and obstruction of the testicular vein. In 25% of cases the primary growth remains silent; the patient presents because of symptoms from secondary deposits, such as a painful enlargement of a bone, or a spontaneous fracture, persistent cough or haemoptysis. Occasionally persistent pyrexia—37.8–38.9°C—is the only symptom, there being no infection to account for the temperature. It is presumably due to the absorption of blood and necrotic material. Such pyrexia usually disappears after nephrectomy, but should it persist after the operation this may indicate that metastases are present. Rarely the patient presents on account of lassitude, and is found to be extremely anaemic, the degree of anaemia being out of proportion to that which would be expected from the haematuria, if such is present. On the other hand polycythaemia occurs in 4% of cases, and this is believed to be due to excess erythropoietin production. The blood sedimentation rate is always raised above the 1–2 mm found in idiopathic polycythaemia vera. The blood count will return to normal after nephrectomy but a return of the polycythaemia has been known to occur with the development of metastases.

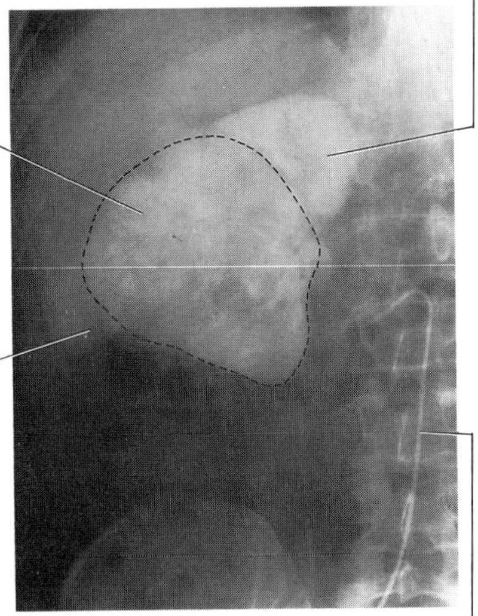

Fig. 39.12 Renal carcinoma. A large tumour has replaced most of the central portion of the kidney, leaving only small parts of the upper and lower poles of normal pattern. Since these tumours are generally very vascular they are easily shown up by selective renal artery angiography—as in the present example—as an irregular mass of disorganized small vessels.

Early diagnosis

By the time a patient has the classical triad of symptoms—haematuria, pain and a palpable renal tumour, he or she nearly always has metastases. It is therefore of paramount importance to endeavour to make an early diagnosis, and any one of these symptoms calls for a thorough renal investigation. Patients with haematuria should be examined cystoscopically while the bleeding is in progress. If blood is seen to be issuing from one ureteric orifice and there is a clear efflux from the other, the information gained is of considerable importance, but is by no means conclusive evidence of renal neoplasm. Ultrasound examination of the kidney should clearly define the tumour, and differentiate between it and a cyst in more than 90% of cases. Intravenous urography is rarely helpful, but does demonstrate the normality of the contralateral kidney.

Differential diagnosis

Other renal lesions may present as a mass in the flank, including hydronephrosis, polycystic disease and single cyst. Radiographic techniques afford differentiation (Fig. 39.12).

Complications

These are usually related to local invasion or metastasis. A few patients develop hydronephrosis from ureteral compression, or hypertension from interference with the renal blood supply. Occlusion of the renal vein may cause findings compatible with the nephrotic syndrome.

Treatment

In the absence of demonstrable metastases, radical nephrectomy is indicated. These tumours are ordinarily radioresistant. As far as chemotherapy is concerned, the administration of medroxyprogesterone (Depo-Provera) 100 mg/week intramuscularly may have some palliative effect, but in general the results have been very disappointing.

Prognosis

About 35% of nephrectomized patients are alive at 5 years, but metastases may become evident even 10–15 years later. The prognosis is poor if the renal vein is involved by tumour. A solitary metastasis should be excised surgically.

Tumours of the renal pelvis

Tumours of the renal pelvis resemble those in the bladder, but are less common. They tend to invade the kidney proper and to take on malignant characteristics. Spread downwards by seeding may give rise to multiple ureteric and bladder tumours. On the other hand a diffuse metaplasia of the urothelium may be the result of some carcinogenic agent in the urine.

Clinical features

Haematuria is the commonest presenting symptom, and is often continued for months at a time. A renal swelling is absent except in rare cases where the pelviureteric junction becomes occluded and a hydronephrosis results, in which event there is lumbar pain. Clot colic may occur. Intravenous urography reveals a characteristic filling defect in the renal pelvis.

Treatment

Nephrectomy with extended ureterectomy is the correct treatment. The intramural portion of the ureter along with the ureteric orifice must be excised in continuity by sleeve resection of the bladder wall. For the pathology of this tumour, see page 453.

Squamous cell carcinoma of the renal pelvis

This is the least common variety of malignant disease of the kidney. In some instances it appears to be preceded by leukoplakia, and in most cases a stone or stones are present. Unless the stone gives rise to symptoms this is the most elusive of all renal neoplasms, for it causes indefinite abdominal pain, which finally becomes localized in the region of the involved kidney. Haematuria is slight, or to be found only on microscopical examination of the urine. Excretory pyelography shows a kidney excreting little or no medium. Retrograde pyelography sometimes reveals a deformed renal pelvis. Owing to diagnostic difficulties, by the time a nephrectomy is performed there are often widespread metastases which are radioresistant. This tumour has the worst prognosis of any renal neoplasm.

Primary neoplasms of the ureter

These are rare, and similar to those of the renal pelvis. The symptoms are identical to those of neoplasms of the renal pelvis although hydronephrosis, haemonephrosis and pyelonephrosis are more frequent accompaniments. Occasionally a portion of the papillomatous growth can be seen protruding from the ureteric orifice. Usually the diagnosis is made by intravenous urography. Papillary tumours of the ureter should be treated by nephroureterectomy as the epithelium frequently shows changes of carcinoma-in-situ at many points along the course of the ureter. The intramural ureter should be removed or the epithelium destroyed by fulguration. Only rarely is it justifiable, because of reduced renal reserve, to perform a resection of the ureter and replacement by an ileal conduit.

VASCULAR ABNORMALITIES AFFECTING THE KIDNEY

RENAL ARTERY STENOSIS

Renal artery stenosis may occur primarily as a consequence of fibromuscular dysplasia, a disease affecting the muscular secondary arteries of the body including the renal arteries, the carotids and the mesenteric vessels. It may affect one or both kidneys and the disease may extend from the origin of the renal artery into its branches. The most common type of fibromuscular dysplasia is fibromuscular hypoplasia which characteristically affects young people under the age of 30, and is associated with alternating strictures and aneurysms along the course of the renal artery, or its branches.

Presentation

The classical presentation is with severe intractable hypertension. As a result of underperfusion of the kidney, hyperplasia of the juxtaglomerular apparatus occurs. Large quantities of renin are released into the circulation, which converts angiotensin I to angiotensin II and stimulates the release of aldosterone. In this way, by a mixture of vasoconstriction and salt retention, persistent severe hypertension occurs, and may result in cerebrovascular accident, retinal detachment, cardiac failure and even, on rare occasions, rupture of major arteries.

Diagnosis

On ultrasound examination the affected kidney is found to be smaller than the other, and on excretion urography the small kidney is seen to concentrate late, but more intensely, than the normal kidney. Radioimmunoassay for circulating renin reveals high levels, with associated high levels of aldosterone. The high renin levels distinguish this form of hypertension from primary aldosteronism (Conn's syndrome).

Treatment

The choice of treatment lies between nephrectomy and reconstruction of the damaged renal artery, the choice depending on judgement of the renal functional reserve of the damaged kidney. Clearly when both kidneys are affected or when renal artery stenosis affects a solitary kidney, reconstruction is the only possibility, offering a life free from dialysis. Reconstruction can be performed in situ by either

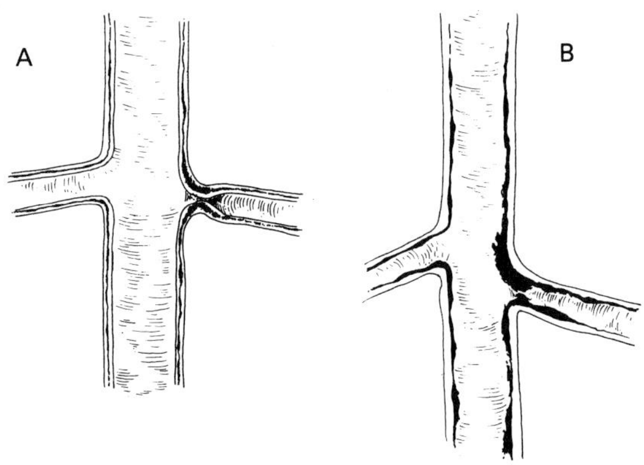

Fig. 39.13 Renal artery stenosis. (**A**) Localized fibromuscular dysplasia affecting origin of renal artery; (**B**) extension of atheromatous plaque on the aorta across or into the origin of the renal artery.

bypass using autologous artery or vein, or alternatively it can be carried out by autotransplantation of the affected kidney, with or without repair of the damaged segment of artery on the workbench.

Secondary renal artery stenosis occurs as a consequence of atherosclerosis affecting either the aorta or the origin of the renal artery (Fig. 39.13). The presenting symptoms are the same, although the patients tend to be in a much older age group, and often have stigmata of generalized atherosclerosis. Treatment once again lies as a choice between nephrectomy to cure the hypertension, or reconstruction of the renal artery, which may be accomplished by endarterectomy, or by bypass, or by autotransplantation.

Aneurysm of the renal artery

This is a relatively rare condition resulting from weakness of the wall of the artery, caused by atherosclerosis, polyarthritis nodosa or trauma. Some renal artery aneurysms are congenital. If the aneurysm causes stenosis of the renal artery hypertension may ensue, secondary to the ischaemia. A plain abdominal X-ray may reveal a ring-like calcification in the wall of the aneurysm. Angiography is usually diagnostic. Because there is a significant incidence of spontaneous rupture of these lesions, their repair or removal must be considered. Nephrectomy may be necessary, particularly if emergency intervention for bleeding is called for. Elective repair of a renal artery aneurysm can usually be accomplished on the workbench, with the kidney cooled and then replaced by autotransplantation.

Renal infarction

Common causes of occlusion of the renal artery are subacute bacterial endocarditis, atrial or ventricular thrombi, arteriosclerosis, polyarthritis nodosa and trauma. Multiple emboli are common and lead to patchy renal ischaemia. Occlusion of the main renal artery will cause atrophy of a portion or all of the kidney. The patient may suffer from flank pain or the lesion may be silent. Haematuria is common. Excretory urograms may reveal no excretion of radiopaque material or may only opacify a portion of the kidney. With complete occlusion of the main renal artery a ureteral catheter will drain no urine, yet retrograde urogram will reveal normal anatomy. Renal angiography makes the diagnosis by revealing occlusion of the artery or arterioles. A renal scan will show similar findings. This disease may be mimicked by ureteral stone, but urograms and angiograms will differentiate them. Following a renal infarction hypertension may develop secondary to renal ischaemia, and this may later resolve spontaneously. If the diagnosis is made promptly endarterectomy should be considered, otherwise anticoagulant therapy may be instituted. If permanent hypertension develops definitive treatment of the arterial occlusion or nephrectomy should be performed.

Thrombosis of the renal vein

Thrombosis of the renal vein affects both infants and adults. In infants it is apt to complicate ileocolitis and dehydration. In the adult it may be secondary to renal infection or ascending thrombosis of the vena cava. There is usually flank pain and a palpable kidney. If it is secondary to infection the patient is septic and urinalysis reveals pus cells and bacteria. The patient with bilateral involvement is bound to have renal insufficiency and a nephrotic syndrome may develop. Excretory urograms show delayed and impaired opacification in an enlarged kidney. The calices are elongated. Later the kidney may become atrophic. Renal angiography reveals stretching and bowing of arterioles, and selective renal venography may demonstrate the thrombus. If the diagnosis of unilateral infected renal vein thrombus can be established, nephrectomy should be done. In bilateral disease anticoagulant therapy is required. A few cases of successful thrombectomy have been reported.

Retroperitoneal fibrosis

One or both ureters may be compressed by a chronic inflammatory process, usually of unknown cause, which involves the retroperitoneal tissues of the lumbosacral area. Patients treated for migraine with methysergide may develop this fibrosis. Sclerosing Hodgkin's disease has been found to be an occasional cause. The symptoms include renal pain, low backache and the syndrome of uraemia. Some patients present with complete anuria. Urinary infection is unusual. If both ureters are obstructed the serum creatinine will be elevated. The only pathognomonic sign is the presence of a palpable firm mass over the sacral promontory. Renal function tests are normal unless both ureters are completely obstructed, in which event anaemia may be found together with uraemia. The diagnosis of retroperitoneal fibrosis is most often made by excretory urography which reveals midline deviation of the ureters involved in the fibrous plaque, usually in the lumbar area. Secondary to the obstruction will be dilatation of the ureter and the renal pelvis proximal to the point of constriction. If the radiographic changes are moderate and the patient is not uraemic, corticosteroid therapy should be started. The condition may respond dramatically to corticosteroids within a matter of weeks. Prednisolone is usually started at 100 mg/day, and reduced as the hydronephrosis declines, by 10 mg every 3–4 days, down to a maintenance dose of 15–20 mg/day. If the degree of obstruction is severe the ureters should be freed from the fibrous plaque, and either transplanted intraperitoneally or displaced lateral to the psoas muscles. Since there is a tendency for the disease to progress, prophylactic corticosteroid therapy should be instituted.

40. Disorders of the bladder and prostate

CONGENITAL ANOMALIES OF THE BLADDER

Ectopia vesicae (exstrophy of the bladder)

Exstrophy of the bladder is a complete ventral defect of the urogenital sinus and the overlying skeletal system. The infraumbilical part of the anterior abdominal wall and the anterior wall of the bladder and urethra are absent. Exstrophy occurs once in every 50 000 births and may be complete or incomplete. In the more common complete variety, because of the pressure of the viscera behind it, the deep red posterior bladder wall protrudes through the defect. The exposed mucous membrane may then bleed, and urine can be seen to efflux from the ureteric orifices on to the pale, wet trigone.

The lot of a patient with ectopia vesicae is particularly unfortunate. A portable urinal seldom keeps him or her dry for long and the odour of urine always pervades. Frequently the extroverted vesical mucous membrane becomes ulcerated and painful. It undergoes metaplastic changes and sometimes becomes the seat of adenocarcinoma. Attempts to prevent recurrent attacks of ascending pyelonephritis by chemotherapeutic and antibiotic agents are only partially successful, and without definitive treatment by diversion of urine to an ileal conduit and/or transplantation, 50% of those afflicted by exstrophy of the bladder will die of renal failure before the age of 30.

Treatment

Diversion of the urine into the colon or into an ileal conduit is undertaken between 4 and 6 years of age. The best results follow diversion into an ileal conduit, with excision of the bladder (see Fig. 40.5). Renal function is likely to be better maintained by this treatment than by ureterocolic anastomosis, and there are no problems of rectal control. Very rarely complicated reconstructive procedures on the abdominal wall and bladder remnant are attempted in the first year of life, but usually with indifferent results.

Persistent urachus

Embryologically the allantois connects the urogenital sinus with the umbilicus. Normally the allantois is obliterated and is represented by a fibrous cord—thc urachus—extending from the dome of the bladder to the navel. Incomplete obliteration sometimes occurs, and if this happens at the superior end, a draining umbilical sinus may be noted. If it in turn becomes infected, the drainage will be purulent. If the inferior end remains open it will communicate with the bladder, but this does not usually produce symptoms. Rarely the entire tract remains patent, in which case urine drains constantly from the umbilicus. This is apt to become obvious within a few days of birth. If only the ends of the urachus seal off the cyst of that body may form and become quite large, presenting as a low midline mass. Should the cyst become infected signs of general and local sepsis will develop. Adenocarcinoma may occur in a urachal cyst, particularly at the vesical extremity and will tend to invade the tissue beneath the anterior abdominal wall. Stones may also develop in a cyst of the urachus and these can be identified on plain X-ray.

Treatment

Treatment consists of excision of the urachus, which lies on the peritoneal surface.

INJURIES TO THE BLADDER

The urinary bladder may be injured during surgery, e.g. accidental incision in pelvic operations, or in the repair of hernia (Fig. 40.1), or during the course of transurethral procedures on the bladder. Rupture of the bladder caused by direct blow presupposes a bladder distended with urine. The bladder can also be perforated by bony spicules from a fractured pelvis.

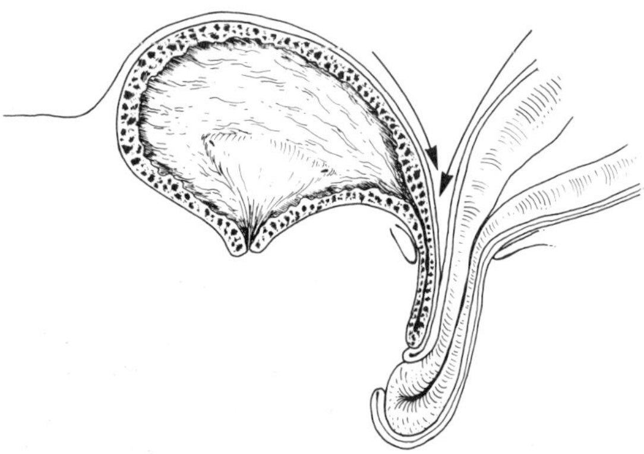

Fig. 40.1 'Sliding' pattern of inguinal hernia, with a portion of bladder wall pushed down along with the peritoneum of the sac. In addition a loop of small bowel is contained within the lumen of the sac. The segment of bladder is vulnerable to damage during surgical repair of the hernia.

Pathogenesis and pathology

A sudden blow to the full bladder causes a sharp rise in intravesical pressure. This may either contuse the wall or split it. With such an injury the extravasation of urine is usually intraperitoneal. If the vesical contents are infected, death from peritonitis will occur unless the laceration is closed surgically, or seals itself spontaneously. If the urine is sterile few symptoms may develop immediately, although anuria with uraemia becomes obvious, and ascites develops as the urine progressively fills the peritoneal cavity. If this urine becomes infected following catheterization or cystoscopy or from bacteria carried there in the blood stream, true peritonitis will supervene. Vesical laceration secondary to fracture of the pelvis causes extraperitoneal extravasation of urine (see Ch. 41). If this urine is infected or later becomes so, a spreading cellulitis develops and death occurs, unless adequate drainage is afforded. Rupture and perforation of the bladder are fatal injuries unless treated promptly.

Clinical findings

A history of an injury or blow to the lower abdomen followed by low abdominal pain and haematuria is strongly suggestive of vesical injury. Fracture of the pelvis is commonly accompanied by injury to the bladder. The finding of suprapubic tenderness or a mass is suggestive. Signs of peritonitis may be elicited. Cystography is the most dependable test. If, however, clinical judgement suggests the presence of vesical trauma, even a normal cystogram should be ignored.

Symptoms

If the patient can urinate, haematuria is to be expected, but he or she may not be able to urinate at all. Pain is present, low in the abdomen, and pain in the shoulder may also be noted if the urine is in the peritoneal cavity, and high fever may suggest infection.

Signs

Shock may be profound, especially if multiple injuries have been suffered. There may be evidence of local trauma, e.g. a bullet or knife wound, or ecchymoses. Marked tenderness in the suprapubic area is to be expected. There may be rebound tenderness if the laceration involves the peritoneum. Spasm of the muscles of the lower abdomen occurs even though extravasation is perivesical. A board-like abdomen suggests intraperitoneal rupture. A large suprapubic mass may be felt or percussed, as the perivesical collection of fluid develops. This will contain blood, urine and even occasionally pus. Rectal examination may reveal a large boggy mass, obliterating the normal landmarks.

Laboratory findings

Urinalysis will reveal haematuria, either gross or microscopic; a midstream urine specimen may demonstrate the presence of bacteria, and the blood urea and serum creatinine levels may be significantly increased. Plain X-ray may reveal fractures of the pelvic bones and an increased greyness from prevesical collection of urine and blood. Excretory urography will be helpful in surveying the kidneys for damage, and for demonstrating extravasation of opaque material into the prevesical tissues. The bladder may or may not be displaced by extravesical blood or urine. A cystogram is the most dependable test for vesical injury. After instilling 300–400 ml of radiopaque fluid, anteroposterior and posterior films are taken, before and after draining the vesical contents. This will reveal small amounts of extravasated fluid lying behind the bladder, or in the prevesical tissues.

Passage of a catheter will detect possible injury to the urethra. If an injured person cannot void he or she should be catheterized. The presence of bloody urine must be investigated. If 300–500 ml of sterile solution can be instilled into the bladder and the full amount recovered, the bladder is assumed to be intact. On occasion, however, this may afford erroneous information, as omentum or blood clot may temporarily plug the laceration. Cystoscopy is usually not very helpful.

Differential diagnosis

Haematuria and signs of injury to abdominal organs can also arise from an injured kidney. A mass and tenderness in the flank and evidence of fractures in the renal area are suggestive of renal injury. Changes on the plain film of the abdomen or on excretory urography should establish the diagnosis. Urethral injury may accompany fractures of the pelvis. Exploration of the urethra with a catheter is helpful, and a urethrogram will show extravasation, if this is the site of the tear.

Treatment

Emergency measures

The patient may need to be resuscitated by replacement of body fluids with saline and blood, relief of pain and ventilatory support if necessary.

Specific measures

1. If the rupture is extraperitoneal the site of injury should be drained surgically. Suprapubic cystostomy is a more reliable method than catheterization for keeping the bladder emptier and at rest. The peritoneum should be opened and intraperitoneal organs explored for associated injury.
2. The repair of an intraperitoneal rupture should be approached transperitoneally. If the point of rupture is inaccessible, suprapubic cystostomy usually permits healing without complications. Extravasated fluid in the peritoneal cavity should be aspirated. Injury to other organs should be looked for.

Prognosis

With diagnosis made and proper treatment instituted within 6–12 h after the injury, morbidity and mortality should be minimal. If treatment is delayed for several days, perivesical infection or peritonitis may develop and may not be controlled.

Injuries to the membranous urethra

The urogenital diaphragm encloses the membranous urethra and the external urinary sphincter. It is strongly attached to the pubic bone. In pelvic fractures this diaphragm may be torn, sheering off the prostate from the membranous urethra. Bony spicules may perforate the urethra and the bladder may also be lacerated. These injuries usually occur in association with trauma to other organs or structures. They occur just above the urogenital diaphragm, and this causes extravasation of blood and urine into the periprostatic and perivesical tissues. Only if the triangular ligament is badly damaged will extravasation present in the perineum (see Ch. 41). Extravasated urine may become infected, and if this is not properly treated early death may ensue from sepsis.

Clinical findings

Urethral bleeding may be noted following a history of injury, usually severe. Pain is present in the perineum or low in the abdomen, and the patient may be unable to void urine.

Signs

Urethral bleeding or haematuria is present, and

there may be a mass in the suprapubic area, which is dull to percussion. Suprapubic tenderness may be marked, and this may be due to extravasation or to fracture of the pelvis with associated haematoma. Rectal examination may reveal a large boggy mass of extravasated blood and urine. The prostate may be dislodged upwards if this has been avulsed from the membranous urethra.

Instrumental examination

If a catheter can be passed to the bladder the urethral injury is minor. If more extensive injuries are present the catheter will be arrested at the site of injury.

X-ray findings

Fracture of the pelvis may be shown on a plain X-ray film. Radiopaque fluid (20–30 ml) should be instilled into the catheter past the point of arrest. An X-ray will show the site of extravasation. If the catheter passes to the bladder a cystogram should be taken to determine whether there is any vesical injury.

Complications

Haemorrhage about the prostate and bladder may be marked in the early stages. Urinary extravasation may occur if the patient is unable to urinate. This may lead to severe sepsis if the diagnosis is late. Urethral stricture is a common late complication, particularly if proper treatment is not instituted early. Sexual impotence—loss of erection—may develop in one-third of men, probably as a result of nerve injury. Impaired control of urination occasionally results. This may be due to direct injury to the external sphincter, or may be secondary to nerve damage.

Treatment

Emergency measures

Resuscitation with blood and fluids and analgesia.

Specific measures

If a urethral catheter of adequate size can be successfully passed to the bladder it should be left in place for 12–21 days. Simple lacerations usually heal well with only this simple splinting. If a catheter cannot be passed into the bladder, surgical intervention is imperative. The principles of treatment include the following:

1. Suture the injured urethra if possible, and then place a splinting urethral catheter in the bladder. The catheter should be left in place for 3 weeks.
2. If repair by suture cannot be done, an indwelling catheter of the self-retaining type should be placed under direct vision. One pound of traction on the external end of the catheter will bring into apposition the ruptured ends of the urethra. The catheter should be left in place for 3 weeks. Drains should be placed down to the site of injury and left in place for 7–10 days.

General measures

If treatment has been instituted late and sepsis is already present, broad-spectrum antibiotics should be used as a life-saving measure, as well as to minimize fibrous reaction. Analgesics and sedation should be used as indicated.

Treatment of complications

It must be assumed that all patients suffering from deep urethral injuries will develop strictures. It is therefore necessary to get urethrograms, or pass urethral sounds periodically, for as long as 6–12 months, in order to discover the development of a stricture. If stricture does occur definitive treatment is required. There is no treatment that will correct loss of erection. Little can be done for patients with impaired sphincteric function.

Prognosis

Unless other serious injuries have been sustained the mortality rate for injury to the membranous urethra is quite low. This is true even though perivesical infection has developed because of delayed treatment. Antibiotics are usually successful in combating this. The most troublesome complication is urethral stricture which may require the periodic passage of sounds for the rest of the patient's life. Surgical correction of the stricture may be necessary. If this is not done, chronic infection of the bladder and even of the kidneys may develop, and vesical and renal stones may form because of stasis.

RETENTION OF URINE

Retention of urine is either acute or chronic, the latter leading ultimately to retention with overflow. The general features of obstruction of the urinary tract, and in particular of the bladder, have been dealt with earlier on, but retention of urine is such a common complaint that more specific details are required here.

Acute retention

Retention is often acute-on-chronic, for, except in postoperative and traumatic cases, it seldom occurs without warning.

Aetiology

The most frequent causes are in the male prostatic enlargement, urethral stricture, or postoperative retention; in the female retroverted gravid uterus, disseminated sclerosis, hysteria; in the male child meatal ulcer with scabbing. Other causes include postspinal anaesthesia, blood clot in the bladder, rupture of the urethra, neurogenic (injury or disease to the spinal cord), faecal impaction in the rectum, acute urethritis or prostatitis, urethral stone, phimosis, certain drugs and muscular atony from advanced age.

Clinical features

The patient has usually not passed urine for some hours, and is unable to do so. The swelling caused by a full bladder can often be seen in a thin person. There is tenderness to palpation and dullness to percussion above the symphysis pubis. Spasms of acute pain occur periodically as the muscle of the bladder contracts. An attempt to elicit the cause of the retention should be made. This is most frequently due to vascular engorgement of an already enlarged prostate in the male.

Early management of acute retention

It is of paramount importance never to relieve or attempt to relieve acute retention and forthwith send the patient home. He or she must always be confined to bed immediately and kept there for at least 24 h after relief has been obtained. Blood urea and serum creatinine should be estimated once the patient is in suitable surroundings. The effect of administering a dose of omnopon to relieve the anxiety and a hot bath to diminish internal congestion can be tried. In some cases the patient will be able to pass urine into the bath. If this fails, catheterization is attempted. This should always be performed with a full aseptic ritual. If the blood urea level is raised the catheter will have to be left indwelling for several days. A small presterilized Foley catheter, 12/14 French gauge, is introduced after the urethra has been dilated by injecting a local anaesthetic jelly. Provided this is done with gentleness and sensitivity the catheter will most often pass beyond the large prostate, and allow relief of the obstruction. If after a reasonable attempt with catheters the bladder has not been entered, one of four options may be adopted according to circumstances:

1. Suprapubic puncture.
2. Suprapubic catheterization.
3. Immediate prostatectomy.
4. Urethral dilatation.

Chronic retention

In such cases the distension of the bladder is painless. Blood urea and creatinine are often very high, and when this is the case the relief of the obstruction must be by slow decompression.

Retention with overflow

In this condition the patient has no control of the urine: small amounts are passed involuntarily from time to time, overflowing from the bladder which is distended to its maximum capacity. It may follow a neglected acute retention or chronic retention. Retention with overflow is referred to also under incontinence, and prostatic enlargement.

Postoperative retention of urine

Retention of urine may be encountered after any surgical operation. It is more common in young people, and after operations on the anal canal and in the perineal region, and is due to reflex spasm of the urinary sphincters. After operations on pelvic viscera retention of urine is so common that it is usual to forestall it by inserting a catheter before or at the conclusion of the operation. When the patient is an elderly male, latent prostatic obstruction should be suspected. Many patients cannot urinate while lying or sitting in bed. Another extremely common cause is sedation; when a sufficient quantity of an analgesic to relieve pain is administered frequently the desire to micturate is suppressed until the sympathetic nerve fibres are stimulated from over-distension of the bladder.

Treatment

If a male patient is permitted to sit on the edge of the bed he is often able to empty his bladder. The sound of running water is often helpful. Parasympathomimetic drugs, such as carbachol, may be prescribed, but they should be avoided after operations on the gastrointestinal tract. If after a reasonable trial the patient cannot pass urine he or she must be catheterized.

Acute retention due to drugs other than sedatives

A number of drugs are prone to induce or precipitate retention of urine. Propantheline bromide, antihistamines, antihypertensives and anticholinergic drugs have all been responsible for producing acute retention of urine.

Retention of urine due to a lesion of the spinal cord

When the nervous control of the bladder is disrupted because of a complete or incomplete lesion of the spinal cord, the bladder passes through various stages of dysfunction.

Atonic neurogenic bladder

Immediately following the injury the detrusor muscles become paralysed, the sphincter vesicae is tightly contracted, and the sphincter urethrae is relaxed. The only factor permitting any evacuation of the bladder is the elasticity of its walls. In lesions situated above S2 to below T4–T6, because the sympathetic innervation of the bladder is intact, the patient can appreciate that the bladder becomes filled to capacity. If allowed to do so the bladder becomes greatly distended and paralytic overflow incontinence ensues. This phase, due to spinal shock, lasts for days, weeks or even months. As recovery from spinal shock takes place, depending on the level of the lesion, automaticity or autonomy of bladder function occurs but, before it does so, it passes through two intermediate phases:

1. The phase of ineffectual emptying contractions, when contractions of the detrusor muscle occur but, because the sphincter remains in spasm, only small quantities of urine are voided frequently. This phase is usually only of a few hours' duration.
2. The phase of hypertonicity—the detrusor passes into spasm, the sphincter vesicae relaxes physiologically and the sphincter urethrae reflexly contracts.

The autonomic reflex bladder

When the lesion is situated above the centre of micturition, the bladder empties reflexly every 1–4 h; the amount of residual urine varies from patient to patient. When the filling reaches a certain point the detrusor muscle contracts reflexly, a condition similar to that seen in early infancy.

The autonomous bladder

This results when a lesion is situated at a level that will destroy the centre for micturition, or in a lesion of the cauda equina. Emptying of the bladder is dependent upon the precarious and inefficient control by the nerve plexus situated between the muscular strata of the bladder wall. Continual dribbling is the outcome, but the bladder can be emptied by manual compression. Residual urine, however, is never absent, and dilatation of the ureters, and eventually the renal pelvis and calices, results.

Treatment

During the period of atonicity the treatment is aseptic catheterization with a silastic self-retaining catheter. A high fluid intake is advised during this period to maintain high urine flow and minimize the risk of infection. Antibiotics are usually withheld in case infection supervenes.

The state of automaticity is heralded by the return of bulbocavernous reflex erections and anal reflexes and, if the catheter tubing becomes blocked, urine will be passed alongside the catheter. With the return of detrusor activity bladder training is commenced. At first the catheter is clipped off and released at regular, but lengthening, intervals. Later the catheter is removed and reflexes are initiated by the patient lifting him or herself in the chair or bed, again at regular intervals by the clock. Drinks are given during the day but none after 7 p.m.

When the autonomic reflex state is reached, manual expression of urine by the patient, if he or she has the use of the arms, plus contracture of the abdominal muscles, if they are not paralysed, is the only but often tolerably successful method of avoiding lifelong urethral or suprapubic catheter drainage.

INCONTINENCE OF URINE

The patient is either unaware that urine is passing, or is aware of it but unable to prevent leakage of urine from the urethra. The history is most important and in many cases will indicate the cause.

Enuresis

This is incontinence of urine due to involuntary acts of micturition in children without detectable neurological or urological disease. Usually the condition presents as failure to acquire normal control, but in about 15% of cases it may commence after control has been acquired. In such instances there is usually an illness or psychological factor which accounts for the condition. In both, the underlying state is a persistence of the infantile pattern of bladder activity, sudden forceful contraction and emptying in response to a certain distension, and impairment of the sensory awareness of the bladder content with lack of inhibitory control from higher centres. Nocturnal enuresis is much more frequent than diurnal. The diagnosis may be made confidently if the history is typical. There is no dribbling between the acts, no abnormality on clinical examination, and the urine is completely normal.

Treatment

Drugs to inhibit bladder irritability, e.g. belladonna, and to strengthen the action of the sphincter, e.g. ephedrine, may help. Diurnal enuretics should be encouraged to pass urine by the clock, and gradually lengthen the duration between acts. At night the child should be wakened regularly. In cases of onset enuresis after a dry period, the social and sociological aspects of the family must be investigated by the paediatrician. Older children may respond to an alarm which is activated by urine passing on to a pad.

Stress incontinence

The leaking of urine on coughing, sneezing, or lifting heavy weights is due to weakness of the urinary sphincters, and is common in women after childbirth. It may also follow operations on the bladder neck or the prostate to relieve obstruction.

Operative treatment

In patients with considerable bulging of the anterior vaginal wall (cystocele) anterior colporrhaphy frequently improves continence. In the absence of any cystocele an operation to rectify the sagging of the bladder neck can be undertaken in cases where there is little or no improvement after a course of exercises.

Total incontinence

In this condition there is complete loss of control. Urine dribbles away all the time and the bladder is usually empty. Excluding all fistulae, the causes of this condition are:

1. Congenital—severe epispadias.
2. Traumatic—damage to the pelvic muscles and nerves postprostatectomy.

3. Infective—acute exfoliative membranous cystitis as in chemical irrigation and chronic tuberculosis.
4. Neoplastic—fixation of sphincters, carcinoma of the prostate, carcinoma of the cervix.
5. Neurological—meningomyeloceles, multiple sclerosis (usually retention and overflow).

Management of incontinence

The aims are to keep the patient dry, free of odour, to lessen the incidence of skin excoriation, and to protect the kidneys from the effects of infection and back-pressure. Appliances in women are usually unsatisfactory, although a new range of implantable sphincters is becoming available. An indwelling catheter drained constantly into a leg urinal is usually a satisfactory solution, although in some instances diversion via an ileal conduit is necessary. In men a condom urinal or a Cunningham penile clamp may be satisfactory, and they avoid an indwelling catheter. Regular pyelographic checks to confirm the absence of retention and back-pressure effects are essential.

Some of the conditions listed above may be amenable to specific surgical treatment, e.g. a gracilis muscle sling may be attempted for epispadias, or a postprostatectomy incontinence, or the bulbocavernosus muscle may be pleated with non-absorbable sutures. Severe contraction of the bladder, if the sphincters are normal, can be helped by cystoplasty, using ileum to enlarge it (see Fig. 40.5). When incontinence is caused by neurological disease it is usually necessary to divert the urine into an ileal loop, if there is evidence of increasing dilatation of the upper tract, particularly in the presence of recurrent infection. The bladder does not need to be removed, but it should be washed out after the operation with 1g neomycin. It should be washed out two or three times in the post-operative period. After this it rarely produces symptoms.

Diverticulum of the bladder

A diverticulum of the bladder must be distinguished from a saccule. Normal intravesical pressure at the commencement of micturition is about 35 cm of water. Pressures as great as 100 cm are reached by a hypertrophied trabeculated bladder endeavouring to force urine past an obstruction. This pressure causes the mucous lining between the inner layer of hypertrophied muscle bundles to protrude, so forming multiple saccules (Fig. 40.2). If one or more—usually only one saccule—is forced through the whole thickness of musculature of the bladder wall it becomes a diverticulum.

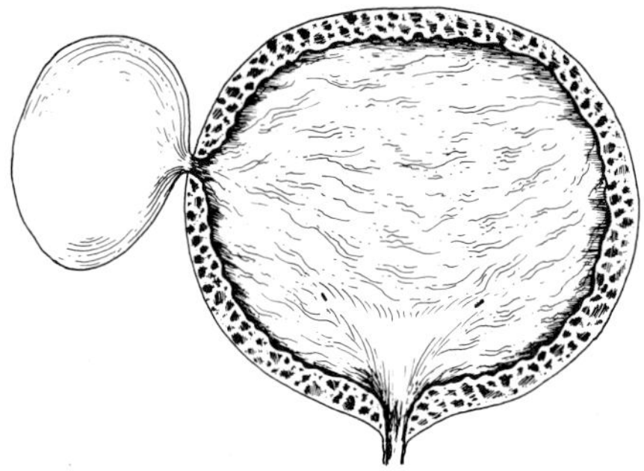

Fig. 40.2 Diverticulum of the bladder. An outpouching of mucosa through a thinned, stretched portion of the muscle wall, resulting from increased pressure within the bladder.

Aetiology

Congenital diverticulum is rare and unimportant. It is situated in the midline anterosuperiorly and represents the unobliterated vesical end of the urachus. The vast majority are pulsion diverticula, caused by obstruction of the bladder neck, benign enlargement of the prostate, fibrous prostate, urethral stricture or congenital valves of the posterior urethra.

Pathology

Usually the mouth of the diverticulum is situated above and to the outer side of one ureteric orifice. Exceptionally it is near the middle line behind the interureteric ridge. The size varies from 2 to 5 cm but may be larger. It is lined by bladder mucosa and the wall is composed of fibrous tissue only. A diverticulum enlarges in a downward direction and sometimes may obstruct the ureter.

Complications

The main ones are recurrent cystitis, vesical calculus, hydronephrosis and hydroureter and neoplasm.

Clinical features

An uninfected diverticulum of the bladder may cause no symptoms whatsoever. The patient is nearly always male and usually over 50 years of age. There are no pathognomonic symptoms of vesical diverticulum other than those of lower urinary tract obstruction, recurrent cystitis and pyelonephritis. Haematuria due to cystitis, vesical calculus or rarely a neoplasm may also occur. In a few cases micturition occurs twice in rapid succession, the second act possibly following a change of posture. When the first specimen is clear but the second cloudy, diverticulum of the bladder should be strongly suspected. In cases of chronic retention of urine two swellings may be recognized rising out of the pelvis, one being the bladder, the other the diverticulum.

Cystoscopy is the usual means of discovering a diverticulum. Most often its orifice is seen as a clear-cut hole about 1 cm in diameter, the depths of which are black and unilluminated. It is sometimes possible to pass the endoscope into a diverticulum and examine its interior. Excretory urography will not only outline the diverticulum but also exclude or reveal implication of the upper urinary tract. A vesical diverticulum usually increases in size, and once infected the infection cannot be permanently eradicated. Therefore, unless the pouch is small and uninfected it should be removed, usually when the associated lower urinary tract obstruction is treated.

Traction diverticulum of the bladder (hernia of the bladder)

A portion of the bladder protruding through the inguinal or femoral hernia orifice occurs in 1.5% of such herniae treated. The condition is relatively frequent in femoral and direct inguinal herniae. The disposition of the diverticulum in the hernia varies and in order of frequency is intraperitoneal, paraperitoneal and extraperitoneal.

Clinical features

In a few cases, in order to empty the bladder completely the patient finds it necessary to exert pressure on the hernia. Suspicion of a bladder hernia can be confirmed by cystoscopy or cystography.

URINARY FISTULAE

A urinary fistula is an abnormal communication between any part of the urinary system and the skin or some internal hollow viscus. The persistence of a fistula on the skin implies the presence of distal obstruction or the presence of chronic infection such as tuberculosis or a foreign body, for example a stone or a non-absorbable ligature.

Congenital urinary fistula

1. Ectopia vesicae, mentioned above.
2. Patent urachus (see above).
3. In association with imperforate anus.

Traumatic urinary fistula

These may be due to a perforating or penetrating wound, damage not recognized during surgery, or poor handling and avascular necrosis following a combination of radiotherapy and surgery. Clot retention occurring after transvesical prostatectomy or diverticulectomy may lead to a dehiscence of the bladder wound and a temporary fistula which will heal quickly provided the bladder is kept empty with an indwelling catheter.

Vesicovaginal fistula

Vesicovaginal fistula is possibly the greatest misfortune that can happen to a woman, more so because she is often condemned to live with it and cannot hope to die from it.

Aetiology

1. Obstetric causes: from time immemorial the usual cause has been protracted or neglected labour.
2. Gynaecological causes: the operations chiefly concerned with this complication are total hysterectomy and anterior colporrhaphy.
3. Radiotherapeutic causes: the commonest cause is radium treatment for carcinoma of the cervix uteri and, less frequently, irradiation of the pelvic viscera for other reasons.
4. Direct neoplastic infiltration may occur, especially by carcinoma of the cervix uteri, ulcerat-

ing through the anterior fornix to implicate the bladder, and carcinoma of the colon or rectum infiltrating the bladder and the vagina.

When a wound of the bladder is recognized and repaired at once leakage is uncommon, but escape of urine will quickly follow if such damage is passed unnoticed. However, most vesicovaginal fistulae are the result of ischaemic necrosis of the bladder wall due to prolonged pressure of the fetal head in obstetric cases. In gynaecological causes the ischaemia is brought about by grasping the bladder wall in a haemostat, including the bladder wall in a suture, or perhaps even by local oedema or haematoma. Leakage due to necrosis of tissue seldom manifests itself before 7 days after the operation. An intractable fistula following radium treatment of carcinoma of the cervix uteri may arise from avascular necrosis years after the apparent cure of the original lesion.

Clinical features

There is leakage of urine from the vagina, and as a consequence excoriation of the vulva. Digital examination of the vagina reveals a localized thickening on its anterior wall. On inserting a bivalve speculum urine will be seen escaping from an opening in the anterior vaginal wall, and it is usually possible to pass a bent probe from the vagina into the bladder. Cystoscopy is often difficult owing to the contraction of the bladder from the cystitis, and the escape of urine from the fistula. However, usually the tip of the probe which has been passed can be seen emerging through an area of granulation tissue. Differential diagnosis between ureterovaginal fistula and vesicovaginal fistula can be made if a swab is placed in the vagina and a solution of methylene blue is injected through the urethra. The vaginal swab becomes coloured blue if the fistula is in the bladder, but in the case of a ureterovaginal fistula the vaginal swab is not so coloured. Ureterovaginal fistula is discussed above.

Treatment

Operations must be postponed until 4–6 months after the development of the fistula, so as to enable viable tissue in the neighbourhood to recover fully and for scar tissue to consolidate. The fistula is exposed via the vagina, the edges are freshened and a longitudinal repair used to traverse the bladder wall (but not the mucosa) and the whole thickness of the vagina. Parallel vaginal incisions may be used to relieve tension on the suture line. The bladder is drained with a fine Foley catheter for 14 days unless the urethra is primarily affected, in which event a suprapubic cystostomy is performed.

Fistulae from the renal pelvis to the skin and gut

Tuberculosis of the kidney may result in destruction of the kidney by caseation and chronic sinus leading to the duodenum or colon and/or the skin, usually in the iliac fossa or in the lumbar triangle. Similarly, pyonephrosis and stone may spontaneously discharge into the gut or by fistula to the skin. Cases of duodenal ulcer penetrating the pelvis of the right kidney are also on record.

Vesicocolic fistula

The commonest cause is diverticulitis of the colon. It may also follow Crohn's disease, appendix abscess or pelvic sepsis in association with acute salpingitis, or as a result of surgery and radiotherapy within the pelvis. The onset may not be dramatic and may well be treated as acute cystitis. The diagnosis can be difficult to make because the acute signs subside, but on cystoscopy a patch of oedema on the left side of the vault is suggestive, and a cystogram may reveal the fistula. However, as the track is not always patent a negative result may be obtained. The passage of gas per urethram in a patient who has cystitis is most suggestive.

Treatment

A defunctioning colostomy is made proximal to the fistula as the first step, and the inflammation is allowed to subside over 2-3 months. At laparotomy the communication is separated, the hole in the bladder being closed and patched with omentum, and the segment of diseased bowel resected. The bladder is drained by urethral catheter. The colostomy is usually closed after about 3 weeks, provided a barium enema reveals no leaks.

Malignant vesical fistula

By the time a fistula between the bowel and the bladder has developed, as a rule the growth is inoperable, or requires pelvic evisceration for its attempted eradication. As so often these patients are unfit for this major procedure it is best to leave the patient with a defunctioning colostomy performed in the first instance. Exceptions do occur and occasionally it is warranted to undertake segmental resection of the colon and partial or complete cystectomy.

Neoplastic fistulae

Primary bladder tumours may fungate through the abdominal wall when neglected. Only palliative treatment is possible in most of such cases. Involvement of the bladder by growths of cervix, uterus, colon and rectum do produce fistulae, as may lymphosarcoma of the small gut. Carcinoma of the prostate rarely produces a rectal fistula. Treatment in most cases is difficult and prolonged, and in most only palliative relief can be given. It is rarely in the patient's interest to divert the ureters.

Tubercular cystitis

This is always secondary to renal tuberculosis, and unless treated early is a particularly relentless form of chronic cystitis. Cystoscopy shows that early tuberculosis of the bladder commences around one ureteric orifice, or in the neighbourhood of the trigone, the earliest evidence being pallor of the mucosa due to submucosal oedema. Subsequently tubercles may be seen, and in long-standing cases there is much fibrosis and the capacity of the bladder is so much reduced that it has earned the name 'thimble bladder'.

Treatment

This usually responds rapidly to antituberculous drugs, but occasionally in cases of advanced renal changes it may not subside until the involved kidney and ureter have been removed. When the bladder is considerably contracted but free from ulceration, remarkable relief from the distressing frequency can be achieved by ileo- or caecocystoplasty, an extremely efficacious method of increasing the capacity of a contracted bladder (Fig. 40.3).

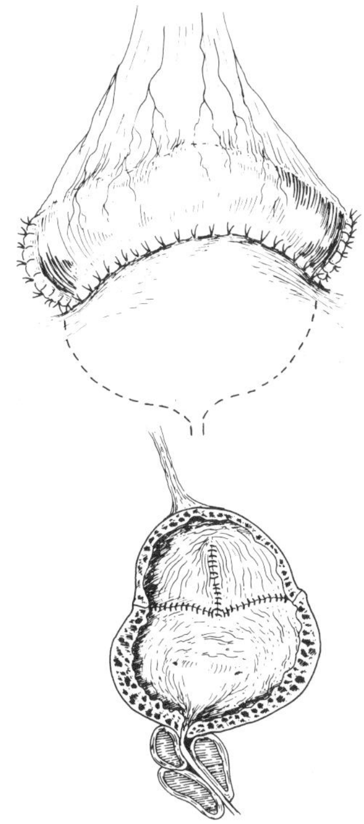

Fig. 40.3 Ileocystoplasty. The capacity of the bladder, reduced by either disease or after deliberate excision, can be greatly increased by isolating a segment of ileum, closing this at both ends, opening it up along its antemesenteric border, and finally anastomosing this 'pouch' to the opened-out dome of the shrunken bladder.

Interstitial cystitis (synonym: 'Hunner's ulcer')

For practical purposes Hunner's ulcer can be said to be a condition peculiar to women. The symptoms commence in the early 40s and can cause more pain, mental anguish and associated neurosis than does carcinoma of the bladder. As a consequence the incessant painful micturition it occasions sometimes leads to drug addiction and even suicide. The aetiology is still obscure, as it was when Guy Hunner described it in 1914. Certainly it does not commence as an ordinary pyogenic infection of the mucous membrane but rather as an infection of the paravesical tissues secondary, it is suggested, to infection of the adnexa, or even to infection of a more distant focus such as the nasopharynx. Some believe that the condition is due to attenuated

Mycobacterium tuberculosis which so far has defied isolation.

Pathology

As a result of the paracystitis, fibrosis of the vesical musculature ensues, leading to contracture of the bladder and areas of avascular atrophy of the mucous membrane. Finally ulceration of the mucosa occurs in the least vascular portion of the bladder, namely the fundus. Often the capacity of the bladder is reduced to 30–60 ml. The characteristic linear bleeding ulcer is a crack due to splitting of the mucous membrane when the bladder is distended under anaesthesia for cystoscopy. Microscopically inflammation of all coats of the bladder is present, with granulation tissue in the submucosa underlying the ulcer. The muscularis is hypertrophied, and the peritoneum in the proximity of the area of maximum disease is thickened.

Clinical features

A large reduction in bladder capacity and increased frequency, eventually every hour, day and night, is the leading symptom. Pain, relieved by micturition, and aggravated by jarring and by overdistension of the bladder, is the second most characteristic symptom. In early cases the urine is crystal-clear and sterile; in later cases it contains ordinary pyogenic bacteria in under half of the specimens examined. In the remainder the urine remains sterile. In 60% of cases haematuria is also present. Treatment is difficult and unsatisfactory. Local hydrocortisone and irrigation of the bladder with various sedatives, including warm water, have proved valuable. Hydrostatic dilatation under light anaesthesia may give relief for some months. Light diathermy of the ulcer may also help. Corticosteroids cause an increase in bladder capacity and often afford complete or partial relief from pain. If corticosteroids fail to afford any relief subtotal cystectomy and enlargement of the bladder by adding a patch of colon, caecum or ileum should be considered.

BILHARZIASIS OF THE BLADDER
(synonym schistosomiasis; see Ch. 15)

Pathogenesis and pathology

The eggs with their terminal spines penetrate the wall of the vein with the assistance of muscular contraction. This allows the eggs to be extruded into the vesical cavity. Healing is by scar formation and the bladder gradually becomes thickened and contracted. The appearance of calcification of the bladder wall is caused by calcium deposition in the shells of the ova. The intramural portions of the ureters may become stenosed with consequent hydronephrosis. With the advent of secondary infection pericystitis may occur. Ulceration and papilloma formation develop on the vesical mucosa, and the major lesion is usually in the trigonal area. Mucosal congestion and oedema is at first the only finding, but as the eggs approach the mucosa tubercles are noted, which are quite similar to the lesions of tuberculosis. The small yellow nodule represents the egg and the specific cellular reaction around it. The egg is surrounded by a zone of hyperaemia. Larger nodular polypoid masses develop later and then break down and ulcerate. At this stage the eggs are easily found in the urine. In the later stages fibrosis may be extreme. The incidence of bulky, squamous cell carcinomas in patients suffering from schistosomiasis is very high.

Microscopic examination of the bladder wall reveals many eggs surrounded by neutrophils, eosinophils and foreign body giant cells. Calcified eggs are seen in the submucosa and in the muscle layer. Later fibroblastic proliferation dominates the picture.

Clinical findings

Symptoms

Intense itching may be present when the parasites are invading the skin. Generalized symptoms develop in about 1–3 months, when the adult flukes begin to lay eggs. The patient may develop backache, headache, chills, fever and profuse sweats. Symptoms of cystitis appear when the bladder wall becomes involved, and terminal haematuria is common. If untreated the bladder symptoms gradually increase in severity as ulcerations develop and these symptoms may be extreme. Secondary infection exacerbates the symptoms. Calcific incrustation and even stones may form, and markedly contracted bladders are sometimes seen. Renal pain may be experienced as ureteric stenosis or reflux leads to hydronephrosis. Death may occur as a result of uraemia or general sepsis.

Signs

In the early stages the physical examination is not helpful. Later urethral stricture and perineal fistulae may be found. A mass in the flank may be discovered if hydronephrosis is present. Rectal examination may reveal fibrosis of the prostate and the base of the bladder.

Laboratory findings

During the egg-laying stage leukocytosis is present, and eosinophils often outnumber neutrophils. Anaemia may be due to blood destruction by the flukes, or may be secondary to non-specific infection or uraemia. The urine contains pus, red blood cells and the eggs of *Schistosoma haematobium*. These findings establish the diagnosis. Non-specific pyogenic organisms may also be found. Renal function may be impaired in the presence of ureteric stenosis and vesicoureteric reflux.

X-ray findings

Calcification of the bladder wall or the lower ureter may be demonstrated on a plain film of the abdomen. Excretory urography may show hydroureters and hydronephrosis due to vesicoureteric reflux. Cystograms may demonstrate a contracted bladder, vesical tumour or reflux. Instrumental examination reveals urethral strictures. Cystoscopy may show varying stages of tubercle formation, nodulation with tubercle formation, widespread ulceration, papillomatous reaction, carcinoma, vesical stones or calcium deposits. Biopsy of the lesions will demonstrate the eggs.

Differential diagnosis

Non-specific cystitis may be differentiated from schistosomiasis in the early stages since, although no bacteria will be found on stain smear, eggs will probably be discovered. Non-specific cystitis will ordinarily respond to antibiotics; schistosomiasis will not. Tuberculous cystitis may be confused with schistosomiasis since the history in both may be the same. Neither responds to the usual antibiotics, and superficially at least the cystoscopic appearance may be similar.

Complications

The main complication is fibrosis of the bladder with contracture, leading to bladder neck obstruction, perineal and suprapubic fistulae, vesical calculus formation, squamous cell carcinoma of the bladder, secondary ureteric obstruction, and uraemia.

Treatment

Treatment is quite satisfactory if the diagnosis is made before complications develop.

Specific measures

See Chapter 15.

General measures

Secondary infection can be combated with antibiotics, and supportive treatment may be indicated,such as blood transfusion for anaemia.

Treatment of complications

If vesical fibrosis is of such a degree that urinary frequency is a problem, colocystoplasty or ileocystoplasty is indicated. Urethral fistulae or strictures will require plastic repair, and vesicoureteric obstruction or reflux may raise the question of ureterovesical reimplantation.

Control

Sanitary measures can do a great deal to reduce the incidence of schistosomiasis in endemic areas. Attempts at control have been made by draining ponds and canals, thus decreasing the population of freshwater snails. Little, however, has been accomplished. Chemicals may be added to water to minimize snail infestation. Intensive chemotherapy of infected persons has so far failed to decrease the incidence of the disease.

Prognosis

If the diagnosis is made early, at the time of initial vesical symptoms, medical treatment is almost always curative. Reinfection may occur in endemic areas. In the latter stages of the disease (fibrosis, secondary infection) the prognosis is only fair. Specific therapy, even if it eradicates the fluke and kills the eggs, cannot reverse the disabling secondary changes. In many epidemic areas schistosomiasis ranks high on the list of fatal diseases.

FILARIASIS

Filariasis is endemic in the countries bordering the Mediterranean, in South China and Japan, the West Indies and the South Pacific islands including Samoa. Limited infection, as has been seen in American soldiers during World War II, gives an entirely different clinical picture from the frequent reinfections usually encountered amongst the native population.

Aetiology

Wuchereria bancrofti is a threadlike nematode about 0.5 cm or more in length, which lives in the human lymphatics. The female in the lymphatics gives off microfilariae which are found particularly at night in the peripheral blood. The intermediate host, usually a mosquito, bites an infected person and becomes infested with the microfilariae which develop into larvae. These are in turn transferred to another human being in whom they reach maturity. Mating occurs, and microfilariae are again reproduced.

Pathogenesis and pathology

The adult nematode in the human host invades and obstructs the lymphatics. This leads to lymphangitis and lymphadenitis. In long-standing cases the lymphatic vessels become thickened and fibrous, and there is marked reticuloendothelial reaction.

Clinical findings

Symptoms

In mild cases the patient suffers from recurrent lymphadenitis and lymphangitis with fever and malaise. Not infrequently inflammation of the epidydimis, the testes and the scrotum and the spermatic cord occurs. These structures then become oedematous, boggy and at times very tender. Hydrocele is very common. In advanced cases obstruction of the major lymphatic channels may cause chyluria and elephantiasis.

Signs

Varying degrees of painless elephantiasis of the scrotum and the extremities develop as obstruction of the lymphatics progresses.

Laboratory findings

Chylous urine may look normal if minimal amounts of fat are present, but in an advanced case or following a fatty meal it is milky. In the presence of chyluria large amounts of protein are to be expected. Hypoproteinaemia is found, and the albumen:globulin ratio is reversed. Both white and red cells are found in the urine. Marked eosinophilia is the rule in the early stages and microfilariae may be demonstrated in the blood, which should preferably be drawn at night. The adult worm may be found by biopsy.

Treatment

Specific measures

Diethylcarbamazine is the drug of choice. The dose is 3 mg/kg orally three times a day for 21 days.

ECHINOCOCCOSIS (HYDATID DISEASE; see Ch.16)

Involvement of the urogenital organs by hydatid disease is relatively rare in Europe. It is common in Australia, New Zealand, South America, Africa and Asia.

Clinical findings

If renal hydatid disease is closed, i.e. not communicating with the pelvis, there may be no symptoms until a mass is found. If communicating, there may be symptoms of cystitis and renal colic as the cysts are passed from the kidney into the bladder. Eosinophilia is the rule. X-ray films may show calcification of the wall of the cyst, and urograms often reveal changes typical of space-occupying lesions. The finding of scolices and hooklets in the urine is pathognomonic. A positive skin sensitivity test (Casoni) is suggestive, and complement fixation tests are positive in 90% of cases. Retroperitoneal (perivesical cysts) may cause symptoms of cystitis, or acute urinary retention may develop secondary to pressure. The presence of a suprapubic mass may be the only finding. It may rupture into the bladder and cause hydatiduria which establishes the diagnosis.

Treatment

Nephrectomy is generally the treatment of choice of renal hydatid disease, although aspiration and marsupialization have also been recommended. Retroperitoneal cysts are best treated by marsupialization and curettage. Echinococcosis of the kidney usually has a good prognosis. The problem presented by perivesical cysts is more troublesome. After surgical intervention drainage may be prolonged, and it must be remembered too that involvement of other organs, especially the liver, is usually present.

NEOPLASMS OF THE BLADDER

More than 95% of primary tumours of the bladder originate in the mucous membrane. The remainder are connective tissue growths, e.g. angiomas, and less commonly, myoma, fibroma and sarcoma. These are too rare to merit further description, as also is phaeochromocytoma arising in the bladder wall from accessory adrenal tissue. Another common benign bladder tumour is endometrioma characterized by localized smooth vascular projections on the bladder wall, sometimes containing chocolate-coloured cysts, at other times translucent cysts of bluish hue. The tumour enlarges and bleeds during menstruation, and the treatment is partial cystectomy. Secondary involvement of the bladder can occur from extension of malignant neoplasms of a neighbouring organ, particularly the sigmoid, colon and rectum, uterus or ovary. On rare occasions the first symptoms of carcinoma of the pelvic colon are those of cystitis. Cystoscopy reveals a circumscribed area of intense inflammation, usually on the left side of the fundus.

Aetiology

The first suspicion of a chemical cause for bladder tumours was raised by Rehn in 1894, when he recorded a series of tumours in workers in aniline dye factories. Subsequent investigation has exonerated aniline itself for the carcinogenic agent was the impurity beta-naphthylamine. It is now recognized that benzedine, alpha-naphthylamine, xylenamine, auramine and magenta are all carcinogens. The particular occupations involved are in the dyeing, rubber and printing industries, and gas workers. Bilharzia, active or inactive, and bladder cancer are commonly found together; probably the former produces chronic irritation and incomplete emptying, which in turn produces metaplasia and squamous carcinoma.

Leukoplakia of the bladder must also be regarded as a precancerous condition. Despite these facts, in the majority of cases the cause of bladder cancer is not determined.

Pathogenesis and pathology

Tumours of the transitional cell mucosa of the bladder are the second most common of all genito-urinary neoplasms; only prostatic tumours occur more frequently. In all 75% are found in men, and most are seen after the age of 50. Papillomatous growths submit readily to transurethral treatment if diagnosed early. Infiltrating transitional cell types constitute one of the most difficult of all urological problems. It is customary to judge it in two ways—the degree of differentiation of the cells, and the depth of penetration of the tumour into the vesical wall.

The grade and stage of the tumour

Grade—the degree of cell differentiation. Grade I tumours are quite well differentiated, and the lamina propria is usually not involved. Most are relatively small, papillary in type, and have a narrow base. These are curable by transurethral means but are radioresistant.

Grade II tumours are papillary in type, show less differentiation of their cells, and are apt to invade the lamina propria, if not the detrusor muscle itself. They tend to be larger than grade I tumours and have a wider connection with the bladder wall. They are often curable by transurethral resection. They do not respond well to radiotherapy.

Grade III and IV neoplasms are poorly differentiated, even anaplastic. They tend to be nodular rather than papillary, and as a rule are quite invasive. They respond poorly to transurethral removal, as well as to cystectomy, but are usually sensitive to radiotherapy.

Stage—the degree of invasion. Stage 0 represents a papillary tumour which has not invaded the lamina propria. Stage A tumours have invaded the lamina propria but not the muscle of the vesical wall. Stage B1 tumours have extended into the superficial half of the detrusor muscle, and stage B2 tumours are found deep in the muscle layers. Stage C tumours have extended into the perivesical fat or have involved underlying peritoneum. Stage D tumours have demonstrable metastases, e.g. in the lymph nodes or the liver.

Type and location

Since 80% of vesical tumours arise on the base of the bladder they may involve one or both ureteric orifices or the vesical neck. Hydroureteronephrosis and pyelonephritis are common complications when the tumours ulcerate, and they bleed and often become infected. Most growths are papillary in type and are malignant. They may be single or multiple. Generalized papillomatosis is not uncommon. Generally speaking, the larger the tumour and the broader its base, the more malignant it is, and nodular tumours are more malignant than papillary types. After successful treatment of even grade I and II types that are superficial, there is a definite tendency for new tumours to develop elsewhere in the bladder. Indeed, the papillary tumour has been described as a florid manifestation of an unstable urothelium. This suggests that the appearance of these tumours is in some way related to a generally increased susceptibility of the mucosa to neoplastic proliferation, perhaps in response to carcinogens. This is true also of renal pelvic and ureteric transitional cell tumours. Vesical neoplasms most commonly metastasize to the vesical, hypogastric, common iliac and lumbar lymph nodes. The bones, liver and lungs are at times affected. Rarely other types of vesical neoplasm may be encountered.

Epidermoid carcinoma. About 5% of vesical neoplasms are of squamous cell variety. These are ordinarily highly malignant, anaplastic, deeply invasive and metastasize early. With very few exceptions they are incurable.

Adenocarcinoma is very rare and may arise in a urachal remnant.

Clinical findings

Symptoms

Gross haematuria is the commonest symptom. As with all tumours of the urinary tract, haematuria is usually intermittent, and often painless. If infection supervenes symptoms of cystitis will usually be present; these include a burning feeling on urination, urgency, frequency and nocturia. Symptoms of bladder neck obstruction may develop if the tumour encroaches on the internal orifice. These include hesitancy and decrease in the force and calibre of the urinary stream.

Signs

In most cases nothing abnormal can be found on physical examination. Renal tenderness or enlargement may be present due to ureteric obstruction and infection. A suprapubic mass may be noted on rare occasions but this is a sign of a large and advanced carcinoma. On rectal or vaginal examination a mass at the base of the bladder may be noted. Less often, rectal examination may reveal an invasive mass in the trigonal area. Bimanual palpation, whether abdominorectal or abdominovaginal, is of the greatest importance in feeling and estimating the size and extent of the growth, and this is best done under anaesthesia. Signs of metastases may be noted. These include palpable abdominal masses involving lymph nodes along the iliac vessels. On X-ray, excretory urograms are usually normal, but may show the tumour itself,

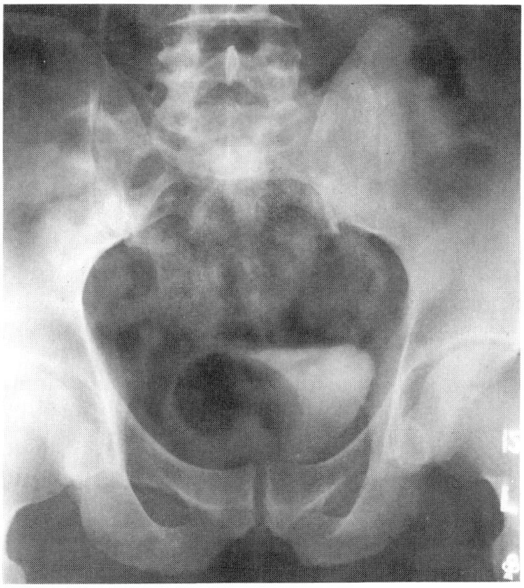

Fig. 40.4 Large rounded mass of carcinoma showing as a radiolucent area on intravenous urogram. While the left lower ureter is clearly visualized, the absence of the right one indicates blockage by the tumour.

evidence of ureteric obstruction or primary tumour of the renal pelvis or ureter as a cause of the primary vesical growth (Fig. 40.4).

Instrumental examination

Cystoscopy almost always reveals the tumour, and biopsy of the lesion should be routine. A few tumours may be missed by this, but these may be visualized if the patient is given tetracycline for a few days before cystoscopy using ultraviolet illumination, as tetracycline causes fluorescence of the tumour.

Cytology

Papanicolaou smear preparations, or preferably the simple methylene blue stain of fresh urinary sediment, will almost always reveal transitional cells shed from the tumour. Well differentiated tumours shed round cells of rather uniform size with large nuclei. When anaplastic tumours are present the urinary sediment always reveals large epithelial cells, often in clumps, with large dark-staining nuclei.

Complications

Secondary infection of the bladder is common when the tumour ulcerates, and this may be severe. Renal infection is not uncommon when ureteric obstruction ensues. Urinary retention may develop if the tumour invades the bladder neck. Hydronephrosis due to ureteric occlusion is common, and if bilateral, uraemia supervenes, and this is the most common cause of death.

Treatment

There is still considerable disagreement about the proper treatment of vesical neoplasm. Certain low-grade superficial tumours lend themselves well to transurethral resection. For the more malignant, invasive tumours the choice lies between radiotherapy and radical surgery, or a combination of the two.

Surgical measures

Most single or multiple papillomas are best treated by transurethral resection, care being taken to saucerize deeply into the wall of the bladder in order to remove the base of the tumour completely. This procedure will cure many of the papillary carcinomas of stage 0, A, B1, B2, grades I and II. However, if the tumour has invaded deeply into the vesical muscle—stage B2 and C—this method will usually fail.

Partial segmental cystectomy is feasible if the malignant tumour does not lie on the base of the bladder, for in this case one or both ureteric orifices may have to be sacrificed. Unfortunately, fewer than 20% of vesical tumours are restricted to areas far removed from the trigone. Total cystectomy is therefore the treatment of choice together with removal of the prostate in the male. It is the preferred procedure for the treatment of papillomatosis, and for many of the more undifferentiated invasive tumours.

Diversion of the urinary stream presents a problem. Ureterosigmoidostomy results in urinary continence, but frequently causes ureteric obstruction or reflux, with hydronephrosis and renal infection. Many of these patients will then die of renal insufficiency rather than of cancer. A few

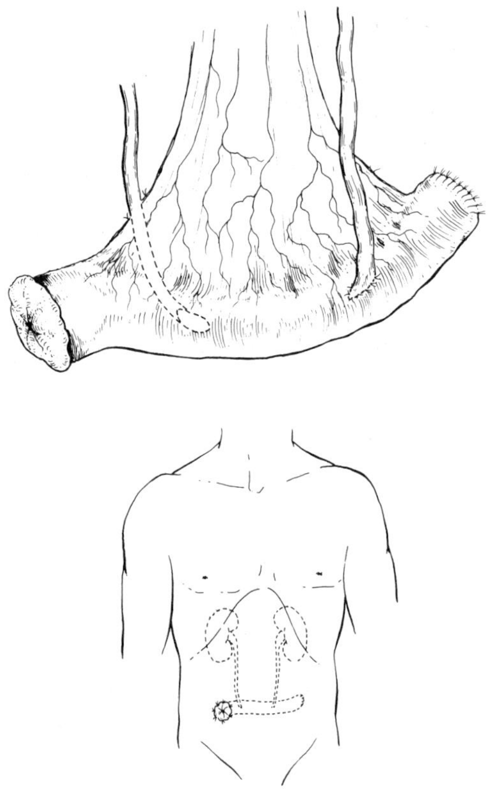

Fig. 40.5 Ileal conduit. After total cystectomy, the lower ends of the divided ureters are anastomosed to an isolated segment of the ileum, which is closed at its proximal end, and brought out to the surface of the anterior abdominal wall as a permanent stoma.

will develop symptoms of acidosis from absorption of hydrogen ions in the urine. Hyperchloraemia may also occur, and the administration of potassium citrate will be necessary to correct these electrolyte defects. The most popular method of urinary diversion today is anastomosis of the ureters to an isolated loop of ileum, or of sigmoid colon, with one end of the loop brought to the skin as a conduit (Fig 40.5). Renal complications and electrolyte problems are minimized in this circumstance.

Radiation therapy

In general, the more undifferentiated the tumour, the more radiosensitive it is. It is therefore most useful in grades III and IV, stage B2 and C lesions. There is mounting evidence that radiotherapy in this type of neoplasm gives at least as good if not better control than radical surgery.

Chemotherapy

Palliation of vesical neoplasms with parenteral anticancer drugs has been reported. With 5-fluorouracil, the effects are not dramatic. The instillation by catheter of 60 mg triethylene ethiophosphoramide (thiotepa) dissolved in 30–60 ml of normal saline has been suggested for the treatment of superficial low-grade papillomas.

Prevention

Employment in aniline dye factories should be restricted to 3 years, during which time periodic urinary Papanicolaou smear studies and cystoscopy are indicated. The clinical significance of endogenous carcinogenic agents has not been established, and it has also been suggested that the administration of ascorbic acid 0.5 g three times a day may prevent the formation of vesical tumours through neutralization of urinary carcinogens. Again, this is not fully substantiated.

Prognosis

The superficial, well differentiated tumours may recur or new papillomas may appear. Constant vigilance with periodic cystoscopy is therefore necessary for at least 3 years. New tumours may also be well controlled by transurethral resection, but if they tend to recur they are apt to become progressively invasive and of higher grade. Cystectomy or radiation therapy must then be considered. Prognosis with any vesical tumour varies in general with the stage and grade. The best results are obtained by transurethral resection of grade I–II, stage 0, A and B1 tumours.

THE PROSTATE AND SEMINAL VESICLES

Benign enlargement of the prostate

Benign enlargement of the prostate usually occurs in men over 50 years of age, most often between 60 and 70. In Indians prostatic enlargement is less frequent, but when it occurs is more often to be found in a younger age group. In Negroes it is rare, while in Asiatics it is exceptional. The reasons for these discrepancies are unknown.

Aetiology

Hormonal theory

Previous castration seems to prevent prostatic hypertrophy in men. However, administration of oestrogens or even castration has little if any effect upon the gross size of the enlarged gland, although microscopically some atrophy of the epithelial structures may be noted. The administration of oestrogens or androgens has little effect upon the amount of acid phosphatase elaborated by the gland. Certainly androgens per se cannot be blamed for this hyperplasia, for the disease occurs at a time when androgenic activity of the organism is decreasing. Therefore, an imbalance between androgens and oestrogens may be the causative factor. It is not clear why hyperplasia of the prostate develops in some men and not in others, and affects different individuals in varying degrees. The enlarged gland produces its harmful effect by obstructing the bladder neck and by upsetting the mechanisms which force open and funnel the vesical orifice. Changes in the bladder and the upper urinary tract have already been described on page 403.

Pathology

The prostate of the young adult may be compared to an apple; its true capsule is thin and entirely attached to the underlying secretory tissue. For this reason intracapsular enucleation of a young man's prostate is impossible. The enlarged gland, on the other hand, is more like an orange (Fig. 40.6); it has a thick surgical capsule, the peripherally compressed external part of the prostate, which is poorly connected to the central obstructing tissue, and this permits easy shelling out of the hyperplastic prostatic lobes, leaving the surgical capsule behind. It should be noted that the posterior prostatic lobe is left as part of the surgical capsule, since it is in this lobe that carcinoma most commonly develops. Intracapsular prostatectomy is not prophylactic against cancer developing later. On section the adenomatous pattern of the prostate is usually obvious, with multiple nodules; the surgical capsule is composed of atrophic true extraurethral prostatic tissue which has been compressed and displaced to the periphery and may be 2–5 mm in thickness.

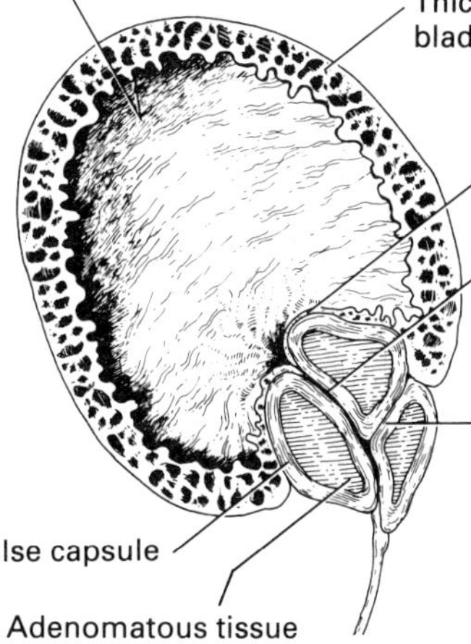

Fig. 40.6 Benign prostatic enlargement. Diagrammatic representation of main gross changes.

This capsule is poorly connected to the hyperplastic lobes which therefore may be easily enucleated.

Clinical findings

Benign prostatic enlargement rarely causes significant symptoms before the age of 50. The complaints are referrable to obstruction, and may increase with infection. Rectal examination may or may not reveal prostatic enlargement.

Symptoms

In the early stages the patient may notice that as the bladder becomes too full there is a little hesitation in starting the stream, and some loss of force and calibre of the stream. Later the symptoms are more persistent and severe.

Bladder symptoms. Hesitancy in starting the stream may be marked, and considerable straining is commonly necessary. Because of the increased urethral resistance, decrease in calibre of the bladder neck, and derangement of the normal mechanism which opens the bladder neck, the stream is small and lacks force. This will be worse if the urge to urinate must be postponed, for the smooth muscle of the bladder becomes overstretched and loses tone.

Towards the end of urination the stream tends to diminish gradually and may end as a mere dribble. Frequency, both day and night, develops, depending on the degree of irritability of the bladder and the amount of residual urine. If infection complicates the picture all of the above symptoms are increased. The inflammatory oedema of the prostate or bladder neck will increase the degree of obstruction, and will cause more residual urine, thereby further increasing frequency. Haematuria is not uncommon and it may be due to rupture of dilated veins of the bladder neck which are apt to develop with straining. Acute urinary retention may develop suddenly in a patient who has had few premonitory symptoms. At other times it occurs after some months or years of increasing symptoms of 'prostatism'. The patient then experiences great suprapubic pain and marked urgency. He is miserable until relieved by catheterization.

Renal symptoms. Hydronephrosis secondary to prostatic obstruction is usually painless until it becomes infected.

Signs

A mass low in the midline of the abdomen, representing the bladder, may be seen, felt or percussed. In acute retention it is quite tender. In chronic urinary retention the bladder may be so flabby that only percussion will reveal it. On rectal examination the prostate may or not be enlarged; one lobe may be larger than the other. The surface is usually smooth, and it may be firm, fibromuscular or unduly soft and adenomatous. Localized areas of induration raise the possibility of cancer of the prostate.

Laboratory findings

Urinalysis may reveal an otherwise completely silent complicating infection. Renal function is sometimes deteriorating, particularly in chronic retention.

X-ray findings

A plain film of the abdomen and excretory urography may show complicating calculi, and often ureterohydronephrosis. This is usually caused by hypertrophy of the trigone which applies increased occlusive pressure on the intravesical and ureteric segments.

Instrumental examination

The amount of urine retained after voiding (i.e. the residual urine) is a measure of the degree of decompensation of the bladder. This is ascertained by passing a catheter into the bladder immediately after voiding. Cystoscopy will show the degree of enlargement of the prostatic lobes, and the secondary changes in the bladder wall, e.g. trabeculation, diverticula and/or infection. It will also reveal complications such as vesical stone or incidental neoplasm. The differential diagnosis is from neurogenic bladder, contracture of the bladder neck caused by chronic prostatitis, cancer of the prostate, acute prostatitis, urethral stricture and sarcoma of the prostate.

Complications

Obstruction leads to infection which may involve the bladder, kidneys, or prostate; from the latter epididymitis may develop; stones may form in the bladder; obstruction may cause vesical diverticula; hydronephrosis may occur from hypertrophy of the trigone.

Treatment

Since benign prostatic hyperplasia is not necessarily a progressive disease, conservative therapy should be initiated where applicable. The problem is to decide which patients can be treated in this manner, and which require surgery. Criteria for operation vary, but the following seems feasible:

1. Impaired renal function due to obstruction—this indication is not debatable.
2. Symptoms which so upset the patient that he requests relief—this may vary, since one man may be distressed at urinating three times during the night, whereas another may not be.

Conservative measures

Regular intercourse is the best means of combating

prostatic congestion. If necessary, this may be replaced or augmented by three or four prostatic massages given at intervals of 14 days. At times the improvement is striking. Prostatitis and cystitis can be treated with antimicrobials, prostatic massage and Sitz baths. If pyuria is present antibiotics or sulphonamides may afford considerable relief.

Catheterization is mandatory for acute retention. If the patient is still unable to void spontaneously and particularly if there have been few antecedent symptoms, a catheter should be left indwelling for 2–4 days. Thus prostatic congestion is relieved and vesical tone re-established, and fairly normal voiding may return after removal of the catheter.

Surgery

There are four operations in vogue at present, but it is impossible to state the indications for each. The choice of operation is a personal matter for the surgeon. Transurethral prostatectomy is most often used; the amount of prostate removed varies from surgeon to surgeon. Usually the whole of the internal prostate is removed down to the prostatic capsule. Mortality from this is 1–2%, and the urinary result is good in most instances. Potency is maintained and hospitalisation is short.

Suprapubic transvesical prostatectomy is still popular when the open method of removal of the prostate is required. Mortality rate, again, is 1–2%. The urinary result is excellent, probably more consistently so than with the transurethral method. Potency is also maintained. Retropubic extravesical prostatectomy also has a mortality rate of 1–2%, the urinary result is excellent and again, potency is maintained. Perineal prostatectomy involves little risk—2–3% mortality—but impotence may occur. There is often some delay in regaining perfect urinary control and on occasion some degree of stress incontinence persists. Rectourethral fistula has a definite incidence of 1–5% and is most distressing.

Some enthusiasm for cryosurgery is being evinced for the poor-risk patient. The instrument is passed down the urethra with a freezing unit placed in the prostatic urethra. Liquid nitrogen is circulated through the probe until the temperature in the prostatic capsule reaches -l0° C. This leads to death and slough of the obstructing tissue. Blood loss is usually minimal, but the result is not as good as with conventional prostatectomy.

Prognosis

Most patients can be given considerable relief by conservative means. If on follow-up their symptoms increase, or renal function begins to diminish, surgical intervention is indicated.

Carcinoma of the prostate

Carcinoma of the prostate is rare before the age of 60 and increases in frequency thereafter, probably afflicting 25% of men in the eighth decade. The disease is rare in Japanese men and Jews. Negroes are more commonly afflicted than whites. There is a significant familial incidence which suggests a genetic component, and multiple cancers are common in these patients. Carcinoma of the prostate metastasizes primarily to the bones of the pelvis, and may damage the kidneys because of the vesical obstruction which ensues.

Aetiology

The true cause of prostatic cancer is not known but it is quite clear that its growth is strikingly influenced by sex hormones. The adult prostate is the major site of elaboration of acid phosphatase. In advanced prostatic cancer, particularly when it has metastasized to bone, three-quarters of patients will have markedly increased amounts of this enzyme in the blood. The administration of androgens usually increases the rate of growth of this tumour and increases the acid phosphatase level in the serum. Oestrogen therapy or orchidectomy slows the growth of these tumours and maintains the amount of acid phosphatase in blood at a normal level. Determination of the amount of acid phosphatase in the serum is, therefore, an index of the extent of the tumour. It also indicates the degree of success of antiandrogen therapy.

Pathogenesis and pathology

Cancer of the prostate is usually associated coincidentally with benign prostatic hypertrophy but does not develop from it. Most malignancies originate in the posterior lobe in the surgical capsule, the compressed peripheral prostatic tissue, although a few may be found within the hyperplastic benign prostatic lobes. These latter tumours are usually very small, occult cancers, and apparently often completely removed by intracapsular enucleation of the enlarged gland. The initial lesion is usually a firm area on the posterolateral surface, which gradually spreads in the capsule and involves the hyperplastic tissue as well. The seminal vesicles may then become involved, and later the tumour may extend through the urethral mucosa to the bladder wall. The rectal wall, however, is singularly immune; only rarely does the tumour invade Denonvilliers' fascia. Cancer spreads in the perineural lymphatics and the vesical, sacral, external iliac and lumbar lymph nodes become involved. When the seminal vesicles are involved, 80% of the patients will have invasion of the pelvic nodes. Metastases also occur by way of the veins, particularly through the vertebral ones. This mechanism accounts for the predilection of this tumour for the bones of the pelvis, the heads of the femurs and the lower lumbar spine. Other bones, including the skull, are occasionally involved. Visceral spread is also seen to the lungs and the liver. Infiltration of the bone marrow is particularly common. On microscopic study the tissue is largely epithelial or may be fibrous. The epithelial elements may assume a papillary pattern or be anaplastic. Invasion of the stroma is usually obvious; mitoses are common, and invasion of the perineural sheaths is an outstanding feature.

Clinical findings

The presenting symptoms in 95% of men with prostatic malignancy are from obstruction to the flow of urine, infection or both. They are similar to those described in the discussion of benign prostatic enlargement.

Signs

Rectal examination is the most important step in the diagnosis of cancer of the prostate. A cancerous nodule is usually not raised above the surface of the gland. Rather, there is a sudden change in consistency between it and the surrounding tissues. Diagnosis may not be possible without surgical biopsy.

Laboratory findings

Urinalysis may show infection, and red cells may be present. Renal function may be impaired. Serum acid phosphatase determinations are important in the diagnosis of prostatic cancer, and when the cancer spreads outside the prostatic capsule and metastases are present 75% of patients will have significant elevation of their acid phosphatase concentration.

X-ray findings

A chest film may show evidence of metastases in the hilar nodes, lungs or ribs. A plain film of the abdomen may reveal typical osteoblastic metastases from the prostatic tumour; common sites include the pelvic bones and lumbar vertebrae. An isotopic bone scan with strontium 85 may reveal involvement of bones, even though plain films are normal.

Biopsy

If the lesion is extensive a positive diagnosis can be made on pathological studies of tissue removed by transurethral resection. In early cases and where the tumour is external to the capsule this method fails, and needle biopsy through the perineum or transrectally is a useful procedure in order to establish the diagnosis.

Complications

Obstruction of the prostatic urethra may cause the formation of vesical diverticula, or stones, followed by infection. Renal damage may be due to functional obstruction of the ureterovesical junction secondary to trigonal hypertrophy. Oedema of the legs may occur from pressure of involved iliac nodes upon the great vessels. Spontaneous fractures may develop at the sites of bony metastases. Sudden spinal cord compression is not uncommon and may require immediate laminectomy.

Treatment

Curative radical measures

If on palpating an indurated nodule in the prostate of a well preserved man under the age of 70 the clinician is unable to say that the patient does not have early malignancy, and unless there is evidence of metastases to bone by X-ray or scan, or elevation of the serum acid phosphatase, perineal exposure and immediate frozen section are indicated. If cancerous the entire prostate including its capsule, seminal vesicles and a portion of the bladder neck can be removed through the same wound. The same radical procedure can be performed retropubically.

Prostatovesiculectomy will cure about half of these favourable cases. Urinary control is usually normal after the operation but impotence is to be expected. Some advise preliminary oestrogen for 3–6 months before radical prostatectomy is performed, in the belief that the overall control is thereby improved.

Palliative measures — antiandrogen therapy

About 85% of prostatic cancers are androgen-dependent. These will show definite regression in size after a few weeks of antiandrogen therapy, and the consistency of the gland tends to approach normal. The degree of urinary obstruction lessens, and bone pain disappears or decreases. The patient gains weight and strength and anaemia tends to correct itself. X-ray films often show healing of the metastatic lesions in bone. The price the patient must pay for this palliation includes impotence, with loss of sexual desire, tender gynaecomastia, and at times oedema of the ankles. There is no doubt that this mode of therapy affords much comfort to patients who formerly suffered greatly. It is also true that the life of these patients is slightly prolonged. Although there is little doubt that antioestrogen therapy has a palliative effect on the surgically incurable prostatic carcinoma, it has been shown that the administration of large doses of oestrogen significantly increases the incidence of death from thromboembolic phenomena, and therefore oestrogen should be withheld until the patient develops symptoms or signs of metastases. When this happens oestrogens can be expected to cause regression of metastases in most patients.

Transurethral resection

If the degree of obstruction is severe, or if anti-androgen therapy fails to afford much relief, transurethral resection of the prostate may be necessary. Since the cancer of the prostate invades the hyperplastic tissue there is no longer any cleavage plane which permits intracapsular enucleation, as is ordinarily practised for benign hyperplasia.

Cryosurgery

This technique has been used in the poor-risk patient instead of transurethral resection, with some measure of successful relief of the obstruction. Irradiation is increasing in popularity, and there is justified enthusiasm for this method of therapy in patients with tumours which do not lend themselves to radical surgery. The local lesion tends to decrease in size, and obstructive symptoms tend to regress. It has been shown that X-ray therapy also acts favourably on metastases to lymph nodes as revealed on lymphangiograms. Whether such therapy can cure some of these tumours is still not known.

Prognosis

Of the 10% of men with prostatic carcinoma whose illness is diagnosed early enough so that radical surgery affords a reasonable hope of cure, at least half are over 70 years and many suffer from other infirmities of old age. For this reason they are not good subjects for radical procedures, and most of them will live more comfortably and just as long with palliative treatment and will die of other causes. The curability rate of prostatic carcinoma is therefore about 2–4 %. The prognosis in young men is the same as that in the older age group.

Palliative treatment offers considerable temporary relief for most patients with advanced prostatic carcinoma. Death usually occurs within 3 years after the diagnosis has been made. A few patients will be controlled for 5 and even 10 years.

Sarcoma of the prostate

Sarcomas may arise in the smooth or striated muscle or the fibroplastic tissue of the prostate gland. It is a disease of young individuals—50% occur before the age of 50 years. It is, however, extremely rare though most sarcomas grow rapidly and all are highly malignant. They may extend into the base of the bladder and finally occlude the urethra. They may compress the rectum and cause constipation.

41. Urethra, penis and scrotum

CONGENITAL ABNORMALITIES OF THE URETHRA

Meatal stenosis

The external urinary meatus, normally the narrowest part of the male urethra, is occasionally the seat of congenital stenosis which is associated with phimosis. In the circumcised, meatal stenosis may also be acquired or increased by fibrosis following meatal ulceration. All degrees of narrowing are encountered; when the opening is reduced to a pinhole, back-pressure effects on the whole urinary system can be anticipated. Pinhole meatus is occasionally a cause of enuresis and at any age it may result in chronic retention of urine.

Treatment

Meatal stenosis sufficient to give rise to symptoms and prevent free drainage of the discharge in cases of urethritis, or which obstructs the passage of the full-sized urethral instruments, or a cystoscope, should be treated by meatotomy. Lesser degrees of narrowing respond to dilatation with Hegar's dilators.

Meatotomy

A fine pointed scalpel is introduced into the urethral meatus and a cut is made in a downward direction (Fig.41.1). In infants and children a metal bougie of suitable calibre is passed into the meatus each day for 4 days, and then weekly for 1 month. In adults it is preferable to unite the edges of the urethra to the skin of the glans penis with one or two absorbable sutures. These stitches control haemorrhage and prevent the lips of the meatus from re-uniting. Usually dilatation on two occasions at weekly intervals is sufficient in this instance.

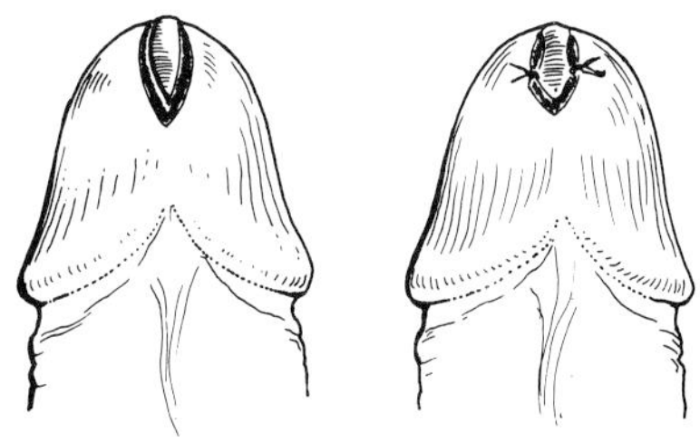

Fig. 41.1 Meatotomy. Using a fine pointed scalpel, the narrowed orifice is slit about 0.5 cm in the directly inferior direction. One or more absorbable sutures is then inserted on each side to unite the mucosa to glans skin, as shown.

Posterior urethral valves

These are often symmetrical and occur usually just below but occasionally above the verumontanum. They allow the ingress of a catheter but obstruct the outflow of urine. In a few instances the valves are incomplete and the patient may reach adolescence or adult life without symptoms. However, in such cases the prostatic urethra is greatly dilated and diverticula of the bladder are usually present. The valves are difficult to see at cystourethroscopy because the irrigating fluid sweeps them into the open position. The most reliable method of confirming the diagnosis is voiding cystourethrography —radiographs are taken during attempts to micturate after the bladder has been filled with contrast medium. Alternatively, pressure above the pubis while the radiograph is taken achieves the same objective. In this way the dilated urethra above the valves is outlined as well as the bladder.

Treatment

Suprapubic drainage of the bladder is life-saving. Several weeks should intervene before attempting to remove the valves. At the definitive operation the valves can be divided with diathermy endoscopically, or the retropubic space can be opened and an incision made into the bladder just above the prostate, and continued downwards into the dilated prostatic urethra. The valves are then removed by diathermy.

Obstruction of the bladder neck (synonym: Marian's disease)

This is analogous to hypertrophic pyloric stenosis of infants, and gives rise to symptoms identical with those of congenital valves. The diagnosis can often be appreciated cystoscopically as a hypertrophied interureteric bar. Voiding cystourethrography demonstrates that the posterior urethra does not fill, and clarifies the differential diagnosis between the two conditions. Treatment consists in opening the bladder and performing a Y-V plasty.

Hypospadias

Hypospadias is the commonest congenital malformation of the urethra and it occurs once in every 350 males. The external meatus is situated at some point on the undersurface of the penis, or in the perineum. There are five degrees of deformity classified as follows:

1. Glandular hypospadias. Here there is an ectopic opening on the undersurface of the glans, separated from a blind depression at the normal site of the external urinary meatus. Sometimes a channel connects the ectopic to the normal meatus.
2. Coronal hypospadias. The meatus is situated at the junction of the undersurface of the glans and the body of the penis.
3. Penile hypospadias. The meatus opens at some part of the undersurface of the penis.
4. Penoscrotal hypospadias. The urethra opens at the junction of the penis with the scrotum.
5. Perineal hypospadias. The scrotum is split and the urethra opens between the two halves. This variety is sometimes associated with bilateral maldescended testes, in which event the sex of the child may be difficult to determine.

Glandular hypospadias is the most frequent variety and is due to a failure of canalization of the glans. The other varieties are looked upon as an absence of the urethra and corpus spongiosum distal to the ectopic orifice, the absent structures being represented by a fibrous cord. In all except the first variety, the penis is curved in a downward direction (chordee). The farther away the opening is from the normal position the more pronounced is the bowing. In all cases the inferior aspect of the prepuce is poorly developed.

Treatment

In glandular hypospadias no treatment is required unless the opening is too small, in which case meatotomy is performed. In other varieties a plastic operation, of which there is a great variety, should be carried out. On this account circumcision during infancy should not be performed in the presence of hypospadias as the redundant skin will prove useful for the plastic procedure.

The operation falls into two stages. Firstly, the penis is straightened: a transverse incision is made on the ventral surface distal to the misplaced external urinary meatus and the skin on either side of the urethra is undermined, exposing the fibrotic corpus spongiosum which is detached from before backwards by severing the fibrous attachment to the corpora. Thus, a coronal hypospadias becomes a penile, penoscrotal or perineal and the penis is no longer tethered. The second stage involves reconstruction of the urethra and is undertaken preferably between 5 and 7 years of age. Diversion of all urine from the seat of the operation can be accomplished by perineal urethrostomy. The urethra is usually reconstructed by creating a tube of skin over a silastic catheter. Denis Browne's operation for hypospadias is shown in Figure 41.2.

Epispadias

Unlike hypospadias, epispadias is very rare, occurring only once in every 30 000 males and in 400 000 females. The defect may be glandular, penile or

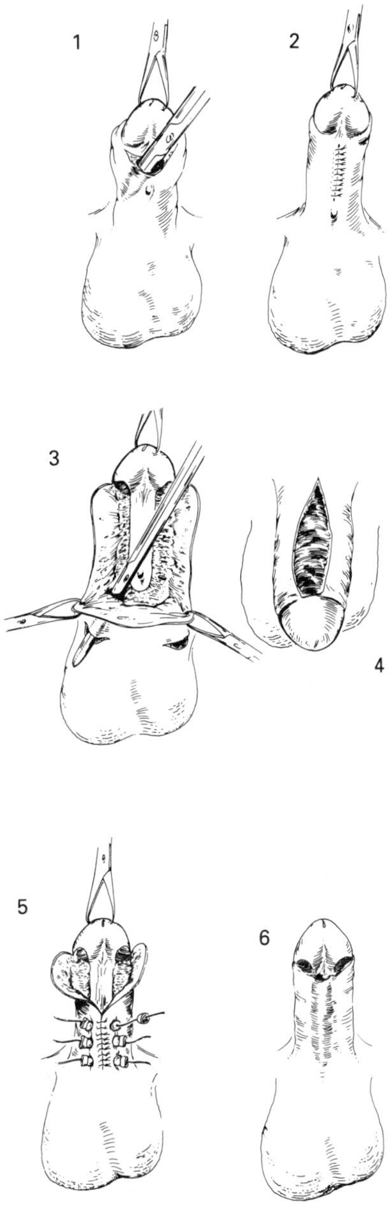

Fig. 41.2 The Denis Browne operations for hypospadias. At the first operation (illustrations 1, 2 and 3), straightening and lengthening of the ventral surface of the distal penis is obtained by undermining flaps through a transverse incision and suturing longitudinally. Any resulting tightness is relieved by a longitudinal incision along the dorsal skin.

The second reconstructive procedure (illustrations 4,5 and 6) is preceded by the insertion of a catheter into the proximal urethra to divert the urine (not shown). The strip of skin between the abnormally sited meatus and the glans is buried by closing the two lateral flaps raised after making the U-shaped incision. Under favourable conditions proliferation from the edges of this new skin 'roof' of the new distal urethra forms a complete epithelial-lined tube.

total, the latter usually associated with ectopia vesicae. In the first two varieties, the urethral orifice is situated on the dorsum and in the second variety the penis curves upwards as well. The operative treatment is similar in principle to that of hypospadias, and is somewhat less difficult to perform.

INJURIES TO THE URETHRA

Rupture of the urethra is divided into two distinct classes—rupture of the bulbus urethra and rupture of the membranous urethra. Each is again subdivided into complete and incomplete, which relates to the circumference of the urethral wall, and total and partial, which relates to the thickness of the wall. Rupture of the bulbus urethra is the more common accident; almost without exception there is a history of falling astride a projecting object. Cycling accidents account for a large number of these cases.

Clinical features

The triad of signs of ruptured bulbus urethra is urethral haemorrhage, perineal haematoma and retention of urine.

Preliminary treatment and investigation

If the condition is suspected, in order to diminish the possibility of extravasation, the patient should be told not to try to pass urine. No attempt should be made to catheterize him until he is fit to be taken to an operating theatre where asepsis can be assured, and the operation can be undertaken in necessary cases. A suitable dose of morphine is given together with antibiotic. When immediate access to such facilities is not available and the bladder is full, it should be emptied by suprapubic puncture. If the patient has passed urine when first seen, and there is no extravasation, then the rupture is partial, and catheterization should be avoided.

Treatment

Under strict aseptic conditions an attempt is made to pass a silastic catheter, 14–16 French gauge. The roof of the urethra is the most likely part to

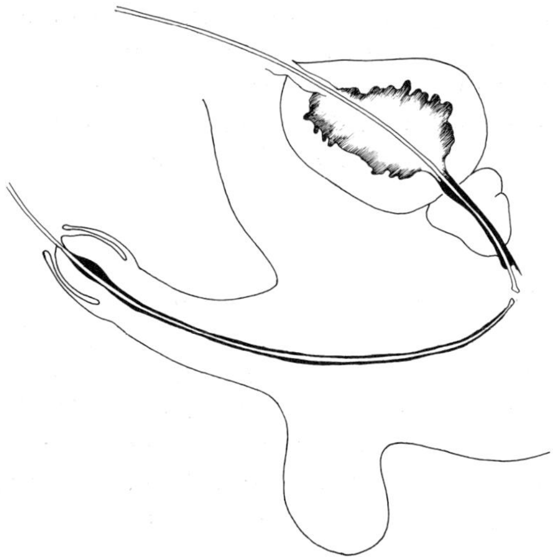

Fig. 41.3 Method of identifying the proximal end of a divided urethra. Where the urethral passage of a catheter or sound has failed to pass into the part proximal to the site of injury, an opening into the bladder is made, and a second sound is passed down through the proximal urethra. By manoeuvring the two sounds, contact can be made and then a catheter 'rail-roaded' across the gap.

be intact, so the tip of the catheter should be directed towards this. If the catheter passes, it should be left in position for 48 h. A perineal haematoma must then be drained and the midline wound packed. If the catheter fails to pass, the site of the obstruction is explored with the patient in the lithotomy position, through a midline perineal incision. If it proves impossible to define the proximal end of the ruptured urethra, a suprapubic cystostomy is performed and a fully curved sound passed down from the internal meatus (Fig. 41.3). The exposed ends of the urethra are then cleaned and the ventral aspects split longitudinally so that the circumference can be sutured with fine absorbable sutures.

Complications

Subcutaneous extravasation of urine occurs in total rupture if the patient attempts to pass urine. Later, a stricture may form and this common complication is due for the most part to infection.

Rupture of the membranous urethra

(see p. 441)

Extravasation of urine

Superficial extravasation of urine occurs after complete rupture of the bulbus urethra. The urine cannot pass behind the mid perineal point because of the attachment of Colles' fascia to the triangular ligament (Fig. 41.4), and it cannot pass into the thigh for the deep layer of the superficial fascia of the abdominal wall, Scarpa's fascia, blends with the pubic portion of the fascia lata just distal to the inguinal ligament, and it cannot pass into the inguinal canals because of the intercolumnar fibres and fascia of the external oblique. It must, therefore, pass into the scrotum beneath the superficial fascia of the penis and up the abdominal wall beneath the deep layer of the superficial fascia.

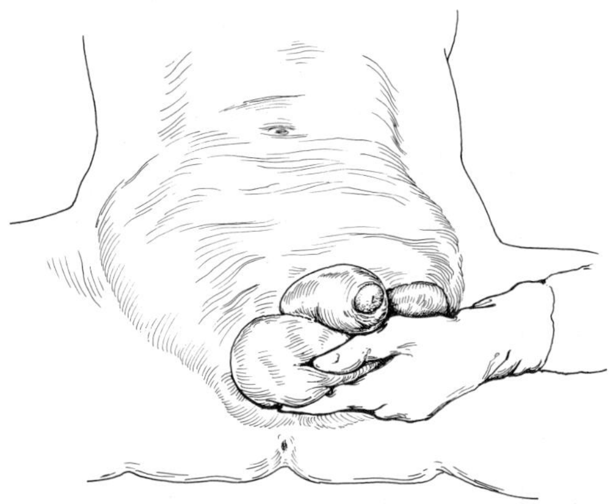

Fig. 41.4 Extravasation of urine. The diagram shows the extent of extravasation, limited in the perineum by the attachment of the posterior edge of Colles' fascia to the triangular pelvic ligament, and in the upper thighs by the fusion of Scarpa's fascia with the fascia lata 2–3 cm below the inguinal ligaments. The leaked urine spreads up the subcutaneous layers of the lower abdominal wall, and over the penis and scrotum.

Treatment

Urgent operation is necessary. Multiple incisions are made in the infiltrated tissue, of sufficient length to penetrate the limiting fascia and to allow free drainage of the collected fluid.

Deep extravasation

Deep extravasation occurs in the case of extraperitoneal rupture of the bladder or intrapelvic rupture of the urethra and after suprapubic puncture when the bladder has been allowed to fill. It can also result from rupture or perforation of a ureter or unnoticed damage to the bladder or prostatic capsule during perurethral resections.

Treatment

When extravasation is proceeding from the bladder it is necessary to drain the prevesical space and to perform a suprapubic cystostomy.

Ulceration of the urethral meatus

This is particularly common in young male children who have been circumcised. Friction of clothing and ammoniacal urine are important secondary aetiological factors. The ulcer causes a scab to form which closes the meatus and the child can only urinate by bursting the scab. This process is usually accompanied by pain and screaming and a few drops of blood may be passed. Ulceration and scab formation alternate and if this is neglected, scarring of the meatus may eventually result in an acquired pinhole meatus.

Treatment

A simple regime of washing the napkins in boric acid crystals after boiling and applying a 5% boric acid ointment locally is usually curative. These measures neutralize the alkaline urine. A few of the children will require meatotomy.

Urethral stricture

Classification

Congenital; traumatic, which can be bulbous or membranous; inflammatory, postgonorrhoeal, posturethral, tuberculous; instrumental—from an indwelling catheter and following the passage of a large-calibre endoscope; postoperatively following prostatectomy, or amputation of the penis.

Postgonorrhoeal stricture, which has become rare since the introduction of antibiotic treatment for gonorrhoea, is most frequently situated in the bulb or at the penoscrotal junction. Multiple strictures are relatively common; when there are two strictures the deeper is usually the narrower; when there are three strictures, the deepest is the narrowest. If a stricture in a penile urethra is very narrow there is seldom another stricture beyond it.

Pathology

Following inadequately treated gonorrhoea, infection persists in the periurethral glands, and spreads to the periglandular tissues, which become infiltrated with round cells and fibroblasts. Gradually the infiltrated periurethral tissues contract with the formation of a scar. Localized thrombophlebitis of the corpus spongiosum may be a part of the disease process.

Clinical features

If a stricture is of large calibre the only symptoms are the occasional passage of desquamated epithelium in the urine, and a varying amount of urethral discharge, most evident in the early morning. Often these symptoms are neglected until the diminished calibre of the urethra causes considerable difficulty in micturition. In contradistinction to obstruction due to enlarged prostate, the patient finds that he must strain to empty the bladder. Another distinguishing feature is the patient's age. He is often considerably younger than the prostatic sufferer. The stream becomes progressively narrower, micturition is prolonged, and after it has seemingly ended, dribbling occurs. This is due to urine trickling from the dilated urethra above the stricture. Increasing frequency of micturition, at first during the day and then both by day and by night, is another common complaint. Urethrography supplies information concerning the length of the stricture, of dilatation or diverticulum formation above the stricture, or failure of the medium to pass a stricture.

Instrumental dilatation

In the majority of cases, provided the patient attends regularly, dilatation at suitable intervals is a satisfactory form of treatment. Before each dilatation the patient should pass urine. The glans penis and the urinary meatus are cleaned and the urethra is filled with a mild antiseptic solution and a local anaesthetic, such as lignocaine, in a methyl cellulose base. Dilatation must be carried out very gently with bougies of increasing size. On no account should the stricture be forcibly overdilated for this will result in traumatization, which induces inflammatory oedema and subsequent formation of more fibrous tissue.

Operative treatment

Urethrotomy

This is the operation of choice when the patient presents with acute retention and the stricture proves impassable. With the patient in the lithotomy position the urethrotome is passed, incising the urethra longitudinally.

Urethroplasty

Surgical cure by means of a two-stage urethroplasty is applicable to all strictures of the bulbar and penile portions and is the treatment of choice.

Neoplasms of the male urethra

Polypi are usually multiple, and occur most frequently in the region of the verumontanum as seen at urethroscopy. Each polypus is a pale, fingerlike projection with blood vessels coursing over it. Polypi are never found without chronic infection. Sometimes if the infection can be cured the polypi will disappear. Conversely, if the polypi are destroyed, chronic urethritis which previously resisted treatment often responds to antibiotic treatment.

From time to time a solitary papilloma occurs, most often within the fossa navicularis, and as it enlarges it protrudes from the external urinary meatus. Multiple papillomas associated with penile papillomas sometimes arise from the mucous membrane just within the external urinary meatus. Papillomatosis of the urethra is most often associated with papillomas of the bladder. The posterior urethra is considerably more often affected than the anterior urethra.

Carcinoma of the urethra is extremely rare.

THE PENIS

Phimosis

While the condition can be acquired as a result of chronic or acute inflammation of the lining of the prepuce, usually it is due to congenital narrowing of the preputial orifice, often associated with an unduly long foreskin. In extreme examples of congenital phimosis, when the patient micturates the prepuce balloons out first and then a thin weak stream of urine flows. Dysuria with residual urine, hydroureters and hydronephrosis is rarely due to phimosis.

Circumcision (Fig. 41.5)

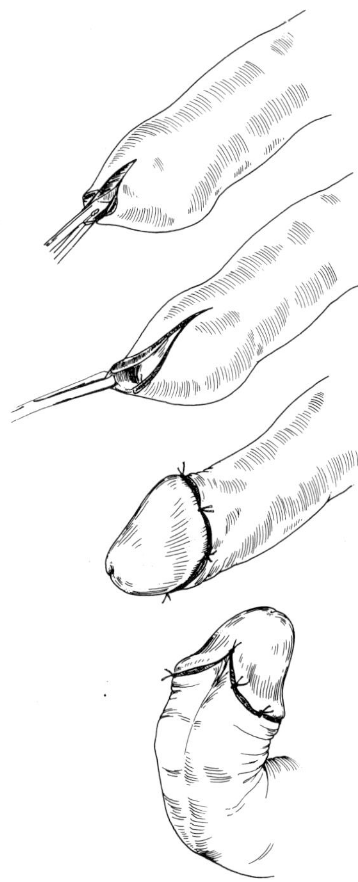

Fig. 41.5 Circumcision: steps in the operation. After ensuring there are no adhesions between the glans and the foreskin, a dorsal division is first made and the line of division is carried to the inferior aspect, taking care to avoid damage to the frenulum. The wound is closed by a series of radially placed absorbable sutures.

Indications

Circumcision is indicated in infants and young boys because of a request by parents on religious grounds, and for personal reasons because of recurrent balinitis with inability to retract the prepuce and, rarely, because of a very long prepuce. Except for the ritual operation most circumcisions are unnecessary purely for medical reasons. It is normal for the prepuce to be long and adherent to the glans at birth and these parts become satisfactorily separated and the prepuce becomes mobile in the first few years of life. Recurrent balanitis and phimosis often follow attempts by parents to retract the prepuce forcibly. In adults, because of the inability to retract for intercourse, or a tight frenum, balanitis and sometimes prior to radiotherapy for carcinoma, a dorsal slit may suffice.

Paraphimosis

The tight prepuce has been retracted but cannot be returned. It is constricting the glans, which is engorged and oedematous. The diagnosis is apparent at a glance.

Treatment

Normal saline (1 ml) containing 150 units of hyaluronidase is injected into each lateral aspect of the swollen ring. Fifteen minutes after the swelling is much reduced and in early cases reduction can be accomplished with ease. If this is unsuccessful a general anaesthetic must be given and the constricting band incised. The narrow cuff of skin which formed the constricting band is then excised (Fig. 41.6). There is now no obstruction to reduction and there remains only to remove a broad cuff of normal skin on the proximal side of the cap and unite the cut free edges, thus performing a circumcision.

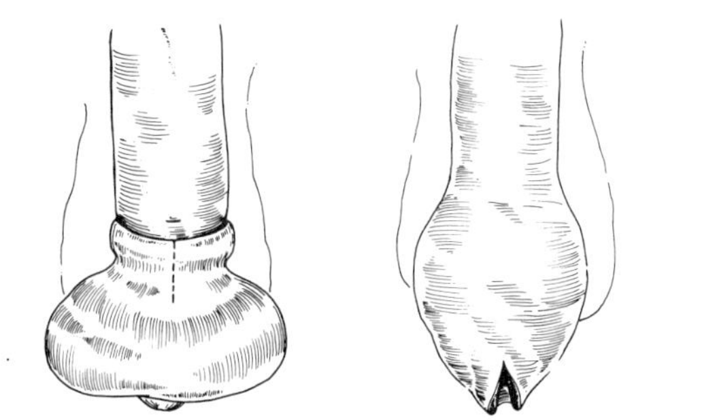

Fig. 41.6 Paraphimosis. The tight band is divided by a short, dorsal slit, which relieves the compression sufficiently to allow the foreskin to be replaced into its normal position. The slit portion now represents the starting point for circumcision.

Injuries to the penis

Avulsion of the skin of the penis

Entanglement of clothing, in rotating machinery accounts for the majority of these injuries. Repair can be carried out by burying the shaft of the penis in the scrotum with subsequent surgical release at a propitious time.

Peyronie's disease

Usually the patient is over 40 years of age, and seldom is there is a history of venereal disease. At the onset pain and curving of the penis on erection cause the patient to seek advice, but after a few weeks the pain disappears. On palpation an indurated plaque can be felt on the dorsal surface of the corpus cavernosum. The condition is slowly progressive and sometimes extends across the midline. Its aetiology is unknown.

Treatment

Treatment is unsatisfactory. Low-dosage X-ray therapy is occasionally valuable. Injection of the plaque with hydrocortisone has been advocated but is not usually effective. Resection of the plaque has been advocated but there appears to be little enthusiasm for this mode of therapy.

Priapism

The penis remains erect and is painful. Most often the erection is due to idiopathic thrombosis occurring in the prostatic venous plexus. Less frequently it is associated with leukaemia or sickle cell anaemia. Secondary malignant deposits in the corpora cavernosa or in the pelvis account for about 7% of cases. In another completely different category are cases due to spinal injury or disease.

Diagnosis

A low spinal anaesthetic will cause priapism of neurogenic origin to ablate temporarily. A blood count is essential to exclude leukaemia.

Treatment

Local applications are useless. Anticoagulant therapy together with adequate sedation for 14 days brings about restitution in the majority of cases. Should this treatment not work after a trial of several days, repeated aspiration of the corpora cavernosa is occasionally of value. When this fails or is unsatisfactory, a small incision into the corpus cavernosum should be made and blood and clot evacuated. A bilateral saphenous vein–corpora cavernosa shunt should be performed. If successful and done early, potency is maintained. Most often, however, the shunt thromboses and the results are equivocal.

Neoplasms of the penis

Papillomata acuminata (synonym: venereal warts)

The commonest benign growth of the penis occurs in both the circumcised and the uncircumcised. Most often they are situated in the coronal sulcus, but they can occur anywhere on the penis, scrotum, perineum and in the anal region. Usually they are moist and attended by an offensive serous discharge. Often they are transmitted by sexual contact and are probably of viral origin.

Treatment

1. Fulguration.
2. Podophyllin.

Carcinoma of the penis

Aetiology

For a reason that is only partially understood, circumcision correctly performed soon after birth confers almost total immunity against carcinoma of the penis. On the other hand, circumcision after early infancy does not provide the same degree of protection. Muslims who are circumcised between the ages of 4 and 9 exemplify this. For practical purposes, then, carcinoma of the penis occurs only in men who have not been circumcised in infancy, and undoubtedly the development of this neoplasm is favoured by chronic balanitis. Furthermore, there are definite precancerous states, viz. leukoplakia of the glans, long-standing penile papillomas and Paget's disease of the penis.

Pathology

There are two types of squamous carcinoma of the penis, the flat or infiltrating and the papilliferous. The former may be associated with leukoplakia and the latter usually commences in a papilloma of long standing. The growth remains purely local for many months, and the earliest spread is to the inguinal and then to the iliac lymph nodes. Direct spread to the body of the penis is prevented for many months by the fascial sheath of the corpora cavernosa, but once this barrier is broken, the growth extends more rapidly, and the iliac lymph nodes become involved. Distant metastatic deposits are infrequent.

Clinical features

It is a mistake to believe that this is a disease confined to the elderly. Forty per cent of sufferers are under 40 years of age. The progress of the disease is slow: the first symptoms are mild irritation and purulent discharge from the prepuce. These symptoms are often neglected and by the time the patient reports, sometimes more than a year after the symptoms have appeared, there is a blood-stained foul discharge. Pain is singularly absent. The inguinal lymph nodes are enlarged in over 60% of cases, but in only half of these is the enlargement due to secondary deposits, the remainder being due to infection.

Treatment

Radiotherapy gives good results—60–70% 5-year survival with small, well differentiated tumours. Partial amputation is needed for larger anaplastic growths, if there is infiltration of the shaft of the penis, or when radiotherapy fails. When an advanced infiltrating or anaplastic lesion is present, total amputation must be performed.

THE TESTIS AND THE SCROTUM

Congenital anomalies

Imperfect descent of the testis

Under this heading are included two conditions: first incomplete descent, the testis being arrested in some part of its path to the scrotum, and second, maldescent of the testis to an ectopic site, where the testis is abnormally placed outside its path.

Incomplete descent. In the neonatal period for a variable number of weeks after birth the cremasteric reflex which is so active in young boys is absent. Imperfect descent is present on both sides in 4% of full-term infants, and in 30% of premature infants (Fig. 41.7). Follow-up of these cases, however, reveals that 50% of the testes reach the scrotum during the first month of life. More often than not, imperfect descent of the testis is not detected during infancy. In later childhood and puberty the incidence is 2%. In adult life it is inconceivable that a man could fail to notice the absence of one or both testes in his scrotum, yet there must be many with this abnormality who do not seek advice about it unless symptoms develop.

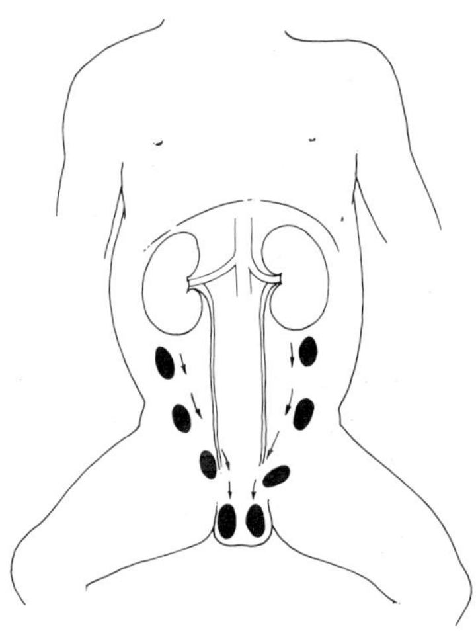

Fig. 41.7 Various levels at which the testis may become arrested during its normal embryological descent.

Pathology

Up to the age of 6 years there are no macroscopical differences between an incompletely descended testis and a normal one. After that time, due, it is believed, to the higher temperature to which the testis is subjected, the development of the incompletely descended organ becomes progressively retarded. By puberty the incompletely descended testis is flabby and hardly more than half the size of its intrascrotal counterpart. Histologically the epithelial elements are grossly immature, and by the age of 16 this is irreversible. The external secretory mechanism of an incompletely descended testis functions only feebly, and often after a few months or years it ceases altogether. Thus its power of spermatogenesis is negligible. Internal secretory activity of an incompletely descended testis is reduced. In bilateral cryptorchidism about half the normal amount of androgen is produced. Notwithstanding, the secondary sexual attributes of a cryptorchid are seldom noticeably in abeyance. If an incompletely descended testis is brought down satisfactorily before puberty it often develops and functions normally.

Clinical features

The right testis alone is affected in 50% of cases, the left alone in 30%, while double arrested descent occurs in 20%. Other abnormalities of the urinary tract may also be present. Major abnormalities have been found in intravenous pyelograms in 13.5% of children with cryptorchidism. The testes may be retained within the abdomen extraperitoneally, usually just above the internal abdominal ring, or in the inguinal canal. Early in life the testis is a soft structure and when, as in this instance, it is submerged in the non-resisting floor of the inguinal canal and shielded by overlying tendinous aponeurosis of the external oblique, it cannot be felt in the superficial subinguinal pouch. Very frequently during childhood the testes are mobile, each being withdrawn by contraction of the cremaster into the superfical subinguinal pouch, a space lined by loose areolar tissue lying beneath Scarpa's fascia, and superficial to the external oblique aponeurosis.

The hazards of incomplete descent

1. Sterility in bilateral cases.
2. Pain — an inguinal testis is liable to oft-repeated trauma.

3. An associated indirect inguinal or interstitial hernia is present in 70% of cases.
4. Torsion.
5. Right-sided epididymo-orchitis occurring in an incompletely descended organ is extremely difficult if not impossible to differentiate from acute appendicitis.
6. Atrophy—even before puberty this sometimes occurs, when the testis is situated in the inguinal canal.
7. Increased liability to malignant disease. All types of malignant testicular tumour have been recorded as developing in undescended testes.

Treatment by orchidopexy

Most surgeons favour performing the operation between the ages of 6 and 8 years. Many choose the earlier age in order to reduce the incidence of thermal damage to the germinal epithelium. After the age of puberty the percentage of successful operations, which at the optimum age approaches 80%, falls considerably. In cryptorchidism one side should be operated upon at a time, with an interval of 6 months between operations.

Ectopic testis

An ectopic testis may be found, in order of frequency:

1. Anchored to the superficial inguinal pouch.
2. In the perineum.
3. At the root of the penis.
4. In the femoral triangle.

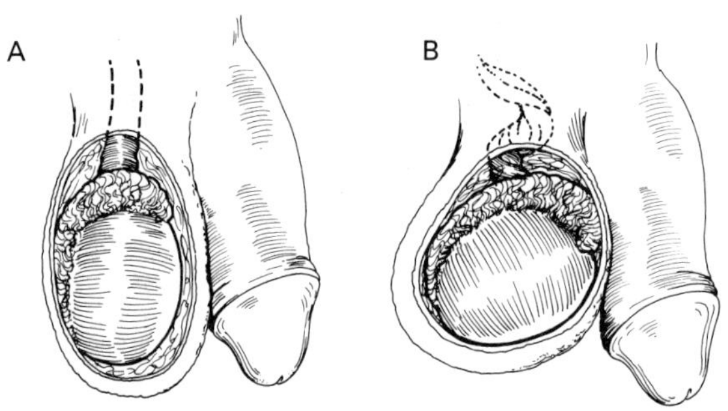

Fig. 41.8 Torsion of the testis. (**A**) The normal disposition of the scrotal contents; (**B**) the testis and epididymis are lying transversely, and the spermatic cord is elongated. Both these factors predispose to rotation, twisting of the cord (as shown) and thus compressive occlusion of the blood supply to the testis.

Injuries to the testis

Closed rupture of the testis from a blow is an uncommon accident, owing to the extreme mobility of the organ within the scrotum. Severe contusion and rupture are each associated with a haematocele, which surrounds the testis. Operation is advisable in these cases in order to evacuate the haematoma, and repair the tunica albuginea if split.

Torsion of the testis

Predisposing causes

Torsion of the testis is uncommon. It does not occur in normally developed fully descended testes, the anchorage of which prevents rotation. Therefore one of several anomalies must be present (Fig. 41.8).

1. Inversion of the testis—this appears to be the commonest predisposing cause.
2. High investment of the tunica vaginalis causes the testis to hang in the tunica like the clapper in a bell. Very occasionally torsion will then be intravaginal.
3. In cases where the body of the testis is separated from the epididymis torsion of the body can occur without involving the cord.

Precipitating factors

Normally the cremaster contracts pari passu with violent contraction of the abdominal musculature, and contractions of the spirally attached cremaster favour rotation round the vertical axis. Straining at stool, lifting a heavy weight, and coitus are all precipitating factors, but often the history fails to reveal any of them. Occasionally torsion may develop during sleep.

Clinical features

The highest incidence is between 15 and 25 years of age, and the second most common age period is during infancy. Symptoms vary with the degree of torsion present. Most commonly the patient experiences sudden and agonizing pain in the groin and lower abdomen, and vomits. Upon theoretical grounds one might think that the diagnosis is simple, but sometimes it is practically impossible to distinguish torsion of an imperfectly descended testis from a strangulated inguinal hernia, until the parts have been displayed at operation.

Treatment

Urgent operation is indicated, as after 6 h of strangulation the chance of the testis recovering is small. In a few early cases it may be possible to untwist the cord under vision, in which case should an improvement in the colour of the organ result, and the testis is fully descended, it can be spared, but it is essential to fix the testis in an anatomically correct position. More usually orchidectomy must be performed. Experience has shown that in cases where torsion occurs the congenital abnormality that permits twisting appertains on both sides. Therefore the contralateral organ should be fixed in the scrotum at the same operation. By failing to observe this precaution patients may lose both testes from torsion.

Torsion of an appendage of the testis

Vestigial structures related to the testis and the epididymis are liable to undergo axial rotation, and most common of these structures to twist is the appendix of the epididymis. Torsion of an appendage of the testis is essentially a lesion occurring before or at the age of puberty. The condition is often mistaken for acute epididymo-orchitis. Immediate operation with ligation of the pedicle and amputation of the appendage cures the condition.

Varicocele

Varicocele is common in young men, and consists of dilatation of the pampiniform plexus above the testis. The left side is more commonly affected. These veins drain into the internal spermatic vein in the region of the internal inguinal ring. This vein passes lateral to the vas deferens at the internal inguinal ring, and on the left side drains into the renal vein. On the right side it empties into the vena cava. The left internal spermatic vein is particularly liable to have incompetent valves. This fact, plus gravity, may lead to poor drainage of the pampiniform plexus, the veins of which undergo dilatation and elongation. At times they are painful, particularly in sexually continent men. Marriage in this instance may relieve symptoms. The sudden development of a varicocele in an older man is sometimes seen as a late sign of renal tumour, when the tumour cells have invaded the renal vein, thereby occluding the spermatic vein.

Examination of a man with varicocele reveals a mass of dilated tortuous veins lying posterior to and above the testis. It may extend up to the external inguinal ring and is often tender. Testicular atrophy from impaired circulation may be present. No treatment is required unless the varicocele is thought to contribute to infertility, or is painful, or so large as to disturb the patient. A scrotal support will often relieve discomfort. Otherwise ligation of the internal spermatic vein at the internal inguinal ring is indicated. The results from this operation are uniformly excellent.

Hydrocele

A hydrocele consists of a collection of fluid within the tunica or processus vaginalis (Fig. 41.9). Although it may occur within the spermatic cord it is most often seen surrounding the testicle. A hydrocele may develop rapidly secondary to local

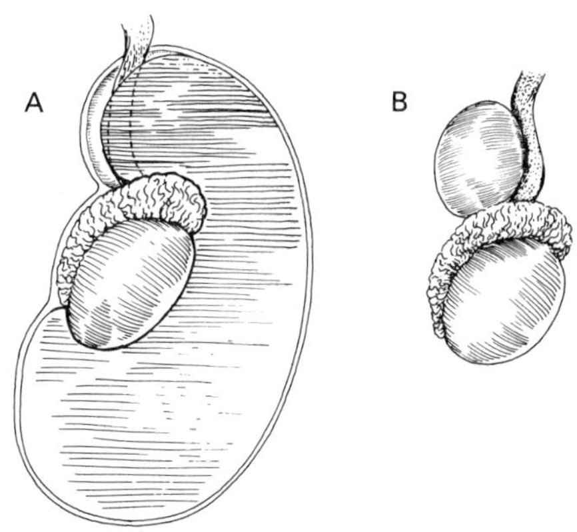

Fig. 41.9 (**A**) Hydrocele: a collection of fluid inside an expanded tunica vaginalis. (**B**) Epididymal cyst arising from part of the tubular network of the epididymis, and located usually above and posterior to the otherwise readily palpable testis.

injury, acute non-specific or tuberculous epididymitis or orchitis. It may complicate testicular neoplasm. Chronic hydrocele is more common, its cause is unknown, and it usually afflicts men past the age of 40 years. Fluid collects about the testis and the mass grows gradually. It may be soft and cystic or even tense, and the fluid is clear and yellow. Hydrocele of the tunica vaginalis is common in the newborn, probably due to late closure of the processus vaginalis which is continuous with the peritoneum. Most of these fluid collections subside spontaneously during the first few weeks of life.

Clinical features

Young boys with hydrocele commonly have a history of a cystic mass which is small and soft in the morning but larger and more tense at night. One can conclude in these instances that a small communication exists in the processus vaginalis between the peritoneal cavity and the tunica vaginalis. Hernia or communicating hydrocele is therefore the proper diagnosis.

Hydrocele is painless unless it is accompanied by acute epididymal infection. The patient may, however, complain of its bulk or weight. The diagnosis is made by finding a rounded, cystic, intrascrotal mass which is not tender unless underlying inflammatory disease is present, and it generally transilluminates quite clearly. If the hydrocele is enclosed within the spermatic cord a cystic fusiform swelling is noted in the groin, or in the upper scrotum. A tense hydrocele must be differentiated from tumour of the testis, which does not illuminate. However, if a hydrocele develops in a young man without apparent cause, it should be aspirated so that careful palpation of the testis and epididymis can be carried out. Haemorrhage into a hydrocele sac following trauma leads to haematocele, or rarely infection complicating an aspiration.

Treatment

Unless complications are present, active therapy is not required. Indications for treatment are a very tense hydrocele which might embarrass circulation to the testis or a large bulky mass which is cosmetically unacceptable. A single aspiration of the hydrocele which is present during the first few months of life is often curative. Periodic aspiration is usually the treatment of choice in chronic hydrocele. Most chronic hydroceles refill slowly over a period of 6–20 weeks. Surgical correction of the hydrocele can be achieved by either excision of the hydrocele, or by inversion of the hydrocele with or without plication of the tunica vaginalis.

Epididymal cyst (spermatocele)

A spermatocele is a painless cystic mass containing sperm. It lies just above and posterior to the testis, but is separate from it. Most spermatoceles are less than 1 cm in diameter, although they are occasionally quite large and may be mistaken for a hydrocele. They may be firm, simulating solid tumour. The aetiology is not entirely clear although they probably arise from tubules that connect the rete testis to the head of the epididymis (the vasa efferentia) or from cystic structures in the upper pole of the testis or epididymis. Since they are relatively small spermatoceles are usually discovered by the physician during routine examination. At times they may be large enough to come to the patient's attention, in which event he may request their excision.

Acute epididymo-orchitis

In many instances inflammation remains confined to the epididymis, in which case it is referred to as epididymitis. When the infection spreads to the body of the testis the condition is known as epididymo-orchitis. In cases where the inflammation is situated mainly, if not entirely, in the body of the testis, the term 'orchitis' is employed.

Mode of infection

As a rule infection reaches the epididymis via the lumen of the vas and affects the globus minor first. It is secondary to infection of the urethra, prostate or the seminal vesicles. Blood-borne infections affect the globus major of the testis primarily.

Clinical features

The initial symptoms are those of acute prostatitis. Some days later an ache in the groin with some increase in fever heralds the onset of epididymitis. Severe pain and swelling of the testis occurs rapidly. The scrotal wall becomes red and oedematous and shiny, and the epididymis may become adherent to the scrotal skin, and may soften and later discharge. Resolution is heralded by scaling of the scrotal skin. Acute epididymitis due to *Escherichia coli*, streptococcus, staphylococcus or pneumococcus is not uncommon. As a rule there is no evidence of urethritis, especially in *Escherichia coli* infection. It is sometimes unaccompanied by infection of the urine. Acute epididymitis may complicate non-gonococcal urethritis, acute gonococcal epididymitis, epididymitis from retrograde passage of urine, acute tuberculous epididymitis and acute epididymo-orchitis of mumps.

Treatment

The patient must be kept in bed until the acute symptoms have abated. A broad-spectrum antibiotic, such as tetracycline, should be given until the resultant urine culture is available. The scrotum is supported on a sling formed by broad adhesive plaster attached across the thighs. Upon this sling is placed a nest of cotton wool and in this the inflamed organ rests. Cooling lotions can be applied. The urine is rendered alkaline and a high fluid intake is necessary. Antibiotic treatment should be continued for 2 weeks, until the inflammation has subsided. If suppuration occurs drainage is necessary. Atrophy of the testis may follow as a sequela in any case of epididymo-orchitis.

Chronic epididymo-orchitis

Nearly 90% of cases of chronic epididymo-orchitis are a result of tuberculosis and the great majority commence insidiously.

Clinical features

Slight ache in the testis or a trivial injury calls the patient's attention to the swelling in relation to the testis. An early manifestation is a discrete, indurated slightly tender nodule in the globus minor, rarely in the globus major. As the disease progresses other nodules appear and eventually the entire epididymis becomes involved and it is felt as a firm, craggy, often painless mass situated behind the testis. In 30% of cases a lax secondary hydrocele is present. Rectal examination reveals a thickened, and later an irregular, indurated seminal vesicle on the corresponding side, and sometimes of the contralateral vesicle as well. The prostate in advanced cases contains one or more discrete nodules. In two-thirds of cases there is either active tuberculosis in the renal tract or evidence of previous disease. In the remainder the patient is apparently healthy. In all cases of chronic epididymitis the urine is examined for tubercle bacilli, if necessary on several occasions, and pyelography should be undertaken. The chest is X-rayed and evidence of previous tuberculous disease will be present in approximately 50% of cases.

Treatment

In tuberculosis epididymitis is secondary; the primary lesion should receive priority. Epididymitis may well resolve during treatment. The treatment of genitourinary tuberculosis has been discussed earlier.

Testicular tumours

Germ cell tumours are the most common form of malignancy occurring in men aged between 20 and 40 years and the incidence appears to be rising, having doubled in the past 15 years. Approximately 900 new cases per year are registered in England and Wales. The risk of testicular tumour is increased in patients with a history of testicular maldescent, although only 10% of germ cell tumours occur in this background. In unilateral maldescent the main risk is to the affected testis. However, there is also a slightly increased risk of germ cell tumour arising in the contralateral testis. Testicular tumours occurring in individuals aged more than 50 years are mainly non-germ cell tumours such as lymphoma, or occasionally stromal tumour.

Diagnosis and staging

The peak age of incidence for testicular tumours is 30 years, with a range from 15 to 45 years. Testicular tumours usually present with a painless swelling of the testis which on examination feels heavy and hard. Some discomfort in the testis or lower abdomen is noticed in 10–20% of patients and occasionally sharp discomfort follows trauma, probably secondary to intratumoural bleeding. Rarely patients present with gynaecomastia as an effect of non-metastatic tumour. Nipple hypersensitivity may occur as a milder form, and there may be symptoms secondary to metastatic disease, such as backache unrelated to posture, which is typical of retroperitoneal lymphadenopathy, and loin pain which may be secondary to ureteric obstruction.

The differential diagnosis of testicular tumour is from epididymitis, torsion of the testis, granulomatous orchitis, tuberculosis, and gumma. Testicular ultrasonography may be helpful in distinguishing epididymitis where clinical assessment is difficult. Diagnosis is confirmed by inguinal orchidectomy. Scrotal incisions are considered to predispose to local scar recurrence.

Pathology

Most testicular tumours occurring in young adults are germ cell tumours. Rare tumours of the testis and adjacent structures include interstitial cell tumours, Sertoli cell tumours, lymphoma, carcinoma of the rete testis, mesothelioma of the tunica vaginalis and paratesticular rabdomyosarcoma. These rare subtypes will not be discussed further in this chapter.

Classification of germ cell tumours

Teratoma

The classification of teratoma used in the UK and the USA recognizes four types:

1. Malignant teratoma—undifferentiated (embryonal carcinoma).
2. Malignant teratoma—intermediate (teratocarcinoma).
3. Malignant teratoma trophoblastic (choriocarcinoma).
4. Teratoma differentiated (teratoma).

The commonest histological subtypes are malignant teratoma undifferentiated and malignant teratoma intermediate. Both subtypes may contain undifferentiated teratoma, but the intermediate variety also has areas of somatic differentiation. A variant of the undifferentiated form of the tumour appears to be entirely composed of a pattern resembling yolk sac. Differentiated teratoma pursues an indolent and usually benign course. Malignant teratoma trophoblastic is usually an aggressive tumour with widespread metastatic potential and rapid growth rate. Different types of teratoma may coexist within the same tumour. Malignant teratomas comprise approximately 35% of all germ cell tumours.

Seminoma

Anaplastic seminoma is a morphological variant of classical seminoma, with the same apparent natural history. Some patients with seminoma have syncytiotrophoblasts, but again these do not appear to change the prognosis. A rare variant in elderly men is spermatocytic seminoma which follows a benign course. About 45% of all germ cell tumours are seminomas.

Combined teratoma and seminoma

Both these elements may be present within the primary tumour, and either or both elements may metastasize. For the purposes of management such tumours are treated as a subgroup of malignant teratoma. Combined tumours comprise approximately 20% of germ cell tumours.

Tumour markers

Either or both of the tumour markers alphafetoprotein (AFP) and beta-human chorionic gonadotrophin (hCG) are expressed in 75% of germ cell tumours. These markers are paramount among tumour markers in oncology because of their sensitivity and specificity. The range of application of AFP and hCG allows them to be used as a diagnostic aid for staging and for prognosis, and also for assessment of the response to treatment and the detection of relapse and for potential immunolocalization.

AFP is an oncofetal antigen, and is the fetal equivalent of serum albumin. It is expressed by yolk sac elements within the tumour and can be detected using immunoperoxidase staining.

The alpha chain of hCG is shared with other

pituitary hormones, but the beta chain is unique. Antibodies to the beta chain are therefore used to detect this marker. HCG is associated in particular with trophoblastic elements within the tumour. In the presence of metastatic teratoma, serum levels may be very high indeed.

Staging, investigation and classification

Following the establishment of the diagnosis, usually by orchidectomy, staging investigations should be performed to determine the extent and volume of metastatic disease, and to define the serum concentration of tumour markers. Standard investigations include an assay of serum AFP and hCG and a computerized tomography scan of the thorax and abdomen. Abdominal computerized tomography scan may occasionally be complemented by lymphangiography in equivocal cases. Thoracic computerized tomography scan is more sensitive than plain X-ray, especially when thin slices are examined.

Staging classification

The Royal Marsden staging classification is widely used and has two main features. First, metastatic disease is divided according to extent such that abdominal nodal metastases are classed as stage II, subdiaphragmatic metastases as stage III and extranodal metastases as stage IV. Second, metastases are subdivided by bulk—abdominal and lung metastases in particular. Abdominal metastases are divided by maximum transverse diameter into categories A, B and C.

Treatment of testicular tumours

Management of teratoma

Stage I teratoma is defined by the absence of metastatic disease radiologically and by the fall of serum tumour markers and beta-hCG to normal levels following orchidectomy. A range of approaches is available for the treatment of stage I teratoma following orchidectomy. Very high cure rates are attained, and the priority is therefore to achieve a cure with minimal morbidity. The option that is now widely practised throughout the UK is to manage the patient by surveillance alone following orchidectomy. About one-quarter of patients classified as having stage I malignant teratoma have subclinical metastatic disease and will relapse. Surveillance detects relapse at an early stage when the results of treatment are excellent.

Metastatic malignant teratoma

There have been major advances in the treatment of metastatic malignant teratoma since the introduction of cisplatin in combination with treatment with vinblastine and bleomycin. With this combination, response rates approach 100% and experience over the past 10 years has shown that 70–80% of patients with metastatic malignant teratoma can be cured. These are, however, very potent drugs and there are a number of toxic side-effects associated with their use, in particular pneumonitis, neurotoxicity, renal toxicity and ototoxicity. Both drugs cause vomiting and depress the bone marrow.

Management of seminoma

Stage I seminoma. Most patients present with stage I disease and management is dictated by two important biological properties of the seminoma. First, the tumour metastasizes in an orderly progression to abdominal nodes, and then to subdiaphragmatic nodes, and thereafter to cxtranodal sites. Second, the tumour is probably the most sensitive of all tumours to radiation. The management of stage I seminoma has therefore consisted of adjuvant irradiation of abdominopelvic lymph nodes for the treatment of subclinical metastatic disease. Surveillance studies suggest that subclinical abdominal nodal metastases occur in approximately 15% of patients with stage I seminoma. The results of management by radiotherapy are excellent.

Metastatic seminoma

Previously metastatic seminoma was managed by radiotherapy alone. More recently, though, the combination schedules used to treat seminoma are the same as those used for non-seminoma. Cisplatin-based combinations are highly effective with long-term survival rates of approximately 90%. Even very large masses of metastatic seminoma can be cured with chemotherapy.

42. Head injury

Head injuries have already acquired an epidemic proportion in most countries of the world. In most advanced countries they are the commonest cause of death in younger age groups, and even in developing countries the incidence is rapidly approaching similar levels. They account for 70% of fatal road accidents.

The term head injury embraces a wide variety of lesions, ranging from an innocuous scalp laceration or minor concussion to gross brain damage resulting in instantaneous death. In a given patient the clinical picture may be confusing because of the coexistence or sequential evolution of concussion, compression due to an intracranial haematoma, cerebral contusion, secondary brain oedema, and foraminal herniation through tentorium or foramen magnum. All may be seen in variable combinations in a single patient at different times. In dealing with a patient after a head injury one is presented with a dynamic, changing clinical picture resulting from an interplay of the immediate consequences of the traumatic forces, nature's attempt at resolution of the same, and secondary phenomena developing at varying intervals after the injury. Notwithstanding this complexity, in the following account an attempt is made to simplify the situation by first considering these lesions individually as distinct entities. This is followed by an outline plan of action for the management of a given patient.

PATHOPHYSIOLOGY

Mechanism of injury

Besides the direct impact of the injuring force, a variety of other mechanical factors play a significant role in determining the type, extent and severity of damage to various structures.

1. A direct blow results in a local distortion of the skull, and also generates a pressure-field within the cranium. The skull distortion may result in local injury to the scalp, skull and the underlying brain. The ultimate result of both factors depends upon the severity of the blow, the nature of impact, and the plasticity of the skull.
2. Acceleration and deceleration forces: in cases of assault the important factor is the acceleration resulting from the stationary head being hit by a mobile object. These forces produce not only linear motion, but also rotational and shearing stresses at sites far removed from the site of impact. In contrast, in the majority of traffic accidents or falls the important factor is the

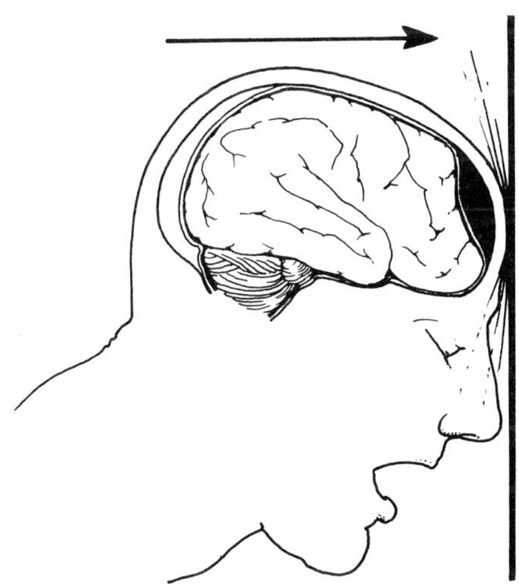

Fig. 42.1 Direct damage to brain and overlying tissues resulting at point of impact from acceleration injury.

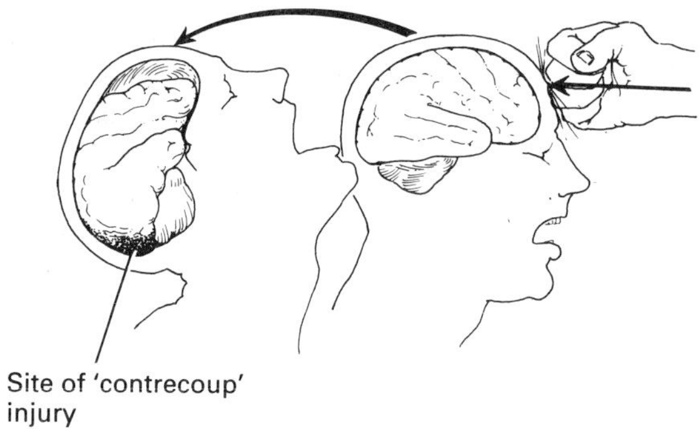

Fig. 42.2 Contrecoup injury: see text.

deceleration resulting from a moving head striking an immovable object, e.g. the road. To produce concussion a greater force is required if the head is fixed and stable than when the head is mobile (Fig. 42.1).

3. Coup and contrecoup injuries: injury occurring on the side of the impact on the skull is designated as coup injury. Not infrequently the diametrically opposite part of the brain also suffers a contusion and this is known as contrecoup injury (Fig. 42.2). Thus contusion of the occipital lobe may follow a frontal impact and vice versa, causing the moving surface of the brain to come into forceful contact with the skull. This is due to the differential movement of the two structures.
4. Differential mobility of various structures: as the elasticity and density of the various structures, i.e. the scalp, the skull, the dura and the brain, are different, any force applied to the head causes variable movement of these in relation to the others, resulting in shearing strains.
5. Existence of intracranial partitions: the brain is neither completely fixed nor freely mobile inside the cranial cavity. The falx cerebri and the tentorium not only restrict the free mobility of the brain during acceleration and deceleration, but also act as rigid structures against which the moving brain may strike and thereby be damaged. Furthermore, these partitions add to the rotational forces, which are mostly centred in the region of the upper brainstem.
6. Configuration of the interior of the skull: the damage to the brain as a result of its mobility within the cranium is further influenced by the existence of jutting bone edges like the lesser wing of the sphenoid, the petrous temporal bones, and the crista galli. Damage is also more likely in regions where the internal surface of the bone is more irregular, e.g. the anterior cranial fossa as compared to the smooth surface of the vault.

PRIMARY LESIONS

Diffuse brain damage

Mild forms of diffuse brain damage (diffuse neuronal injury) are responsible for cerebral concussion, whereas more severe forms result in prolonged unconsciousness, perhaps followed by mental disturbance if the patient recovers. The underlying pathological lesion responsible for these states is diffuse damage to neurocytes and axons. This later may lead to widespread degeneration of the white matter, as has been shown in both experimental and human material. Secondary hypoxia or anoxia may contribute to these changes. There is reasonable evidence to suggest that at least for cerebral concussion, the primary site of neuronal dysfunction is in the rostral brainstem, i.e. the pons and medulla.

Trauma

Trauma may result in gross macroscopic disruption of continuity of the brain tissue (laceration), or damage without actual separation of tissues characterized by bruising, a gelatinous-looking stain, or reddish-blue discoloration due to subpial haemorrhage (contusion).

Blood vessel injury

Associated injury to blood vessels may produce haemorrhage into the extradural, subdural, subarachnoid, subpial or intracerebral spaces. The main danger of this occurrence is that the collection of blood may compress vital brain tissue in the confined space of the skull.

SECONDARY LESIONS

Brain swelling

Brain swelling or oedema may supervene on any

of these lesions. Cerebral contusion, laceration and intracerebral haemorrhages are surrounded by a zone of oedema which may acquire such a magnitude as to cause a dangerous increase in intracranial pressure. As a result of the combined effects of the shed blood and oedema the increased bulk of the intracranial contents inside the rigid skull may cause herniation of brain tissue through the skull apertures.

Foraminal or tentorial herniation

The two principal sites at which herniation (also referred to as Coning) can occur are the tentorium, against which the uncus may be pressed, and the foramen magnum, through which the cerebellar tonsils may be forced. The herniated brain tissues are compressed, displaced and distorted, and both secondary haemorrhage and ischaemic necrosis may result. As a consequence there may be pressure on the midbrain, the oculomotor nerves and the posterior cerebral arteries, in the case of uncal herniation, and on the medulla in the case of tonsillar herniation.

CLINICOPATHOLOGICAL MANIFESTATIONS

Scalp injuries and haematoma

The scalp consists of five layers—skin, subcutaneous tissue, aponeurosis, loose areolar tissue and pericranium. It has a very rich vascular supply. As a rule the arteries run vertically from the base of the skull towards the vertex. In an open wound fibrous septa criss-crossing the subcutaneous tissue layer hold the ruptured vessels open. On the other hand if a haematoma develops in this layer, it produces a small rounded localized swelling 2–3 cm in diameter. In contrast to this, if bleeding occurs deep to the galea aponeurotica, in the layer of loose areolar tissue, a large amount of blood can accumulate, limited only by the attachment of the aponeurosis to the supraorbital ridge anteriorly, zygomatic arch inferiorly and the occipital crest posteriorly. Loss of blood in this layer may even be severe enough in a child to result in shock and anaemia. Haematoma deep to the pericranium—the classical cephalhematoma seen in birth injury—acquires the outline of the underlying bone due to attachment of the pericranium at the suture lines.

Bleeding from a scalp wound can easily be stopped by applying pressure to the edges of the wound or at operation by everting the edges by artery forceps applied to the galea. Attempts to catch individual bleeding points are unnecessary and often unrewarding.

Fracture of the skull

Like fractures in other parts of the body, skull fractures may be simple or compound. They may become compound not only as a result of an associated scalp wound but also by involving the paranasal sinuses or mastoid air cells.

The pattern of fracture may be:

1. linear (Fig. 42.3), stellate or comminuted (Fig. 42.4);

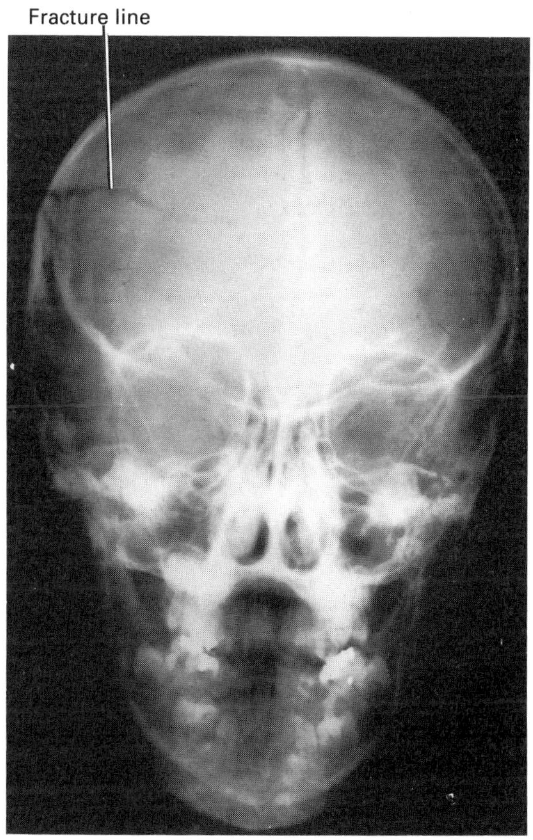

Fig. 42.3 X-ray showing simple linear fracture of the vault of the skull, with no displacement.

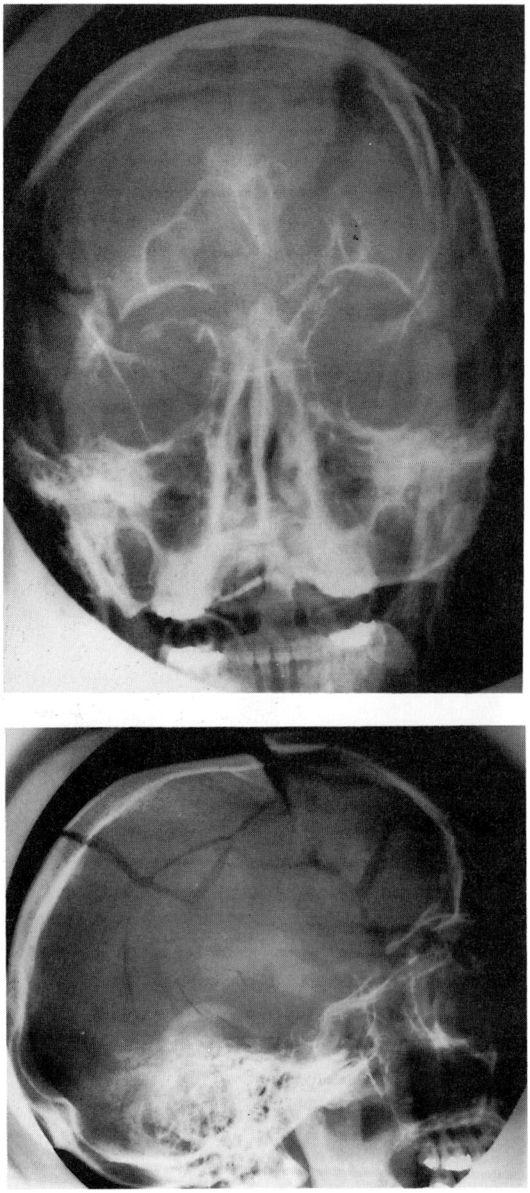

A

B

Fig. 42.4 (A) Anteroposterior and (B) lateral views of a grossly comminuted compound fracture of the skull. There is considerable displacement of the various fragments, and disruption of the frontal air sinuses and orbits.

2. depressed (Fig. 42.5), either as a well defined disc of bone—the so-called pond fracture—or a more irregular spiked depression giving a rosette outline;
3. rarely, elevated, due to the prising up of a segment of bone secondary to a tangential injury.

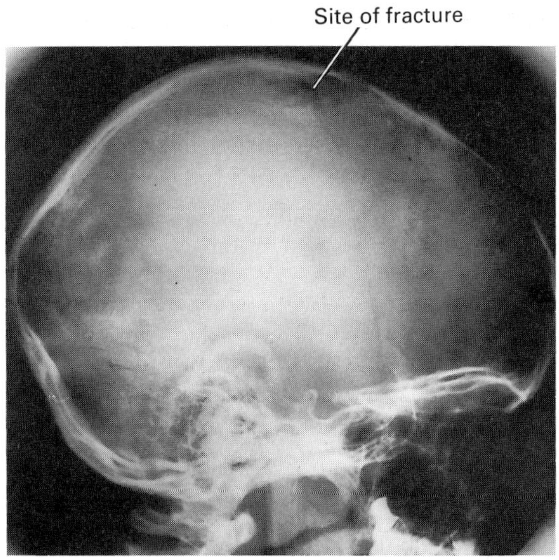

Fig. 42.5 Small localized depressed fracture following impact with small rounded hammer head.

Fracture may involve the vault, the base or both. Linear fractures acquire special significance when they cross vascular markings (e.g. the middle meningeal artery groove) or the paranasal sinuses. In the former case, the risk of an associated extradural haematoma injury due to damage to the dural vessels is high. As mentioned above, a fracture through an air sinus is to be treated as compound.

Depressed fractures

These are of special importance as they are likely to be associated with damage to the underlying brain. In this respect a smooth depression is less dangerous than a sharp jagged depressed fragment, the latter being more likely to pierce the dura and lacerate the brain. A blow with a large rounded object is more likely to result in the former pond type of depressed fracture. This is usually closed, with bruising of the overlying scalp, but the underlying dura remains intact and the underlying brain surface may or may not be contused. The so-called ping-pong ball fracture seen in birth injuries belongs to this category. In contrast, a blow from a small round object or a sharp heavy object usually produces a compound depressed fracture. Depending upon the force and nature of injury, irregular depressed fragments of bone may pierce the dura and lacerate the underlying brain. It is this type of injury which is associated with an increased risk of infection in the initial stage, and epilepsy as a late sequel.

Fracture of the base of the skull

These are usually associated with more severe injury to the brain. As they often involve the various foramina in the base of the skull, they are likely to result in cranial nerve injuries. Involvement of the paranasal sinuses or mastoid air cells may result in cerebrospinal fluid (CSF) rhinorrhoea or otorrhoea and predispose to intracranial infective complications like meningitis and abscess. These fractures are difficult to visualize in routine X-rays of the skull, but can often be suspected from clinical examination alone.

Fracture in the anterior cranial fossa

Leakage of CSF or brain matter through the nose is a sure sign of a fracture through the anterior cranial fossa. Delayed development of periorbital haematomas and fan-shaped subconjunctival haemorrhage with the apex towards the limbus and an undefinable posterior limit are signs strongly suggestive of such a lesion. There may be unilateral or bilateral exophthalmos. Injury to the olfactory and optic nerves may also be associated. X-ray of the skull may reveal opacity of the ethmoid air cells.

Fracture in the middle cranial fossa

Escape of CSF or brain matter through the ear is a sure sign of fracture of the middle fossa. Delayed development of ecchymosis of the skin over the mastoid (Battle's sign) or infranuclear facial nerve palsy is commonly present. Plain X-ray of the skull may reveal opacity of the sphenoid sinus or the mastoid air cells.

Fracture in the posterior cranial fossa

Damage to the lower cranial nerves (IX – XII) or delayed development of suboccipital ecchymosis should arouse suspicion of a fracture in this fossa.

INTRACRANIAL HAEMORRHAGE

Subarachnoid haemorrhage

This is a frequent occurrence following a head injury. It results from a tear of a bridging vein, a surface vessel or, more frequently, secondary to a contusion or laceration of the brain (Fig.42.6). Depending upon the amount of blood leaked out, it results in varying degrees of meningeal irritation. Clinical manifestations are throbbing headache, pain behind the eyes and in the neck, neck stiffness, photophobia, vomiting, and positive Kernig's sign (painful neck rigidity on attempting passively to flex the head forward). A lumbar puncture may be required to differentiate it from meningitis.

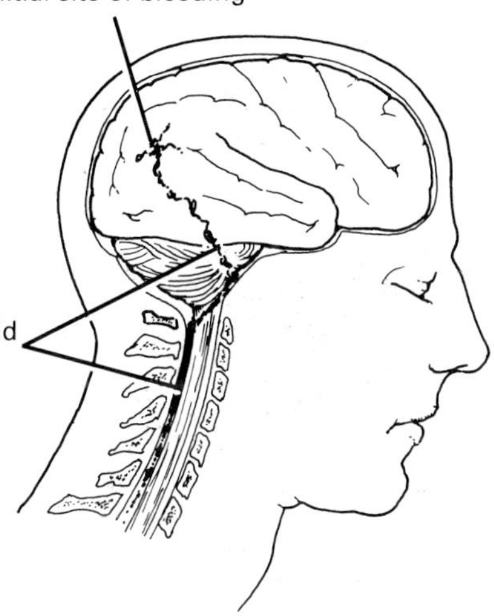

Fig. 42.6 Subarachnoid haemorrhage: blood which has leaked out into the space can trickle down along the continuation of this space along the spinal cord and therefore be detected on lumbar puncture of the subarachnoid space.

Extradural or epidural haematoma

Anatomically there is no true extradural space in the calvarium since the dura is closely applied to the inner table of the skull. Hence for an extradural haematoma to develop, there must be stripping of the dura from this inner table. Since the dura is more densely adherent to the skull at the extremes of ages, extradural haematomas are uncommon in infancy and early childhood and in aged persons.

Extradural haematoma results from injury to the middle meningeal vessels (not necessarily the artery

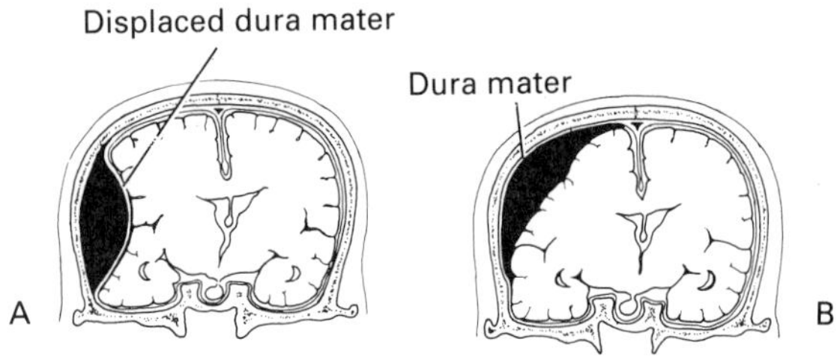

Fig. 42.7 (**A**) Extradural haemorrhage, usually from a tear of the middle meningeal vessels; the escaped blood strips the dura from the inner surface of the skull. (**B**) Subdural haemorrhage is into the loose space below the dura mater, which remains attached to the inner surface of the skull.

only), or to the dural venous sinuses (Fig. 42.7). A variable amount of extradural blood generally accompanies any fracture, but it forms a significant haematoma if a major diploic channel is involved. The commonest site of extradural haematoma is the middle cranial fossa, but it can occur anywhere in the cranial cavity, and is rarely bilateral or both supra- and infratentorial. Associated direct injury to the brain is relatively much less frequent as compared to subdural haematoma.

The clinical picture will depend upon the severity and site of the injury, and the source of bleeding, i.e. arterial or venous. The classical sequence of events is of a relatively minor injury (hit with a ball, fall from a bicycle, etc.) followed by initial loss of consciousness (concussion), recovery of consciousness, during which time the patient may appear to recover fully and continue with whatever he or she was doing—the lucid interval, followed by progressive development of symptoms and signs of increasing cerebral compression. This phase is characterized by increasing headache, vomiting, rapidly deteriorating consciousness, progressive ipsilateral third-nerve palsy (dilatation of pupil, ptosis, and ophthalmoplegia), and contralateral hemiplegia. If the haematoma is not evacuated promptly this leads to deep coma, decerebration, arrest of respiration and death. The march of these events can be extremely fast. As a rule, once the symptoms of cerebral compression set in the progress is in minutes and hours rather than days.

The so-called classical picture is, however, observed in less than 50% of cases. In the majority, the clinical course is very variable. The initial injury itself may be severe enough that the patient does not recover from the initial concussion before the signs of compression set in. On the other hand, in some cases, especially if the source of haemorrhage is venous or the haematoma is located in the anterior or posterior cranial fossa where there are no large meningeal vessels, the clinical course evolves more slowly with a prolonged lucid interval. Rarely an extradural haematoma may have a chronic course. Even the classical picture is not necessarily diagnostic of extradural haematoma. An identical clinical picture may be seen in acute subdural haematoma, intracerebral haematoma, or even cerebral contusion and laceration with brain oedema.

It is important to have a high degree of suspicion of the lesion, with careful and repeated observation to detect at the earliest moment the symptoms and signs of increasing cerebral compression. A boggy swelling in the temporal region, bruising or contusion of the skin in this area and detection on X-ray of a fracture crossing the groove for the middle meningeal vessels should alert the surgeon to such a possibility.

Subdural haematoma

There is a potential subdural space between the dura and the arachnoid. The superficial cerebral veins cross this space before entering the dural sinuses. Movement of the brain during acceleration or deceleration not only opens up this space, but also predisposes to rupture of these bridging veins, leading to extravasation of blood into this space (Fig. 42.8). In other cases a surface contusion or laceration of the brain with a tear in the arachnoid mater may be responsible for haemorrhage into

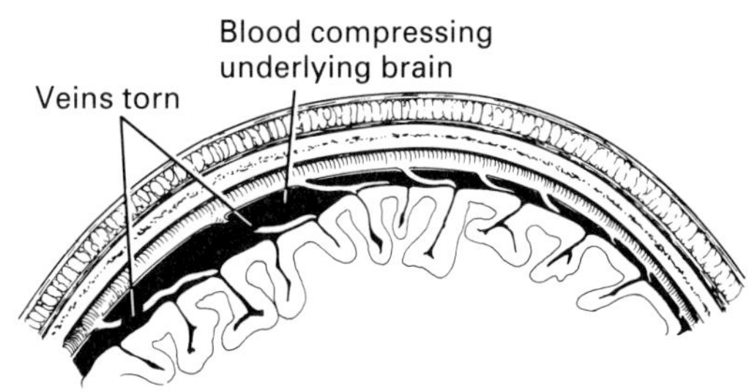

Fig. 42.8 Subdural haemorrhage: veins crossing from the brain surface into the large venous sinuses are torn, and the leaked blood collects, exerting pressure on the underlying brain.

the subdural space. Unlike the case of extradural haematoma, associated direct injury of the brain is a rule rather than an exception in a patient with acute subdural haematoma. In the large majority of such cases the clinical picture and outcome are determined by the extent of the associated parenchymatous damage rather than the compressive effect of the subdural blood.

Classically subdural haematomas are classified as acute, subacute and chronic. There is some confusion regarding the definition of these categories, but it is generally agreed that an acute subdural haematoma should be manifest within 3 days and the subacute within 3 weeks. Chronic subdural haematoma, which really is a distinct entity in itself (see later), becomes symptomatic more than 3 weeks after the injury, which is often a trivial one.

Acute subdural haematoma. A thin film of subdural blood overlies most cerebral contusions and lacerations. This is usually of little clinical significance. Occasionally, due to rupture of a major draining vein or venous sinus, the subdural collection may become large enough to act as a compressive lesion. The common sites of such haematomas are parietal, anterior temporal and inferior frontal. In an elderly person with a relatively atrophic brain the collection may become hemispherical.

There is no characteristic clinical picture. It may mimic an extradural haematoma. However, on account of the associated brain damage, most patients remain unconscious from the time of injury and follow a steadily deteriorating course. Sometimes it is not so much a perceptible deterioration as failure to improve which arouses suspicion of such a lesion. Angiography or computerized tomography (CT) scan may establish the diagnosis or, if these are not available, exploratory burr-holes may be necessary.

Subacute subdural haematoma. In a small percentage of cases of subdural haematoma, the clinical picture may evolve more slowly. The patient continues to be drowsy and disoriented or even in stupor. There may be fluctuations in the degree of responsiveness. Symptoms and signs of increased intracranial pressure and focal neurological signs developing during this period should alert the clinician to such a possibility.

Chronic subdural haematoma. This lesion is usually seen at the extremes of ages, i.e. in infancy and old age. The history of injury is often trivial, or may have been forgotten.

It is postulated that a minor leak in the subdural space results in a localized haematoma. During the process of organization it becomes encapsulated. The outer layer of this capsule is derived from the dura mater and is thick and vascular, whereas the inner layer derived from the pia arachnoid is thin and avascular. In due course the clot liquefies and the outer membrane becomes vascularized and increasingly thick. The high osmolarity of the contents of this enclosed cavity encourages absorption of CSF across the semi-permeable inner membrane. The vascular outer membrane may further add to the haematoma through repeated small leaks. Not all haematomas enlarge in size. The lesion is usually hemispherical, and in a large number of cases, bilateral. It is uncommonly found in the posterior fossa. Some, however, are gradually completely absorbed, and an occasional one may calcify.

The classical history is that of an elderly person who had a minor bang on the head against a door or getting out of a car. He or she soon forgets about it and weeks or even months later, develops symptoms and signs of increasing intracranial pressure or focal neurological deficit. Increasing forgetfulness, mental confusion and a varying degree of disorientation may progress to stupor and coma, and in addition specific neurological disturbances such as progressive hemiparesis, dysphasia and apraxia may develop.

In cases of chronic subdural haematoma of infancy, usually a result of birth injury, the presenting features are enlargement of the head, bulging fontanelle, difficulty in feeding and failure to thrive. This has to be differentiated from hydrocephalus. The diagnosis can be established by a CT scan, but if this is not available a diagnostic subdural tap may be required.

INTRACEREBRAL HAEMORRHAGE

Post-traumatic haemorrhage in the brain parenchyma may be classified as petechial, cortical and subcortical, and intracerebral.

Petechial haemorrhages

These are small, pinpoint haemorrhages irregularly

scattered within the brain substance, frequently in the white matter, basal ganglia, corpus callosum and the brainstem. They are characteristically seen in severe cases of diffuse axonal injury. Prolonged unconsciousness in the absence of any demonstrable haematoma or cerebral contusion is the classical clinical manifestation of such lesions. It is likely that many of these resolve spontaneously in those who survive the initial injury. Some may coalesce and leave behind small gliotic cavities as tell-tale evidence of old injury.

Cortical and subcortical

Most contusions and lacerations of brain are associated with some leakage of blood. The contusion, unless situated in an eloquent area of the brain, i.e. the sensory–motor strip, the speech area, or the brainstem, may itself remain silent. In some cases, especially with a large contusion or laceration, there may be a progressive increase in pressure on the affected part of the brain due to oedema, coalescence of haemorrhages, necrosis and further bleeding. This may then act as a space-occupying lesion indistinguishable from the next group of cases—intracerebral haematomas.

Intracerebral haematoma

In contrast to what has been described above, intracerebral haemorrhage may be seen as a distinct, circumscribed collection of blood in the subcortical white matter, usually underlying a surface contusion. When it is more than 2-3 cm in diameter it is described as a definite intracerebral haematoma.

There is controversy as to whether it is appropriate to differentiate between cortical and subcortical intracerebral haematomas. Instead of entering this debate, for clinical purposes it is correct to say that all such cases which present as a progressively increasing space-occupying lesion should be considered as a distinct entity. The most common sites for such lesions are the temporal and frontal lobes, although they may occur anywhere in the brain, including the brainstem and the cerebellum. A variety of names, eg. pulped temporal lobe, burst temporal lobe, temporal lobe contusion syndrome, intratemporal haematoma or simply post-traumatic temporal lobe lesion, have been given to this entity when the lesion involves the temporal lobe.

Clinically such cases present with the usual symptoms and signs of progressively enlarging intracranial haematoma. The clinical course may mimic an acute, or less commonly subacute, extradural haematoma. The diagnosis is established by CT scanning or angiography. The treatment is surgical evacuation if the patient fails to show progressive improvement or if there are any signs of deterioration.

With this background knowledge of the pathogenesis, pathology and clinical features of individual lesions, it is appropriate to outline a plan of management which should guide the surgeon to institute appropriate investigations and therapy when faced with a patient with head injury. The first step in the management is clinical assessment.

Assessment

History-taking. A careful record of the history, looking particularly for the following points, must be obtained before any eye-witness or attendant disappears.

Nature of the injury. As detailed a description of the accident as possible should be obtained from the patient (if conscious) or from eye-witnesses. This may give some idea of the severity, nature and direction of the injuring force, and indirectly indicate the nature of possible damage to the skull and the brain. The account may also help to differentiate those patients who receive an injury to the head as a result of a fall secondary to a cerebrovascular accident, epileptic seizure, or Stokes–Adams syndrome.

Interval since the time of injury. It is important to ascertain the interval between the time of injury and the examination of the patient. The same clinical picture may have completely different significance 30 min, 2 h or 24 h after the injury. Thus stertorous respiration, thready pulse and irregularities of the pupils noted within a few minutes of the accident are likely to be innocuous transitory phenomena, but the same signs if present several hours after injury are of ominous import. Similarly a patient found to be comatose shortly after the injury may simply be concussed, whereas one still unconscious 24 h later will have suffered more serious damage.

Effect of the injury on consciousness. A careful record should be made of the observed state of consciousness of the patient from the moment of injury till the time of examination, and of course from that time onwards until the patient is discharged fully recovered. On this basis patients can be divided into three groups:

1. Those unconscious after injury but already showing signs of recovery or who have completely recovered by the time of the examination. This group of patients requires only periodic clinical check-up over the next 48–72 h. It is possible that an occasional patient belonging to this group may develop serious complications even after 72 h but, as a rule, there would be enough warning symptoms to arouse suspicion of impending trouble. Thus every such patient at the time of discharge from hospital should be warned to report back immediately if there is increasing headache, vomiting, convulsions, or the appearance of a new neurological deficit.
2. Unconsciousness persisting since the time of injury: if already some time has elapsed between the injury and the time of evaluation, and the patient continues to be unconscious, the possibility of an intracranial haematoma should be entertained. However, frequently patients belonging to this group have suffered diffuse brain damage which requires no more than careful observation rather than surgical intervention.
3. Patients whose conscious state shows deterioration either following initial improvement, or without this preliminary phase are strongly suspected of having intracranial haematoma, and appropriate investigations should be pursued.

If a careful history is not recorded the intervening period of improvement (lucid interval) may be overlooked and the patient's unconsciousness may be considered to be either due to concussion or to diffuse brain damage.

Convulsion. A focal or generalized convulsion is not an infrequent occurrence following head injury, especially in children. Immediately after a seizure the clinical picture of the patient may be considerably altered, thereby making assessment difficult. Deep coma, dilated fixed pupils, noisy respiration, and bilateral extensor plantar response are grave signs, if observed in the absence of a convulsion. However, the identical clinical condition may be seen immediately after a seizure, and yet all these abnormal signs return to normal within a short period of time. Evidence of progressive recovery should be observed from minute to minute in such cases. If the history of convulsion is not directly sought from the relatives or other witnesses, a wrong assessment may be made of the patient's condition.

Examination of the patient

General physical examination. Baseline observations of pulse, blood pressure, respiration and temperature should be made and recorded. Any changes in these may be the first signs indicating intracranial pathology or any associated injury elsewhere in the body. A slowing of the pulse rate and increase in blood pressure are frequently, though not always, observed in cases developing an intracranial haematoma. On the other hand, tachycardia and a fall in blood pressure should arouse suspicion of an associated closed injury, e.g. of abdomen, chest or pelvis. Shock is uncommon in head-injured patients and when present implies either a very severe injury or an associated injury elsewhere in the body.

The neck should be examined for stiffness and for Kernig's sign. These indicate meningeal irritation due to subarachnoid haemorrhage.

Local signs suggestive of extradural wound or haemorrhage are sought.

Evidence of injury elsewhere in the body must be searched for, especially at sites likely to be overlooked, e.g. fracture of the cervical spine, fractured pelvis, closed-injury of the abdomen or chest.

Neurological examination

Consciousness. By far the most important single observation in a case of head injury is that of the level of consciousness. It should be assessed and recorded in detail rather than in single words like coma, stupor or semi-coma, which have different meanings for different persons. Minor alterations in the conscious state provide the most vital information regarding the progress of the patient. As long as the degree of consciousness improves, the patient is on the way to recovery. The moment consciousness stops improving or deteriorates, a warning is sounded that demands prompt action.

The most generally accepted method of recording the state of consciousness is the one provided by the so-called Glasgow coma scale. This consists of recording the best response obtained following graded stimulation, as shown in Table 42.1. Each response has been given an arbitrary number, which can then be added to quantify the conscious state.

Table 42.1 The Glasgow coma scale

Response	Degree of response	score
Eyes open	Spontaneously	4
	To speech (verbal command)	3
	To pain	2
	To neither stimulus	1
Verbal response	Oriented	5
	Confused	4
	Inappropriate words	3
	Incomprehensible sounds only	2
	Nil	1
Motor response	Obeys commands	6
	Localizes	5
	Flexor withdrawal	4
	Abnormal flexion	3
	Extends	2
	Nil (flaccid)	1

Thus a patient who opens eyes spontaneously (4), whose verbal response is oriented (5), and who obeys command (6), has the best score—15—which is equivalent to full consciousness. At the other extreme a patient who manifests no eye-opening (1), no verbal response (1) and no motor response (1) has a score of 3 which indicates a state of deep coma. In between these two extremes there is a range of disturbance of consciousness. All scores below 8 are considered to indicate unconsciousness. It may be added that if there is closure of the eyes due to swelling or chemosis of the lids, or if the patient has a tracheostomy, it may be difficult to ascribe an accurate rating.

Eye signs.

1. *Pupils:* The size and reaction of the pupils to light are a sensitive index of the presence of an intracranial haematoma. Whenever an initially normal-sized pupil is seen progressively to dilate, one should strongly suspect an enlarging intracranial haematoma until and unless proved otherwise. The classical sequence of events (described as Hutchinson's pupils) is (1) constriction on the side of the haematoma; (2) dilatation on the side of the haematoma; (3) constriction on the contralateral side; (4) dilatation of both pupils (Fig. 42.9). It must, however, be pointed out that the initial phase of constriction is not always noted, and in some instances may not occur. As the pupil starts to dilate, its reaction to light also becomes progressively impaired.

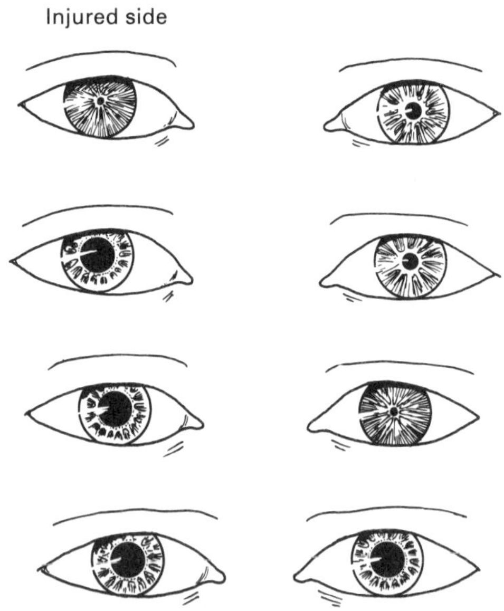

Fig. 42.9 Hutchinson's pupils: sequence of changes of pupil size and reaction during increased intracranial compression on injured side—see text.

Although the above is the usual pattern, the following should be borne in mind:

a. A fatal intracranial haematoma may develop without manifesting pupillary abnormality.
b. Pupillary abnormality may be due to recent or previous local injury to the eyeball, the visual pathways or the third nerve itself. Where such damage is the result of the most recent injury, the pupillary dilatation will be observed immediately after the injury.
c. As a rule the haematoma is on the side of the dilated pupil, but contralateral haematoma cannot be excluded on the basis of this sign alone.
d. By the time both pupils become dilated and fixed the chances of recovery of the patient even after successful evacuation of the haematoma are very remote.

   e. Bilateral constricted, pinpoint, non-reacting pupils are also of grave omen.
2. *Corneal reflex:* This is one of the last reflexes to be abolished, and its absence signifies a terminal state.
3. *Oculocephalic reflex:* In an unconscious patient sudden turning of the head to one side results in conjugate deviation of the eyes to the opposite side. The presence of this reflex indicates that the neural pathways subserving it, which traverse the brainstem, are intact. Absence of this reflex points to damage of the brainstem.
4. *Vestibulo-ocular reflex:* Stimulation of the labyrinth by infusion of ice-cold water into the external auditory canal, after excluding a perforation of the drum by visual inspection, results in nystagmus in normal individuals. In an unconscious patient it may produce conjugate deviation of the eyes (with or without nystagmus) to the side of stimulation. By eliciting this reflex one can get valuable information, not only regarding the vestibulo-ocular pathways, but also indirectly of the integrity of the brainstem. An absent vestibulo-ocular reflex is of grave significance.
5. *Funduscopy:* This should be done at regular intervals in every case of head injury under observation. It is important to have a baseline record on admission. Developing papilloedema may then provide early evidence of an enlarging intracranial haematoma, especially of the subacute and chronic varieties.

Evidence of motor weakness. Even in an unconscious patient it is usually possible to detect monoparesis or hemiparesis by observing the spontaneous movements, the response to painful stimuli, and the tone of various muscle groups. The following facts should, however, be noted:

1. Hemiplegia present from the moment of injury is most likely to be due to cerebral contusion.
2. A fatal haematoma may develop without ever manifesting hemiplegia or any other focal (localizing) neurological deficit.
3. Usually the haematoma is on the side opposite to the hemiplegia, but in 10% of cases it may be on the same side.
4. By the time hemiplegia develops as the result of a haematoma, the patient's conscious state will normally have deteriorated. Therefore, hemiplegia in association with a normal state of consciousness is unlikely to be due to a haematoma.

Reflexes. Alterations in the superficial and deep reflexes may help in localizing the side of a lesion.

Clearly, if the patient is conscious and co-operative a full neurological examination should be done. If, however, a complete neurological examination was not possible at the initial assessment, it should be done as soon as the patient's condition permits. It is then possible to detect newly developing neurological signs, should they develop.

Continued observations

As a rule, after the initial examination most patients with head injury require an additional period of careful observation to detect, at the earliest possible moment, signs and symptoms of an enlarging intracranial haematoma or any other secondary complication. A careful record is maintained of all the factors mentioned in the preceding account. Even at the risk of repetition it must be emphasized that the most important single sign is the *slightest deterioration of consciousness.* Certainly alteration in the size of the pupils, slowing of the pulse rate, rise in the blood pressure and change in the rate and rhythm of the respiration are important, but these signs are frequently absent or may not develop till a very late stage of compression.

Investigations

Plain X-ray of the skull

This provides valuable information in all cases of head injury, and is required for medicolegal purposes. Good-quality films are necessary. However, X-ray examination should not take precedence over the institution of proper first aid and resuscitation measures. In a restless, struggling patient it may not be possible to get proper pictures. Finally, if the patient's condition is deteriorating rapidly and there is a strong clinical suspicion of a rapidly enlarging intracranial haematoma, it would be foolhardy to waste time on obtaining X-rays.

A number of views have been recommended for routine use in cases of head injury. The practice of doing a conventional lateral X-ray of the skull, requiring rotation of the neck, can only be condemned. It is generally sufficient to have antero-posterior (Towne's) and translateral films, all taken with the patient in the supine position. Special views like basal, tangential or Water's may be taken if required. X-rays should be scrutinized for the following information:

1. Is there a fracture present? In the case of a linear fracture its site, extent and its relation to any vascular markings, to the paranasal sinuses, mastoid air cells or large foramina should be ascertained. Any separation of its edges should be noted. If there is evidence of depression its extent should be assessed, if necessary with the aid of tangential or stereoscopic views.
2. The paranasal sinuses and mastoid air cells should be looked at to see if there is any evidence of opacity or fluid level, suggesting the presence of blood or CSF. Such a finding gives indirect evidence of a basal fracture which should be considered compound.
3. If the pineal body is calcified its displacement from the midline provides a useful sign of the presence of a supratentorial haematoma.
4. The presence of any intracranial air may be detected.
5. The presence of any radiopaque foreign body intracranially may be seen.

Echoencephalography (a scan)

This is a very useful bed-side investigation which may provide reliable information with minimal disturbance to the patient. A shift of the midline structures can be rapidly ascertained. However, the absence of a demonstrable midline shift should not be accepted as an unequivocal evidence of the absence of a haematoma.

Carotid angiography

This is the most direct way of outlining the intracranial vessels and localizing a haematoma. One should look for the following in an angiogram:

1. Shift of the midline vessels—the anterior cerebral arteries and the internal cerebral vein are normally midline structures. A shift across the midline of more than 2 mm should be considered abnormal, and implies the presence of a supratentorial space-occupying lesion. As in the case of pineal shift, its absence should not be accepted as unequivocal evidence of the absence of a haematoma.
2. The presence of an avascular area between the inner table of the skull and the outlined vessels provides evidence of an extracerebral (extra- and /or subdural) haematoma. The shape of this avascular area may even indicate the precise nature of this haematoma.
3. Elevation of the middle cerebral artery (especially in the lateral view) indicates the presence of a temporal lobe or middle cranial fossa haematoma.
4. Stripping of the sagittal sinus or the middle meningeal artery away from the inner table of the skull points to an extradural haematoma.
5. Extravasation of contrast medium is a direct sign of leakage of blood.
6. Any other abnormality, e.g. a vascular thrombosis or traumatic carotid–cavernous fistula, may be detected.

CT scanning

This is by far the safest, quickest and most informative investigation to determine the presence or absence of an intracranial haematoma, parenchymatous lesions or brain oedema. Figure 42.10 provides examples of such lesions. Very precise details of the site, shape, location, density and relations to other structures can be obtained. Each type of lesion tends to have its own particular pattern. For example, an extradural haematoma usually presents as a biconvex, high attenuating lesion just under the inner table of the skull; a crescentic lesion with the concavity parallel to the surface of the brain indicates a subdural haematoma, and an intracerebral haematoma is seen as an irregular, high attenuating lesion in the substance of the brain.

The absorption values of blood change with the passage of time. Thus a high attenuating lesion may after some days become isodense with the brain, and later still be low in attenuation. This, at

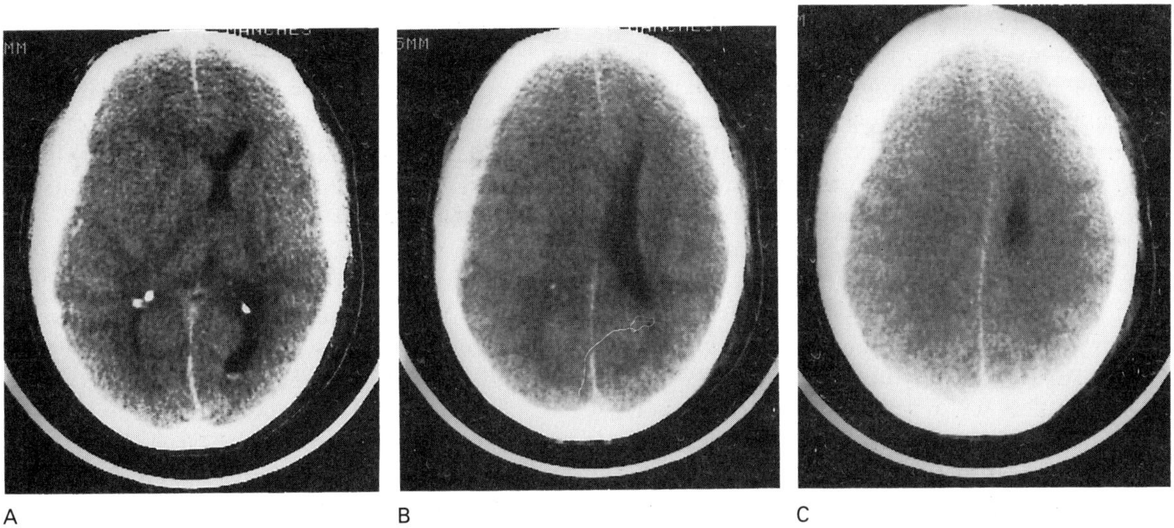

Fig. 42.10 Computerized tomography scans of a skull with a subdural haematoma on the left side. (**A**) This view is taken at deepest level, near to the base of the skull; (**B**) and (**C**) are taken at progressively higher levels approaching the vault. The most striking finding is the absence of any sign of the cisterna magna on the left at any of the three levels, due to compression by the haematoma. There is also widening of the opacity on the left side of the bony skull—part of which is due to the blood collection.

times, causes some difficulty in the diagnosis of a subacute or chronic subdural haematoma.

Besides the actual demonstration of blood, the presence of a haematoma could be suspected from the displacement of the ventricular system, which should be clearly seen in a CT scan. This shift, however, may not be present in bilateral haematomas or in those in the vertex or the base of the skull.

The estimation of the size of the lateral ventricles provides indirect evidence of the existence of brain oedema, or in later stages may identify hydrocephalus. In addition, intracranial air and foreign bodies are easily seen in a CT scan.

Isotope encephalometry and electroencephalography

These are not of much help in evaluating patients with acute injury to the head.

Inspection burr-holes

In the absence of facilities for modern diagnostic aids, exploratory burr-holes still serve as a useful investigation in cases of head injury where there are strong clinical indications of the presence of intracranial haemorrhage.

Management

First aid

After head injury the first step is to protect the victim from further damage—the so-called second accident, the commonest of which is anoxia, due either to inadequate or obstructed respiration or shock. To prevent this it is desirable to have first aid available at the spot and an efficient ambulance service to transport the patient quickly to an emergency station. Ambulance staff should have training and equipment to provide the necessary first aid and promptly institute resuscitative measures.

General principles of management

1. No case of head injury is considered too trivial to be ignored, or too severe to be despaired with.
2. On admission, even before an assessment of the neurological status is made, attention should be paid to the following:
   a. The securing and maintenance of a satisfactory airway.
   b. The detection of signs of shock.
   c. The arrest of any external haemorrhage.

On the basis of the initial examination and immediate subsequent course, patients may be divided into the following four main groups with regards to management.

1. *Those requiring no treatment:* By far the largest number of patients fall into this group, which comprises mainly those with uncomplicated concussion. Most of these patients already show evidence of rapid recovery, even by the time they are first examined. Depending upon the severity of the injury, the duration of unconsciousness, the length of post-traumatic amnesia and evidence of any external injury or fracture of the skull, they should be kept under observation for a period varying from 24 to 72 h. As a rule no patient should be discharged unless already fully conscious, normally oriented, and completely asymptomatic.
2. *Those requiring surgery:*
   a. All open wounds, irrespective of their extent, require primary debridement as soon as the patient's general condition permits.
   b. Patients with evidence of increasing intracranial pressure—most likely due to an enlarging intracranial haematoma—require prompt confirmation of the diagnosis and surgical evacuation.

   An intracranial haematoma is suspected in patients manifesting the following:

   i. Progressive deterioration in the level of consciousness or failure to show the expected improvement.
   ii. The development of pupillary dilatation.
   iii. Slowing of the pulse rate and rise in blood pressure (though not a constant occurrence).
   iv. The appearance or progression of neurological deficit, hemiparesis, aphasia, etc.
   v. Persistent headache and vomiting.

   Notwithstanding the descriptions in many textbooks there is no typical clinical picture of an intracranial haematoma. One should not hesitate to take steps to exclude one by appropriate investigations, if there is any suspicion.
3. *Those requiring conservative management:* Most patients who fall into this group are those who manifest varying degrees of impairment of consciousness and other neurological signs and symptoms which cannot be ascribed to an intracranial haematoma, or those who are left with these signs and symptoms after a haematoma has already been evacuated. Some may remain unconscious for days or weeks, others pass into a state of irritation, while the remainder have a relentless downhill course, as a result of severe damage to the brain. The management, therefore, has to be tailored to the needs of the individual patient, but the following general principles are helpful in planning treatment:
   a. Maintenance of a free airway: It is important to ensure this throughout the period of unconsciousness. The patient is preferably nursed on the side; oropharyngeal secretions are removed as and when required by suction, and oropharyngeal or intratracheal intubation may be necessary to prevent any mechanical obstruction. If a patient remains unconscious for more than 24 h it may be advisable to perform a tracheostomy.
   b. Prevention of secondary infection: Antibiotics are administered to all cases with open wounds, with bleeding from the nose or the ear, with a fracture through a paranasal sinus or mastoid air cell, and to those who remain unconscious for prolonged periods.
   c. Control of pyrexia: In all cases of head injury the temperature should be monitored regularly. As far as possible it should be kept within the normal range and if there is any tendency to hyperpyrexia, this may be countered by sponging, fans or antipyretic drugs, e.g. aspirin and phenacetin. In severely injured patients elective hypothermia may be instituted.
   d. Control of pain and restlessness: As a rule sedatives are undesirable for head-injured patients. Analgesics (aspirin, phenacetin, paracetamol) should be given in adequate doses. Morphia is contraindicated. Restlessness may be an early sign of a developing haematoma, and administration of sedatives to relieve it will only delay the discovery of its cause. If an intracranial haematoma has been positively excluded, and the patient is unmanageable because of restlessness, chlorpromazine may be administered. Physical restraint by tying the hands and legs often increases the restlessness. If it is feared that the patient is in danger of falling out of bed,

it may be better to nurse him or her on the floor.

e. Attention to nutrition: All patients remaining unconscious for more than a day or two require intragastric tube-feeding of adequate quantities of fluids, minerals and calories.
f. Attention to bladder and bowel: It is desirable to institute a closed urinary drainage system to prevent soiling. A condom drainage is usually adequate for males, but for females catheterization is generally required. If the bowels do not move regularly, enemas may be required to prevent faecal impaction. Inadequate emptying of either bladder or bowel may contribute to restlessness.
g. Arrest of seizures: Any patient who manifests local or generalized epileptic attacks should be given adequate doses of antiepileptic medication, e.g. Luminal 60–100 mg 8-hourly. An attack of status epilepticus should be aborted by intravenous diazepam, or if necessary pentothal drip. The role of routine anticonvulsant medicine for all seriously injured patients is debatable.
h. Measures to reduce brain oedema: Mannitol as a 20% solution,100–300 ml administered intravenously over 20–30 min, appears to be a satisfactory agent to reduce undesirable brain oedema. It may be repeated once or twice a day. It should, however, never be used unless an intracranial haematoma has been unequivocally excluded. Other means of obtaining the same objective include intravenous urea, hypothermia, corticosteroids or barbiturates. Though corticosteroids are valuable in the management of brain oedema associated with a tumour or an abscess, there is no certain evidence of their usefulness, even in high doses, for alleviation of post-traumatic oedema. Lumbar puncture, once generally recommended for relieving increased intracranial pressure, is not only useless but also dangerous. Controlled artificial respiration, carefully monitored, has its advocates.
i. General nursing care: Proper nursing care of an unconscious patient may be the most decisive factor in the ultimate outcome of any treatment, whether medical or surgical. Proper positioning of the patient in bed, care of the skin, bladder and bowel, active or passive exercises of the paralysed limbs—all go a long way towards accelerating the convalescence.

4. *Those requiring surgery for sequelae:*
   a. Cranioplasty: This may be required for patients who have lost pieces of the cranial vault, either as a result of the injury or surgery following it. It may also be necessary in growing fracture of the skull in childhood, or the so-called craniocerebral erosion. This occurs when a linear fracture of the skull in a child, usually below 2 years of age, associated with separation of the edges and tearing of the underlying dura, tends to enlarge with the passage of time. To prevent this progressive damage duraplasty and cranioplasty are advisable.
   b. Surgery for post-traumatic inflammatory lesions: Osteomyelitis and intracranial abscess are not uncommon sequelae of open injuries of the skull, especially if primary debridement has not been thorough.
   c. CSF rhinorrhoea and otorrhoea: Leak of CSF, through either the nose or the ear, may require craniotomy and duraplasty to prevent spread of infection intracranially. The indications for surgery are as follows:
      i. When the CSF leak persists for more than 2 weeks after injury.
      ii. When there is clinical or radiological evidence of extensive damage to the paranasal sinus.
      iii. When the patient has already had an attack of meningitis.

Some neurosurgeons advocate prophylactic duraplasty whenever a CSF leak or fracture compound into an air sinus is detected.

   d. Recurring focal cerebral seizures (post-traumatic epilepsy): Recurrent seizures developing after a head injury may require surgical excision of the epileptogenic area if an adequate trial of medical therapy fails; if the epileptogenic focus can be clearly demarcated clinically, radiologically and electroencephalographically, or if the focus is situated in an area which can be sacrificed without any damage to vital functions.
   e. Carotid–cavernous fistula: This is characterized by pulsating exophthalmos, chemosis of

the conjunctiva, oedema of the lids and a loud bruit, and is an uncommon sequela of head injury. The aim of operation is to obliterate the fistula.

Surgery for sequelae requires specialist neurosurgical expertise and equipment.

SOME SURGICAL CONSIDERATIONS

Scalp wounds

The general principles of management of scalp wounds are the same as of any other wound. Owing to the rich vascularity, scalp wounds bleed profusely, but they also heal well. Before embarking on the debridement of a scalp wound it is essential to rule out an underlying skull fracture or an associated intracranial haematoma by the appropriate investigations described earlier. Attention must be paid to the following:

1. Shave the skin for several centimetres around the wound.
2. The wound must be cleaned and washed thoroughly to remove all foreign bodies.
3. Remove all debris, displaced hair, and badly damaged tissue from under the skin edges.
4. Look carefully for any underlying fracture, CSF leak or herniation of brain matter.
5. Debride the margins of the wound sparingly. However, it serves no useful purpose to retain contused, ragged, crushed, badly contaminated edges.
6. The edges of the wound should be approximated without tension. Extension of the original wound, undermining and mobilization of the flaps suffice in most cases. In the event of extensive loss of skin, a releasing incision, rotation of a flap or skin-grafting may have to be resorted to.

Exploratory burr-holes

Where facilities do not exist to carry out definitive diagnostic investigations like angiography or CT scan, exploratory burr-holes may be required for diagnostic purposes. In such an event the whole head must be shaved and prepared. The location of the burr-holes is planned taking into consideration any clinical evidence of the site of impact; the demonstration of a fracture on the X-ray skull and the presence of any localizing signs. If some localizing feature is present, the first burr-hole is made at that site. If this reveals the suspected lesion capable of explaining the patient's clinical condition, it should be dealt with by adequately increasing the exposure either by enlarging the hole or raising a flap (Fig. 42.11). If, on the other hand, no lesion is encountered, burr-holes at other sites on the same side and if necessary, the opposite side, should be made. The usual sites are:

1. frontal: 3–4 cm, lateral to the midline and just in front of the coronal suture, i.e. one-third the

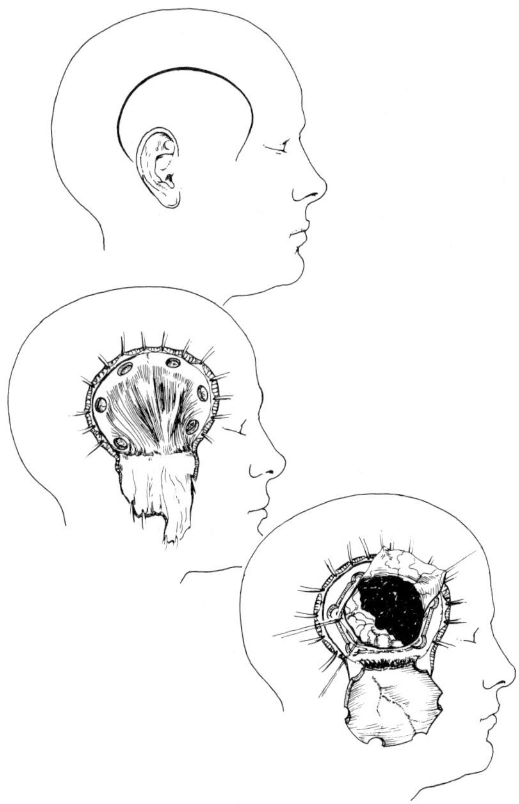

Fig. 42.11 A formal temporal bone flap for proper exploration of damaged brain and haematoma. **Top:** the skin incision; **centre:** a series of burr-holes in a horseshoe pattern; **bottom:** the bone flap bent downwards with the intact temporalis muscle as its pedicle. A large extradural haematoma is represented bulging from under the anterior edge of the opening of the skull.

distance between the nasion and external occipital protuberance;
2. temporal: 2–3 cm in front of and above the zygomatic arch in the temporal bone;
3. parietal: 3–4 cm from the midline and 8–9 cm above the external occipital protuberance.

Compound depressed fractures

Surgery for compound depressed fractures should be undertaken with full preparations for a major operation. General anaesthesia is desirable. Arrangements must be made for blood transfusion.

In most cases appropriate extension of the existing scalp wound permits adequate exposure. If the existing wound is small and the fracture rather extensive, it may be better to turn a formal scalp flap exposing the whole extent of the fracture. Before attempting to remove the bone, the scalp and the overlying tissues should be thoroughly cleaned and debrided.

In some cases the loose pieces of bone may be easily lifted off. However, more often these fractured pieces are locked with each other. Under such circumstances, a burr-hole should be made at the edge of the fracture and if necessary nibbled into it (Fig. 42.12). The locked fragments can then be disengaged by means of a periosteal elevator, and lifted out with a bone-holding forceps. One must be careful in lifting off a fragment overlying a major venous sinus. For an inexperienced person, it is best to leave such fragments alone. The bone pieces should be carefully preserved, washed and cleaned thoroughly and unless badly contaminated, these are replaced at the end of the operation.

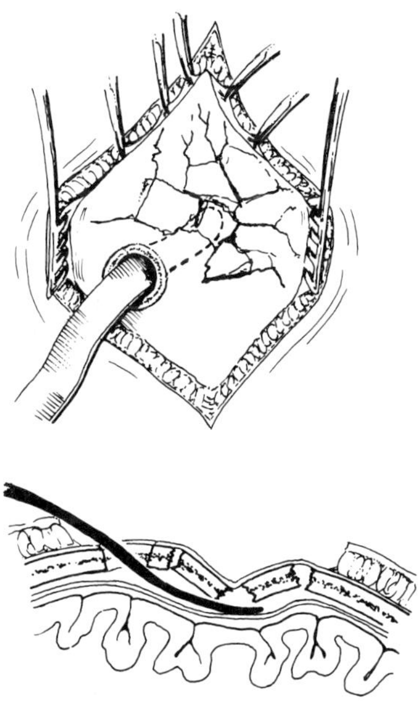

Fig. 42.12 Elevation of small depressed fracture. Through a burr-hole made to the side of the fracture, an elevator is introduced to lever up the depressed fragments.

Following removal of the bone fragments any extradural clot is sucked away and the tear in the dura outlined. It is best to enlarge the opening in the dura to be able to inspect the underlying brain. Any subdural collection of blood is removed. If the brain surface is undamaged or only bruised and the brain is lax, nothing further needs be done. On the other hand any lacerated, necrotic softened brain needs to be carefully sucked away till one has reached the bottom of the wound. Haemostasis is achieved by cauterizing any bleeding points. At the end of the operation the edges of the wound must be clean and the brain lax and pulsating.

All efforts should be made to close the dura completely. In case of difficulty a pericranial or fascial graft may be used to bridge the defect.

Extradural haematoma

If the diagnosis and location of the haematoma are established by preoperative investigation, and the patient is not deteriorating rapidly, it is best to plan a formal flap overlying the haematoma. On the other hand if the diagnosis or site of the haematoma is not established, it is best first to explore the temporal region (the commonest site of such a haematoma) through a vertical incision starting from the zygomatic arch, 2–3 cm in front of the tragus and extending up for 8–9 cm. The temporalis muscle is split and held retracted with a mastoid retractor. A burr-hole is then made in the squamous temporal bone. The haematoma may be seen as the burr-hole is completed.

Depending upon the expertise and facilities available, one may decide either to enlarge the hole by craniectomy (a quicker procedure which, however, leaves a cranial defect) or to convert it into a formal flap. The liquid extradural clot is sucked away, but most of the haematoma is usually clotted and adherent to the dura. This is gently scraped and lifted off piecemeal. It is advisable to leave a thin film of clotted blood adherent to the dura, for over-enthusiastic scraping may unnecessarily start fresh bleeding which may be difficult to control. Any bleeding points encountered are coagulated by diathermy. There is seldom any need to pursue exposure of the middle meningeal artery at the base of the skull, or plug the foramen spinosus. In the event of bleeding from a venous sinus, usually the application of a haemostatic cellulose preparation such as Surgicel or Gelfoam, held in place by gentle pressure with a sucker, will control the haemorrhage. To prevent re-accumulation of blood it is best to apply hitch stitches between the dura and the pericranium all around the bone edges. Oozing from the surface of the dura can usually be controlled by further Gelfoam. The wound is then closed in layers.

If a haematoma is not found at the site of the first burr-hole, further burr-holes will have to be made to exclude haematoma at other sites. The next burr-hole may be made at the site of any boggy or contused area of the scalp, or where a fracture has been seen in the X-ray of the skull.

In the absence of adequate preoperative investigations multiple burr-holes may have to be made to rule out a haematoma (see above).

Acute subdural haematoma

As mentioned earlier, this is seldom an isolated lesion. However, if a large subdural collection is seen on an angiogram or CT scan, or revealed by an exploratory burr-hole, it can be evacuated through appropriately placed burr-holes. The space between the burr-holes should be carefully washed by means of a soft catheter till the return is clear.

Most acute subdural haematomas are coincidental findings associated with more serious parenchymatous lesions of the brain. To deal with such lesions, a formal craniotomy is necessary, not only to evacuate the subdural haematoma but also to attend the underlying damaged brain. This procedure requires experienced neurosurgical expertise.

Chronic subdural haematoma

Once the diagnosis is established it is usually a straightforward procedure to drain this through one or more suitably placed burr-holes, often in either the parietal or frontal regions, located as described in the section on exploratory burr-holes above. The dura is opened through a cruciate incision and just under the dura a bluish-grey membrane is encountered. This is incised and a piece taken for biopsy. Dark-brown liquid haematoma drains out on its own. The residual collection may be evacuated by means of a catheter mounted on a suction tip. A second burr-hole may be made to permit through and through washing of the cavity. The brain, covered by a thinner membrane, is usually depressed away from the surface, and it is desirable for it to expand so as to obliterate the cavity. Repeated washing of the cavity with saline and Valsalva manoeuvres performed by the anaesthetist can be helpful.

It must be remembered that chronic subdural haematoma often tends to be bilateral. It may, therefore, be desirable to make an exploratory burr-hole on the opposite side also, especially if definitive diagnostic investigations have not been carried out preoperatively.

43. Vascular surgery

ARTERIAL DISEASE

The management of peripheral artery disease, particularly its surgical management, has been transformed by the development of good arterial imaging techniques. Intra-arterial angiography, by injecting radiopaque contrast medium either directly into the aorta by a long translumbar needle or via a special catheter passed retrograde into the aorta through a puncture in the common femoral artery in the groin, can give a good outline of the vessels supplying the lower limbs and trunk. More proximal manoeuvring of retrograde catheters can permit visualization of the main branches of the aortic arch. Although these procedures are relatively safe in experienced hands, there are nonetheless risks of dislodging atheromatous material or damaging the artery wall, and they should not be undertaken unless there is a strong clinical indication that the patient is a serious candidate for operation.

Less invasive means of visualizing the arterial tree include digital subtraction angiography, in which the contrast medium is injected into a peripheral vein, and Doppler ultrasound imaging which does not involve any injection. Although the clarity of definition of pictures obtained by these latter two techniques is not generally as good as with good–quality intra-arterial angiography, it is likely that improvements will follow. One particularly useful application of ultrasound scanning is the precise measurement of aneurysms.

ATHEROSCLEROSIS

The commonest disease affecting the peripheral arteries is atherosclerosis, an increasingly prevalent condition in most western societies, which tends to produce symptoms in middle and later life. It is the principal cause of coronary artery disease, strokes, gangrene of the lower limbs and the formation of aneurysms in large arteries.

Pathology

Initially lipids are deposited in the intima, with secondary changes in time affecting all the layers of the arterial wall. Lipids deposited initially in the deeper layers of the intima increase in size to form atherosclerotic plaques (Fig. 43.1). Soon there is disruption of the internal elastic lamina and replacement of the muscle in the media by fibrous tissue, which may also be deposited in and around the adventitial coat of the artery. The internal plaque may become calcified. When the plaque has ulcerated through the endothelium, platelets and fibrin are deposited on the rough surface, forming platelet or fibrin thrombus. Gradual occlusion of the vessel, which had arisen firstly on account of the narrowing caused by the atheromatous material, may thus suddenly become complete when thrombus forms.

There are many theories to explain the recent increase in the incidence of atherosclerosis which has apparently affected western countries more than eastern ones. Much of the evidence points to the

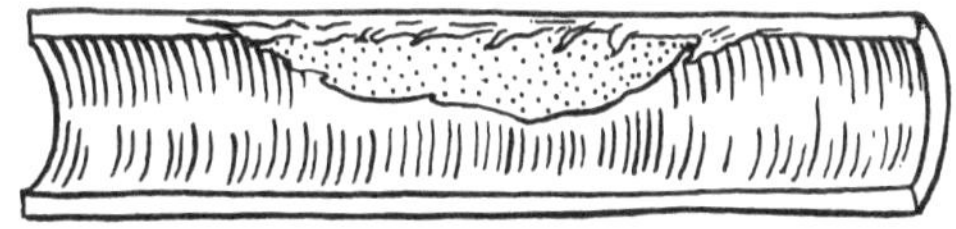

Fig. 43.1 Diagrammatic representation of atheromatous deposit arising subintimally and extending to involve the other layers of the vessel wall.

role of environmental factors, e.g. a diet rich in saturated fats, lack of exercise and cigarette smoking. The disease may well be associated with the additive effects of many factors commonly occurring in modern life. However, there is a group of individuals who have genetically determined high levels of fat in their blood, i.e. primary hyperlipidaemia or hypercholesterolaemia, and these patients tend to be more subject to atherosclerosis occurring at an earlier age than the normal population.

On the whole, men are more liable to the disease than women, and diabetics develop atherosclerosis earlier and to a more severe degree than the non-diabetic population. Although the distribution of atheromatous disease along arteries is usually patchy and irregular, it is commonly found at sites of origin of branches and at bifurcations, e.g. of aorta or common carotid, common iliac or popliteal arteries, and also in the superficial femoral artery as it passes through the distal part of the adductor (Hunter's) canal. The effects on the circulation are mainly caused by narrowing of the lumen of the artery and eventually occlusion of the narrowed artery by thrombosis. On the other hand disruption of the elastic lamina and fibrosis of the arterial wall may predominate, weakening the arterial wall so that the pulsatile arterial pressure tends to cause dilatation of the wall and thus the formation of an aneurysm.

OCCLUSIVE ARTERIAL DISEASE

Lower limb

Atherosclerosis

Ischaemic symptoms in the leg may arise from stenosis or occlusion of any segment of the lower limb arterial tree from the common iliac artery to the anterior or posterior tibials. In general the larger arteries tend to be more often affected, the smaller ones remaining relatively free of the disease, which is fortunate as far as patients are concerned for there is more hope of successful arterial surgery, e.g. graft insertion, with larger than smaller vessels. Also, with more proximal blockage there is usually a better chance of a reasonable collateral arterial supply developing. For example, a patient with a completely blocked common iliac artery may complain of only some limitation in walking capacity, whereas another with a short blockage in the distal popliteal artery may develop gangrene of the foot and require amputation.

As has been mentioned, the superficial femoral artery is one of the commonest to be occluded by the disease. Fortunately the profunda femoris often escapes so that through its several muscular branches it can provide the main source of collateral flow to the distal parts of the limb via anastomoses with geniculate and other arteries. When occlusion affects more than one segment the effects are, not surprisingly, more severe, and also the chances of a successful outcome to reconstructive surgery are less.

Clinical features

Most patients are over the age of 50, but may present at an earlier age if there is a background of strong family history of the disease or one of the predisposing conditions, e.g. diabetes or lipid disorder.

Intermittent claudication (Latin *claudicare:* to limp)

This is the commonest presenting (initial) symptom and the description given by the patient is usually quite clear and indeed classical (easily recognized). He or she complains of pain, often described as gripping, tight or vice-like, in the calf muscles on walking a fixed distance. Resting for a few minutes relieves the pain; the patient is able to walk again, either the same distance or perhaps slightly less, and the cycle of walking, onset of pain, rest, relief, and ability to walk again is repeated. The distance the patient is able to walk before the start of pain gives some idea of the severity of reduction in arterial flow, and is referred to as that patient's claudication distance. If he or she walks more quickly or goes up an incline or stairs the claudication distance will shorten.

On exercise the muscles greatly increase their metabolic rate with, among other effects, the production of acidic metabolites, e.g. lactic acid. The local accumulation of these products causes pain, and if the reduced arterial inflow is not sufficient to wash them out into the venous side of the circulation, claudication occurs. Rest, by stopping or slowing down the further production of painful metabolites, allows the gradual clearance of the accumulated materials to levels below pain threshold until the next period of further exercise increases the output once more.

The onset of claudication may be either gradual or sudden; sudden claudication probably results from thrombus formation in an atheromatous segment completing the occlusion of a vessel.

The constancy, increase, or decrease in the claudication distance between the time of onset and assessment by the doctor gives helpful information. If it has steadily shortened, the occlusion is progressively affecting more segments of the arterial tree, and operative measures to improve arterial flow, if technically feasible, may well be needed in the near future. If, on the other hand, the walking distance increases even slightly, this suggests that reasonable collateral arterial supply is developing, and there may be no need to consider operative treatment.

Although the calf is the commonest site for claudication pain, it can also be experienced in the thigh or buttocks, the latter distribution indicating occlusion of the lower aorta or iliac arteries. The more proximal the site of pain, the higher is the blockage in the arterial tree.

Rest pain

This is almost invariably located in the foot or part of it, and not in the same sites as intermittent claudication. It has quite a different origin. It is due to ischaemia affecting the skin, soft tissues, and sensory nerves, rather than muscles. It is often worse if the patient lies flat, and is particularly troublesome in bed at night. Indeed the patient often soon learns that it is more comfortable with the foot hanging out over the side of the bed and left uncovered. The explanation for this is partly that warmth below the bedclothes increases the metabolism of the skin and superficial tissues, and partly that gravity assists the sluggish arterial flow more with the lower leg dependent than horizontal.

Other symptoms

Various disorders of sensation in toes, foot or leg are fairly common, and probably result from ischaemia affecting the sensory nerves. Paraesthesia (pins and needles) numbness, or feelings that the limb or part of it is like wood, or lead, or woolly are frequent complaints. The affected foot is often noted to be colder, and pallor or cyanosis may be observed, particularly on removing socks and shoes at the end of a cold day.

A reduced arterial supply increases the risk of infection following trivial injury to a toe or any other part of the foot, and any infection may be very slow to heal. The occurrence of such an infection or a protracted healing course should alert the doctor to the possibility of underlying arterial disease, particularly in a middle-aged or elderly male.

If the arterial flow becomes insufficient to maintain tissue viability, gangrene develops. Gradual reduction in the absence of gross infection will lead to dry gangrene—patches of firm, black, dead tissue usually demarcated from the proximal surviving tissue by a clearly defined line (Fig. 43.2). As long as the area remains free from infection the gangrene will remain dry, but superadded infection will lead to pus formation and therefore a wet type of gangrene (Fig. 43.3). This latter type is usually encountered in diabetics.

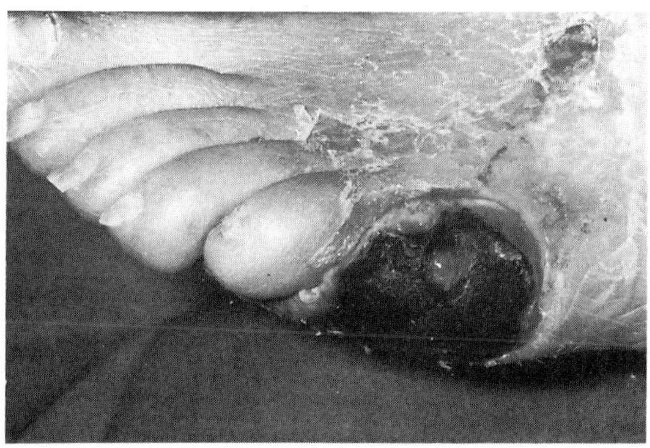

Fig. 43.2 Dry gangrene: well defined area of blackened dead tissue over the head of the metatarsal of the little toe in a patient with atherosclerosis.

Examination findings

The legs may look completely normal in patients presenting solely with intermittent claudication, but signs of wasting in the muscles of calf and/or thigh should be looked for, as should changes in the skin

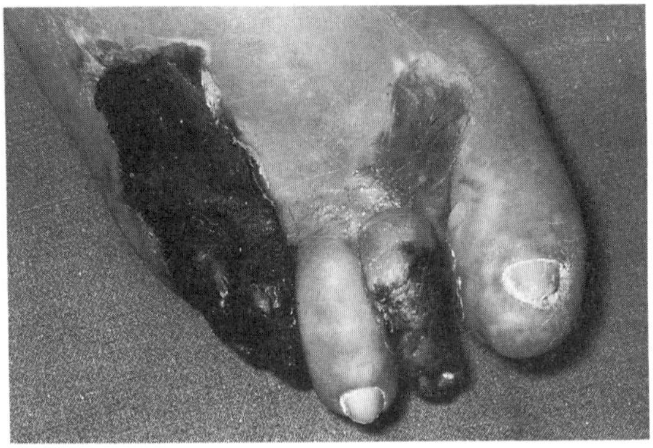

Fig. 43.3 More extensive patches of gangrene, with complete ischaemic death of most of the second toe, the entire fourth and fifth toes and the dorsal skin proximal to them. The viability of the skin in the space between the first and second metatarsals is also doubtful.

of the lower leg, e.g. pallor, cyanosis, "thinning", shiny appearance, and scaliness. The veins may be darker blue than normal and more easily seen through thin skin (Fig. 43.4).

Particular attention should be paid to the toes and heels to detect any breaks in the skin at pressure areas, infection, especially around the nails, or patches of dusky cyanosis heralding gangrene. Arterial deficiency per se does not, of course, lead to oedematous swelling in the region of foot or ankle. In the presence of infection, however, there may well be local inflammatory oedema. In the absence of obvious infection, oedematous swelling may indicate the presence of concomitant deep vein occlusion. There may be reduction in the hair distribution on the skin of the affected limb.

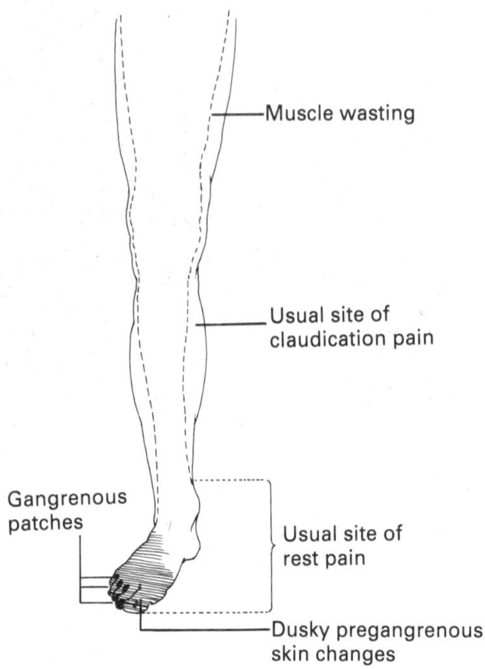

Fig. 43.4 Main signs and symptoms in atherosclerosis of the leg arteries.

Palpation for pulses in both common femoral arteries at the groins, the popliteal behind the knee, posterior tibial and dorsalis pedis vessels should give information as to which segment of the arterial tree is involved. For example, if only the femoral pulse is palpable on one side there is blockage in the superficial femoral artery with or without more distal disease. On elevating the ischaemic leg the veins may empty completely and the skin become pale. Allowing the leg then to hang down over the side of the examination couch may produce an exaggerated red blush in the skin of the foot and lower leg—the so-called dependence rubor.

It is important also to examine the abdomen for aneurysm of the aorta and for bruits which, if present, would indicate stenosis in the aortoiliac segments or other intra-abdominal main branches.

Assessment of the patient presenting with symptoms and signs of ischaemic disease of the limb is not complete without measurement of the blood pressure to detect any hypertension, a urine test for sugar—as this may be the first manifestation of diabetes mellitus—an electrocardiogram to assess whether there are signs of myocardial ischaemia and chest X-ray in case of concomitant infective or neoplastic lung disease or cardiac enlargement.

Management

One of the main anxieties harboured by a patient presenting with impaired circulation to the leg is whether he or she is likely to lose the leg. The majority of those presenting with intermittent claudication will not come to amputation, and some cautious reassurance on this point may be offered. However, those with rest pain or patchy areas of skin duskiness or other trophic damage have a much higher risk of losing toes, the lower leg or the entire leg up to thigh level.

Since atheroma is a generalized disorder, all patients presenting with any pattern of ischaemic symptoms and signs in the lower limb will have a higher than normal risk of myocardial infarct and cerebrovascular accident, and these are the commonest causes of death in this group of patients.

General measures

If diabetes mellitus is present good control is required. Gross hypertension may need appropriate medication. If the patient is overweight, reducing weight will be helpful. Any anaemia should be corrected.

The skin of an ischaemic limb is more vulnerable to damage, infection and delayed healing of any injury. Therefore, care is needed to keep the foot and leg clean, dry, free from constricting or irritating clothes and to avoid crowds where accidental knocks may be sustained. Those whose complaint is solely of intermittent claudication should be encouraged to take frequent walking exercise within the limits of their claudication distance, as this encourages the expansion of collateral vessels.

Many pharmacological agents are available which possess vasodilating properties, but these are generally of little or no real benefit to arteries which are hardened by atheromatous deposits or completely blocked.

Where rest pain is present the care of the skin is particularly important. The foot should be exposed to cool air as much as possible and any pyogenic infection treated by systemic antibiotic. If a small area of dry gangrene tissue shows signs of separating spontaneously from the neighbouring surviving tissue it should be allowed to do so gradually. All attempts at local avulsion or local amputation should be resisted, as opening up new planes in tissue where the blood supply is reduced gives a very high risk of introducing further infection, leading to extensive destruction of tissue and the urgent need for higher amputation. There is also the danger of anaerobic gas gangrene organisms gaining entry, with disastrous consequences.

Surgical procedures

Patients to be seriously considered as possible candidates for operation are those with rest pain or signs of imminent gangrene of even a small patch of foot or toes; those with progressive reduction in claudication distance, and those whose occupation is made difficult or impossible in view of limited walking capacity.

The mere presence of an easily operable block in an accessible artery is not sufficient grounds for surgery. It is wise not to consider operation in someone with very recent onset of claudication, for often with the passage of a few weeks there is considerable improvement in walking as collateral arteries open up. The patient may, therefore, become much less troubled by the symptoms.

As mentioned previously, arteriography, or other available methods of imaging should only be requested if there is a clear indication to advise operation. There is always a risk—albeit a small one—of damage to a diseased artery from puncture and cannulation to obtain pictures. Such injury to the vessels may precipitate blockage of a distal vessel or cause local haemorrhage or the formation of a false aneurysm, and may call for urgent operative intervention and possibly jeopardize the affected limb. Arteriography should therefore not be done just for curiosity or where there is clearly no likeli-

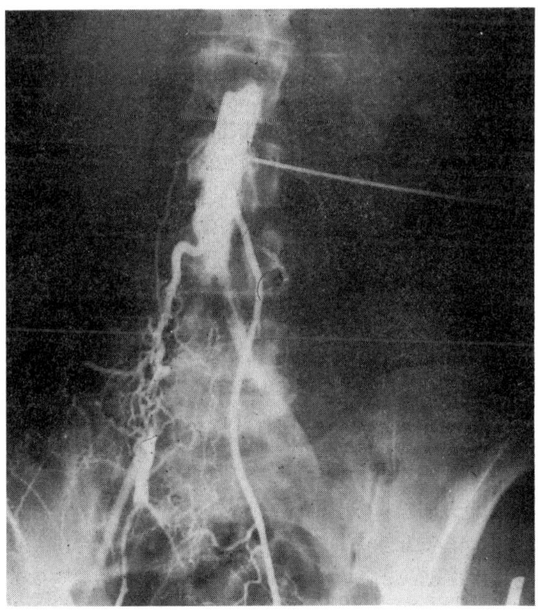

Fig. 43.5 Translumbar aortoarteriogram showing a complete atheromatous block at the lower end of the aorta. Short segments of both right and left iliac arteries show up as still patent; these are filled only by collateral circulation. The inferior mesenteric artery is still patent.

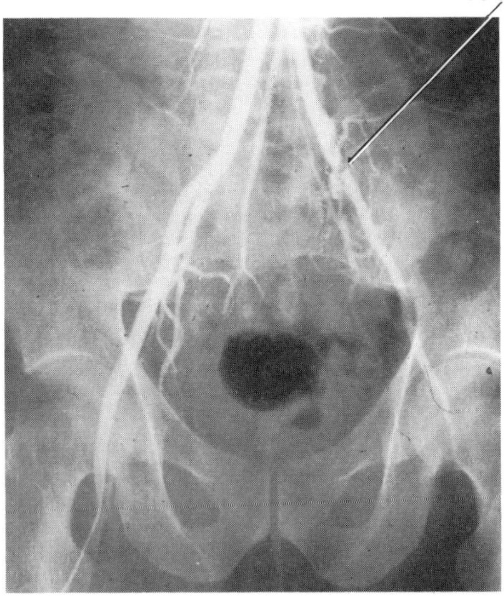

Fig. 43.6 Retrograde Seldinger technique: arteriogram showing a very short localized and almost complete occlusion at the origin of the left external iliac artery, but good re-filling just distal to this lesion. The left internal iliac artery also fills poorly.

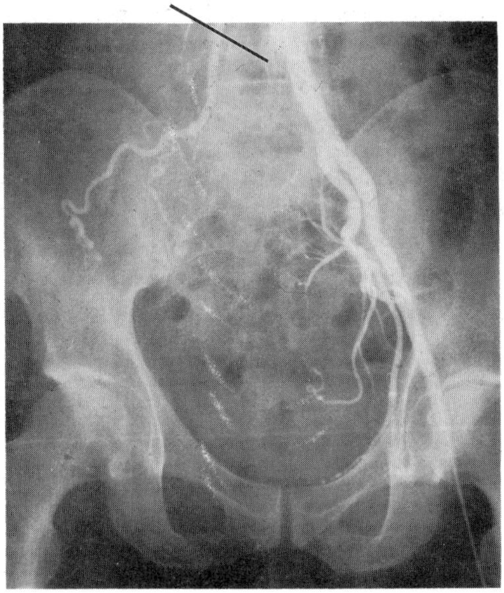

Fig. 43.7 Aortoarteriogram showing complete occlusion of the entire right iliac arteries from the point of origin of the common iliac.

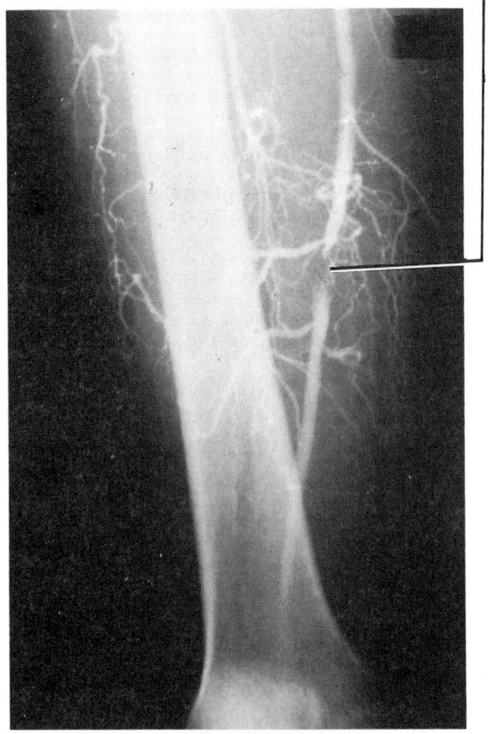

Fig. 43.8 Peripheral arteriogram demonstrating a short occlusion in the superficial femoral artery, as well as numerous small vessels forming collateral links across the blocked segment.

hood of operation being seriously considered. Where there are good grounds, however, it can give vital information about the presence of completely blocked segments, their location, extent, and the state of patency of the vessels both proximal and, every bit as importantly, distal to the block (Figs 43.5–43.8). Occlusions which are single, short, and more proximal larger vessels are more amenable to direct arterial surgery than are multiple ones affecting more distal, smaller segments.

Direct arterial procedures

The main procedures used to overcome the effects of complete blockages are bypass grafting and endarterectomy (Fig. 43.9); the former is now in general much more frequently employed than the latter. Apart from very short occlusions in large

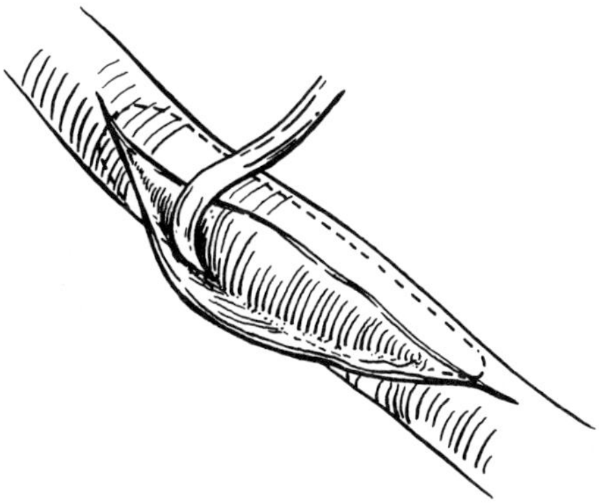

Fig. 43.9 Endarterectomy: after application of occlusion clamps above and below the blocked segment, an arteriotomy is made and the occluding segment of atheroma is dissected from the outer coats of the artery wall by means of a small dissector. The arteriotomy is then sutured after ensuring adequate return of flow.

vessels, e.g. the common iliac artery, with virtually normal artery wall both proximal and distal where endarterectomy may prove easy to perform and beneficial in restoring good flow, it is usually better to insert a graft to bypass an appreciably longer stretch of the arterial tree. Common grafting procedures are from lower abdominal aorta to external iliac or common femoral arteries for blockage of aortic bifurcation, common and/or external iliac segments (Fig. 43.10), and from common femoral

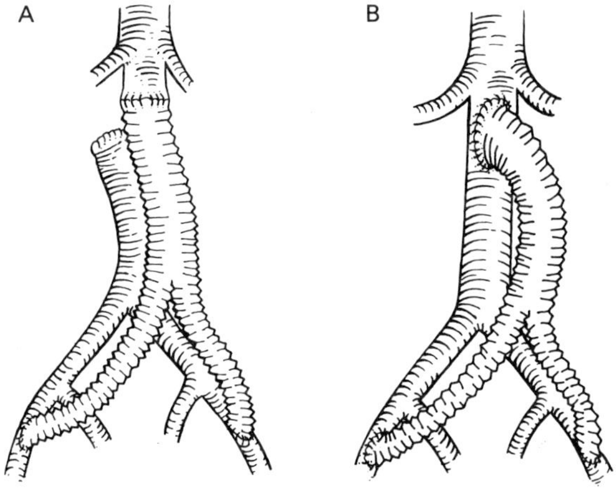

Fig. 43.10 Aortoiliac bypass graft, using synthetic Y-graft. The proximal anastomosis may be either (**A**) end-to-end, after transection of the aorta and suture closure of distal end, or (**B**) end-to-side. The distal anastomoses may be at the distal part of the external iliac artery or, more often, with the common femoral artery just distal to the inguinal ligament.

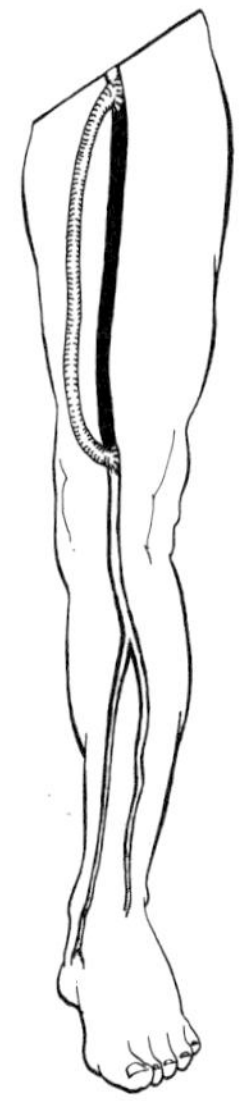

Fig. 43.11 Femoropopliteal bypass graft: this can be with either the patient's own long saphenous vein, reversed, or a thin-walled synthetic graft, e.g. PTFE. The upper anastomosis is with the common femoral artery, and the distal at whatever level in the popliteal artery is sufficiently patent.

to popliteal arteries for blockage of superficial femoral or upper popliteal segments (Fig. 43.11). Synthetic materials, e.g. Dacron or Teflon, are frequently used, either as straight tubes or Y-grafts for aortoiliac bypasses, and the reversed long saphenous vein, if of suitable calibre, is preferred for femoropopliteal grafts. An adequate alternative, if the vein is insufficient, is the synthetic material PTFE (Goretex).

The success of grafting depends on the freedom from early complications such as thrombosis from inadequate local or systemic heparinization, or irregularities in the anastomosis, or local infection which can be especially serious in the presence of a synthetic graft, since it will persist as long as the foreign material is present and may cause erosion at the anastomosis and consequent dramatic haemorrhage. If none of these mishaps arises the graft should remain patent for many years. However, when groups of grafted patients are followed up, year by year, there is a progressive loss of patency due mainly to the progression of atheromatous blockage at or near to the anastomoses. Approximately 60% of femoropopliteal bypass grafts should remain patent at 5-year follow-up.

Lumbar sympathectomy

In situations where it is not possible to perform either a graft or endarterectomy benefit can sometimes be obtained from sympathetic denervation. In keeping with the theoretical consideration of the fact that the sympathetic system is vasoconstrictor to skin and superficial arterioles and not to muscle vessels, sympathectomy does not help intermittent claudication, and indeed may slightly worsen it. However, when the main problem is rest pain, or trophic changes in the skin—even imminent gangrene—the improvement in blood flow to the skin may be sufficient to relieve symptoms and promote healing.

The sympathetic chain is approached through an oblique incision in the lumbar region, by reflecting the peritoneum with its contents forwards and dissecting along the paravertebral region close to the vertebral bodies. A segment of 5–7 cm of lumbar sympathetic chain, including two or three ganglia, can usually be excised (Fig. 43.12).

The arteries of the upper limb are much less often affected by atherosclerosis than the lower limb and even when obstruction occurs it may be comparatively symptomless because of the very adequate collateral circulation available in the upper limb. When atherosclerotic occlusion occurs in the axillary and subclavian arteries, the symptoms are often more severe than with a more distal occlusion because the collateral circulation available at the level of the axillary and subclavian arteries is relatively poor. When symptoms do occur they fall into the two types seen in the lower limb: intermittent claudication which occurs during the course of repetitive movements of the arm, and ischaemia in the form of gangrene or pregangrene leading to loss of tissue usually only at the fingertips. In the hand, gangrene when it occurs is usually much less extensive than is found in the leg.

Embolism

An embolus is a foreign body in the blood stream and embolism is the occlusion of a vessel by this foreign body (Fig. 43.13). The foreign body is usually a thrombus. Such emboli arise in a variety of

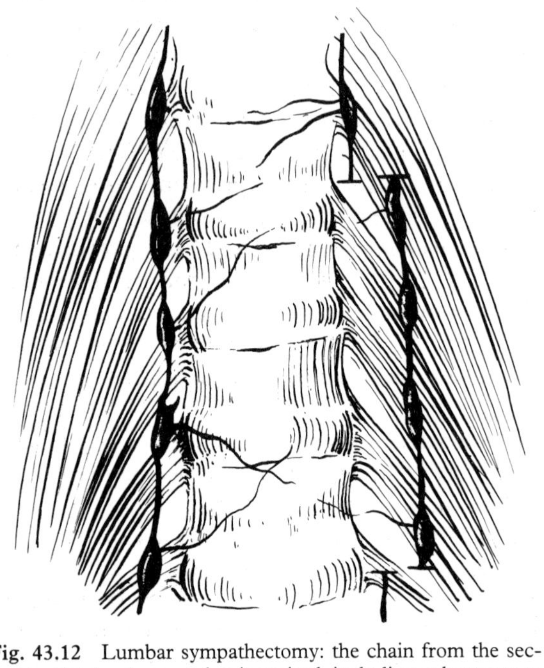

Fig. 43.12 Lumbar sympathectomy: the chain from the second to fifth lumbar vertebra is excised, including at least two to three ganglia.

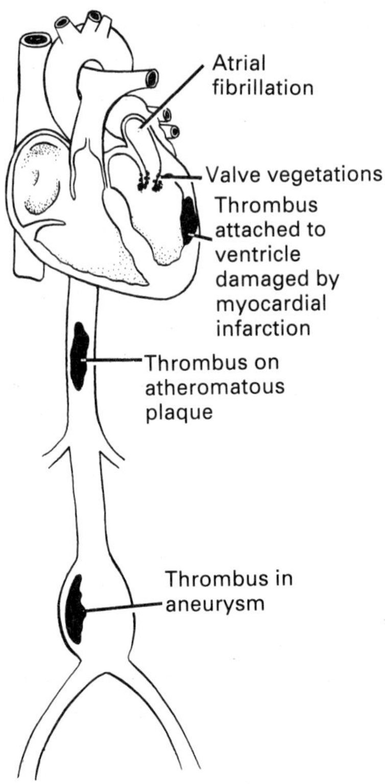

Fig. 43.13 Various sources of arterial emboli.

situations. One of the commonest sites is the atrium in a patient with auricular fibrillation. When the contractions of the atrium become inco-ordinated, thrombus may form in the atrial appendages or on the wall of the atrium, and particularly if the auricular fibrillation ceases or changes in any way, a piece of this thrombus may be dislodged and enter the arterial circulation. In myocardial infarction thrombus may form on the wall of the damaged ventricle, and pieces of thrombus may be thrown off as emboli. When an atheromatous plaque, particularly in the aorta, becomes ulcerated either portions of the plaque, or of adherent thrombus may become dislodged to form emboli. Finally, a further possible source is the laminated thrombus which forms on the wall of an aneurysm, again particularly in the aorta. In subacute bacterial endocarditis, bacteria lodge on the valves as vegetations and these may be dislodged as emboli. Unlike other emboli these contain bacteria and tend to cause infection where they end up—the so-called mycotic or infected embolus.

The clinical effects of an embolus depend to some extent on the size of the embolus and on the size of the artery which is occluded. Sometimes an embolus breaks up on impaction at the first site of hold-up and the fragments pass onwards to block a more distal smaller artery. When the embolus lodges, the blood in the artery beyond the embolus may clot because of the stasis, forming the so-called secondary or consecutive thrombosis. Usually the blood in the arterial tree distal to the embolus is squeezed out, the affected tissues become pale and blood may only reach them by whatever collateral circulation is available. However, in many patients who have atherosclerotic lesions before the incidence of embolism, a collateral circulation may have already developed and the results, therefore, are somewhat less spectacular. If the embolus lands in an end artery, for example, to the spleen or the kidney, thrombosis occurs distal to the embolus and irreversible damage occurs very rapidly, certainly within 10–12 h.

The symptoms and signs of embolism vary according to the organ affected. When embolism occurs in a limb, the patient usually complains of very severe bursting pain due to the acute ischaemia. The limb becomes pale and cold, the muscles become paralysed and there is loss of sensation to touch in the distal part of the limb. The site of the embolus can be deduced from the pulse pattern, being beyond the most distal pulsating artery, and a rough guide is given also from the level of coldness, paralysis and anaesthesia. The pulse immediately proximal to the embolus often feels stronger than its fellow on the opposite side.

The common sites of embolism affecting the leg are at the main bifurcations—aortic, common iliac, common femoral, or popliteal. The aortic bifurcation one, the so-called saddle embolus, commonly breaks up, and may then lead to blockage of either both iliac arteries or both femoral arteries. If the embolus is not removed, the leg becomes white, then livid and blue as stagnant venous blood fills it, and finally gangrene develops. Tissues die at different rates. Muscles will only survive about 6 h of total arterial occlusion whereas nerves, although losing conductivity early, can recover after 24 h of ischaemia. Skin commonly survives up to 48 h.

Treatment

The ideal treatment is removal of the embolus by operation, ideally within the first 4–6 h, and this usually results in complete recovery of the tissues, but embolectomy may still be worthwhile even after this time if the collateral circulation is sufficient to maintain the viability of the limb. As soon as the diagnosis of embolism has been made, the patient should be anticoagulated with intravenous heparin—starting with an initial dose of 10 000 iu. The operation in the leg can be performed under either local or general anaesthesia.

After passing slings around both proximal and distal to the intended site of opening the artery, the arteriotomy is made at or near to the site of the embolus and the embolus removed. If the opening is directly over the embolic plug this may be a simple matter of gently expressing or sucking out the embolus, with the immediate restoration of good pulsatile forward and back-bleeding. During removal, traction on the distal sling will prevent accidental dislodging of fragments into the more distal, smaller vessels. Where the embolus is not easily removed by these straightforward manoeuvres the passage of a Fogarty catheter in the appropriate direction will often easily dislodge the embolic material and permit it to be pulled out through the

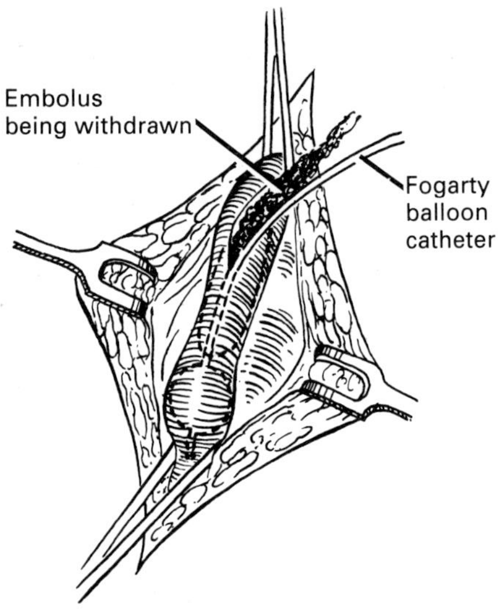

Fig. 43.14 Embolectomy: with proximal and distal slings in place, a Fogarty balloon catheter is introduced distally beyond the lower end of the embolus, and after inflation of the balloon it is drawn upwards, dislodging the embolus as it moves.

arteriotomy (Fig. 43.14). Even when good clearance has apparently been achieved, it is wise to pass a Fogarty catheter as far distally as it will go, inflating the balloon and pulling steadily back, to ensure that no distal fragments have been overlooked.

NON-ATHEROMATOUS OCCLUSIVE DISEASE

Thromboangiitis obliterans (Buerger's disease)

This is an uncommon chronic vascular occlusive condition affecting mainly young male smokers of European and American origin. It is characterized by:

1. occlusion of medium and small-sized vessels of the limbs;
2. thrombophlebitis in the veins accompanying the affected arteries;
3. Raynaud's phenomenon in the hands.

The first of the above three components is always present; the second or the third and sometimes both may be absent.

Pathology

This is a progressive disease which is usually more rapid in progress than atherosclerosis. There may be periods when the progress is comparatively slow or the disease may appear to be stationary, but this is usually followed by a period of accelerated progress of the disease.

Arteries of the lower limbs are most commonly affected, and both the arteries and the accompanying veins show inflammatory changes with thrombosis leading to the occlusion of the vessels. Sometimes recanalization of the thrombus may occur.

Thrombophlebitis may occur in superficial veins of the body and as one segment dies down, another in a different area of the body may develop, thus giving a so-called migratory pattern. In addition spasm may occur in the vessels of the digits of the hand, resulting in painful colour changes in the digits on exposure to cold. This is called Raynaud's phenomenon and will be described later.

The arterial occlusions lead to intermittent claudication, rest pain, ulceration and gangrene of the toes. The gangrene is usually at first of the dry type.

Clinical features

The patient usually complains of one lower limb to begin with, but the opposite limb is involved sooner or later and sometimes the hands are also affected.

There are two main groups as far as clinical presentation is concerned. In the first, intermittent claudication is the main symptom. In the second advice is sought because of pain in the foot at rest, ulceration of the toes or even gangrene.

On examination, there may be evidence of wasting of the calf muscles and the skin of the leg may be pale or cyanosed, cold, thin, atrophic and shiny with loss of hair.

Pulsation is usually absent in the dorsalis pedis and posterior tibial arteries. Later in the progress of the disease the popliteal or even the femoral pulsation may also be absent.

There may be obviously active segments of thrombophlebitis in the superficial veins with longitudinal raised, red, tender patches, or evidence of recently subsided thrombophlebitis in non-tender, firm, cord-like segments of the veins.

Ulcers, when present, are often confined to the toes and are very painful and tender. Gangrene of one or more toes may be present and is most commonly of the dry type with black skin over a shrivelled digit or digits.

Management

The patient must be strongly exhorted to give up smoking altogether. Stopping will slow down or temporarily arrest the progress of the disease. Continuing will certainly accelerate it.

Those who complain of intermittent claudication usually learn to live within their claudication distances.

Surgery has little to offer. First, since the pattern of the disease is to occlude smaller, distal vessels, direct arterial procedures such as grafting and endarterectomy are rarely if ever feasible. Lumbar sympathectomy may give some relief to rest pain, and may assist in achieving healing of ulcers or limitation of digital gangrenous changes, but the benefit is often temporary. Amputation of toes or larger portions of the limb is usually required sooner or later. Although there is a tendency to make these somewhat conservative distal amputations, there is regrettably often a need to perform steadily more proximal revisions as the arterial damage progresses.

Cystic disease of the popliteal artery

This is a rare condition of unknown aetiology which tends to occur in young males and is characterized by a local collection of mucin within the media of the popliteal artery. The collection of mucus compresses the lumen of the artery, usually causing intermittent claudication. The diagnosis can be made from an arteriogram, and the treatment is quite simple. It consists of opening the outer wall of the artery and evacuation of the mucoid material. This is very successful provided the arterial lumen has not become obliterated by thrombus.

The popliteal entrapment syndrome

This also is a very rare syndrome. The popliteal artery, which normally passes between the heads of the gastrocnemius muscle, passes instead through the medial head so that when the muscle is contracted the artery is compressed. When this has been going on for some time local thrombosis results and the artery becomes occluded, leading to intermittent claudication. Before thrombosis occludes the artery the problem can be relieved by a simple division of the offending muscle fibres, so releasing the popliteal artery. If thrombosis has already taken place the segment of artery may be replaced by a graft, preferably of endogenous vein.

Cervical rib

A cervical rib is an extra rib which articulates with the last cervical vertebra and extends forward to a variable extent. It may be complete, passing forward to articulate with the first rib, or it may be only a short proximal bony stump, ending either abruptly with a rounded knob of bone or cartilage, or being continued forwards by a dense fibrous band which in turn is inserted into the upper surface of the front portion of the true first rib (Fig. 43.15). The brachial plexus and subclavian artery pass over the top of this abnormal structure as they travel to the arm and symptoms may ensue due to pressure on

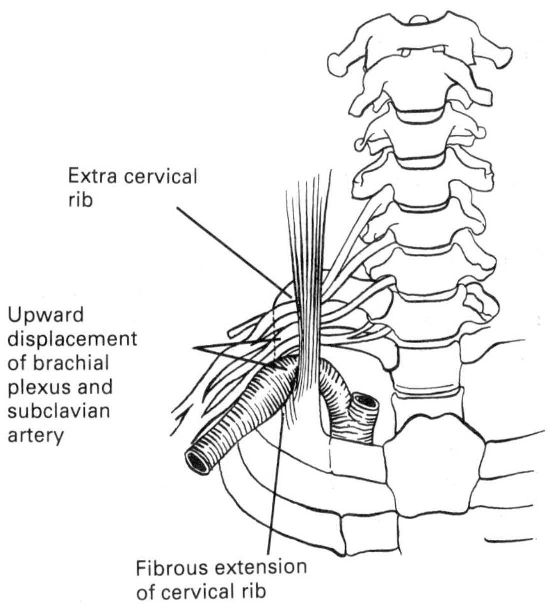

Fig. 43.15 Cervical rib, with a fibrous extension running forward to attach to the proper first rib. The vessel and nerves are elevated and arch over the rib and/or fibrous band.

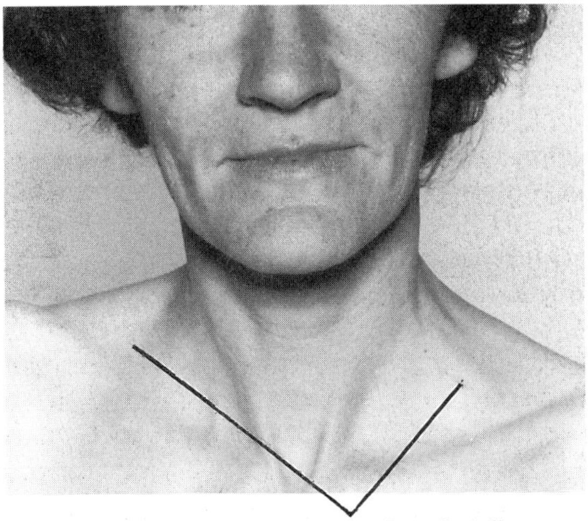

Fig. 43.16 Bilateral cervical ribs, with a prominent bulge in the left supraclavicular fossa. The hard extra bony ridge was easily palpable.

or stretching of either of these structures. The most common symptoms are due to nerve involvement, the lower parts of the plexus being compressed between the scalenus anterior muscle and the cervical rib (Fig. 43.16). Symptoms may occur only when the arm is placed in certain positions, e.g. elevated above the head, or when carrying heavy loads. Arterial compression may lead to a stenosis of the artery, with dilatation of the artery distal to the stenosis (poststenotic dilatation). Mural thrombosis may occur in the compressed or dilated segments and give rise to distal emboli. A more dramatic and serious arterial complication from a cervical rib is complete occlusion of the subclavian artery by thrombus. This may cause gangrene of fingers or part of the hand if not promptly dealt with.

If the extra rib or rudimentary part of one is a completely incidental finding, causing no symptoms whatsoever, it should be left alone. However, if either neurological or vascular symptoms are present it is wise to advise surgical excision. This is accomplished by a supraclavicular approach, taking care to free the brachial plexus and subclavian artery of all compression or displacement by removing all bony and fibrous elements of the supernumerary structure.

Raynaud's disease and phenomenon

There has been considerable discussion about the existence of a specific disease called Raynaud's disease since Raynaud first described the colour changes in the hand after exposure to cold in 1826. Most workers would, however, agree that there is a primary and a secondary Raynaud's phenomenon. Whether the primary Raynaud's phenomenon should be called Raynaud's disease or not is debatable, but the behaviour of the hand on exposure to cold is identical in both types. The sequence of colour changes on exposure to cold from pallor of the hand, followed by a dark blue discoloration and then by fiery red colour is characteristic. As these colour changes take place the patient complains of pain in the fingers, which are also felt to be clumsy, numb, difficult to use especially for fine tasks, e.g. fastening buttons, picking up small objects, etc. After a variable period of time—usually some minutes after moving to a warmer environment—both the colour and sensory changes gradually revert to normal.

Although exposure to cold is by far and away the commonest triggering factor, in some patients typical attacks can be precipitated by emotional stress.

Examination of the hands between attacks and in a comfortably warm environment may show no

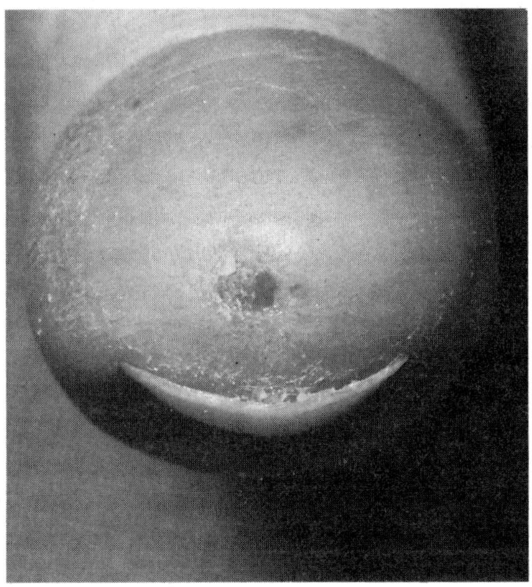

Fig. 43.17 A small healing infarct at distal end of finger-pulp, typical of microembolism in Raynaud's disease.

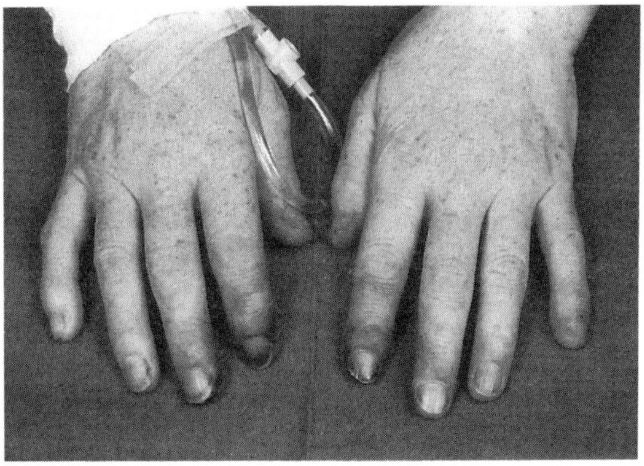

Fig. 43.18 Ischaemia of several fingers of both hands in a patient with Raynaud's syndrome. Gangrenous patches in several finger-tips are due to small emboli from the partly compressed and dilated subclavian arteries.

obvious abnormality. In the more severe cases the pulps of affected fingers may show some loss of substance, giving a tapered rather than rounded appearance. This is due to repeated minute infarcts of pulp substance from the prolonged blockage of small digital arterioles (Fig. 43.17). Occasionally discrete gangrenous patches are encountered on the fingertips (Fig. 43.18). Peripheral pulses, e.g. brachial and radial, are usually normal and easy to feel.

In the primary form of the disorder, usually in young females, there is no apparent associated cause, but there may be a family history of the condition.

Secondary Raynaud's phenomenon, on the other hand, has an underlying cause such as systemic sclerosis, a cervical rib, injury or rheumatoid disease. It may also present in patients who use vibrating tools for long periods. These latter cases may show extensive occlusion of the digital arteries.

The treatment of secondary Raynaud's phenomenon is therefore either the removal of the incapacitating factor or the treatment of the underlying cause.

The mainstay of treatment for primary Raynaud's phenomenon is for the patient to avoid, as far as possible, exposure to rapid changes of temperature, particularly to cold—and this applies to all parts of the body, not just the hands. The less often attacks are precipitated, the less likely severe progression will occur, and there is a chance that the frequency and severity of attacks will lessen with the passage of time. Vasodilators may be prescribed, particularly over the colder seasons, but usually afford little or no benefit. For those whose symptoms worsen, and where disability is compounded by damage to the pulps or gangrenous patches threaten, the operation of upper thoracic sympathectomy should be considered (Fig. 43.19). Immediate improvement in all symptoms is usually very impressive, but unfortunately it is nearly always temporary and the symptoms gradually return as bad as ever over months or 1 or 2 years. The operation is, therefore, only recommended for those who are most badly troubled and the patient should be warned that the benefit may not be permanent.

Allied to Raynaud's phenomenon is acrocyanosis, where the patient's extremities simply go blue and cold on exposure to cold. The blueness is blotchy and the patients often have thickened ankles and wrists. It is usually confined to young females living in colder regions and, as with primary Raynaud's phenomenon, there is no very adequate treatment, although vasodilator drugs occasionally help.

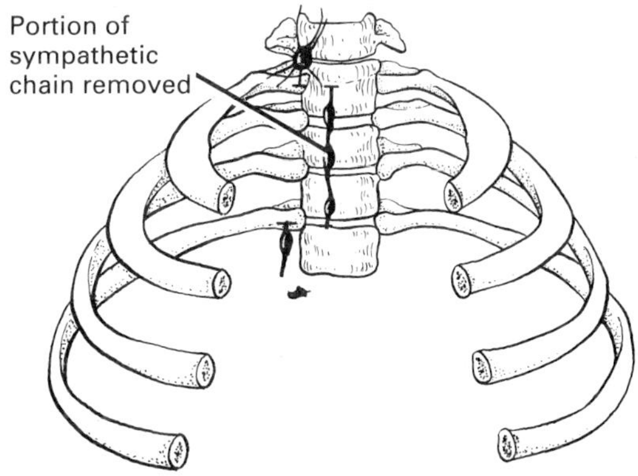

Fig. 43.19 Cervical—or more correctly upper thoracic—sympathectomy. Through either an anterior supraclavicular, or a transaxillary approach, the upper three or four thoracic ganglia are dissected and excised, taking care not to damage the stellate ganglion which may lead to a Horner's syndrome.

Arterial aneurysms

An aneurysm is a blood-containing sac connected with an artery. It may be a true aneurysm, of which the wall comprises the stretched tissues of the

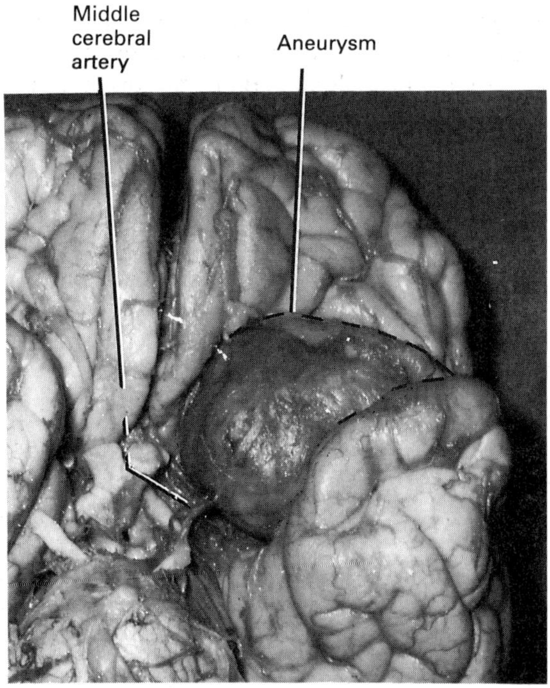

Fig. 43.20 Large aneurysm of the middle cerebral artery, displacing the temporal from the frontal lobes of the brain.

arterial wall itself, or a false aneurysm, which is a cavity in the soft tissues around an artery connecting with the lumen of the artery. A true aneurysm may be saccular, where one wall of the artery dilates to form a sac connected to the vessel by a wide mouth, or it may be fusiform with almost symmetrical dilatation of the arterial wall (Fig. 43.20). Aneurysms may be:

1. congenital in origin, e.g. the intracranial aneurysms on the branches of the circle of Willis;
2. traumatic, where the artery is punctured and a false aneurysm forms around the puncture site (Fig. 43.21);
3. infective, e.g. syphilitic or mycotic aneurysms;
4. atherosclerotic in aetiology—the vast majority.

The commonest site at which atherosclerotic aneurysms develop is in the abdominal aorta below the renal arteries. The aorta becomes elongated, dilated and tortuous. Calcium is often deposited in its wall and layers of thrombus form on the inner wall of the sac, leaving a central channel surrounded by laminated thrombus through which the blood flow is maintained. If the aneurysm is untreated, increasing dilatation will almost invariably lead to rupture and the patient will die of massive haemorrhage unless operated on as an emergency. The common iliac arteries are often aneurysmal either separately or in continuity with an abdominal aortic aneurysm. Aneurysms may also occur in other vessels, e.g. the femoral or popliteal arteries, the aortic arch, the thoracic aorta or the visceral arteries.

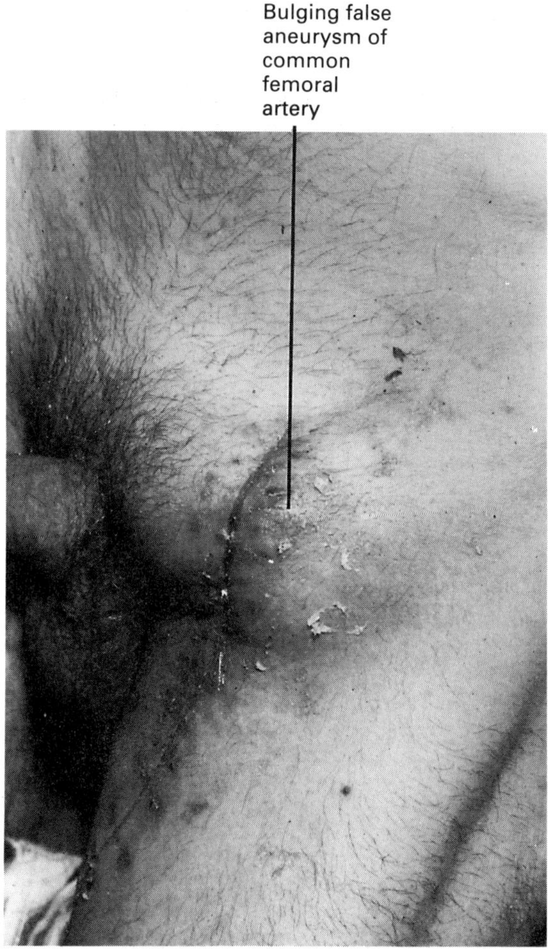

Fig. 43.21 False aneurysm of common femoral artery. This is secondary to local infection at the site of the proximal anastomosis in a femoropopliteal bypass graft. The wall of the false aneurysm is simply layers of fibrous tissue laid down in response to the infection, and into which the leaking blood from the damaged anastomosis pulsates. Operative correction is needed.

Abdominal aortic aneurysms

The majority of abdominal aortic aneurysms occur in the older age groups, around 60 years of age.

Presentation may be simply as a pulsating lump in the upper abdomen found either by the patient or by a doctor during routine examination, as the patient has no other complaint. On the other hand, the patient may complain of mild symptoms such as abdominal discomfort or back pain, particularly if the aneurysm erodes the front of the vertebral bodies. Since atheromatous disease commonly presents with intermittent claudication and other ischaemic problems affecting the legs, and atheroma is also the main cause of aneurysms, a significant number are detected in the physical examination of the patient presenting with these leg symptoms. If a portion of the blood clot from the aneurysm becomes detached, it may block a distal artery as an embolus, and this may be the episode which brings the diagnosis to light.

Palpation of the abdomen, unless there is very gross obesity, will reveal the tense rounded swelling exhibiting truly expansile pulsation, as distinct from the transmitted pulsation of a solid mass overlying the normal aorta. The examining fingers, placed as laterally as possible around the mass and gently compressing it, are pushed apart from each other by each beat. If desired, more precise definition of its width and longitudinal extent can be obtained by the non-invasive technique of ultrasound. Arteriography is potentially very dangerous, unnecessary, and should be avoided.

The correct advice to most patients with an aortic aneurysm is to have it surgically replaced by a synthetic graft because of the high risk of fatal rupture. The only two groups where an exception might be made are where the aneurysm is less than 5 cm in diameter: in this case it is reasonable to keep under review, assessing the size by repeat ultrasound measurements and advising operation if there is clear evidence of progressive enlargement, and in patients with even greater risks to their lives, e.g. from recent large myocardial infarcts or cerebrovascular accidents.

The operation, through a long longitudinal or transverse abdominal incision, involves application of clamps proximal and distal to the aneurysm, opening it along its length and inserting either a straight or inverted Y-shaped graft of Dacron or Teflon, anastomosing this to the proximal aorta above and either distal aorta or the two common iliac arteries below, depending on the distal extent of the aneurysm. On completion of the anastomoses and restoration of blood flow the walls of the original sac are usually sutured around the graft.

In experienced hands a mortality of less than 5% can be expected and long-term patency is good.

Ruptured aneurysm

Complete rupture will, of course, lead to fatal exsanguinating haemorrhage within a few seconds. Often, however, there is a limited escape of blood initially into the retroperitoneal tissues, which for a while may be contained, giving a brief opportunity for surgical correction, before going on to the otherwise inevitable fatal bleed. The clinical picture presented by this initial limited leak is dramatic, with the sudden onset of severe encircling pain around the upper or mid abdomen, distress and the symptoms and signs of blood loss, e.g. rapid pulse and breathing, faintness, sweating and anxiety. Emergency operation is the only hope for the patient. It is essential to control the bleeding and replace the aneurysm with an appropriate graft.

Resection of a ruptured abdominal aortic aneurysm is one of the few operations where time is of the essence, and the patient must be taken to the theatre as soon as possible. It is important not to begin the operation until blood is available because the induction of anaesthesia can inactivate the important mechanisms compensating for the hypovolaemia, and furthermore on opening the abdomen fresh bleeding is often induced. Once the abdomen is opened the diagnosis is usually obvious because of the presence of a large, retroperitoneal haematoma and free blood in the peritoneal cavity. The aneurysm is exposed rapidly and the aorta below the renal artery is defined with a combination of sharp and finger dissection so that a clamp can be placed across it. Once this clamp has been applied, the danger of massive bleeding is controlled and at this stage sufficient blood should be transfused to restore normal blood pressure. The remainder of the procedure is little different to that of an uncomplicated aneurysm.

In order to replace the lower aorta, the inferior mesenteric artery has to be sacrificed and although this has usually little or no effect on the viability of the sigmoid colon, it is essential to inspect the colon before the abdomen is closed. As the majority of patients presenting with a ruptured abdominal aortic aneurysm are elderly they often have many other vascular and cardiorespiratory problems which appear during recovery.

The operative mortality for ruptured abdominal aortic aneurysm is between 50 and 60% in most centres. Since this is 10–20 times greater than the mortality risk for elective grafting, this emphasizes the wisdom of elective surgery to avoid this danger.

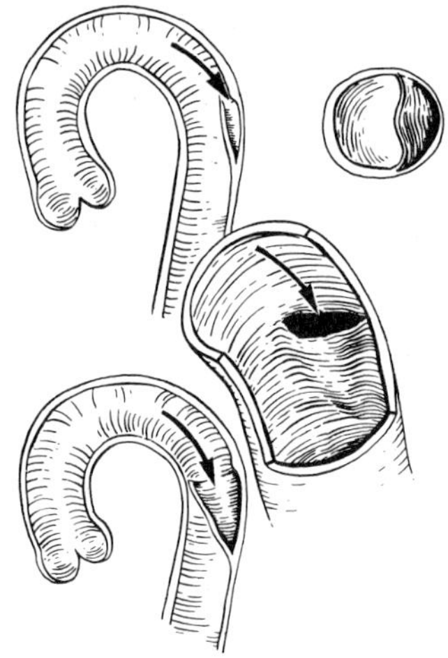

Fig. 43.22 Stages in the development of a dissecting aneurysm. At first a small split in the intima appears and then the force of each pulse beat, represented by the arrows, further peels the inner layer away from the outer ones in the arterial wall, until finally the raised flap completely occludes the original lumen.

Aneurysm of aortic arch

Aneurysms of the aortic arch were previously associated with syphilis but these are now uncommon. Atherosclerotic aneurysms are also relatively uncommon but when they occur they cause symptoms, usually from pressure on the trachea or the oesophagus, or the erosion of the sternum. There may also be pressure on the recurrent laryngeal nerve causing paralysis of the vocal cord and hoarseness. There may in addition be abnormalities of the aortic valve. The diagnosis of aneurysm is usually made when a chest X-ray demonstrates an increased width of the mediastinum with sometimes a globular shadow in it. Surgical replacement by synthetic graft usually requires cardiopulmonary bypass after careful and full cardiac and arteriographic assessment.

Dissecting aneurysms

Dissection occurs where blood driven by the intra-arterial pressure forces a way through a split in the friable diseased intima to find a plane within the damaged, weakened media (Fig. 43.22). It then forces a longitudinal split distally along this plane so that the inner layer of intima plus media is pushed across the lumen to block both the artery distal to this point and the branches arising from the segment. At the distal end of the dissection the blood may escape outwards to cause fatal haemorrhage, or it may re-enter the artery lumen through a 'window' back through the inner layer of intima and media. Dissecting aneurysm is one of the causes of sudden death. It is associated in the majority of cases with atherosclerosis and occurs usually in the region of the ascending aorta or the aortic arch, but may occur lower down in the descending or abdominal aorta.

The patient with dissection presents with sudden severe pain in the chest or abdomen associated with severe back pain, a fall in blood pressure and a rising pulse rate. It is often possible to detect a difference in the force and volume of the radial and the femoral pulses, and this is an important clue in clinical diagnosis. It is helpful to get a firm diagnosis of the origin of the dissection and its extent by aortography. The only exception to this rule is where the viability of the legs is at hazard from a dissection which has reached the lower abdominal aorta. In this situation urgent operation is required, with the aim of creating a 'window' in the inner layer of the aorta proximal to the lower end of the dissection and suturing the lower flap of the media back into position below the 'window'. The aorta is then closed. As far as lesions in the aortic arch or descending thoracic aorta are concerned, considerable judgement is required to decide between conservative management with hypotensive drugs if necessary, or surgical repair or replacement by graft under bypass.

Coarctation of the aorta

Coarctation of the aorta is a fairly common congenital abnormality where the arch is narrowed, usually just distal to the left subclavian artery, by a congenital failure of complete canalization of the aorta. Blood tends to pass to the distal part of the body through an extensive collateral circulation which includes the intercostal arteries, the internal mammary artery and the parascapular arteries (Fig. 43.23). The patient becomes hypertensive in the upper part of the body proximal to the narrowed segment and relatively hypotensive in the lower part of the body. The hypertension occurs because the heart attempts to force blood through the increased peripheral resistance caused by the narrowing in the aorta. The patient presents, therefore, with features of hypertension, such as headaches, or with signs of left ventricular failure. Physical examination shows a diminution or even absence of the femoral pulses. There may be an increase in blood pressure in the arm with a reduced blood pressure in the lower limbs, and sometimes abnormal vessels can be felt, particularly along the medial border of the scapula. X-ray examination of the chest shows notching of the ribs caused by the very much enlarged intercostal arteries and aortography confirms the presence of the coarctation. Under the usual circumstances of it being distal to the left subclavian artery, it can therefore be dealt with without cardiopulmonary bypass because of the presence of the very large collaterals, maintaining an adequate supply of blood to the lower part of the body. However, in much rarer cases, the arch itself is affected and these patients may indeed need a cardiopulmonary bypass.

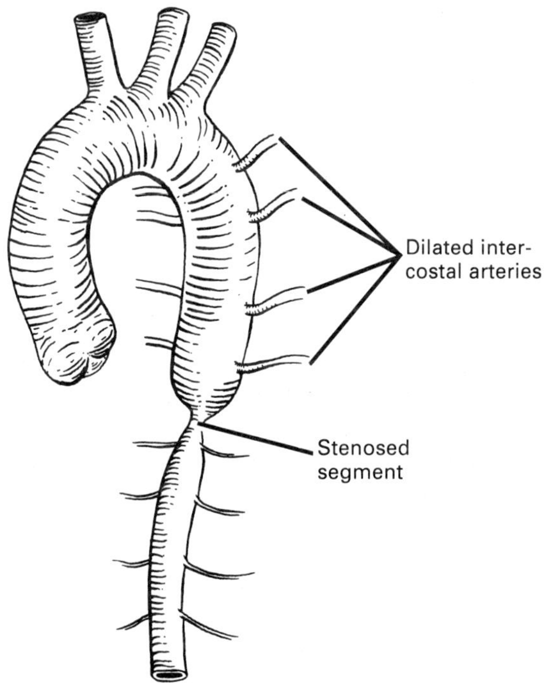

Fig. 43.23 Coarctation of the aorta: above the congenitally stenosed segment the aorta and its branches dilate, and distally there is poor low-pressure filling. The intercostal arteries may palpably pulsate.

Management

Coarctation of the aorta is treated by the excision of the stenosed segment and end-to-end anastomosis. If the narrowed segment is very large, the gap is bridged by a Teflon or Dacron graft.

Occlusion of the great vessels

The vessels arising from the aortic arch are the innominate, the left common carotid and the left subclavian arteries. Any of these may be affected by atherosclerosis of the aortic arch itself or, much more commonly, they are affected from about 1 cm or so from their points of origin. Usually the narrowing is slowly progressive and a collateral circulation develops so that the occlusion itself may be without symptoms; the first indication that a great vessel has been occluded may be the recognition of a disappearing pulse in the radial artery or any pulse in the arm. Nearly always this occlusion is atherosclerotic but a rare condition which affects young patients in their 20s or 30s is a form of non-specific arteritis known as Takayasu's disease. Isolated atherosclerotic lesions in these large vessels rarely require operative treatment.

Lesions of the carotid and vertebral arteries

These vessels arise from the aortic arch or its branches and are quite often the seat of symptomatic lesions. It will be recalled that the blood supply to the brain comes from the two internal carotid arteries and the two vertebral arteries, all of which enter the circle of Willis which is formed by anastomosing channels at the base of the brain. The internal carotid artery is one of the two main branches of the common carotid which on the right side arises from the innominate artery and on the left directly from the aortic arch. The vertebral arteries arise from the subclavian arteries and pass upwards alongside the vertebral column to reach the posterior part of the brain. On the whole, cerebral ischaemia does not develop from occlusion of only one artery and usually two or more arteries are involved. However, a solitary lesion in the internal carotid artery may cause cerebral problems because of the formation of thrombus, either of platelets or of fibrin on the plaque and portions breaking off to form small emboli which may block intracranial vessels.

The common site for atherosclerotic lesions in the internal carotid artery is at its origin, and this may cause narrowing or, much more commonly, an ulcerated plaque at this site. In nearly all patients before a major stroke there are transient episodes which may act as a warning. These symptoms are called transient ischaemic attacks and as approximately 30% of major strokes are associated with lesions of an extracranial artery, it is very important that these transient ischaemic attacks should be taken seriously. They may occur as attacks of headache, dizziness or, more commonly, temporary disturbances of vision or of speech, with or without transient limb or facial weakness. The episode may involve one or all of these symptoms and it is very important that, once these are recognized, the patient should be fully investigated. Patients sometimes experience 'drop attacks', in which they lose consciousness so that they fall to the ground. In addition to lesions of the carotid arteries themselves, occlusion of the subclavian or the innominate artery may lead to episodes of transient cerebral ischaemia because of interference with the blood flow through the vertebral artery. This is the so–called subclavian steal syndrome which occurs when the innominate artery or the subclavian artery is occluded at a point before the origin of the vertebral artery. A collateral circulation develops from the normal side via the subclavian and vertebral arteries and when the arm is exercised, blood flow in the vertebral artery on the side of the obstruction reverses its direction and flows down the arm. This reduces the cerebral blood flow and the subclavian is said to be stealing the blood from the brain to supply the arm.

If there is any reason to suspect a vascular anomaly in the extracranial arteries, the patient should be investigated. If the episode takes the form of transient ischaemic attacks attributable to a lesion in the carotid arteries, one has the choice of an arch aortogram or direct carotid puncture. The problem about arch aortogram is that it may not demonstrate adequately the details of the internal carotid artery and if the suspicion exists that there is such a lesion and this is not demonstrated by the arch aortogram, then direct-puncture carotid angiography should be performed. On the other hand, if there is evidence of subclavian steal syndrome then obviously an arch aortogram is required.

The treatment of carotid artery atherosclerosis is by endarterectomy. In this procedure, the obstructing or ulcerating material is removed and usually the arteriotomy can be closed by simple suture or if there is anxiety about any narrowing, by adding a vein patch. The operation can be performed under local anaesthesia, when the patient's cerebral functions can be monitored throughout. If done under general anaesthesia it may be wise to employ some form of arterial bypass shunt to maintain an adequate blood flow to the brain during the procedure. Patients with subclavian steal syndrome can be dealt with either by removing the obstruction in the innominate or subclavian arteries directly or, more commonly by creating a shunt between one of the normal arteries and the obstructed subclavian artery. This shunt can be by means of vein graft or sometimes it is possible to use a Dacron graft. The operations are successful in reducing the number of strokes that follow transient ischaemic attacks. Recent figures suggest that if a patient has a transient ischaemic attack, he or she is very likely to have a major stroke within a period varying between 6 and 18 months. After carotid endarterectomy only a minority experience further problems.

Intestinal ischaemia

Intestinal ischaemia is caused by lesions affecting an arterial supply to the gut. There are three main arteries—the coeliac axis which supplies the stomach and the upper part of the small bowel; the superior mesenteric artery which supplies the middle portion of the gut, i.e. the small intestine and the large bowel up to the distal part of the transverse colon, and the inferior mesenteric artery which supplies the remainder. Occlusion or stenosis of these vessels may produce ischaemia of the bowel which may be acute or chronic, depending on how quickly the interference of the blood supply takes place. The syndromes associated with the disease of the mesenteric arteries therefore vary between the sudden occlusion leading to gangrene of large parts of the alimentary tract and the slower occlusion resulting in problems with absorption and digestion. It is clear that, like the extracranial circulation, symptoms rarely occur from disease of one artery alone, apart from sudden occlusion of the superior mesenteric artery, and certainly in chronic intestinal ischaemia it is usually necessary for two or all three arteries to be involved by the atherosclerosis.

Acute intestinal ischaemia

Sudden occlusion of the superior mesenteric artery cuts off the blood supply to the small intestine, the ascending colon and the transverse colon and if the circulation is not restored within a very short time, gangrene of the bowel with peritonitis will develop and, although the gangrenous area can be removed, survival is very unlikely. There are two main causes of occlusion of the superior mesenteric artery—embolism and thrombosis. Whatever the cause, once the superior mesenteric artery is occluded, the arterial tree beyond the block empties, though it may refill rapidly with blood from neighbouring channels, or alternatively by backflow from the mesenteric veins. If thrombosis occurs in the distal arteries, it is impossible to restore normal circulation, and gangrene of the bowel is inevitable.

The clinical features of acute infarction of bowel are the same whether the occlusion occurs from embolus or from thrombosis. The patient is usually middle-aged or elderly. There may be a known source of possible emboli or, more likely, concomitant evidence of atherosclerosis elsewhere. The main symptom is abdominal pain, often severe, and associated with very few physical signs if examined at an early stage. The pain is accompanied later by symptoms and signs of blood loss and toxaemia. Sometimes the onset may be quite insidious, with ill defined pain and only a gradual deterioration in the patient's general state. Vomiting is common and occasionally diarrhoea, possibly with evidence of blood passed with the stool, is present. The patient's condition deteriorates because of the loss of fluid and blood into the gut. Later, distension appears and vomiting becomes even more frequent as gangrene of the bowel and peritonitis ensue. It can be difficult to make the appropriate diagnosis in the early stage, and this may lead to undue delay before operation is decided upon. It is sometimes possible to resect the bowel, particularly if the gangrene is limited to less than the whole area supplied by the superior mesenteric artery, but this is often not successful and further gangrene develops. If seen early enough it is rarely possible to restore the blood supply to the superior mesenteric artery by a bypass graft or sometimes by removal of the embolus or thrombus from the origin of the artery.

Chronic intestinal ischaemia

If the blood supply is reduced slowly enough, a collateral circulation may develop which allows sufficient blood to flow through these vessels to maintain the viability of the bowel, but not enough to permit normal digestion and absorption. It should be noted that it is not uncommon to find intestinal arteries occluded on arteriography for another purpose, as the patient may be totally symptom-free. Quite often, however, symptoms do occur, the principal one being pain which may come on after eating, particularly if the meal is a large one, but which often does not appear to have a direct relationship with meals. This is the so-called intestinal angina. Almost always the patient loses weight due partly to knowledge that small meals produce less pain than large ones, and also to defective absorption. Evidence of this may be seen in the passage of bulky stools with excess fat. The diagnosis may be quite difficult to make, as the symptoms are often atypical. The occlusion or stenosis of the vessels can usually be confirmed by a *lateral* aortogram. This is necessary in order to visualize properly the origin of the bowel arteries. The aim of surgery is to restore the blood supply to the bowel, and this can be done in several ways, depending partly on the findings on aortography. The various possible approaches are:

1. endarterectomy of the occluded part of the superior mesenteric artery;
2. reimplantation of the patent part of the artery into the aorta;
3. bypass Dacron or vein graft between the aorta and the superior mesenteric artery;
4. anastomosing the ileocolic artery to the right common iliac artery.

A form of ischaemic colitis can affect the colon, usually of elderly patients. The brunt of the change falls on the region of the splenic flexure, at the point furthest from both the middle colic and inferior mesenteric contributions to the marginal arterial arcade, and therefore the part most vulnerable to any overall reduction in arterial flow into this arcade.

The clinical picture often begins with abdominal pain and diarrhoea, and as these symptoms subside a localized fibrous stricture may form, giving rise to subacute obstruction symptoms, or being detected as an incidental finding on barium enema examination. Local excision of the affected segment of colon may be necessary.

Renal artery stenosis and hypertension

Hypertension may be due to a wide variety of conditions, and renal artery stenosis is one of the rare causes. At least, however, if detected, there is often a good chance of alleviating the disorder by either vascular reconstruction, or if unilateral, by nephrectomy. The usual cause of stenosis is atherosclerosis, often occurring in patients younger than usual. Less commonly, fibromuscular dysplasia of the media causes the narrowing of the renal artery. If a hypertensive patient is suspected of having renal artery disease then the investigations which may be helpful are intravenous pyelography, an isotope renogram, renal function studies, differential renal estimations if possible and arteriography. The initial screening test in these patients is a dehydration intravenous pyelogram. When unilateral renal artery stenosis is present excretion of the dye on the affected side is delayed due to reduced glomerular filtration and as there is increased absorption of water in the renal tubules the concentration of the dye on the affected side is increased. This finding on intravenous pyelogram is presumptive evidence of unilateral renal artery stenosis. If the other kidney is healthy in the presence of the delayed excretion and increased concentration on the pyelogram, an isotope renogram can be performed if the equipment is available. This is done by giving 2-8 μg radioiodine and scanning the kidneys. However, in the absence of facilities for performing the renogram, differential renal function studies are a good substitute. In this test both ureters are catheterized and urine from each catheter is collected separately. The patient is given a diuretic to produce a large urine flow and the urine is collected from each kidney separately.

In the patient with renal artery stenosis there is a reduction in the volume of urine from that side, a reduction in sodium and chloride and an increase in the creatinine and urea concentrations. With strongly supportive evidence from one or more of these initial investigations, it is then necessary to proceed with aortography to make a direct diagnosis and evaluation of the pattern of stenosis or occlusion. A stenosed artery usually shows as a constriction near its origin, with often a poststenotic dilatation beyond it. Sometimes, particularly in the patient with fibromuscular dysplasia, the constriction extends into many or all of the branches of the renal artery. Often, when the lesion is due to atherosclerosis, other atherosclerotic lesions can also be seen in the aorta.

If the arterial lesion affects most of the renal artery or the kidney is small and the other kidney is normal, it is probably best to remove that kidney. However, if the kidney is of reasonable size and function, and the arterial lesion is localized on one side, surgical restoration of normal blood flow to that kidney should be attempted. This procedure may be an endarterectomy directly to remove the obstructive lesion from the renal artery or, more likely, the lesion may be bypassed by vein or synthetic graft, or the unaffected segment of the renal artery re-implanted directly on to the aorta.

The results are good when the remaining kidney has not been severely damaged by hypertension and the blood pressure reverts to normal in about two-thirds of the patients. Unfortunately, the so-called normal kidney may be so damaged by the hypertension that this may persist even after successful surgical relief of the stenosis.

ARTERIAL TRAUMA

Vascular trauma is often part of the picture in the multiply injured patient, and may take priority over other bony and soft tissue injuries. As a result of injury, the blood vessel may be completely sectioned; partially severed, i.e. ruptured without complete section, or contused without any gross break in continuity.

Completely sectioned blood vessels

Completely sectioned blood vessels sometimes do not bleed because of the occlusion of the lumen by the infolding of the intima at each cut end of the artery, and the spasm of the muscular coat of the artery closing the lumen. If these two processes are not sufficient profuse bleeding ensues.

Partially severed blood vessels

Incompletely divided arteries usually bleed profusely because contraction of the arterial wall increases the size of the opening in the artery. Sometimes the extravasated blood becomes organized with the development of a fibrous envelope around it, thereby creating a false aneurysm.

In other circumstances the adjoining vein may also be ruptured and a direct arteriovenous fistula forms, pulsatile arterial pressure being transmitted to the vein. This is more liable to occur in sharp stab wounds rather than lacerations.

Contused blood vessels

In contusion the intima and possibly the media are injured to varying degrees. This may serve as a starting point for thrombus formation which may extend both proximally and distally (Fig. 43.24). Indeed, the intima of the contused artery may be completely torn and the two ends may infold to block the lumen. Ischaemia of the tissues supplied by the contused artery may produce catastrophic results, e.g. in Volkmann's ischaemic contracture which develops following contusion of the brachial artery in fractures and dislocations round the elbow (Fig. 43.25).

This is a particular hazard in supracondylar fracture of the humerus in children. Any suspicion of arterial compromise which persists after good reduction of this fracture should lead to prompt

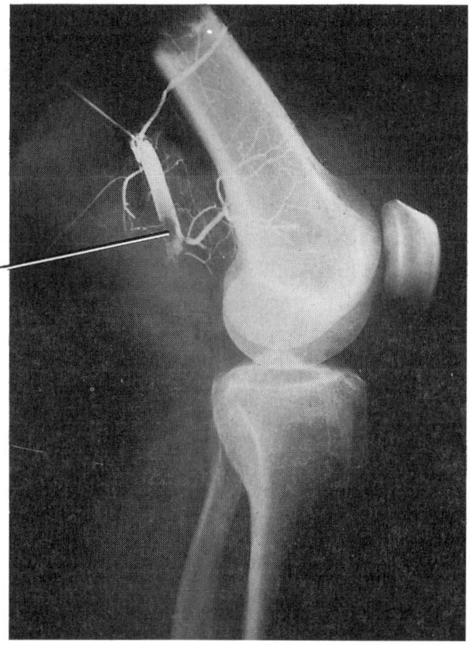

Fig. 43.24 Road traffic accident: patient presenting with clinically ischaemic lower leg. Preoperative arteriogram shows complete interruption of the distal popliteal artery. Exploration revealed thrombosis over a 6 cm segment distal to the point of occlusion demonstrated. Saphenous vein graft was required to replace the damaged segment.

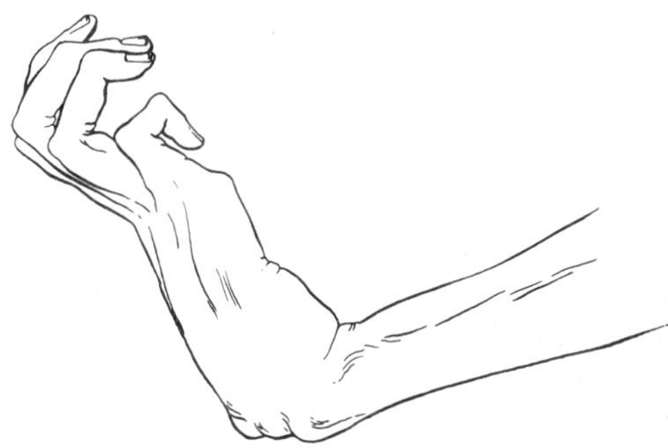

Fig. 43.25 Volkmann's ischaemic contracture of the forearm. The flexors of both wrist and fingers—the more powerful muscle groups—are most affected. The metacarpophalangeal joints remain extended.

surgical exploration of the brachial artery and excision of any damaged segment with either direct re-anastomosis or grafting.

Clinical features and management

Bleeding from an injured vessel is most conveniently and effectively controlled by direct pressure on the vessel as a first-aid measure. On exploring a wound, judgement is exercised in deciding whether to ligate the bleeding artery or to attempt to re-establish continuity. In general, injuries of the internal carotid, the common femoral, popliteal, axillary and brachial arteries should be dealt with by end-to-end anastomosis if possible. If the gap between the end segments is too great, a graft, preferably from the long saphenous or some other suitable superficial vein, is used to bridge it. In the case of most of the other arteries of the limbs the two ends can safely be ligated.

It may be possible to repair a partial severance of a major artery after the application of suitable clamps if the cut is small and clean, and the wound is not grossly contaminated. If this is not feasible an approach similar to that for completely severed arteries is used.

Traumatic false aneurysms will require surgical excision after proximal and distal temporary control, and either direct repair of the damaged portion of the artery or graft replacement of the segment.

A traumatic arteriovenous fistula will also need to be repaired by an operation, at which it may be fairly straightforward to divide the communication and repair both artery and vein. Failing this, quadruple ligation, i.e. of artery and vein both proximal and distal to the fistula, may be used.

VENOUS DISORDERS

The three venous disorders which will be considered in this section are congenital arteriovenous fistula, varicose veins and venous thrombosis.

CONGENITAL ARTERIOVENOUS FISTULA

This is a rare condition which may present in any part of the body but in surgical practice is most frequently seen in the limbs.

There are multiple connections between arteries and veins: the number of the vessels involved is variable but sometimes very numerous indeed.

The structure of the veins involved with the fistula is changed because of the increased quantity of blood at high pressure which is carried by them. These become arterialized, i.e. their calibre increases and there is hypertrophy of the venous wall.

The artery proximal to the fistula may become tortuous and dilated. If the total volume of blood shunted from the arterial to the venous side is large, the greatly increased venous return to the heart puts a considerable strain on it, the left ventricle hypertrophies and eventually the patient goes into heart failure.

The affected limb is enlarged in all directions as a result of an increased rate of development during the growth phase. All the tissues—the skin, muscles and bones—take part in the process. Although the total flow of arterial blood to the limb is increased, paradoxically, as the optimum quantity of blood is not passing through normal capillaries, there are varying degrees of hypoxia of the superficial tissues supplied by the affected artery, giving rise to small patches of necrosis of skin or even gangrene of the part.

Clinical features

There may be an obvious difference in the size of the limbs on the two sides, the affected one being larger than the normal. Dilated veins may be visible and pulsating. There may be evidence of necrosis of skin and ulceration in the distal distribution of the affected artery. The local skin temperature is usually raised, venous pulsation can be clearly felt, a thrill may be felt in the artery and on auscultation a bruit is heard both over the artery and the involved veins.

Arteriography or venography usually demonstrates a honeycomb appearance of multiple minute fistulae.

In most cases attempts at surgical or any other methods of trying to obliterate enough of the communications to make any significant improvement fail. Generally there are so many communicating branches and even if a few are left the overall condition of the limb appears to remain much the same. Occasionally, however, when there are clearly only one or two localized fistulae it is worthwhile dividing these surgically. Rarely, if severe heart failure threatens as a direct result of the large amount of shunting and severe trophic disturbances are present distally on the limb, amputation may be merited.

Many are managed simply by wearing elastic support garments, and any degree of heart failure is treated by the appropriate medical measures.

VARICOSE VEINS

Varicosities may develop in the superficial veins of the leg either as a primary disorder, possibly associated with some congenital weakness in the venous valves, or as a complication of some other condition, e.g. deep vein thrombosis, increased pressure on the veins by a gravid uterus or by a pelvic tumour, or the hormonal changes during pregnancy. Primary varicose veins are commoner in those whose occupations involve prolonged periods of standing.

Normally, the direction of venous blood flow in the limbs is from the superficial to the deep veins. This unidirectional flow is maintained by the valves present in the superficial veins, the deep veins, and in the perforating veins connecting the superficial and deep venous systems. From the deep veins, the blood is squeezed up by the contraction of the muscles of the calf; flow is prevented in the reverse direction by the intact valves. During inspiration blood is furthermore sucked into the heart by the negative thoracic pressure. This may also be helped by the increase in intra-abdominal pressure due to the descent of the diaphragm.

In varicose veins, as a result of reversal of blood flow, the superficial veins dilate and become tortuous (Fig. 43.26). Once one proximal valve fails, a relatively greater hydrostatic pressure will be exerted on the next most distal and therefore it will likely soon also become incompetent, and in turn each of the more distal ones will be more easily damaged. The blood tends to stagnate in these veins and there is congestion of the capillaries draining into them. The area of skin drained by these veins therefore becomes relatively hypoxic. Some capillaries at the most dependent part of the column may rupture and blood then extravasates into the skin and subcutaneous tissues, giving rise to a characteristic patchy brown discoloration.

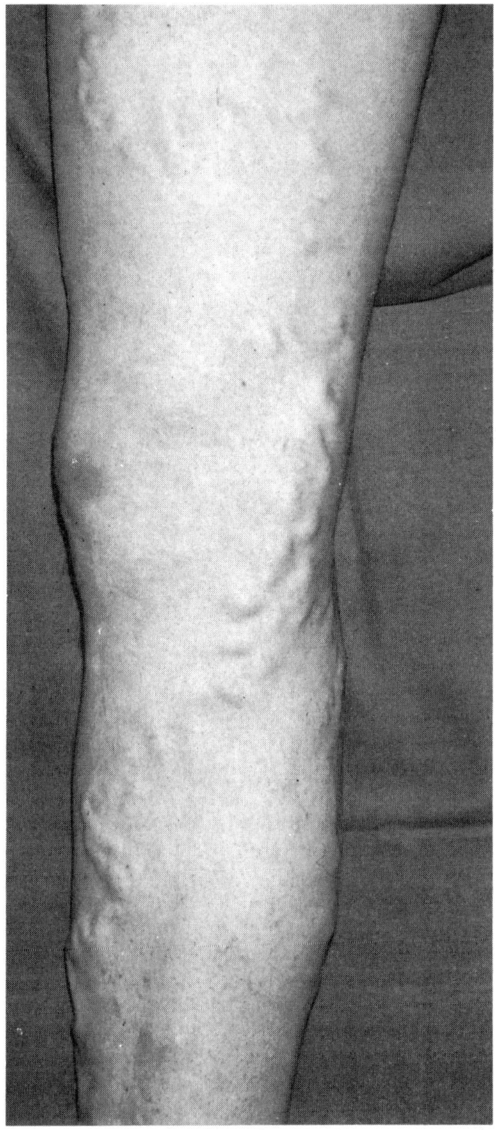

Fig. 43.26 Typical appearance of varicose veins, mainly affecting the long saphenous system of superficial veins.

Subcutaneous hypoxia also encourages ulceration of the skin. The commonest site for these changes and of ultimate ulceration is the area just proximal to the medial malleolus.

Varicose veins become thin-walled and the skin over them thin and stretched. Slight trauma may give rise to bleeding which may be profuse because of the absence of the valves. This can be easily controlled by laying the patient flat and elevating the leg. Light local pressure over the bleeding point may then suffice.

Clinical features

The main reasons for seeking medical advice are:

1. simply because of the unsightly appearance of the varicose veins;
2. the presence of some aching or other local discomfort, often made worse after prolonged periods of standing;
3. anxiety regarding patches of discoloured skin usually near the ankle;
4. frank ulceration, again commonly at this same site.

Assessment

The patient is first examined in the standing position with the entire leg exposed. Simple inspection will usually reveal whether the varicosities are in the long or short saphenous systems, or whether both are involved (Fig. 43.27). The state of the skin is examined; particular attention is paid to the inner aspect of the ankle, looking for areas of the discoloration mentioned above. Attention is next turned to the groin, to see if there is evidence of a saphena varix—the dilated upper end of the long saphenous vein just before it passes deep through the cribriform fascia to join the femoral vein. A significant varix will show as a smooth oval swelling and there may be a cough impulse clearly visible in it. At this stage the opportunity is taken to palpate over any such swelling either to confirm an impulse seen or to detect one which may not have been visible. The presence of a cough impulse signifies that the valve almost constantly present at the saphenofemoral junction is incompetent (Fig. 43.28).

The sites of incompetence in communications between the superficial and deep systems may be indicated by prominent bulges along the varicose veins, especially along both medial and lateral borders of the tibia. Again, with the patient still standing, it may be possible to feel rounded or oval pit-like depressions in the deep fascia at the sites of these incompetent perforators.

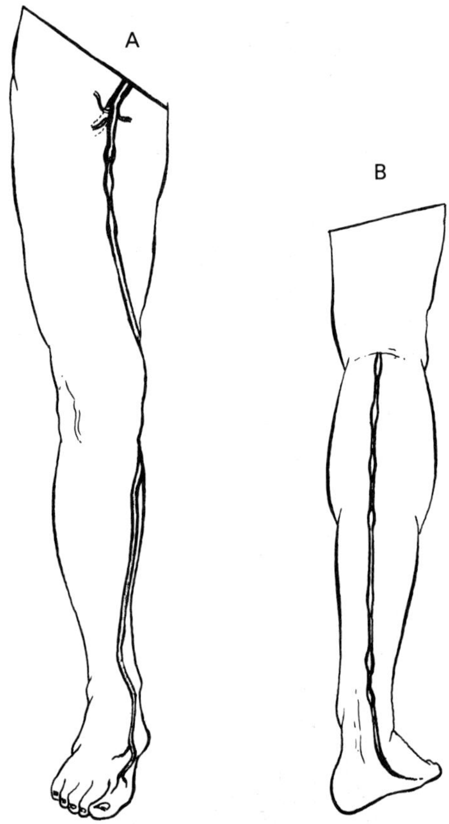

Fig. 43.27 Two main systems of superficial veins in the leg: (**A**) long and (**B**) short saphenous.

More precise identification of points of incompetence between the varicose veins and the deep veins can be made by the Trendelenburg test, and more distal variations of it in the lower parts of the leg (Fig. 43.29). The varicose veins are first emptied by laying the patient supine, elevating and proximally massaging the leg, and then temporary occlusion of the vein at the site of a suspected incompetent perforator is achieved either by pressure from the examiner's fingers or a piece of rubber tubing encircling the limb. With the temporary occlusion being maintained the patient stands upright. If no filling of the varicose veins is observed for at least 30 s, but rapid retrograde filling follows immediately on release of the temporary occlusion, it is concluded that the main defect is the incompetence at the site tested. If, on the other hand, when the patient stands up, with the temporary occlusion still in place, the distal veins fill up immediately or within a few seconds, there are clearly further more

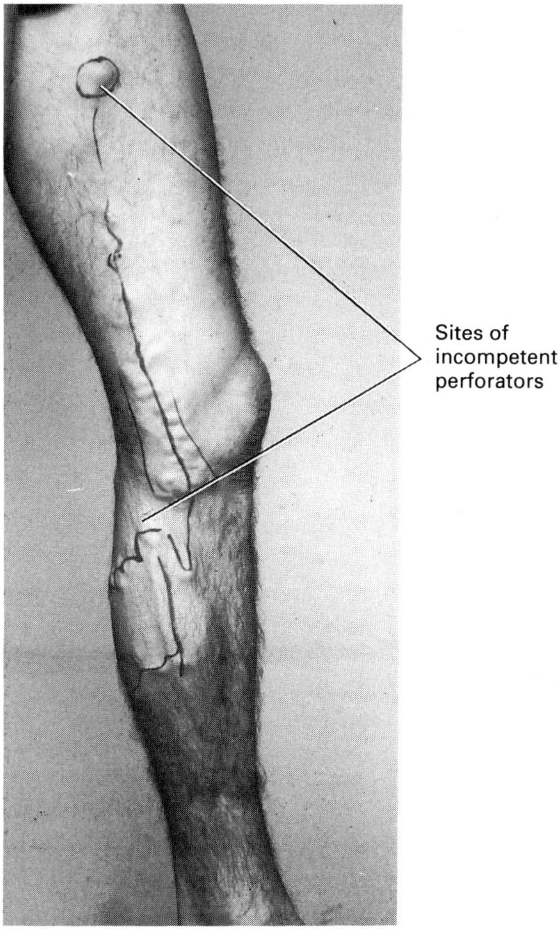

Fig. 43.28 Varicose veins marked prior to operation. The circle at the top of the leg indicates a prominent incompetent perforator—the valve normally impeding backflow from the deep veins into the superficial long saphenous is defective, and a clearly visible and palpable cough impulse was present. A further incompetent perforator is seen about 7.5 cm below the knee, and is marked by the horizontal part of the line. Preoperative marking is most helpful, as when the patient is supine and relaxed under the general anaesthetic the veins will be collapsed and difficult to see.

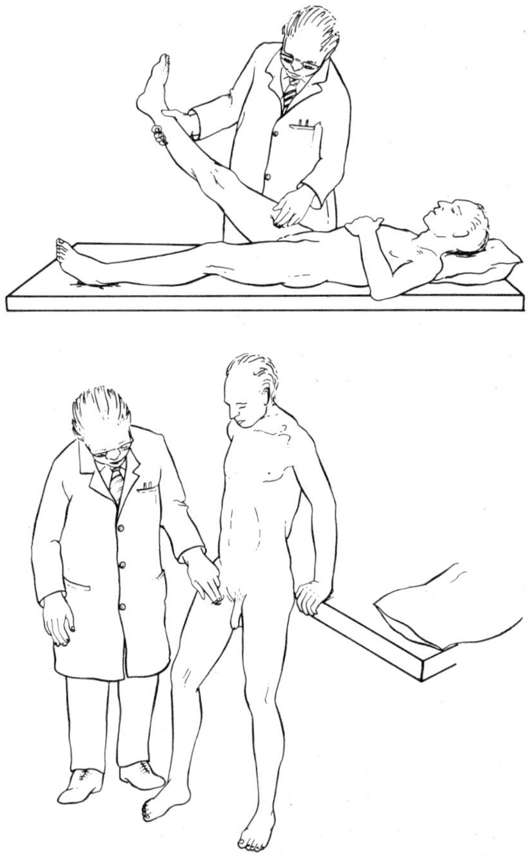

Fig. 43.29 Testing for incompetence of the saphenofemoral valve: Trendelenburg test. The veins are first emptied by elevation of the leg and proximal massage and then with temporary occlusion at the upper end of the long saphenous vein, either by a tourniquet, or more simply by the examiner's finger, the patient stands up. If the varicose veins remain empty the main defect is the valve incompetence at the saphenofemoral junction.

distal incompetent perforators. The test can then be repeated at a series of lower levels, to detect each incompetence in turn. When the test is performed with the pressure applied at the saphenofemoral junction this is the true Trendelenburg test, and at more distal levels various other eponyms are appropriate. The principle is the same, however, at all levels.

Although these simple clinical methods are helpful, they may not give a completely accurate and comprehensive location of all incompetent perforating veins. Venography would be more precise but it is not justifiable, or indeed necessary to submit varicose vein patients to this invasive investigation routinely. Where, however, there is a past history suggestive of a previous deep vein thrombosis, there may be reason to have a venogram to determine whether the deep veins are patent or not. If not, there should be hesitation about offering ablative treatment for the varicose veins, as these may to some extent be compensatory to the occluded deep veins, and removing them may worsen the venous drainage of the leg and aggravate symptoms.

Treatment

The two main options to rid the patient of his or more likely her varicose veins are injection of sclerosants and operative division and ligation, avulsion or stripping. First, of course, it is necessary to ensure that there is no contraindication to treatment, as discussed above, and no known allergy to any of the agents likely to be used.

Injection sclerotherapy is suitable for localized segments of varicosity mainly limited to below the knee. It is less satisfactory for veins in the thigh, mainly on account of the difficulty in keeping bandages in position at this level while remaining fully ambulant. The treatment is most effective if the site of injection of sclerosant, such as 5% ethanolamine or 3% sodium tetradecyl sulphate, is precisely at an incompetent perforator. Once this site is detected, by the method described above, and marked on the skin, the segment is isolated by firm finger pressure both proximally and distally about 1–1.5 ml of sclerosant is injected into the vein lumen; the site of injection is immediately compressed, to empty it of blood and press the anterior and posterior walls of the vein together and a small piece of latex foam pad is applied (Fig. 43.30). If further veins are to be injected at the same session, temporary finger pressure over the pad can be maintained by an assistant until the others are dealt with in the same fashion. When the injections are completed, an elastic webbing support bandage is firmly applied from the forefoot to above the site of the highest injection. The patient is asked to walk several miles each day, to remain active and avoid long periods with the legs resting. All these measures are aimed at reducing the chances of any thrombosis in the deep leg veins. The longer the bandages stay in place without loosening, the more likely it is to obtain satisfactory obliteration of the varicosity. The patient should be reviewed in 3–4 weeks, by which time it should be apparent whether repeat injections or further ones at other sites are required. If the veins are very numerous it is reasonable at the first sitting to inject perhaps only two or three, and deal with the rest at subsequent sessions.

Varicose veins clearly associated with incompetence of the saphenofemoral valve or involving the entire length of the long saphenous system will require some form of operative treatment (Fig. 43.31). This will almost always involve high ligation, by which is implied dissection of all the tributaries to the upper end of the long saphenous vein, and the division and ligation of all these tributaries and of the long saphenous itself—flush with but taking care not to narrow the femoral vein.

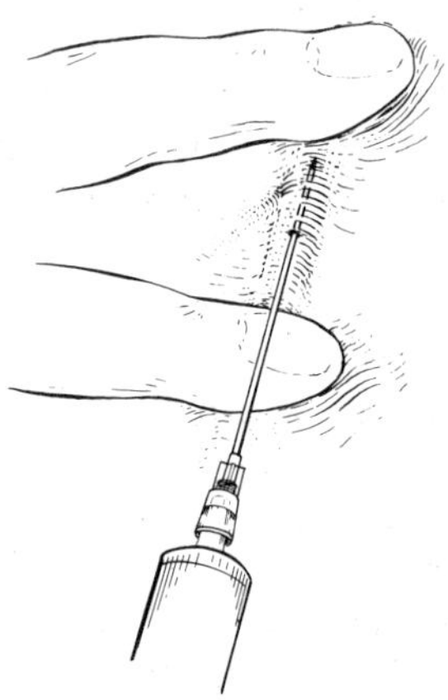

Fig. 43.30 Injection compression sclerotherapy. The sterile sclerosant is injected directly into the lumen of the segment isolated by a finger proximal and distal to the site, and the compression pad and bandage are applied immediately thereafter.

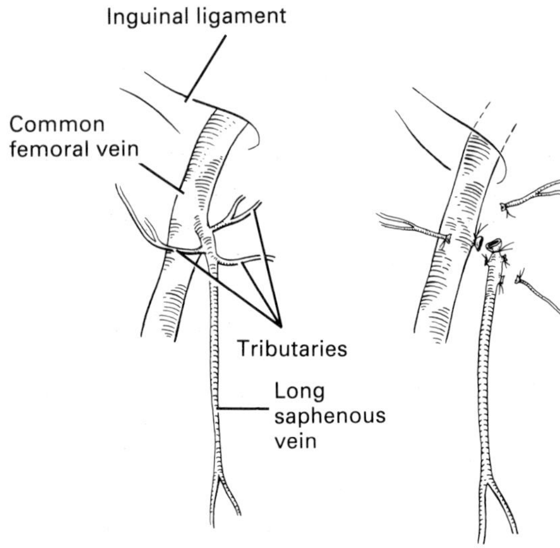

Fig. 43.31 High ligation: Trendelenburg operation. The upper end of the long saphenous vein is ligated and divided just proximal to its junction with the femoral vein. It is also important to ligate and divide the several tributaries which join the long saphenous vein in its last few centimetres, otherwise collateral venous flow may lead to recurrence of the varicosities.

The remainder of the operation may be a choice of:

1. stripping the entire length of the long saphenous vein, by introducing a specially designed long wiry stripper at the ankle and passing it proximally to the groin wound, where it is pulled forcibly out. The objectives are not only to remove the main defective vein, but also to divide across any incompetent tributaries of the long saphenous itself.
2. a series of more distal low ligations at sites of the other incompetent perforators.
3. avulsion of segments of the varicosities through appropriately sited small incisions.

For the less common varicosities of the short saphenous system division and ligation of the upper end of this vein as it passes deep through the popliteal fossa behind the knee are usually effective.

For those who are totally unfit for any of these procedures, or who refuse them, it is customary to advise the wearing of some form of elastic support, preferably a proper-fitting graduated compression stocking. However, if this is not available or acceptable to the patient, any form of support is probably better than none at all.

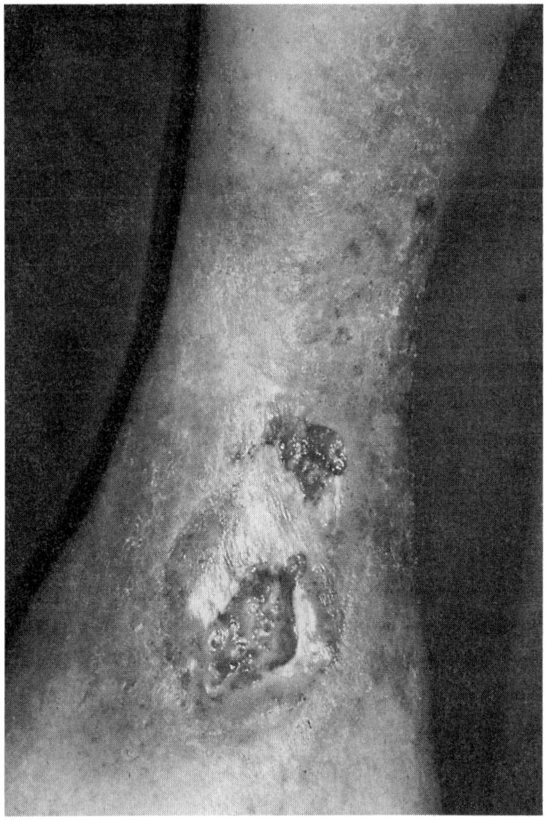

Fig. 43.32 Gravitational (venous) ulcer: typical site and chronic indolent appearance.

Management of varicose (gravitational) ulcer (Fig. 43.32)

As has been mentioned, these ulcers nearly all arise just above the medial malleolus, and are due to stagnant anoxia affecting the skin and superficial tissues. Once the skin breaks, secondary infection is virtually inevitable, and the combination of the underlying venous impairment and the infection makes them difficult to heal (Fig. 43.33).

Very often there are incompetent perforators proximal to the ulcer and all endeavours to get and maintain healing are likely to fail unless these perforators are dealt with. The basic approach, therefore, to the management of gravitational ulcer is first to improve the local venous drainage to the area by rest in bed with the leg elevated, or if this is not possible for one reason or another, to apply a firm, evenly supporting bandage which, as the patient walks, will be pressed against by each muscle contraction and thereby assist vein emptying in a proximal direction. If there is heavy contamination by bacteria, however, this method of treatment may be difficult or impossible. There is no doubt that the most rapid and satisfactory initial healing is obtained by the former approach. Moderate infection may be treated by simple non-irritant antiseptic washes, while more severe infection, especially if there is accompanying cellulitis, will need systemic antibiotic administration.

Once the ulcer is freed of infection and new skin has closed over it consideration has to be given to either operative ablation of all the responsible perforators and varices, or the permanent wearing of a properly fitted graduated-compression elastic support stocking while the patient is ambulant. If neither of these courses is followed, the ulcer will most surely recur whenever the patient resumes normal activities.

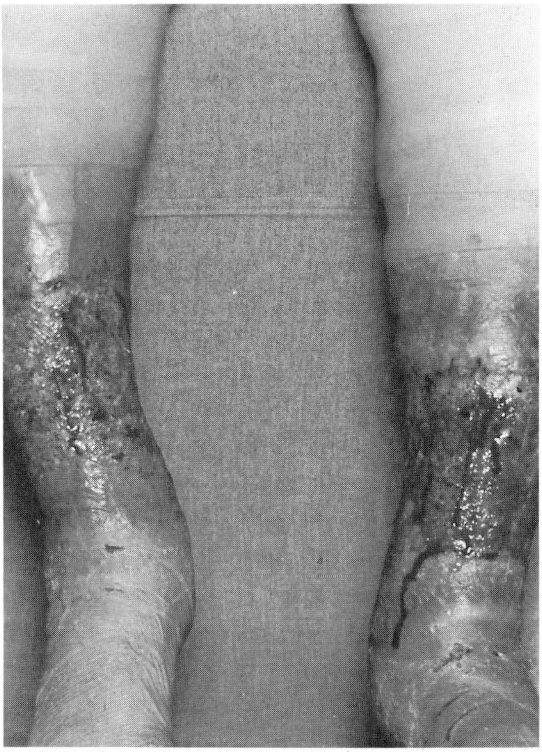

Fig. 43.33 Severe bilateral long-standing venous incompetence leading to circumferential, raw weeping ulceration in the gaiter area. Both lower legs show oedematous swelling, accentuated by the cross-markings left by the elastic support bandages which were removed immediately before this photograph.

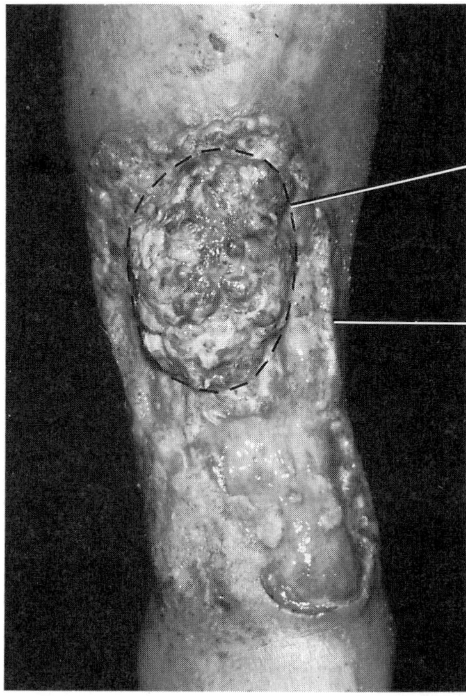

Fig. 43.34 Curling's ulcer: the development of a frank squamous cell carcinoma in a chronic gravitational ulcer. The tumour—raised, nodular and itself ulcerated—has already reached a large size, having started to grow in the upper part of the original venous ulcer.

Rarely, in a long-standing gravitational ulcer, a squamous carcinoma may arise—so-called Curling's ulcer (Fig. 43.34).

VENOUS THROMBOSIS

Superficial thrombophlebitis

This usually arises in a segment of varicose veins in the leg, and is probably due to local stagnation and/or mechanical pressure. The condition presents as a raised, red, firm, tender cord in the affected segment, and although the term thrombophlebitis is traditionally used, it is not a truly infective condition, but rather a sterile inflammation. The disorder, though locally painful and troublesome to the patient, is nearly always self-limiting, resolves spontaneously over a few days, usually leaving a much improved situation as far as the varicose veins are concerned, and there is virtually no risk of embolism arising from it. The treatment is to prescribe an appropriate analgesic and encourage normal mobility.

If superficial thrombophlebitis occurs in the absence of varicose veins, and particularly if there have been previous similar episodes, the possibility of some intra-abdominal malignancy should be borne in mind.

Deep vein thrombosis

This occurrence is quite a different matter and should always be regarded seriously. The veins draining the legs and lower part of the body are most commonly affected, at any level from small tributaries in the calf muscles to the inferior vena cava.

Three main factors (Virchow's triad) are known to contribute to the formation of a thrombus inside a vein. These are a reduced rate of blood flow through the vein, increased coagulability of the blood and damage to the endothelial lining of the vein.

Of particular surgical relevance is the well known increased risk of a deep venous thrombosis in the postoperative period, particularly after prolonged operations in the abdomen or on the hip-joint; also in older patients, those with malignancy, dehydrated patients and those with a previous history of venous complaints. In these patients all three factors may be operative. Under general anaesthesia the venous flow will be reduced and local pressure in the abdomen and on the calves may further diminish local flow. Platelets may become more adherent to each other and to any damaged intima. The latter damage may be caused by direct pressure, e.g. of operating table edge on paralysed leg muscles.

For these reasons it is now virtually routine to take preventive measures in patients coming to operation, such as mobilization right up to the time of operation and as soon as possible after it, avoidance of all pressure on the legs on the operating table, keeping anaesthetic and operating time down to a minimum, and giving to patients who are at special risk prophylactic low-dose heparin (5000 u 8-hourly) or intravenous dextran to discourage thrombus formation.

Although there is some increased risk of deep venous thrombosis after any operation, it is commoner after some than others. For example, it is rare after operations on the neck, yet commoner after abdominal and major orthopaedic procedures. It is more likely after splenectomy (with its subsequent increase in the platelet count) than after parotidectomy.

Other precipitating factors include taking the contraceptive pill, pregnancy, when it is most likely to occur immediately postpartum, pelvic sepsis, in patients with polycythaemia, and in any who have to remain recumbent for any length of time.

As the result of extensive surveys of the various groups at risk it is evident that the incidence of thrombosis mainly in the smaller veins within calf muscles is higher than the number who present with symptoms, particularly with respect to postoperative venous thrombosis.

Clinical features

Observations which raise the suspicion of deep venous thrombosis are pain in the leg, mostly in the calf; oedematous swelling, which may be obvious in the foot or ankle, but if minimal may be limited to the webs between the toes, and an unexplained sharp increase in body temperature or pulse rate.

If it is a postoperative complication these usually appear about the 8th–10th day after the procedure. Very gross swelling of the leg suggests occlusion at iliac vein or even caval level. On the other hand, sometimes even major vein thrombosis can occur without any obvious symptoms or signs in the leg, and the first indication of the serious problem may be a pulmonary embolus with sudden chest pain, haemoptysis, respiratory difficulty, or maybe even sudden death from blockage of the main pulmonary artery.

In the clinical examination of the leg, constant localized tenderness in the calf muscles is a strong pointer to the diagnosis, and if the tenderness is aggravated by dorsal flexion of the foot at the ankle this is additional supportive evidence. The latter sign alone, however, is not completely reliable.

If the clinical suspicion is strong, systemic anticoagulation of the patient is advisable, starting with intravenous heparin, preferably by continuous infusion, and converting to an oral anticoagulant over the next few days. The objective is to discourage further extension of the clot and reduce the chances of further loose fragments becoming dislodged as emboli. Probably the anticoagulants should be continued for 3–6 months, with proper regular haematological control.

Where a small pulmonary embolus has already occurred, consideration can be given to inserting one or other of the filters which are available to place in the inferior vena cava, to limit the size of any further emboli which may be conveyed to the heart.

If there is uncertainty about the diagnosis of deep venous thrombosis the veins can be outlined by venography; the radiologist injects a suitable radiopaque medium into a vein in the foot after blocking the superficial veins with a tourniquet at the ankle. Doppler ultrasound is an alternative technique which may give adequate information, though it is not usually so precise.

Another problem which may follow an episode of deep vein thrombosis of the iliac or caval segments is persisting troublesome swelling of the leg. In spite of collateral venous drainage the overall venous return may be insufficient so that gross pitting oedema develops. Usually the amount of swelling diminishes after rest in bed each night and becomes progressively larger during the day with normal walking activity. The oedema can be partly or sometimes almost completely controlled by wearing a graduated-compression elastic support stocking. This should be put on before rising from bed in the morning and not removed until returning to bed at night. Unfortunately attempts at venous grafting or other reconstruction are almost always unsuccessful.

44. Cardiac surgery

ANATOMY AND PHYSIOLOGY OF THE HEART

Both anatomically and physiologically the heart comprises two halves. The right half receives venous blood from the body as a whole through the superior and inferior vena cavae and pumps it into the lungs. The left half receives oxygenated blood and pumps it to the systemic circulation. Each half of the heart is built to the same pattern, having a collecting chamber or atrium and a ventricle which discharges blood through one of the two great arteries (Fig. 44.1). The inlet and outlet of each ventricle are controlled by one-way valves, the tricuspid and the pulmonary valves on the right and the mitral and aortic valves on the left. The heart contracts as a whole and each half pumps the same amount of blood per minute. The output of each ventricle is called the cardiac output and amounts to approximately 3.2 litres per square metre of body surface per minute at rest. The right ventricle has the easier task of pumping blood through the pulmonary circulation whereas the left ventricle has to produce a high pressure to pump through the systemic circulation. As a result, the left ventricle is the larger and more muscular of the two ventricles and pressure on the left side of the heart is much higher than on the right.

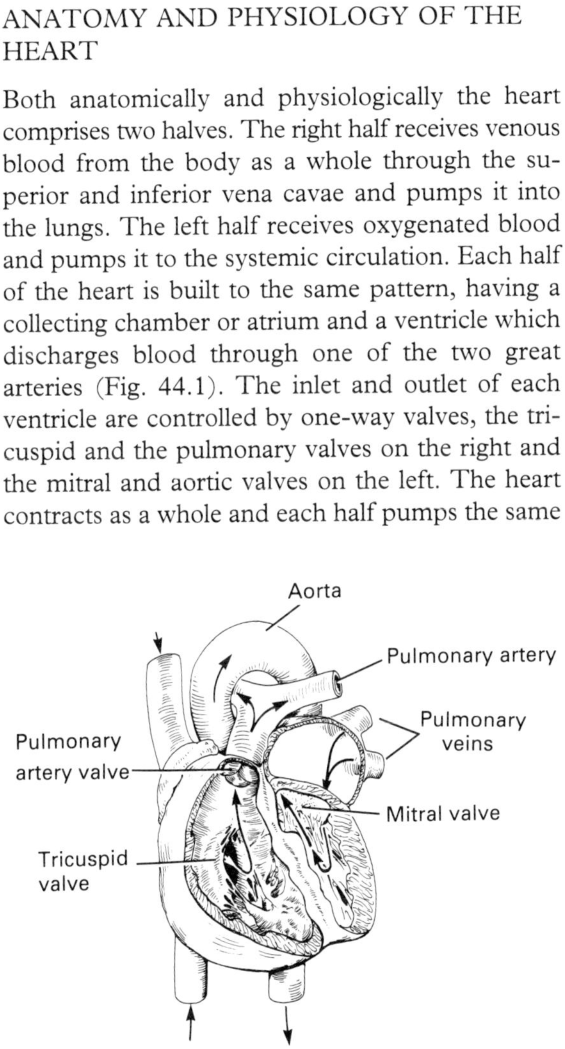

Fig. 44.1 Normal heart: cutaway diagram, showing both ventricles and left atrium opened from the front. The aortic valve, similar in situation to the pulmonary valve, is not shown as it is concealed by the overlying structures. Arrows indicate the normal directions of blood flow.

The blood pressure, whether in the pulmonary or systemic circulation, is directly related to the peripheral vascular resistance in the vascular bed and the quantity of the blood flow. In the systemic circulation the vascular resistance maintains a blood pressure during systole of between 120 and 130 mmHg in a young adult.

The distribution of the output in the systemic circulation is regulated by local changes in vascular resistance and in fact were all the arterioles of the body to dilate together, the blood pressure would fall to injuriously low levels. This is the situation when shock occurs due to bacterial toxaemia. The maintenance of the blood flow and tissue perfusion is dependent on the integrity of the left ventricle. If the ventricle fails, the blood pressure falls to a low level no matter what changes are made in the peripheral resistance. For example, in coronary thrombosis the area of the ventricle deprived of its blood flow dies and becomes an infarct. The peripheral arterioles constrict in an attempt to maintain the blood pressure but this increases the load on the left ventricle which may fail to maintain a reasonable output and blood pressure falls. The combination of low cardiac output and high peripheral resistance is called cardiogenic shock.

In the pulmonary circulation on the other hand, the principal feature is a low resistance to blood flow, the resistance being approximately one-sixth of the systemic resistance. The pulmonary vascular bed is also more elastic than the systemic bed and will accept a fourfold increase in the blood flow without any serious rise in the pulmonary arterial pressure.

The coronary circulation

The coronary arteries arise as the first branches of the aorta at the level of the cusps of the aortic valves, and they run round the heart in the groove between the ventricles and the atria. The left anterior descending coronary artery arises from the left main coronary artery just beyond its origin and runs down the front of the heart between the right and the left ventricles. The other main branch of the left coronary, the circumflex, follows the left atrioventricular groove to end on the posteroinferior surface of the heart. The right coronary artery, arising from the front of the aorta, runs in the right atrioventricular groove and terminates by anastomosing with branches of the left coronary artery.

The coronary veins accompany the arteries and join to form the coronary sinus which empties into the right atrium. The coronary arteries carry between 300 and 500 ml of blood per minute when the body is at rest.

In order to understand fully congenital heart diseases it is essential to know something of circulation before birth and the changes that take place after birth. While in the womb, the baby's blood is oxygenated by the placenta and the lungs are collapsed and airless until birth takes place. The pulmonary circulation in the fetus carries only a very small blood flow and the oxygenated blood passes along the umbilical vein from the placenta to the ductus venosus, bypassing the liver to join the inferior vena cava (Fig. 44.2). The oxygenated blood then enters the right atrium and passes through an opening in the interatrial septum, the foramen ovale, to reach the left atrium. From there it goes to the left ventricle which pumps it to the systemic circulation. The superior vena cava carries venous blood from the head, neck and arms to the right atrium and this stream of blood flows through the tricuspid valve into the right ventricle. The right ventricle pumps the blood through the pulmonary artery but it bypasses the lungs by going along the ductus arteriosus into the aorta where it joins the flow from the left ventricle. At birth or soon after the ductus venosus, the foramen ovale and ductus arteriosus are normally closed. If the latter fails to do so, it gives rise to one of the congenital heart diseases—patent ductus arteriosus.

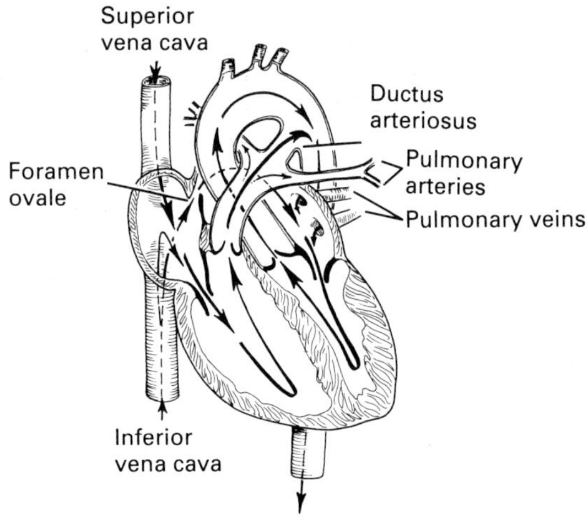

Fig. 44.2 Fetal cardiac circulation—see text.

The symptoms in heart disease are difficult to understand without some idea of the changes from the fetal type of circulation to the postnatal circulation and without knowledge of changes in the physiology in heart disease.

Left-to-right shunts

Defects in either the atrial or ventricular septum, or a patent ductus arteriosus, lead to an abnormal movement of blood from one side of the heart to the other. The direction of the flow depends on the pressure differentiation between the two chambers connected by the defect. The pressure in the left heart and aorta is normally much higher than that in the right heart and the pulmonary artery, therefore the blood flows from the left to the right through an atrial septal defect or a patent ductus arteriosus. These shunts increase the amount of blood which flows through the pulmonary circulation. The right side of the heart and the pulmonary artery have to cope with the normal venous return from the venae cava as well as the oxygenated blood flowing through the shunts. This increases pulmonary blood flow, and as a result there is an increase in the musculature of the pulmonary vessels which leads to a rise in the pulmonary peripheral resistance. Eventually the pulmonary blood pressure rises and the right ventricle hypertrophies, as if trying to overcome this pressure. Small left-to-right shunts produce few symptoms but large shunts can produce pulmonary flooding, recurrent respiratory infection, and finally cardiac failure.

Right-to-left shunts

These occur when venous blood enters the systemic arterial circulation to produce cyanosis. Cyanosis only occurs where there is more than 5 g of reduced haemoglobin per 100 ml of blood. Generally right-to-left shunts occur where there is obstruction in the right heart associated with a septal defect. The common example is Fallot's tetralogy in which pulmonary stenosis and a ventricular septal defect occur together. Pulmonary stenosis leads to obstruction to the outflow from the right ventricle and diverts blood through the septal defect into the left ventricle. A similar result occurs if there is tricuspid atresia and an atrial septal defect. A right-to-left shunt may also occur if pulmonary hypertension develops as a result of obstructive changes in the pulmonary vasculature secondary to left-to-right shunt, which is then reversed, causing cyanosis.

Stenosis of the valves

This may be congenital or as a result of endocarditis, the commonest aetiology being rheumatic. There is partial fusion of the valve leaflets resulting in an increased resistance to the blood flow through the valves, and therefore the cardiac chambers are affected. In mitral stenosis, for example, the left atrium becomes large and more thick-walled, and the right ventricle, which pushes the blood through the valve via the pulmonary circulation and left atrium, becomes much more muscular and a condition of right ventricular hypertrophy develops.

When a valve is incompetent, on the other hand, part of the blood pushed through the valve during ventricular contraction leaks back during the systole. There is thus a net loss of output from the ventricle. The left ventricle normally ejects about 70 ml of blood at each stroke; one-half may leak back in the presence of aortic incompetence and only 40 ml may reach the systemic circulation. To compensate for this the left ventricle enlarges so that it can eject about 110 ml during systole and although 40 ml of this may leak back, a proper output of about 70 ml per beat is maintained.

Heart failure may occur suddenly if the amount of contractile ventricular muscle is reduced by a coronary occlusion, or it may occur slowly if the myocardium has reached the limit of its power of compensation. Usually acute failure is superimposed on a long-standing chronic failure because of a minor insult to the heart which has no reserve left. Right heart failure is the common end-point in patients with advanced pulmonary disease, and pulmonary hypertension, secondary to mitral and aortic valve disease. The right ventricle is unable to cope with the systemic venous return so the veins in the neck become engorged and visible and the liver is enlarged and congested, and finally oedema of dependent parts of the body results. Congestion of the portal venous system also leads to ascites.

Left heart failure may result from coronary artery occlusion, systemic hypertension or aortic valve disease. As the left ventricle is unable to cope, blood accumulates in the lungs and gives rise to pulmonary venous congestion with dyspnoea. If the situation becomes acute, pulmonary oedema develops and the patient coughs up pink, frothy sputum due to extravasation of blood into the alveoli.

Symptoms of heart disease

Dyspnoea is the commonest symptom of heart disease, and is usually associated with overfilling of the pulmonary vascular bed. Initially it occurs only after exercise but as the disease progresses or the heart begins to fail, the patient becomes breathless at rest and has to sit up to feel comfortable. This is the state of orthopnoea.

In peripheral oedema there is excessive fluid in the tissues to a degree sufficient to cause swelling. The site of its collection depends upon gravity so that in bed-ridden patients the sacrum and the hips swell while in those who are ambulant, it is the ankles and feet which swell. Bilateral ankle oedema can occur due to kidney or liver disease, or hypoproteinaemia, but in the presence of heart disease, it is due to right ventricular failure. Pulmonary oedema occurs due to left heart failure when oedema fluid enters the alveoli and interferes with oxygen exchange and the patient may drown in his or her own blood.

Haemoptysis is caused by the rupture of a small blood vessel into the air passages. It is commonly seen early in mitral stenosis because of the engorgement of the pulmonary circulation but the volume of blood is usually small and there are no sequelae. If it is accompanied by dyspnoea and chest pain, haemoptysis is usually due to a pulmonary infarct.

Palpitation occurs when the patient complains of an awareness of the heart beat. It may be caused by extra systoles or by attacks of paroxysmal tachycardia but in a patient with known heart disease, it is often a prodromal sign of the onset of arrhythmias.

Angina is a severe pain caused by a lack of oxygen to the heart. It is a crushing kind of pain and often patients say that they feel a tight band round their chest. It often spreads to the neck and down the left arm or even both the arms. It occurs whenever the myocardium is overworked in the presence of an inadequate coronary blood supply, usually during exercise when the heart has to do extra work.

INVESTIGATION OF THE PATIENT FOR CARDIAC SURGERY

Every operation on the heart is a serious matter and the result of the surgery depends very much on careful selection of patients and precise diagnosis of the cardiac state. The assessment of the patient also includes assessment of pulmonary, hepatic and renal functions. The patient should undergo a careful physical examination for the presence or absence of cyanosis, oedema, distension of the jugular veins and enlargement of the liver. The state of the peripheral pulses should also be noted. The heart should be auscultated in order to try to reach a clinical diagnosis.

Posteroanterior X-ray of the chest is important, for it gives an impression of the size and shape of the heart and X-ray screening will give some information about the movements of the heart, particularly the presence or absence of excessive pulsation in the main pulmonary arteries and calcification of valves.

Electrocardiograms at rest should also be done as a routine to give information about the cardiac rhythm and the size and workload of the cardiac chambers. Electrocardiogram after graded exercise is required to establish the diagnosis of ischaemic heart disease.

M-mode and two-dimensional echocardiography is a non-invasive test based on the principle of ultrasound and has revolutionized the bedside diagnosis for valvular heart diseases such as mitral, tricuspid and aortic stenosis, aortic regurgitation and several congenital lesions such as atrial and ventricular septal defect, tetralogy of Fallot, transposition of great vessels, etc.

However, cardiac catheterization and angiocardiography, i.e. X-ray of the heart using radiopaque media, is essential in most complex cases before cardiac surgery. It involves passage of a small catheter along a vein into the right heart or along an artery into the left heart. This catheter can be used to measure the pressure in the cardiac chambers or the great vessels. It allows blood samples to be obtained from different sites in the heart. Radiopaque dye can be injected to outline the cardiac chambers and the great vessels. For right heart catheterization the medial antecubital vein is commonly used, and for left heart catheterization, percutaneous puncture of the brachial or femoral artery by the Seldinger technique is usually adopted. However, sometimes it is necessary to cut down on to the artery or vein.

GENERAL POINTS ABOUT HEART OPERATIONS

Surgery of the heart is undertaken in three types of diseases—congenital defects, chronic rheumatic disease of the heart valves and coronary artery disease—but surgery for lesions of the great vessels such as coarctation of the aorta, aneurysms of the aortic arch and patent ductus arteriosus is also carried out by the cardiac surgeon. Wounds of the heart and constrictive pericarditis also come within the scope of the cardiac surgeon.

The heart may be operated upon while still maintaining the circulation, so-called closed heart surgery, or while the circulation is maintained by a heart–lung machine—open heart surgery. The commonest operation performed by closed heart surgery is mitral valvotomy, which is done for cases of isolated mitral stenosis.

Open heart surgery, on the other hand, is used for the repair of intracardiac and congenital defects, the repair and replacement of damaged cardiac valves and for direct coronary artery surgery.

Basically all heart–lung machines take over the function of the heart and the lung for varying periods. The machine both oxygenates the blood and pumps it through the systemic circulation (Fig. 44.3). This is made possible by total heparinization of the patient so that there is no clotting in the machine. Most heart–lung machines are connected to cannulas or catheters placed in the superior and inferior vena cavae to collect venous blood. This blood is diverted through a venous line to an oxygenator and the drainage from the venous side is usually by gravity.

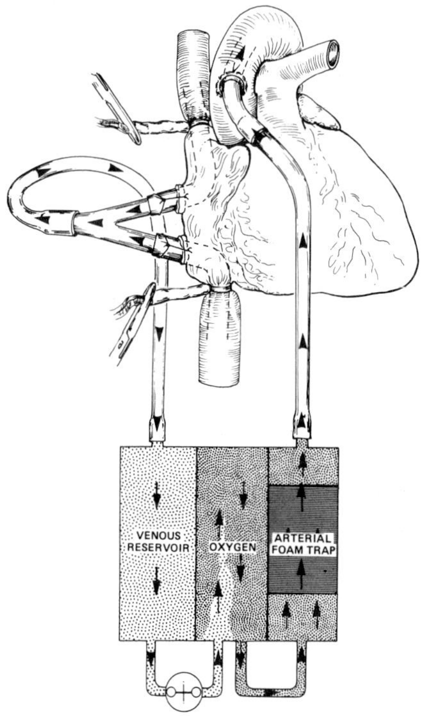

Fig. 44.3 Heart–lung bypass machine. The venous reservoir may be either before the oxygenator and foam trap, as shown here, or after these two compartments, as described in the text. Oxygenation of the blood can be achieved either by bubbling oxygen through the blood, or by means of a membrane oxygenator which allows oxygen to pass across a permeable membrane into the blood flowing past it.

The most widely used oxygenators nowadays are usually a specially designed portable plastic bag or rigid plastic chamber divided into three compartments. In the first compartment, oxygen is bubbled into the blood to oxygenate it; in the second compartment there is an antefoam preparation usually in a fine mesh of nylon or sponge so that the oxygenated blood leaves this compartment free of bubbles, and the third compartment acts as a reservoir to collect the blood which goes to the pump. The pump forces the blood through an arterial cannula, usually placed into the patient's ascending aorta. This type of heart–lung machine is filled prior to use with an electrolyte solution rather than blood. Although this dilutes the patient's blood, the kidneys rapidly compensate for this later by diuresis.

The bypass is started by releasing the clamp on the venous lines and starting the pump so that the venous return from the heart flows out into the oxygenator, emptying the heart. Tapes are then tightened around the caval catheters. The aortic blood pressure closes the aortic valves so that the heart remains empty except for the blood passing through the coronary circulation into the right atrium and the bronchial circulation into the left atrium. This blood is removed by a special sucker when the heart is open and returned to the heart–lung machine via a special side-branch in the venous line. Since the coronary arteries arise above the aortic valve, circulation to the heart can be maintained by the pump while the heart is being operated upon. If on the other hand, the ascending aorta has to be cross-clamped, the myocardiac preservation is maintained by intermittently releasing the clamp for coronary perfusion or by continuous direct coronary perfusion. Since 1975 cold chemical cardioplegic arrest is being increasingly used by injecting cold balanced electrolyte solution or cold blood containing potassium chloride intermittently into the ascending aorta or coronary circulation to achieve a flaccid relaxed heart during surgery. This procedure has resulted in marked reduction in bypass time and has improved the results of surgery.

An additive to cardiopulmonary bypass is hypothermia which means lowering the temperature of the body so that its metabolic rate falls and the tissues therefore require less oxygen to survive. After being anaesthetized the patient is initially cooled by ice-packs to 25° C before bypass begins. The main use of hypothermia is as an adjunct to the heart–lung machine. In more complex operations, if required, total circulatory arrest of up to 45–60 min can be achieved when the body temperature is lowered to 15° C.

Prostheses for cardiac surgery

The main prostheses used in cardiac surgery are made of fabrics which are physically, chemically and biologically relatively inert, and these are mainly Teflon, Dacron and polypropylene. Their main function is to form a scaffold or framework into which fibrous tissue can grow. The artificial valves bear little resemblance to the valves they replace as attempts to manufacture more natural-looking valves failed because the repeated flexion or hinging action causes them to break up. Mechanical valves still fall short of the ideal substitute because no one can predict exactly how long they will last. Moreover, thrombosis on mechanical valves with subsequent embolism remains a major problem. For this reason, fresh or preserved human aortic valves taken from the cadaver have been used in some centres. However, fibrosis, calcification and bacterial or fungal endocarditis are the major problems of allografts. At present glutaraldehyde preserved porcine aortic xenografts or pericardial xenografts mounted on flexible frames are being increasingly used because of the low incidence of thromboembolic complications. With new designs of artificial disc valves with pyrolite carbon discs the incidence of thromboembolic complications is also reduced although the patient requires to remain on lifelong anticoagulation therapy.

Heart transplantation

In 1967 Dr Christiaan Barnard successfully transplanted a human heart and this has certainly introduced new possibilities for the treatment of incurable heart disease. In the USA there are now quite large series of patients operated by Dr Norman Shumway who have survived cardiac transplantation for significantly long periods. The methods of suppressing the immune rejection have improved but this operation is only possible in those countries which have legally permitted removal of a beating heart from cadavers who have undergone brain death. An artificial heart to replace the human heart has been used clinically by Dr Denton Cooley and others. The design, however, needs further modifications to prevent thromboembolic and other associated complications.

CONGENITAL HEART DISEASE

Approximately 2 out of every 1000 babies have some form of cardiac defect. Some of these die shortly after birth, whereas in others symptoms are delayed until later childhood or even adolescence. The causes of congenital heart disease are largely unknown, but the association between it and German measles in the mothers during early pregnancy has been established. The congenital defects which tend to cause death in early infancy are severe tetralogy, transposition of the great vessels, total anomalous pulmonary venous return, severe pulmonary, aortic, tricuspid stenosis or atresia and large ventricular septal defects. A prompt diagnosis and an emergency operation in these babies can save lives but it may not be possible to correct fully the defect and very often only palliative operation to allow the baby to survive is possible and a definitive operation is performed later. In advanced clinics one-stage correction operations are being increasingly performed successfully. Minor defects do not usually cause symptoms until late childhood because of natural compensatory devices and the surgery can be safely delayed.

Congenital cardiac lesions are best divided into two groups—cyanotic and acyanotic. As has been stated earlier, in congenital heart disease persistent cyanosis is usually due to a shunt of venous blood from the right to the left side so that it passes into the systemic circulation without being oxygenated in the lungs.

Acyanotic congenital heart disease

Ventricular septal defect

This is the commonest single lesion of the heart seen in infancy and childhood. The defect may be large or small. If the defect is small the heart is not enlarged and, as the shunting of blood is small, surgery may never be necessary. Spontaneous closure of a small ventricular septal defect can occur usually before the age of 2 years but sometimes during childhood. With the larger defects, however, there is often a history of repeated respiratory tract infection in the early years. Frequently there is a definite thrust over the pulmonary area with a praecordial bulge, a loud systolic murmur and a thrill at its maximum in the fourth and fifth left intercostal space. A chest X-ray shows enlargement of the pulmonary arteries and screening demonstrates a marked hilar pulsation. Pulmonary vascular markings are increased. The electrocardiogram usually shows left ventricular hypertrophy. A large defect with a big shunt of blood from the left side of the heart causes an increase in the pulmonary arteriolar resistance which raises the pressure in the pulmonary circulation and may even reverse the shunt.

The treatment for such ventricular septal defects is closure of the defect under direct vision. This is best undertaken using a cardiopulmonary bypass. The defect is exposed through the right atrium or the right ventricle and large defects are closed with a Dacron patch. The chief hazard of surgery is the production of heart block because the bundle of His, running along the lower edge of the defect, may be picked up by the sutures. If there is any evidence of heart block during surgery, pacemaker wires should be inserted at the time of surgery and connected to the pacemaker.

Patent ductus arteriosus

This is the second most common acyanotic lesion. Classically there is a continuous machinery-like murmur which is maximal over the first and second left intercostal spaces. However, in young infants where the pulmonary and systemic blood pressures may almost equal one another, and in patients with hypertension, the murmur may be systolic only. Often there is an accompanying thrill and a bounding pulse. There is usually an increase in the pulmonary vascular markings on X-ray and screening which may also demonstrate increased pulmonary vascular pulsations. The electrocardiogram shows left ventricular preponderance but evidence of right ventricular hypertrophy may either indicate pulmonary hypertension or that the ductus is complicated by other lesions.

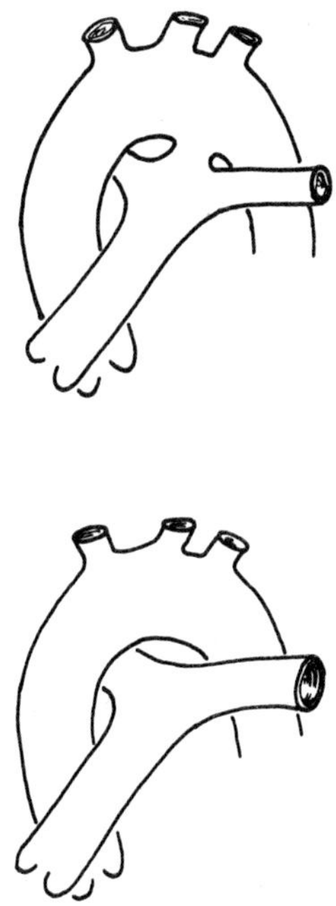

Fig. 44.4 Patent ductus arteriosus: simple division and ligation restores circulation to normal.

The treatment of choice is surgery, preferably between the ages of 3 and 4 years, but if there is severe pulmonary hypertension or congestive cardiac failure it should be done much earlier. The operation is performed through a left fourth or fifth rib thoracotomy and the ductus can be closed by ligation and transfixation if it is less than 0.5 cm in diameter (Fig. 44.4). If larger than this, it should always be divided between clamps and the cut ends oversewn. If the ductus is not closed surgically the child tends to develop progressive pulmonary hypertension. Moreover, as long as the ductus is open there is always a risk of bacterial endocarditis.

Atrial septal defects

These present with an ejection systolic murmur of moderate intensity which is at its maximum over the second and third left intercostal spaces, often coupled with wide and fixed splitting of the pulmonary second sound. Electrocardiography often shows an incomplete right bundle branch block.

Chest X-ray usually shows some degree of cardiac enlargement with increased vascular markings and increased pulmonary pulsation on screening. Echocardiography is most useful in establishing the diagnosis of atrial septal defect. There are two varieties of atrial septal defects: the first is an ostium primum defect which occurs low down on the interatrial septum and may be associated with a split mitral or tricuspid valve or some degree of ventricular septal defect. In these patients symptoms and pulmonary hypertension result much earlier. The ostium secundum defect, on the other hand, involves the atrial septum only. The principal effect of both forms of atrial septal defect is a left-to-right shunt so that blood from the left atrium joins the normal venous return from the superior and inferior venae cava in the right atrium. Because the right ventricle has to cope with an increased volume of blood it becomes hypertrophied, the pulmonary artery becomes dilated and the pulmonary blood flow increases.

Patients with secundum atrial septal defect tend to be free of symptoms until their teens. It is important to close the defect in childhood or early adolescence to prevent the onset of pulmonary hypertension in middle life. The operative treatment depends on the type of defect. Both the ostium primum and ostium secondum defects are closed under open heart surgery using a heart–lung machine. The ostium primum defect may require repair of the mitral or tricuspid valve and closure of an associated ventricular septal defect as well.

Coarctation of the aorta

Coarctation of the aorta is usually diagnosed if examination of the femoral artery is made part of the routine examination of children. In the presence of coarctation of the aorta the femoral pulses are diminished or absent and the blood pressure is higher in the arms than in the legs. There are no characteristic murmurs but a systolic murmur may be present, heard particularly at the apex of the heart and between the scapulae. In the older patients collateral vessels along the edge of the scapula can often be palpated. There are two main types of patients, those with a long narrow segment who get into severe trouble in early infancy and those with a short narrow segment who often present later in life, frequently with a previously undiagnosed hypertension. In most patients the narrowing tends to lie just distal to the left subclavian artery at about the level at which the ductus arteriosus joins the aorta. The important thing to remember in the surgical repair is the presence of an abundant and very large collateral circulation in the thoracic cage which may well lead to large blood loss during the exposure of the aorta. In young children with a short defect it is often possible to resect the defect and carry out an end-to-end anastomosis of the aorta, but in older patients the defect is often so large or the vessel so inelastic that a graft has to be inserted to achieve continuity of the aorta. At present the operation of choice in both children and adults is to carry out widening of the aorta at the site of the coarctation by doing an aortoplasty. In children the proximal segment of the left subclavian artery can be turned down as a patch, while in adults a Dacron patch can be used to achieve the necessary widening.

Pulmonary stenosis

These patients are not cyanosed until they are in terminal cardiac failure. They usually have a very harsh murmur and a thrill maximal over the pulmonary area. The heart size may be normal and even in advanced cases they often have clear lung fields on X-ray. The electrocardiogram demonstrates right ventricular hypertrophy. If treatment is not undertaken, the right ventricle ultimately fails. In most patients symptoms are very few until childhood or adolescence when attacks of dyspnoea and sometimes angina of effort occur.

Surgical correction is performed under heart–lung bypass, the pulmonary valve being cut to give a normal opening, with access to the valve through the pulmonary artery itself. This operation may lead to pulmonary valve incompetence. The atrial and ventricular septa are inspected at operation and any defect, if present, is closed.

Congenital aortic stenosis

Congenital aortic stenosis used to be considered an uncommon defect but it is now clear that the majority of cases of isolated stenosis of the aortic valve found in adults are usually congenital in origin and not due to rheumatic fever. The symptoms are very insidious and do not usually arise until the ventricular muscle has outstripped its coronary artery blood supply and the lesion may then lead to sudden death from ventricular fibrillation. The diagnosis can be made by echocardiography but for the demonstration of a pressure gradient between the left ventricle and the aorta, cardiac catheterization and angiography is necessary. It also distinguishes whether the stenosis is supravalvular, subvalvular or valvular. Operation is performed with heart–lung bypass. In children, if adequate valve leaflets are present, incisions are made which tend to restore a normal opening without making the valve incompetent. In adolescents and adults the leaflets are usually so deformed and calcified that replacement of the valve by either a mechanical or bioprosthesis is required.

Supravalvular stenosis resembles coarctation of the ascending aorta except that the coarctation is just above the aortic sinus. This condition can be relieved by putting a Dacron patch into the ascending aorta to increase its diameter.

Cyanotic heart disease

Tetralogy of Fallot

In this condition there are four abnormalities—pulmonary stenosis which is usually infundibular; an over-riding aortic root; a ventricular septal defect and right ventricular hypertrophy (Fig. 44.5). The important abnormalities from the functional point of view are the pulmonary stenosis and the ventricular septal defect. Because of obstruction from the narrowed pulmonary valve or infundibulum, the right ventricle hypertrophies until it becomes more powerful than the left ventricle and so venous blood is pumped through the large ventricular septal defect into the aorta, producing a right-to-left shunt. The patient becomes blue or cyanosed due to this shunt. Cyanosis increases markedly during exercise.

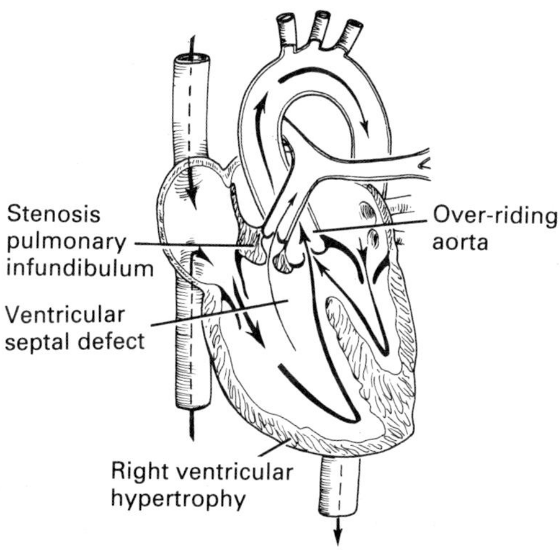

Fig. 44.5 Fallot's tetralogy: the four main components of this congenital malformation.

These children develop symptoms early in childhood and a third of them die during the first 2 years of life. The ones who survive tend to have attacks of deep cyanosis, and exercise intolerance and dyspnoea on exertion are common. By the time they become toddlers they frequently assume a squatting position which appears to ease their discomfort. They usually have a systolic murmur in the third left intercostal space. On X-ray examination and on screening the outline of the heart is altered to a characteristic boot shape. The pulmonary vascular markings are diminished and there is a concavity in the region of the pulmonary artery. The electrocardiogram demonstrates right ventricular hypertrophy.

Echocardiography is helpful in the diagnosis. Cardiac catheterization and angiocardiography is essential for the accurate demonstration of right ventricular outflow obstruction and the ventricular septal defect. The original palliative operation for the relief of this condition was Blalock's left subclavian-pulmonary artery anastomosis, which is now only used in sick infants and small babies. The infundibular stenosis and ventricular septal defect can be corrected directly under a cardiopulmonary bypass. It is the operation of choice in large babies, children and adults as the results of one-stage total correction of Fallot are now excellent. In sick infants and babies total correction is carried out after the palliative shunt procedure.

Transposition of the great vessels

In this condition the aorta arises from the right ventricle and the pulmonary artery from the left, so that both circulations are completely separated one from the other except through the presence of a septal defect through which blood can be short-circuited. The defect is incompatible with life and few survive beyond 1 year. It may be possible to obtain correction of the defect by using an intra-atrial baffle in such a way as to direct venous blood from the right atrium to the left ventricle and the oxygenated blood from the left atrium to the right ventricle. More recently an arterial switch operation has been made possible by implantation of the coronary arteries into the proximal pulmonary artery arising from the left ventricle; the proximal part of the pulmonary artery is sutured to the distal segment of the aorta. In cases where pulmonary stenosis complicates transposition, a conduit has to be used to restore pulmonary circulation.

Tricuspid atresia

These patients have stenosis of the tricuspid valve and there is marked left ventricular hypertrophy which is observed on the electrocardiogram. These children are severely cyanosed and rarely survive for long. For palliation Glen's operation is sometimes used, in which the superior vena cava is anastomosed end-to-end to the right main pulmonary artery, allowing venous blood from the upper half of the body to reach the right lung. Palliation can be also achieved by using Blalock's subclavian-to-pulmonary-artery shunt.

Total anomalous pulmonary venous drainage

Anomalous venous drainage is another condition which causes severe cyanosis. The diagnosis of the commonest supracardiac variety is made on the demonstration of a double shadow in the upper mediastinum and total correction can be achieved under cardiopulmonary bypass.

ACQUIRED CONDITIONS

Rheumatic heart disease

Although rheumatic fever is now less common in advanced countries, there are still quite a large number of patients with lesions of the mitral, aortic or tricuspid valves who require surgical relief of their valvular disease. Heart disease occurs in rheumatic fever because of an abnormal immunological response to infection with a haemolytic streptococcus.

Children or adolescents are principally affected, and about two-thirds of children who have rheumatic fever develop permanent valve damage. At the time of the acute illness the leaflets of the valves are inflamed and swollen and become partially adherent, with involvement of the chordae tendineae. Following this there is a slow process of scarring which distorts the valve and its leaflets and after varying periods of time symptoms and signs appear. The changes are slow enough for the myocardium to hypertrophy so that decompensation may take a long time to make its appearance. The mitral and aortic valves are the ones most commonly damaged.

Mitral valve disease

Mitral stenosis is the commonest rheumatic valvular disease. As the valve narrows the left atrium enlarges and its wall hypertrophies in an attempt to force the blood through the narrow opening, but the main effect of the narrowing is on the right ventricle which hypertrophies in an effort to pump blood through the lungs and indirectly through the narrowed valvular orifice. In mitral incompetence the valve fails to close because the distorted leaflets lead to ineffective apposition of the valve and blood leaks back into the left atrium with each contraction of the left ventricle. This produces the same effects on the left atrium and the right ventricle as in pure mitral stenosis but in addition, the left ventricle enlarges and hypertrophies in an attempt to compensate for the leak back of the blood through the valve. In both stenosis and incompetence the pulmonary circulation is affected and the pulmonary arterioles hypertrophy and become narrow so that eventually pulmonary hypertension develops. As the valvular disease progresses, the patient gets breathless on exertion and this tends to increase in severity. Breathlessness may first be precipitated by pregnancy because of the increased demand on the heart.

Many patients present initially with haemoptysis which is common in early stages of the disease and associated with a raised pulmonary arterial pressure. The patient may also experience palpitations and by far the commonest disorder of cardiac rhythm in mitral valve disease is atrial fibrillation. In this condition the normal regular progressive contractions of the atrium are replaced by irregular fibrillating contractions of the atrium. Patients with mitral valvular disease often complain of being easily tired. Systemic emboli may occur because pieces of blood clot which form in the left atrium may break loose and be pumped out into the systemic circulation.

The operations available for the relief of this condition are mitral valvotomy or mitral valve replacement (Fig. 44.6). For pure mitral stenosis closed mitral valvotomy is still the treatment of choice unless the valve is calcified. Closed mitral valvotomy was the first intracardiac operation to be commonly practised. However, if the valve is incompetent or heavily calcified, it is usually necessary to replace it by an artificial one.

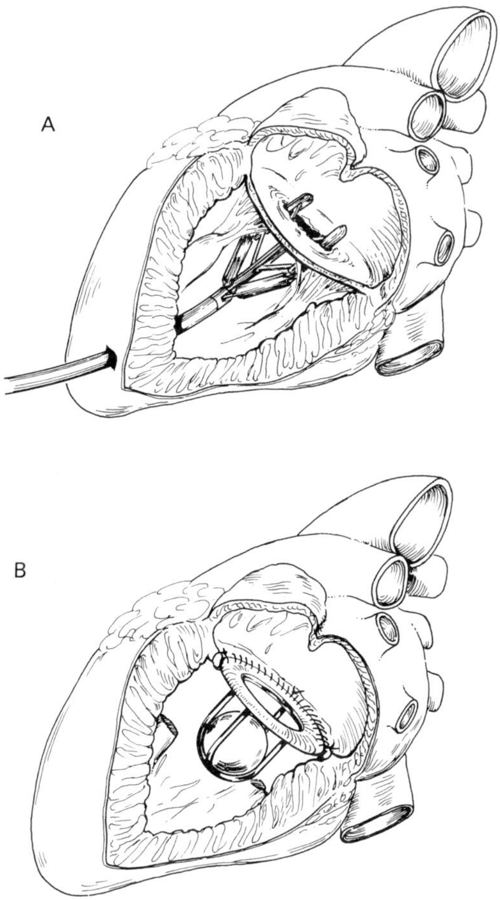

Fig. 44.6 Operations for mitral stenosis: (**A**) Valvotomy—the dilatation of the narrowed valve by means of a Tubb's dilator introduced through a small incision in the apex of the ventricle. A finger is usually also introduced through a small incision in the atrial appendage, to guide the instrument and assess the size of the opening. (**B**) Replacement of the damaged valve by one pattern of artificial valve. This is a much more common procedure nowadays than valvotomy. Several different types of valve have been developed.

Closed mitral valvotomy is a simple operation. The adhesions between the leaflets are divided blindly, usually with instruments, while the heart is still beating. However, it has been found on long-term follow-up that about 50% suffer from recurrence of symptoms after about 10 years. It is possible to do a second valvotomy in some of these patients. At present the majority of surgeons with facilities for heart-lung bypass prefer to do open mitral valvotomy, during which they are not only able to achieve valvar separation but also separation of subvalvar apparatus, namely the papillary muscles, by splitting them. The haemodynamic correction is far more complete as compared to closed valvotomy and the incidence of residual stenosis and re-stenosis is insignificant.

Mitral valve replacement is required only if the valve is heavily calcified, fibrosed or leaking.

The aortic valve is less commonly affected by rheumatic fever than the mitral, but once symptoms occur in aortic valve disease, the progress is more rapid because incompetence of the aortic valve overloads the left ventricle. In patients with aortic stenosis there are usually blackouts on exertion. Angina is another common symptom. The diagnosis of aortic stenosis can often be made from the presence of a harsh systolic murmur, often preceded by an aortic click in the aortic valve area, but the firm diagnosis is made by echocardiography and angiography. In older patients the aortic valve is almost always calcified. Diagnosis of aortic regurgitation can be made from a collapsing pulse, low diastolic pressure and early diastolic murmur in the mitral area. Echocardiography and cardiac catheter and angiocardiography are useful to grade the degree of incompetence and left ventricular function. Nowadays the standard treatment for aortic stenosis or incompetence is replacement of the diseased valve by either an artificial valve or by a xenograft.

Sometimes the tricuspid valve is affected by rheumatic fever as well, but it is unusual for patients with rheumatic heart disease to suffer from tricuspid disease alone. In some of the patients correction of a mitral valve lesion results in a reduction in the right ventricular hypertrophy and the functional tricuspid regurgitation is relieved. However, if the triscuspid valve has been directly affected by rheumatic disease, then valvotomy or tricuspid valve replacement is required.

Coronary artery disease

Coronary artery disease is the leading cause of death in the western world, with a rapid increase in its incidence in recent years. The cause in virtually all cases is coronary atherosclerosis affecting the main coronary arteries or their principal branches. Often the patient presents with angina of effort, but in any stage of the coronary artery disease, either before or after the onset of angina, occlusion of the artery may occur from thrombosis superimposed upon the atheromatous narrowing. The result of this occlusion varies depending on the site and extent of the block, and on how well the collateral circulation in the heart may have developed. The patient may die suddenly and without warning due to ventricular fibrillation, or blockage of a coronary artery may lead to death of a segment of myocardium (myocardial infarction) which may lead to progressive heart failure, or the patient may survive with a large dilated section of the ventricle, known as a cardiac aneurysm. Finally, the conduction system of the heart may be affected, leading to heart block.

In patients who survive the first or subsequent heart attack, selective coronary angiography usually reveals blocks or narrowing in the main coronary arteries but the distal vessels are often relatively free from disease. As approximately one-third of the patients who have had one attack of myocardial infarction have a second attack within 5 years, this fact has been a great stimulus towards the development of surgical treatment to prevent these recurrent attacks. However, before undertaking surgery for coronary artery disease, it is very important to have a firm diagnosis. Initially this is made from the clinical symptoms and the electrocardiogram, which shows typical changes in the ST segments in some of the leads, although these changes may not appear until late in the disease. Often the electrocardiogram gives better information if it is repeated after exercise. However, if surgery is contemplated it must depend on the accurate delineation of the coronary arteries by coronary arteriography.

The main indication for surgery is severe angina, particularly if it is thought that an attack of myocardial infarction is imminent. If coronary angiography reveals significant left main coronary artery occlusion, three-vessel occlusion (right coronary, left anterior descending and circumflex coronary branches of the left coronary) or severe occlusion of two coronary arteries, operation is strongly advised. If there is a single-vessel disease, operation is not advised unless the occlusion is in the proximal portion of the left anterior descending branch of the left coronary artery. The left ventricular function must be studied during angiography. The commonest operation performed at present is the

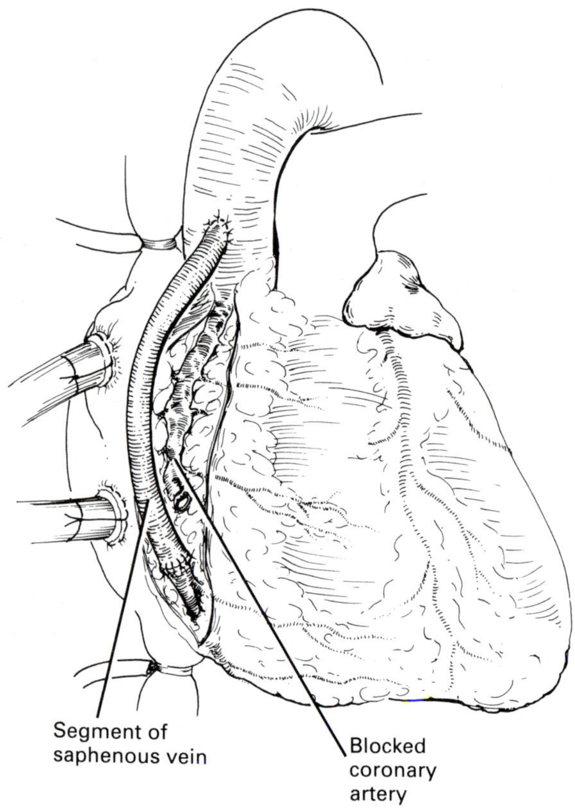

Fig. 44.7 Coronary artery bypass operation: a reversed segment of usually the long saphenous vein removed from the leg is shown here anastomosed proximally to the root of the aorta, and distally to the patent part of the coronary artery, distal to the atheromatous occlusion. Often several grafts are required to bypass multiple blocked vessels.

insertion of an autogenous bypass graft using the reversed saphenous vein which is sutured to the ascending aorta proximally and to the coronary arteries beyond the occlusion (Fig. 44.7). Depending on the number of segments of significant coronary occlusion the number of bypass grafts varies. In a few cases it is necessary to carry out local endarterectomy before the bypass is performed.

Cardiac aneurysm

One of the problems after an episode of coronary thrombosis is aneurysm of the left ventricle. This occurs when a large area of muscle has infarcted and is replaced by fibrous tissue which stretches to form an aneurysm. This can be diagnosed on X-ray of the chest, echocardiography and by left ventriculography. The treatment consists of excision of the aneurysm and suture of the normal ventricular wall under cardiopulmonary bypass.

POSTOPERATIVE MANAGEMENT

It is important to be aware of the problems which are common in the postoperative period after any form of direct or indirect surgery on the heart. Haemorrhage is much more common after cardiac surgery than in most other operations, because the use of the heart–lung bypass tends to deplete the circulation of platelets and clotting factors, and this may interfere with the normal haemostatic process. Haemorrhage is particularly dangerous because blood collects within the pericardial cavity and with an inefficient drain a small amount of blood can cause pressure on the heart resulting in tamponade, leading to a progressive fall in blood pressure and rise of venous pressure. It is a very dangerous complication and must be dealt with immediately on diagnosis. Another complication common to both cardiac and intrathoracic operations is the situation where blood or clot collects in the pleural cavity causing compression and collapse of the underlying lung. If the blood is fluid, it can be aspirated but if clotting has occurred it is best removed by drainage surgically at an early stage. Collapse of part or the whole of the lung is common after any thoracic operation, despite the presence of an underwater seal drain. Collapse may occur because the patient does not breathe as deeply as is desirable. Cerebral complications are comparatively uncommon but one complication to be feared is air embolism, because during the intracardiac part of any open-heart operation the chambers of the heart are filled with air and great care must be taken to remove this air before the circulation is restored at the end of the operation.

Two other complications may occur, particularly associated with closed mitral valvotomy. Clots may be dislodged during the manipulations in the left atrium and peripheral embolism may be produced. This may also occur in other forms of cardiac surgery, though much less frequently. A second complication is renal tubular necrosis which is the result of hypotension. A severe constriction of the peripheral vessels is produced, resulting in a severe reduction in renal blood flow, which in turn leads to necrosis of the renal tubular epithelium. There is a reduction or abolition of urine secretion, with a resultant increase in the levels of blood potassium and urea. It is much easier to prevent this happening than to treat it, and hypotension should be avoided if at all possible during the operation. Routinely, more and more often, agents such as mannitol or frusemide are given intravenously to maintain a high level of secretion during all forms of major surgery.

45. Thoracic surgery

RESPIRATORY PHYSIOLOGY

The main function of the respiratory system is to add oxygen to and remove carbon dioxide from the mixed venous blood perfusing the lungs.

Ventilation

Ventilation is produced by the rhythmic contraction of the inspiratory muscles, which causes expansion of the thoracic cavity and lowers the intrathoracic pressure to a subatmospheric level. As this occurs air flows from a region of higher pressure (atmospheric) to one of lower pressure (subatmospheric). In ventilating the lungs the inspiratory muscles must overcome the elastic forces of the lungs and thorax, and the resistance of the airways to the flow of air through them. Both the lungs and the thoracic cage contain tissues which have elastic properties, i.e. the ability to return to their original shape after they have been expanded by the inspiratory muscles. Expiration during quiet breathing is by passive elastic recoil of the lungs and thorax. Inspiration against abnormal resistance may bring accessory muscles such as the sternomastoid and scaleni into play; expiration, if forced or performed against airway resistance, is accomplished with the aid of the accessory muscles of expiration, chiefly those of the abdominal wall. Not all of the volume of the inspired air takes part in gas exchange in the lungs. Some of each breath ventilates the conducting airways down to the respiratory bronchioles, which constitute the anatomical dead space because it is not exposed to the gas-exchange part of the lungs, i.e. the alveoli.

Distribution of ventilation and perfusion of the inspired air

Even in healthy persons ventilation is not distributed uniformly. In the normal upright adult breathing slowly, more inspired air is distributed to the lower part of the lungs than to the upper regions, because of the differences in pleural pressure caused by gravity. As with ventilation gravitational forces also affect the distribution of the pulmonary blood flow; it is normally greatest in the dependent lower regions in an upright subject and least in the upper regions of the lung. Because of the uneven distribution of ventilation some of each breath is wasted in ventilating underperfused parts of the lungs. This portion of the inspired air is therefore like the air in the conducting passages, and can be regarded as dead space or wasted ventilation. The anatomical dead space plus the volume of this dead space-like air is referred to as the physiological dead space. Thus the effective ventilation is the volume of air reaching the alveoli where gas exchange takes place each minute. It is called the alveolar ventilation, and equals the tidal volume minus physiological dead space and then multiplied by the respiratory rate. The areas of lung with ventilation but which are not perfused cannot contribute to gas exchange, and thus form a physiological right-to-left shunt, or venous admixture effect.

In most forms of lung disease the distribution of ventilation and perfusion is impaired. An increase in the physiological dead space means that greater total ventilation is needed to achieve a given alveolar ventilation. Any increase in physiological shunting causes arterial hypoxaemia.

Diffusion of gases in the lungs

Diffusion can be defined as the movement of molecules from a region of higher to one of lower concentration, and is a passive process. In the lung oxygen moves by diffusion from alveolar gas into the pulmonary capillary blood. Carbon dioxide also moves by diffusion, but usually in the direction opposite to that of oxygen. Both oxygen and carbon dioxide undergo chemical reactions in the blood stream at the start and finish their journeys between the lungs and the peripheral tissues; oxygen reacts solely with haemoglobin and carbon dioxide reacts in part with haemoglobin and in part to form bicarbonate.

LYMPHATIC DRAINAGE

The pleura and all the lung substance with the possible exception of the alveoli are richly supplied with lymphatic vessels which are located beneath the pleura, around the vessels and bronchi and also within the bronchial wall. Aggregations of lymphoid tissue are found in the angles of bronchial branches from the periphery inwards. Hilar glands are found around the main lobar bronchi and are also clustered around the lung root. The glands lying lateral and inferior to the tracheal bifurcation are the upper and lower tracheobronchial groups. On the left side the glands along the aorta are called para-aortic glands. Paratracheal glands lie on either side of the trachea.

Pulmonary lymph drainage is as follows:

1. Upper two-thirds of the right upper lobe to the right tracheobronchial glands.
2. Lower one-third of the right upper lobe to hilar glands.
3. Middle lobe to the hilar glands.
4. Right lower lobe to the hilar and glands in the tracheal bifurcation.
5. Apex of the left upper lobe to para-aortic glands.
6. The rest of the left upper lobe to the hilar glands.
7. The left lower lobe is the same as the right lower lobe.
8. Lower lobes also drain to glands in the posterior mediastinum and through the diaphragm to the retroperitoneal lymph nodes.

CHEST INJURIES

Management of trauma to the thoracic cage and contents is becoming an increasingly common problem with the increase in the volume of road traffic and a sharp rise in road traffic accidents. Chest injuries are classically divided into two major categories—non-penetrating or blunt injuries and penetrating injuries.

Non-penetrating injuries may occur as the result of an automobile accident or by a fall or crushing injury. Blast injuries are usually the result of military combat or aerial bombardment. In addition to its direct effect on the chest wall, it may cause disruption of lung tissue by the high-energy shock waves. Stabbings and gunshot wounds are responsible for the majority of penetrating thoracic wounds.

Initial assessment

This should be directed towards relieving immediate life-threatening situations. The main requirements are to ensure adequate ventilation and restore the circulation. A quick but thorough examination of the patient must be made to assess the extent of all injuries, but the initial assessment—the most important factor—is the degree of anoxia. Simultaneously, the circulation should be grossly assessed. This should include pulse, blood pressure, examination for fullness of the neck veins and the quality of the heart sounds.

The aims of treatment

1. Maintain a clear airway.
2. Relieve pulmonary compression by air or blood.
3. Restore the mechanical respiratory efficiency of the thoracic cage.
4. Blood volume replacement.
5. Control of major life-threatening haemorrhage.
6. Pericardiocentesis for cardiac tamponade.

Surgical repair of injuries to the heart, aorta, bronchi, oesophagus and diaphragm can usually be delayed until initial resuscitative measures have been achieved.

Maintain a clear airway

At the site of the accident, upper airway obstruction

may quickly progress to asphyxiation and a patent airway must be established at all costs. The mouth should be cleared of blood, secretions, false teeth, and debris. If the patient is unconscious and the tongue is slipping back and obstructing the air passages it may have to be held forward or the head turned into a more prone position. An airway, if available, should be inserted, and emergency endotracheal intubation may be necessary. If intubation is impossible puncture of the cricothyroid membrane is rarely required to establish a patent airway.

Relieve pulmonary compression by air or blood

Immediate relief of a tension pneumothorax is mandatory. The insertion of an intravenous needle into the involved pleural space will quickly eliminate the lethal potential of a tension pneumothorax. Signs such as shift of the trachea and apex beat are unreliable in the presence of a flail chest but a unilateral fixed hyperinflated hemithorax may provide a diagnostic clue. The release of air under pressure when the needle is inserted confirms the diagnosis.

An open chest wound results in an open pneumothorax. A wound larger than the glottic opening will produce complete lung collapse and marked shifting of the mediastinum with each respiratory effort. The resultant hypoventilation and diminishing cardiac output will threaten life. An open chest wound should be covered immediately with any material readily available, in order to convert the condition from an acute emergency to that of a closed pneumothorax.

A massive haemothorax should be evacuated with an intercostal chest drain.

Restore the mechanical respiratory efficiency of the thoracic cage

Flail chest results when trauma produces double fractures of three or more adjacent ribs or when frontal impact separates the sternum from the ribs. The flail segment is unstable and can be seen to suck in on inspiration and push out on expiration. The mechanical effect on the function of the heart and lungs results in hypoxia and low cardiac output, hence the flail segment should be stabilized (see below).

Blood volume replacement

Patients with massive blood loss into the pleural space require immediate restoration of blood volume. Infusion fluid should consist of whole blood, packed cells and plasma (plasma protein fraction). Overzealous crystalloid administration should be avoided.

Control of major life-threatening haemorrhage

Intrathoracic vascular or major cardiac injury may demand very urgent or even desperate surgical intervention.

Pericardiocentesis for cardiac tamponade

Cardiac tamponade should be suspected in a chest injury when a low cardiac output occurs in association with venous congestion and high central venous pressure. The diagnosis of cardiac tamponade must be made on the basis of rapid, thorough patient evaluation. Pericardiocentesis, i.e. withdrawing the blood from the pericardial sac by a needle introduced at the xiphisternal junction, is a life-saving procedure.

Indications for early thoracotomy

1. Massive or continuous intrapleural haemorrhage.
2. Cardiac tamponade, initially or after its recurrence following pericardiocentesis.
3. Aortic transection—widened mediastinum with left haemothorax and aortogram confirming aortic transection.
4. Ruptured oesophagus.
5. Open pneumothorax with a major defect of the chest wall.
6. Ruptured bronchus.
7. Traumatic diaphragmatic hernia.
8. Valvular or septal cardiac injury.

Specific injuries

Rib fractures

A simple rib fracture is a trivial injury in most patients. However, elderly patients and those with chronic respiratory disease may have significant problems if lung collapse, pneumonia or both supervene. It is important to exclude associated intrathoracic and intra-abdominal injuries. The treatment of rib fractures consists mainly of adequate relief of pain to allow the patient to cough and deep-breathe frequently. Narcotics in small doses given frequently or intercostal nerve blocks are frequently adequate. Strapping of the thoracic cage with adhesive plaster or other materials is contraindicated, especially in the elderly, because it will restrict chest wall expansion and ventilation leading to lung collapse.

Flail chest

This causes respiratory difficulty because the segment of chest wall is unstable, moving inward with inspiration and outward with expiration (Fig. 45.1). The development of negative intrathoracic pressure is limited and thus the patient cannot move air in and out of the trachea normally. This reduces ventilatory efficiency and this plus underlying lung contusion often leads to progressive respiratory insufficiency. Hypoventilation due to the chest pain adds to the difficulty.

Management

Providing the arterial oxygen can be maintained above 8.0 kpa (60 mmHg) with physiotherapy, effective pain relief and oxygen therapy should be continued. Pain relief can be obtained with low doses of opiates, intercostal nerve block or thoracic epidural block.

If there are other early indications for thoracotomy, an opportunity should also be taken to stabilize the chest wall by internal fixation.

Intermittent positive pressure ventilation (IPPV) remains the most practical form of management

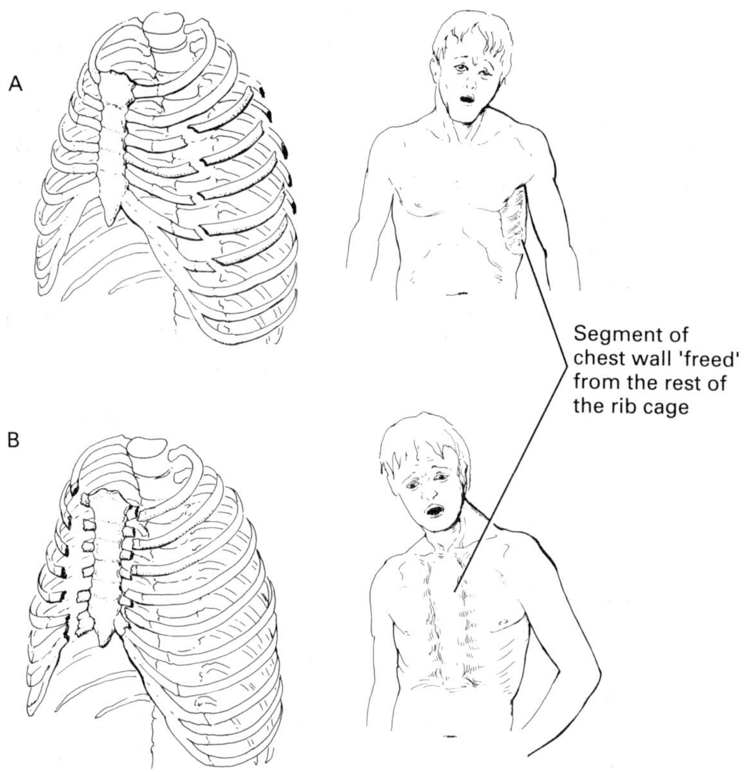

Fig. 45.1 Flail chest: a segment of the chest wall is freed from the chest cage, and therefore is displaced (**a**) outwards on expiration and (**b**) inwards on inspiration: so-called paradoxical respiration. Two patterns of flail segment are represented here: (**A**) of the lateral chest wall, and (**B**) the sternum plus anterior portions of the ribs.

of a flail chest. Endotracheal intubation is often inappropriate if ventilation is likely to be required for at least 10–14 days to stabilize the chest wall. In these circumstances elective tracheostomy should be carried out.

Haemothorax

A massive haemothorax usually results from injuries to the aortic arch, pulmonary hilum or systemic vessels such as the internal mammary or intercostal artery. Rupture of the large vessels is usually incompatible with survival. Early placement of an intercostal drain in a patient who has evidence of a haemothorax is important.

Surgery should be considered in:

1. Any patient who continues to bleed in excess of 300 ml/h over a period of 2–3 h.
2. Any patient who on initial placement of the chest drain had blood loss in excess of 1.5 l.

Pulmonary contusion

Contusion of the underlying lung may follow non-penetrating blunt trauma to the chest; it may affect the opposite lung, a so-called contrecoup effect. Pulmonary contusions are usually localized to a segment or lobe of the lung, and can usually be seen on the initial chest X-ray film. Pulmonary contusion can result in serious complications, the most common being infection. Management involves physiotherapy, fluid restriction and using plasma protein fraction to maintain plasma osmotic pressure, if necessary.

Injuries to the trachea and major bronchi

An interruption of the tracheobronchial tree can result from either blunt or penetrating chest injuries. The presence of tracheobronchial rupture should be suspected whenever there is major chest trauma. Findings requiring further investigation include massive haemoptysis, airway obstruction, progressive mediastinal emphysema, tension pneumothorax, persistent air leak and pneumothorax. Atelectasia of one lobe or an entire lung that does not respond to treatment should also arouse suspicion of major bronchial rupture.

The most reliable means of establishing the diagnosis and determining the site and nature of the tear is bronchoscopy. Thoracotomy will be needed to repair the tear.

Traumatic rupture of the diaphragm

When closed rupture of the diaphragm is associated with a large tear, the abdominal contents may herniate through into the thorax. It is most often on the left side when secondary to blunt trauma, although it can occur in either hemidiaphragm when penetrating trauma is the cause. The common presenting symptoms include dyspnoea and chest pain. Physical findings include decreased breath sounds on the side of herniation, contralateral shift of the mediastinum and the presence of bowel sounds in the chest. Chest X-ray confirms the diagnosis.

Immediate operative repair is indicated.

Injuries to the heart

Myocardial contusion, closed rupture of the interventricular septum, heart valves and traumatic rupture of the aorta are complications that follow blunt trauma to the chest. Penetrating wounds of the heart causes haemopericardium and cardiac tamponade.

DISORDERS OF THE CHEST WALL

Deformities

Pectus excavatum (funnel chest)

This is the most common deformity in which the body of the sternum, often only its lower end, is curved backwards (Fig. 45.2). The heart may be displaced to the left and compressed between the sternum and the vertebral column. Some patients with this deformity have symptoms of dyspnoea, pericardial pain, palpitation, syncope on moderate exertion and repeated lung infections.

When the deformity is severe it should be repaired so that chest wall growth and development will be normal and to alleviate any pulmonary or cardiac function impairment. Cosmetic concerns alone are not sufficient justification in themselves for repair of pectus excavatum.

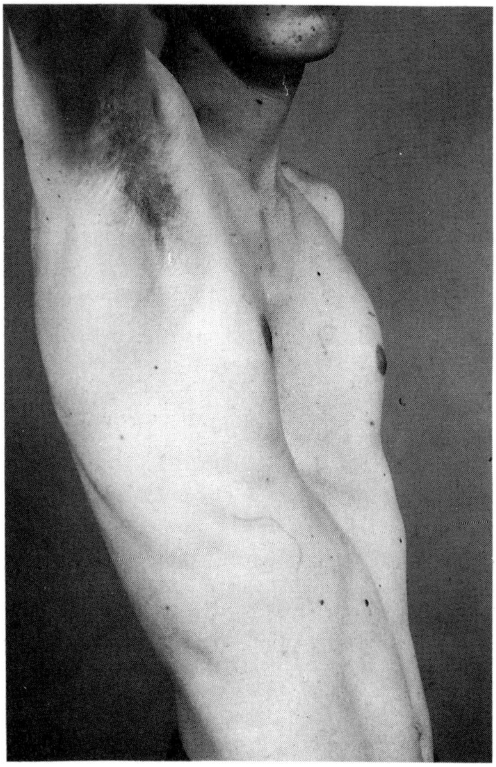

Fig. 45.2 Pectus excavatum. This patient, in spite of a moderately severe degree of the deformity, had no symptoms.

Pectus carinatum (pigeon chest)

This is a much rarer chest wall deformity. In this condition the sternum is prominent, forming an anterior ridge with the ribs falling steeply away on either side. This is purely a cosmetic deformity.

Tumours of the ribs and sternum

Metastatic tumours are much more common than primary tumours of the rib. The tumours that commonly metastasize to the ribs are from the lungs, breasts and kidneys. There is usually local pain and tenderness but they are sometimes painless. A lump may be felt. In the early stages there may be no radiological change; often there is rib destruction and pathological fractures may occur.

Primary chest wall tumours

Among primary tumours, malignant tumours are as common as benign ones. The common benign and malignant tumours are given in Table 45.1.

Table 45.1 Common tumours of the chest wall

Benign tumours	Malignant tumours
Chondroma (enchondroma)	Chondrosarcoma
Osteochondroma (exostosis, ecchondroma)	Ewing's tumour
Fibrous dysplasia	Solitary plasmacytoma
Aneurysmal bone cyst	
Eosinophilic granuloma of bone	

Clinical features

Pain and the presence of a mass are the two commonest complaints of patients with chest wall tumours. One in 10 is asymptomatic, the tumour being discovered during a routine chest X-ray examination. A tumour of the first or second rib may lead to brachial plexus compression producing pain, muscle weakness and atrophy of the upper extremities. Malignant tumours may lead to a pleural effusion. Preoperative differentiation between benign and malignant lesions cannot usually be made with certainty.

Treatment

All primary chest wall tumours should be treated by radical excision. This is necessary not only for adequate diagnosis but also to provide the best chance for a cure in both benign and malignant lesions.

THE PLEURA

Anatomy and physiology

The pleura is a serous membrane which consists of two layers, the visceral and parietal. The visceral layer forms the outer covering of the lung which it encloses completely except at the hilum where it is reflected over the structures entering the lung and becomes continuous with the parietal layer. The parietal layer lines the interior of the chest wall and the upper surface of the diaphragm. In health, the parietal and visceral pleura are in close contact, separated only by a thin film of serous fluid which acts as a lubricant so that the two surfaces can glide smoothly over each other during the act of breathing. There is a potential space between the layers which is termed the pleural cavity.

The mean pressure within the pleural cavity is below atmospheric, fluctuating between 8 and 9 mmHg during inspiration and 3 and 6 mmHg during expiration. There is a constant movement of fluid through the pleural cavity from the parietal to the visceral pleura where absorption occurs. The amount of fluid that traverses the pleural space each day is 5–10 l. The passage of protein-free fluid through the pleural membranes is dependent on the hydrostatic and colloid osmotic pressure across them.

Pneumothorax

Pneumothorax is the presence of air in the pleural cavity. Air may enter the pleural cavity through either a hole in the visceral or parietal pleura. There are three principal types of pneumothorax, based on their aetiology:

1. Spontaneous.
   a. Primary.
   b. Secondary.
2. Traumatic.
3. Iatrogenic.

Pneumothorax of whatever type may be:

1. Open when the air moves freely in and out of the pleural space during respiration.
2. Closed when no such movement of air takes place.
3. Valvular when air enters the pleural cavity during inspiration but is prevented from escaping during expiration—a tension pneumothorax results.

Primary spontaneous pneumothorax

This is a disease of young adults; males are affected more frequently than females. The patient is usually tall, thin and in the 20–30 year age group. The air escapes from an area of the subpleural bed or from bullae (cysts). These are usually in the apical part of the lung and may be bilateral. The cause of these lesions is unknown.

Secondary spontaneous pneumothorax

In patients over 40, spontaneous pneumothorax is due to the presence of underlying lung disease, such as chronic bronchitis, asthma and emphysema. Pneumothorax also occurs as a complication of any condition with generalized fibrosis of the lungs. Tuberculosis, carcinoma and hydatid disease can also be complicated by pneumothorax.

Recurrent spontaneous pneumothorax

Some patients with primary spontaneous pneumothorax have a tendency to have recurrent episodes. This tendency increases in frequency after every episode.

Traumatic pneumothorax

Penetrating wounds of the chest, rib fractures, and rupture of the bronchus complicating closed chest injuries are the common causes of traumatic pneumothorax.

Iatrogenic pneumothorax

Transbronchial biopsy and needle biopsy of the lung or pleura may be followed by pneumothorax. Inadvertent pleural and pulmonary puncture may result from paracentesis of the pericardial sac or liver biopsy. Pneumothorax is well recognized as a complication of ventral venous catheterization when it is introduced through the subclavian route.

Clinical features

Clinical features in patients with spontaneous pneumothorax depend largely on the extent of lung collapse and the presence of pre-existing lung disease. In a few patients it is asymptomatic and only found on a routine chest radiograph. In the majority of patients initial symptoms occur at rest or during normal activity. The onset is usually sudden. Common clinical features are:

1. Pain—sharp and pleuritic in nature.
2. Dyspnoea—the degree depends on the size of the pneumothorax and according to whether the lungs are healthy or not.

3. Cough—when present it is short and unproductive.
4. Cyanosis—in patients with underlying lung disease.

Tension pneumothorax

This is associated with increasing anxiety, restlessness, respiratory distress and shock when increasing pleural pressure impairs venous return. Unless the condition is relieved, death will occur from a combination of respiratory and cardiac failure.

Physical signs

Physical signs depend essentially on the degree of pulmonary collapse. When the pneumothorax is greater than 30%, the physical signs are reduction of movement on the affected side, diminished vocal fremitus, hyper-resonant percussion note and diminished or absent breath sounds. Tracheal deviation and displacement of the apex beat away from the affected side can be elicited if the pneumothorax is large (Fig. 45.3).

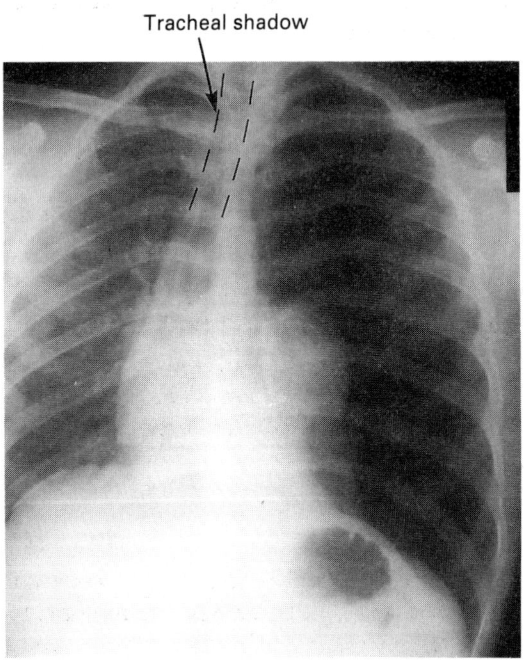

Fig. 45.3 Pneumothorax: complete absence of lung markings in the left side of the patient's chest, and displacement of the tracheal shadow to the right.

Radiographic features

The characteristic radiographic appearance in pneumothorax is the sharply defined lung edge separated from the bony cage by a clear zone devoid of lung markings. If the pneumothorax is small those features may escape detection unless a radiograph is taken in full expiration. The chest radiograph should also be examined for underlying pulmonary abnormalities.

Complications

1. Respiratory failure in patients with chronic lung disease.
2. Tension pneumothorax—death from circulatory failure.
3. Infection.
4. Haemopneumothorax.

Treatment

A small pneumothorax in a healthy individual can be managed by bed rest and observation as air will be gradually absorbed. A pneumothorax that is greater than one-quarter of the hemithorax is usually treated by intercostal tube drainage. Even a small pneumothorax has to be treated by intercostal tube drainage in patients with severely embarrassed respiratory function.

Initial treatment of tension pneumothorax should be by needle puncture of the involved hemithorax in the second intercostal space at the mid clavicular line. This procedure converts the tension pneumothorax into a simple one, and then it can be managed by the insertion of intercostal tube drainage.

Indications for active treatment in spontaneous pneumothorax

1. Persistent air leak.
2. Failure of the lung to expand fully.
3. Recurrent pneumothorax (second episode).
4. Specific surgical indications for conditions causing secondary spontaneous pneumothorax (hydatid disease, carcinoma).
5. Bilateral pneumothorax.
6. Special circumstances—occupational indications: pilots, seamen and divers.

The objectives of surgical treatment are to relieve symptoms and to prevent further recurrences. Two approaches are possible: chemical and surgical pleurodesis.

Chemical pleurodesis is the installation of an irritant substance (tetracycline in 20 ml saline or 100 mg mepacrine in 20 ml saline) into the pleural cavity to cause sterile pleural irritation and subsequent pleural adhesions. This mode of therapy is frequently very painful and often ineffective in stimulating adequate adhesions.

Surgical pleurodesis is a more effective method of preventing recurrent pneumothorax. This procedure, which can be done through a small thoracotomy, involves stripping off the parietal pleura from the chest wall and the upper mediastinum so as to leave a raw surface to which the visceral pleura can adhere.

Pleural effusion

A pleural effusion is an accumulation of fluid in the pleural space and is a sign of underlying disease, and not a disease in itself. It is clinically useful to classify pleural effusions as either transudates or exudates. The distinction between them is made chiefly on the protein content of the fluid: transudates contain less than and exudates more than 3g/100 ml. A transudate occurs when the systemic factors influencing the formation or absorption of pleural fluid are altered, such as plasma oncotic pressure or hydrostatic pressure in the pulmonary or systemic circulation. There is no pleural disease in transudate effusions. In contrast, exudates result from disease of the pleura or lymphatics, such as tumour and infection.

Causes of pleural effusion

Transudate. A collection of transudate fluid in the pleural cavity is known as hydrothorax.

1. Congestive cardiac failure.
2. The nephrotic syndrome.
3. Hypoproteinaemia.
4. Constrictive pericarditis.
5. Meig's syndrome (ovarian fibroma, ascites and hydrothorax).

Exudate.

1. Primary pleural malignancy—mesothelioma.
2. Pleural metastasis, e.g. from lung, breast, ovary, pancreas, colon or stomach.
3. Lymphoma.
4. Infection—tuberculosis; pyogenic: bacterial pneumonia.
5. Pulmonary infarction.
6. Subphrenic abscess.
7. Asbestos exposure.
8. Collagen disorders.

Clinical features

Clinical presentation of pleural effusion depends on the cause, the rate of accumulation and the size. The principal symptom from the effusion is dyspnoea.

Physical findings

The effusion may be either in the general pleural space or loculated in the general pleural space, or interlobar fissures.

If the pleural effusion is in the general pleural space and is sufficiently large, the characteristic physical signs are:

1. Restriction of respiratory movements on the affected side.
2. Diminished or absent breath sounds.
3. Marked (stony) dullness on percussion.
4. At the upper level of dullness, bronchial breathing may be heard.
5. Large effusions will displace the trachea and apex beat to the opposite side.

An effusion loculated within the tissues may not be detectable on physical examination. With small effusions the signs are usually best elicited at the base posteriorly.

Radiography

The radiographic density of pleural fluid is the same whether it is serous, purulent (empyema) or blood. A very small amount of effusion is represented by obliteration of the costophrenic angle. A moderate-sized effusion appears as a triangular lateral opacity with the base obscuring the hemidiaphragm and

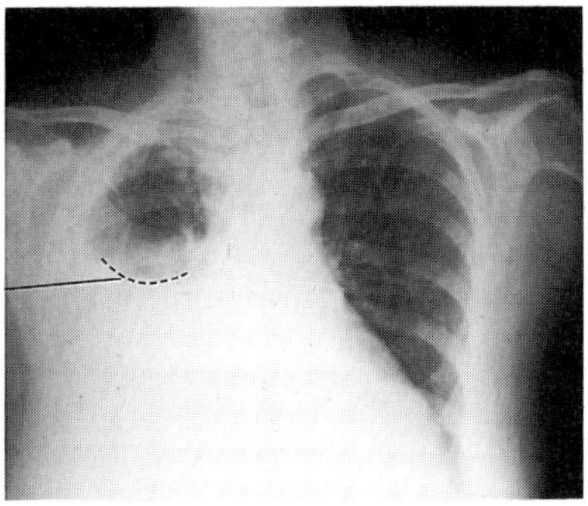

Fig. 45.4 Large right-sided pleural effusion with characteristic crescentic upper edge.

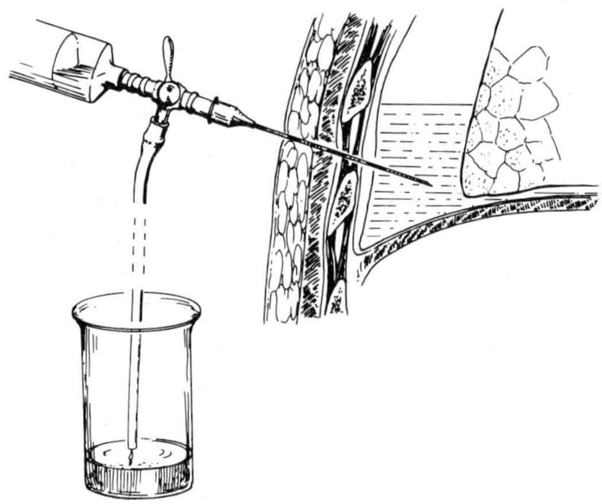

Fig. 45.5 Aspiration of pleural effusion (pleural tap). Under local anaesthesia a rigid, large-calibre needle is introduced, passing just above the upper border of a rib into the pleural space. A three-way tap allows emptying of each aspirated syringeful into a receptacle, without altering the position of the needle.

with a curved upper border, concave medially, extending upwards in the axilla. A large effusion may obscure the whole hemithorax and displace the heart and trachea to the opposite side (Fig. 45.4). The effusion may be distinguished from pleural thickening by the simple technique of comparing the chest X-rays taken with the patient in the upright and lateral recumbent positions, since fluid will gravitate to the dependent part of the pleural space. Transudates are often bilateral, while exudates are usually unilateral. Ultrasound is useful for differentiating between pleural thickening and fluid.

Diagnosis

It is important to identify underlying causes such as infection, embolism, cardiac failure, the nephrotic syndrome and constrictive pericarditis. When the cause of an effusion is unclear, diagnostic aspiration of a sample of the fluid is performed to determine the aetiology (Fig. 45.5). This is usually accompanied by pleural biopsy. Following aspiration the fluid is subjected to the following examinations.

Macroscopic appearance

Pleural transudates are clear or faintly yellow, whereas exudates are dark yellow or amber, often slightly cloudy and frequently clot on standing in a specimen jar. Blood-stained pleural effusions are usually due to trauma, pulmonary infarction or malignancy. A yellow or tan creamy fluid (pus) is diagnostic of empyema.

Biochemical examination

The significance of the protein content in distinguishing transudates and exudates has been mentioned already. A low glucose level in the pleural fluid relative to its serum level is observed in rheumatoid arthritis, empyema, tuberculosis and malignant tumour.

Bacteriology

Bacteriological culture is essential for a precise aetiological diagnosis of those effusions complicating infections.

Pleural fluid cytology

The numbers of lymphocytes, neutrophils, eosinophils, mesothelial cells and erythrocytes are noted, as well as the presence of any malignant or atypical cells.

Pleural biopsy

Biopsy of the pleura using an Abram's biopsy needle, is helpful in establishing two common causes of pleural effusion—tuberculous pleuritis, and tumour involving the pleura.

Management

Small or asymptomatic effusions do not warrant immediate treatment unless the removal is necessary for diagnostic reasons. If the effusion is not due to malignancy, it usually responds to treatment of the underlying disease. Malignant effusions causing severe distressing respiratory symptoms will require local treatment. Pleural tap (thoracentesis) is the primary therapy. Sufficient fluid should be removed to make the patient comfortable. However, care should be taken to limit the initial aspiration to about 1.5 l, otherwise pulmonary oedema may occur. If the pleural effusion rapidly reaccumulates an attempt to secure pleurodesis may be made by the intrapleural infusion of a sclerosing agent, e.g. tetracycline, mepacrine, bleomycin, thiotepa or talc. The results, however, are often disappointing.

Empyema

Empyema thoracis is defined as pus in the pleural cavity. An empyema may involve the whole pleural space, i.e. total empyema, or only part of it, a loculated or encysted empyema. It is almost always unilateral.

Pathology

The American Thoracic Society has classified empyema into three phases based on its natural history, and this scheme is useful in planning therapy.

Exudative or acute phase

This is the earliest phase. Infection of the pleura results in exudation of protein-rich fluid of low viscosity and a low cellular content. The lung is still expandable.

Fibrinopurulent or transitional phase

Untreated empyema progresses into this stage, which is characterized by thicker, more turbid fluid due to increase in the polymorphonuclear leukocytes. Fibrin is deposited on both pleural surfaces, forming adhesions limiting the empyema. The lung also begins to be trapped by this restrictive fibrin peel during this phase.

Organizing or chronic phase

The fibrin peel becomes organized with ingrowth of capillaries and fibroblasts. The pleural peel finally becomes almost avascular and can be stripped off the pleura at operation (decortication). Organization may begin as early as 7–10 days after the onset of the disease and usually by 4–6 weeks the process has entered the chronic stage.

Aetiology

Causes of empyema are:

1. Extension of infection from the lung, e.g. pneumonia primary or secondary to bronchial neoplasm, bronchiectasis, lung abscess secondary to bronchial foreign body or bronchial carcinoma, or tuberculosis.
2. Penetrating chest wounds.
3. Complication of thoracic surgery.
4. Subphrenic abscess.
5. Perforation of the oesophagus, either spontaneous or iatrogenic.
6. Pyaemia or septicaemia.

The commonest infecting organisms are *Staphylococcus pyogenes*, the pneumococcus, group A beta-haemolytic streptococcus, anaerobic streptococci and *Bacteroides* species. Gram-negative organisms such as *Pseudomonas*, *Klebsiella pneumoniae*, *Escherichia coli* and *Proteus* are the next most common causative organisms.

Complications

Empyema may be complicated by rupture of pus into the bronchus giving rise to a bronchopleural fistula or into the chest wall resulting in the so-called empyema necessitatis.

Reasons for an empyema becoming chronic are:

1. Failure to recognize an acute empyema or ineffective drainage.
2. Chronic forms of infection such as tuberculosis or of actinomycosis.
3. Chronic bacterial lung infections such as bronchiectasis or lung abscess which result in shrunken fibrotic lung that cannot expand to fill the cavity.
4. Lung cancer.

5. Bronchopleural fistula.
6. Foreign body in the pleural cavity.

Clinical features

Empyema should be suspected in patients with pulmonary infection if there is a recurrence of pyrexia which fails to respond, or responds only partially, to the continued administration of appropriate antibiotics. In addition to the clinical features of the primary condition the following are characteristic of empyema:

1. Fever with rigors.
2. Sweating, anorexia and loss of weight.
3. Leukocytosis in the range of 15 000–20 000 per mm^3.
4. Pleuritic chest pain, mostly in the early stages.
5. Dyspnoea.
6. Anaemia and finger-clubbing, which may develop within 2–3 weeks of onset.
7. An abscess of the chest wall, commonly in relation to the costochondral junction of the fifth rib.
8. Bronchopleural fistula, heralded by increase in cough and sputum which may be blood-stained.

Physical examination and radiological features

These are those of a pleural effusion (see above).

Diagnosis

Empyema may be suggested by the history and physical examination, but the diagnosis is made on the basis of chest X-ray films and pleural aspiration (Fig.45.6). The pleural aspirate should be sent for cytological and bacteriological examination, including anaerobic culture and sensitivity tests of any organism isolated.

Management

The aims of the treatment of empyema are:
1. Control of systemic and local infection.
2. Evacuation of the pus.
3. Re-expansion of the lung with obliteration of the empyema cavity.

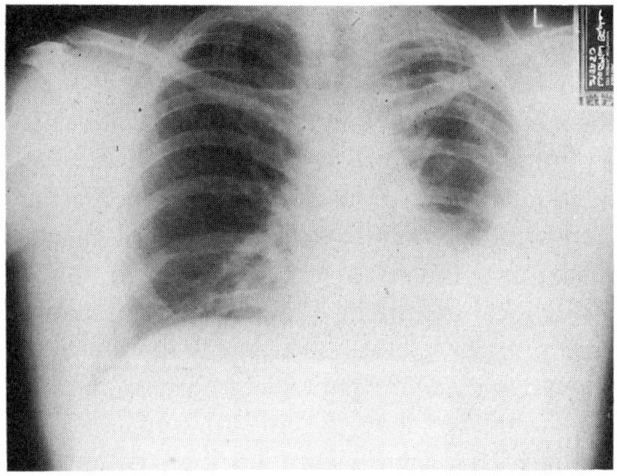

Fig. 45.6 Large left-sided empyema, with some collapse of the underlying lung.

Control of infection

This should be effected by the oral or parenteral administration of appropriate antibiotics as determined by culture and sensitivity. These antibiotics may also be injected into the pleural cavity.

Evacuation of the pus

Pleural aspiration. If the empyema is in the exudative phase and pleural fluid is thin and can be aspirated completely, pleural aspiration with appropriate antibiotics will be curative. Repeated aspiration may be used as long as the pus remains thin.

Intercostal tube drainage. If complete evacuation of the pus cannot be accomplished, or rapid reaccumulation occurs and also the pus remains thin, then treatment by intercostal drainage through an underwater seal should be carried out. The tube is placed on suction until closure of the empyema cavity occurs. This may take several weeks provided the lung is not enclosed in a thick fibrin coat. The tube is then converted into an open drainage. Premature removal will lead to loculation of pus and recurrence of the empyema. After the early stages, underwater seal is unnecessary because the rigid walls of the empyema cavity prevent the lung from collapsing. The size of the cavity should be checked regularly (weekly) by instilling lipiodol and taking radiographs (sinogram) in several planes. If the cavity is decreasing in size then the intercostal tube is gradually shortened (withdrawn) over the

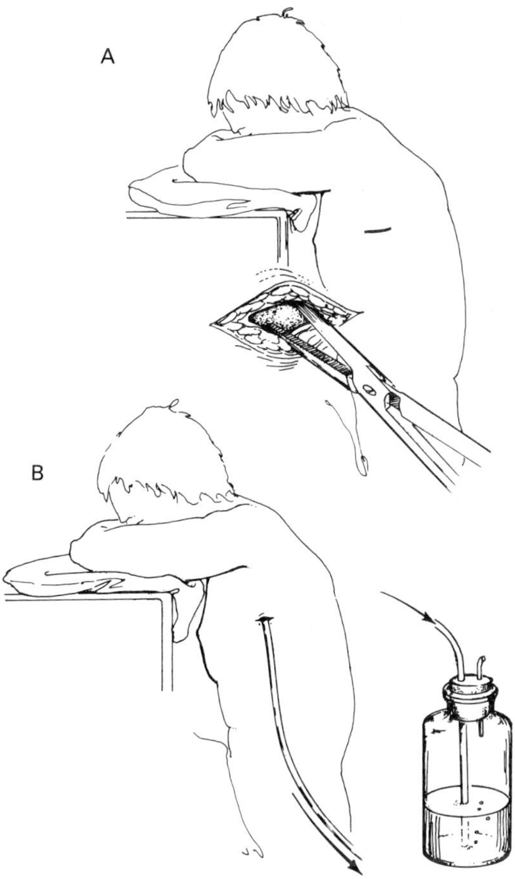

Fig. 45.7 Technique of rib resection and drainage. (**A**) Under local anaesthesia, a short incision is made over the selected rib, and after stripping the perichondrium, a short segment of the rib is removed by bone shears. This enables the creation of an adequate-sized hole through the rib bed, into the pleural cavity for the insertion of a large-diameter drainage tube (**B**) This is fixed by sutures to the skin, and connected to an underwater seal drainage bottle.

next 1–3 months until only a tube track remains; only then should the tube be removed.

Rib resection and drainage. A chronic empyema containing thick pus, with the lung enclosed by thick fibrous peel, needs more aggressive surgical treatment. Drainage with a short segment rib resection must be performed in patients too ill to withstand decortication (Fig. 45.7). This has the advantage of being more comfortable than intercostal tube drainage and avoids the danger of intercostal artery haemorrhage as the intercostal bundle is ligated proximally and distally during the rib resection, and a larger tube can be inserted into the empyema cavity.

Decortication. This is carried out through a posterolateral thoracotomy. The fibrous 'peel' covering that traps the lung, diaphragm, mediastinum and pleural surface of the chest wall is removed. This allows full expansion of the lung. Rarely is thoracoplasty required to obliterate an empyema cavity.

Tumours of the pleura

The commonest pleural tumour is a metastasis and the commonest source is a primary tumour of the lung, but others that are fairly common are from the breast, ovary, pancreas, colon and stomach. These usually present with a pleural effusion.

Primary pleural tumours

These are rare.

Benign tumours

Localized fibrous mesothelioma (pleural fibroma). These are well encapsulated and firm but may be nodular or pedunculated, attached to the visceral or parietal pleura by a narrow vascular pedicle. They are usually asymptomatic and found on routine chest X-ray; some patients present with dyspnoea, chest pain and cough. Treatment is surgical resection. Lipomas, angiomas and cysts of the pleura have also been reported. These tumours arise from the subpleural tissue. Treatment is also by surgical excision.

Malignant tumours

Mesothelioma. This tumour arises from mesothelial cells lining the pleura.

Aetiology

There is a strong aetiological association with exposure to asbestos. Some 5–7% of individuals exposed to asbestos may develop mesotheliomas. Furthermore, there is a latent period of 20–40 years from the period of exposure until the emergence of the tumour. The age incidence is therefore at its maximum in the sixth and seventh decades.

Pathology

The tumour grows as a diffuse sheet of thick rubbery, yellowish-grey tissue encasing and infiltrating into the lungs. Direct extension occurs to the pericardium, heart, contralateral pleura and also through the diaphragm. Characteristically the tumour gives rise to a massive effusion, which may consist of necrotic or fibrinous material. As the lesion advances the space becomes obliterated by neoplasm. Local invasion of the chest wall may occur. Spreading of the tumour along the track of healed operation wounds and needle biopsy tracts is a particular hazard in malignant mesothelioma. Patients usually succumb to local complications of the primary lesion.

Clinical features

Chest pain is the most outstanding symptom. Breathlessness, cough and loss of weight are also common. The disease usually runs a 2-year course from the onset of symptoms. Radiographic features are those of a massive pleural effusion.

Diagnosis

A characteristic biochemical feature of the aspirated fluid is a high content of hyaluronic acid, though not all samples may show this. Cytological examination of pleural fluid is often difficult; more confident histological diagnosis often depends on pleural or open biopsy.

Treatment

Mesothelioma is a diffuse tumour, so its total removal is not feasible even when the diagnosis is made early. The tumours are unresponsive to irradiation and chemotherapy. Only rarely have pleurectomy, pleuropneumonectomy or decortication been performed, but there is no evidence to suggest that this prolongs life. Hence, on the whole, treatment is symptomatic to alleviate distressing symptoms.

Mediastinal tumours

Many different neoplasms and cysts may arise from the multiple anatomical structures present in the mediastinum. There are numerous lymph nodes in this area. Metastasis secondary to lesions in other parts of the body are also frequently found. The mediastinum is regarded as having four compartments, and the tumours most often encountered in each compartment are as follows:

Superior mediastinum

1. Thymic tumours.
2. Teratoma.
3. Retrosternal goitre.
4. Parathyroid adenoma.
5. Lymphoma.

Anterior mediastinum

1. Thymic enlargement, tumours or cysts.
2. Teratoma.
3. Pericardial cyst.
4. Lipoma.
5. Lymphoma.

Middle mediastinum

1. Pericardial cyst.
2. Bronchogenic cyst.

Posterior mediastinum

1. Neurogenic tumours and cysts.
2. Gastroenteric (enterogenous) cysts.

Pathology

Thymoma

This is one of the common neoplasms originating in the anterior and superior mediastinum. Thymoma occurs with equal frequency in male and female patients, and has a peak incidence between the ages of 40 and 60; it rarely occurs in children. It is either encapsulated with no evidence of local invasion at operation, or invasive when the lesion infiltrates the pericardium, pleura, heart or great vessels. It is difficult to establish the diagnosis of malignancy microscopically, and hence all thymomas should be considered malignant and removed.

About half of all patients with thymic tumours

have myasthenia gravis, and about 10% of patients with myasthenia have thymic tumours. Thymic tumours may also be associated with red cell aplasia, hypogammaglobulinaemia, thyrotoxicosis, collagen vascular disease and Cushing's syndrome.

Thymic cysts

These are rare and are usually small, multiple and embedded in the gland; most are asymptomatic.

Teratoma

This is a neoplasm composed of multiple tissues foreign to the part in which the tumour is found. When the tumour consists only of ectodermal tissues it is called a dermoid cyst. When it contains ectodermal mesodermal and endodermal tissues it is called a teratoma. A dermoid cyst is benign and a teratoma is malignant and presents most commonly in young adults or in middle age.

Retrosternal goitre

An intrathoracic extension of a goitre is most frequently from the lower pole or isthmus, and lies in the upper part of the anterior mediastinum.

Parathyroid adenoma

A parathyroid adenoma may occasionally occur in the anterior mediastinum. Its usual presentation is by clinical or laboratory evidence of hypercalcaemia.

Lymphoma

Mediastinal lymph nodes usually in the anterior mediastinum are frequently involved with disseminated lymphoma. Rarely is it confined only to the mediastinum.

Pericardial cysts

These are well defined, ovoid or round opacities which lie adjacent to the sternum, more frequently on the right side. They are continuous with and adherent to the pericardium. They are asymptomatic.

Neurogenic tumours

These are the commonest masses to arise in the posterior mediastinum. They include all benign and malignant neoplasms arising from the intercostal nerves, sympathetic ganglia and chemoreceptor cells. They occur mainly in the paravertebral gutter, causing local splaying of the ribs, and may produce rib erosion and very rarely spinal cord compression when they grow through the intervertebral foramina to produce a 'dumb-bell' tumour. The four main histological types are neurilemmoma, neurofibroma, ganglioneuroma and neuroblastoma.

Neurilemmoma. This arises from the sheath of Schwann cells of an intercostal nerve. It commonly occurs in the third to fifth decade.

Neurofibroma. This tumour arises from a fibrous nerve sheath of an intercostal nerve. A neurofibroma may be associated with neurofibromatosis (von Recklinghausen's disease). Both neurolemmoma and neurofibroma can undergo malignant degeneration.

Ganglioneuroma. This is a benign tumour arising from one of the sympathetic ganglia.

Neuroblastoma. This is a malignant neoplasm of the sympathetic nervous system.

Clinical features

Whether or not malignant change occurs, tumours and cysts of the mediastinum tend to enlarge and compress adjacent structures. Cough and dyspnoea may be caused by pressure on the bronchi and trachea, dysphagia by pressure on the oesophagus, distension of the neck veins and the development of collateral circulation by superior vena caval obstruction, and tachycardia by displacement of the heart, limiting diastolic filling. Neurogenic tumours may give rise to a pain which may be intercostal or vaguely distributed in the chest. Those with dumb-bell extensions into the vertebral canal may result in symptoms due to spinal cord compression. Recurrent laryngeal nerve involvement may result in hoarseness, and Horner's syndrome from involvement of the cervical sympathetic ganglia.

Some patients manifest systemic symptoms.

Thymic tumours may be associated with myasthenia gravis, hypercalcaemia secondary to a parathyroid adenoma, systemic hypertension due to a neurogenic tumour and thyrotoxicosis due to an intrathoracic goitre. Nearly a third of the lesions are asymptomatic and are discovered on a routine chest X-ray.

Investigation of a mediastinal mass

1. Posteroanterior and lateral chest radiographs demonstrate the size, density, presence or absence of calcification and the anatomical location of the mass.
2. Barium swallow demonstrates invasion, extrinsic compression or displacement of the oesophagus.
3. Tomography is useful in outlining the lesion more clearly and will also identify any erosion of the posterior ribs, vertebral bodies and widening of intervertebral foramina by dumb-bell extensions.
4. Computerized tomography scanning is of great value in demonstrating mediastinal abnormalities. It can often precisely define a mass and determine its density.
5. Iodine 131 thyroid scintiscan will provide a diagnosis of retrosternal and intrathoracic goitre.
6. Mediastinoscopy and anterior mediastinotomy provide biopsy material from the lesion and also give an estimate as to the resectability of the lesion.

Treatment

Fifty per cent of symptomatic mediastinal masses are malignant, whereas 90% of asymptomatic masses are benign. An aggressive surgical approach should be taken in all patients with a newly diagnosed mediastinal lesion, since benign tumours may enlarge and compress mediastinal structures or may produce haemorrhage, rupture, infection or malignant degeneration. Moreover, early diagnosis and treatment are accompanied by the most favourable prognosis in those patients with malignant tumours. All these tumours are approached via a median sternotomy incision.

CONGENITAL LESIONS OF THE LUNGS

Congenital abnormalities of the lung are uncommon. Those that require surgical attention are: pulmonary sequestration, bronchogenic cyst and pulmonary arteriovenous malformation.

Pulmonary sequestration

The condition is defined as an area of embryonic lung tissue that is supplied by an aberrant artery or arteries arising from the aorta (descending thoracic or abdominal) or one of its branches and which is drained, as a rule, by the pulmonary veins. Two forms are recognized:

1. Extralobar—Abnormal lung tissue is separated from the normal lung by a separate lining of pleura.
2. Intralobar—Abnormal lung tissue is incorporated into the normal lung and shares a common covering of visceral pleura.

Intralobar sequestration is seen more frequently than extralobar sequestration. Extralobar sequestration is associated with other congenital abnormalities (such as congenital diaphragmatic hernia, congenital heart disease and pectus excavatum) in about 50% of cases. Pulmonary sequestration commonly involves the lower lobes, the left side being affected more commonly than the right.

Clinical features

The condition may remain asymptomatic and may simply be detected on a routine chest X-ray examination. Symptoms typically appear in the first decade of life and onset is rare after the age of 40.

Respiratory symptoms

The presence or absence of respiratory symptoms is determined by whether or not there is a bronchial communication to the sequestrated segment and if so, common symptoms are cough and sputum and those related to recurrent pneumonia.

Cardiovascular symptoms

These are symptoms of heart failure due to shunting

of blood through the sequestrated segment, i.e. a left-to-right shunt from the systemic arterial side to the pulmonary vein.

On chest X-ray common appearances are those of cystic lesions with or without air fluid levels. Extralobar sequestration typically demonstrates a triangular density with the costophrenic angle. Bronchograms usually demonstrate the lack of connection to the bronchial system and displacement of terminal branches by the space-occupying sequestrium. It is uncommon to fill the sequestered segment even in the presence of bronchial communication. Retrograde aortography is essential to demonstrate the abnormal arterial supply. The treatment of all pulmonary sequestration is resection of the involved area.

Bronchogenic cysts

Embryologically, these cysts arise from nests of cells that become isolated from the main pulmonary branching when the lung bud is separating from the foregut. Bronchogenic cysts are thin-walled and occur characteristically near the tracheal bifurcation, and may be attached to the oesophagus. The cyst wall contains cartilage and respiratory epithelium.

Clinically bronchogenic cysts are frequently asymptomatic and discovered as incidental findings on a routine chest X-ray. In children they can cause wheezing, stridor, cough, dyspnoea and recurrent infection due to tracheobronchial compression by a large cyst. If bronchial communication is present cough, fever, purulent sputum and haemoptysis may occur due to infection.

Chest X-ray and tomography will show a smooth, round or oval opacity in the superior or middle mediastinum. The presence of a fluid level in the cyst indicates communication with the tracheobronchial tree. A barium swallow may show displacement of the oesophagus posteriorly.

Surgical removal is the treatment of choice for both infected and uninfected cysts.

Pulmonary arteriovenous malformation

This abnormality consists of one or more communications between the arterial and venous sides of the pulmonary circulation, bypassing the pulmonary capillary bed. In 50% of cases this condition is associated with hereditary haemorrhagic telangiectasia (Rendu–Osler–Weber disease). The malformation is often multiple and is more common in the lower lobes.

The lesion may be asymptomatic. When there is a major shunt of unoxygenated blood from the right to the left side of the heart through the malformation there will be dyspnoea, cyanosis, polycythaemia and finger-clubbing. Local complications from the malformation may occur, and these include spontaneous haemothorax, pleurisy and haemoptysis.

Chest X-ray may show a round or lobulated opacity in the middle or lower zones of the lung field. A pulmonary angiogram should always be carried out to demonstrate the lesions and to assess operability.

The treatment is surgical excision. However, in patients with widespread malformations surgical resection will be impossible and for these patients, embolization of the fistula via pulmonary angiogram catheters has proved useful.

FOREIGN BODY IN THE TRACHEOBRONCHIAL TREE

Any object, edible or inedible, that finds its way into the mouth may be inhaled. Inhalation of foreign bodies occurs more frequently in children and most often in the right side. Foreign bodies cause bronchial inflammation at the site of impaction and infection distally, leading to lung abscess, bronchiectasis and empyema.

Clinical features

The history of an inhaled foreign body is important. The history of cough, wheezing and fever in a young child should always suggest the possibility of a foreign body in the tracheobronchial tree. A foreign body lying in the trachea or major bronchi causes extreme distress with cough and stridor. Dyspnoea is present when there is lung collapse or obstructive emphysema. Occasionally the patient is symptomless.

Diagnosis

Posteroanterior and lateral chest radiographs of the chest are essential in suspected cases. The diagnosis is simple when the foreign body is radiopaque. If the foreign body is not opaque, its presence is indicated by a lobar or segmental collapse or obstructive emphysema (when the foreign body acts as a small ball-valve). Chest films should be taken in both inspiration and expiration to detect emphysema and mediastinal shift. However, the X-ray is sometimes completely normal.

Treatment

Bronchoscopic removal

Bronchoscopic removal of a foreign body should be carried out in a theatre capable of undertaking a thoracotomy. Only rigid bronchoscopy under general anaesthetic should be used (Fig. 45.8).

Thoracotomy and removal of foreign body

In a minority of cases, when the foreign body cannot be removed with the bronchoscope, thoracotomy will be necessary. At operation the foreign body is felt and located in a large bronchus which is exposed, opened and carefully resutured after its removal. In very rare instances when lung abscess or bronchiectasis is involved a lobe may have to be removed.

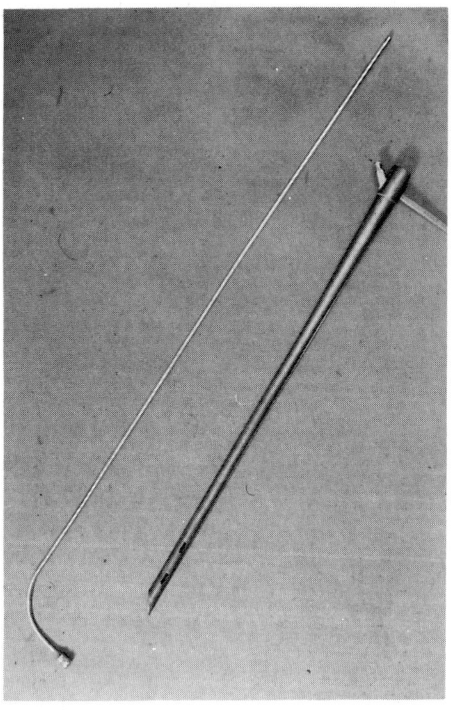

Fig. 45.8 A rigid bronchoscope (Negus pattern). Suction of secretions and other fluid can be performed using the long tube shown alongside the bronchoscope.

LUNG INFECTIONS

Bronchiectasis

Bronchiectasis is a condition in which there is abnormal and often permanent dilatation of the bronchi. Today, with effective antibiotic therapy its overall incidence has decreased significantly.

Pathology

Three major patterns of dilatation are recognized on bronchogram:

1. Cylindrical: the bronchi are uniformly dilated.
2. Varicose: there is a greater degree of dilatation, irregularity in outline and absent peripheral filling.
3. Saccular or cystic: there is gross dilatation of the bronchi, increasing toward the periphery, causing cyst formation. There is no communication with the peripheral bronchial tree.

Bronchiectasis commonly involves the basal segments of the lower lobes. The disease is bilateral in one-third of patients. The lingular segment of the left upper lobe is also often affected in patients who have bronchiectasis of the left lower lobe. Upper lobe bronchiectasis is usually a sequel to apical pulmonary tuberculosis. Because of efficient drainage of the upper lobes by gravity, secondary infection of these is relatively unusual and clinical symptoms of bronchiectasis rarely develop. The right middle lobe is also vulnerable to bronchiectasis, particularly when this lobe is involved in a primary tuberculous complex. The walls of the bronchiectatic cavities are characteristically thin, with no muscle or cartilage and a minimum of elastic tissue, being composed predominantly of fibrous tissue. The epithelium lining affected bronchi is variable in appearance, but focal areas of squamous metaplasia are often prominent.

Aetiology and pathogenesis

The aetiology of bronchiectasis is still uncertain and different factors may well be involved in different patients. The two main factors of major importance are infection and pulmonary collapse.

Infection can produce bronchiectasis by irreversible damage to the bronchial wall. This is most likely to follow pneumonia in childhood complicating measles, whooping cough or influenza and particularly if treatment is inadequate. Infant bronchiolitis or bacterial pneumonia may also lead to bronchiectasis.

Pulmonary collapse is found when a large bronchus or numerous small bronchi are occluded, and the air in the distal lung parenchyma is absorbed by blood with resultant alveolar collapse. This is associated with bronchiectasis. Infection of the secretions that accumulate behind the obstruction causes damage to the bronchial wall and ultimately leads to dilatation of the bronchial wall.

Other factors include bronchial asthma, any condition which gives rise to severe lung fibrosis, and a variety of congenital factors. Among these latter are:

1. Cystic fibrosis due to abnormal mucus production.
2. Alpha-antitrypsin deficiency.
3. Poor ciliary activity in Kartagener's syndrome (sinusitis, situs inversus and bronchiectasis).
4. Structural deficiency in the bronchial cartilage.
5. Reduced immunity to infection in congenital hypogammaglobulinaemia.

Clinical features

Bronchiectasis most commonly begins in childhood but may not produce severe symptoms until some years later.

Symptoms

There is a chronic cough which is usually worse in the morning and is often induced by a change in posture.

There may be purulent sputum which in advanced cases is copious. There is, however, a pattern of dry bronchiectasis (bronchiectasis sicca) in which sputum production is minimal.

Haemoptysis is common. It usually consists merely of streaks of blood in the sputum but occasionally is very severe.

Dyspnoea and wheeze may occur, depending on the amount of generalized bronchitis and on the amount of lung damage.

Signs

The most important physical sign is the presence of medium or coarse crepitations on auscultation.

Radiology

In a plain X-ray of the chest the dilated bronchi themselves may not be visible. Occasionally cystic spaces, sometimes with a fluid level, may be seen. The diagnosis can only be made with certainty by bronchography (Fig. 45.9), but this should not be performed during an acute exacerbation of the disease. Special effort should be made several days before bronchography to clear the infection with antibiotics and postural drainage.

Pulmonary function tests show no specific pattern in bronchiectasis, but should be performed to assess the fitness of the patient for lung resection.

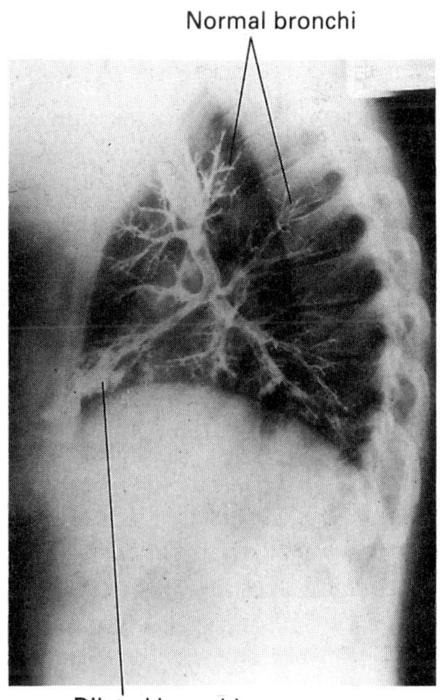

Fig. 45.9 Bronchogram showing a group of bronchiectatic bronchi in the right middle lobe.

Bronchoscopy should be performed to exclude bronchial tumour or a foreign body.

Complications

1. Recurrent pneumonia.
2. Pleurisy, pleural effusions and empyema.
3. Sinusitis.
4. Haemoptysis.
5. Brain abscess—a classic complication of bronchiectasis. The infection reaches the brain by means of the blood stream.
6. Amyloidosis—this is now rare. Nevertheless, the possibility should be borne in mind.

Treatment

Medical treatment aims to relieve or reduce the symptoms of bronchiectasis, while surgical treatment aims to eliminate the disease itself. This latter is preferable, but often not practicable.

Medical treatment

Postural drainage. The bronchiectatic bronchus has lost its elasticity, its muscle tone and its cilia, all of which are important factors in clearing the normal bronchus of secretion. Therefore, gravity has to be used to keep the dilated bronchi emptied of secretion and thereby reduce the secondary infection and toxaemia caused by such infection.

The position the patient should adopt for postural drainage depends on the site of the affected bronchi. Having adopted the appropriate position the patient should take deep breaths to aid the emptying of the segmental bronchi into the main bronchi and trachea, and then cough to clear the larger air passages.

Chemotherapy. Antibiotics should be chosen based on culture and sensitivity data, and should be continued until production of sputum is minimal. *Haemophilus influenzae* and pneumococcus are the two most important organisms encountered.

Prophylactic treatment. Suppressive chemotherapy is used to control chronic infection and to prevent exacerbations.

Surgical treatment

The use of antibiotics and postural drainage has greatly reduced the need for surgical treatment.

The chief indications for operation are:

1. Bronchiectasis localized to a single lobe or segment.
2. Very severe bronchiectasis in one segment, thought to be responsible for most of the symptoms in a patient with some disease elsewhere.
3. Severe haemoptysis, or if haemoptysis has occurred more than once in a young but otherwise fit patient.
4. Bronchiectasis distal to a bronchial adenoma, a foreign body in the bronchus or a bronchial carcinoma, if resection is feasible.

Prevention

As bronchiectasis starts in childhood, good treatment of severe lower respiratory infections in childhood should prevent the disease. The early recognition and prompt treatment of bronchial obstruction is also important in this respect.

Lung abscess

A lung abscess is defined as a localized area of suppuration and cavitation in the lung. Lung abscess may be divided into the following three general categories based upon the underlying aetiology: aspiration, post pneumonic and secondary lung abscess.

Aspiration lung abscess

This is the commonest form of lung abscess. Because the right main bronchus is more in line with the trachea than the left, aspirated material tends to pass from the trachea to the right lung. Aspiration abscesses are therefore more common in the right lung and are characteristically situated in the posterior segment of the right upper lobe or the apical segment of the lower lobe, these being the dependent parts of the lung when the patient is supine.

The predisposing factors for this category of lung abscess are:

1. Upper respiratory tract infection, e.g. sinusitis,

oral infection and infected laryngeal tumour.
2. Oesophageal disorders such as achalasia and carcinoma of the oesophagus.
3. Tonsillectomy and dental operations.
4. Aspiration of vomitus either during the induction of anaesthesia or when unconscious.

Postpneumonic lung abscess

Staphylococcal and klebsiella pneumonias are more commonly and pneumococcal pneumonia less commonly complicated by lung abscesses.

Secondary lung abscess

Lung abscess is found in association with a variety of other pathological processes as a secondary complication. The most frequently seen condition leading to lung abscess of this type is bronchial neoplasm, specifically squamous cell carcinoma.

A tumour obstructing a bronchus may be the cause of a lung abscess if the stagnant secretions in the obstructed segment become infected. Secondary lung abscess may also develop following infection of pre-existing lung cysts.

Clinical features

These depend to a large extent on the pathogenesis of the lesion. The onset of the illness may be acute with fever, cough, purulent sputum, haemoptysis and chest pain. On the other hand, many patients will have prolonged symptoms for more than 4–6 weeks with weight loss and general ill health.

Signs

It is unusual for the classical signs of cavitation to be elicited over a lung abscess. Signs of consolidation are the most frequent finding.

Laboratory findings

The white cell count is almost invariably increased and is usually in the region of 20 000–30 000/mm^3. The sputum contains pus, and culture of the sputum gives the nature of the organism and an indication of appropriate antibiotics.

Radiological examination

The chest radiograph at first shows a pneumonic opacity, and only later does this opacity develop a cavity in which a fluid level may appear, indicating that the abscess has established connection with a bronchus (Fig. 45.10).

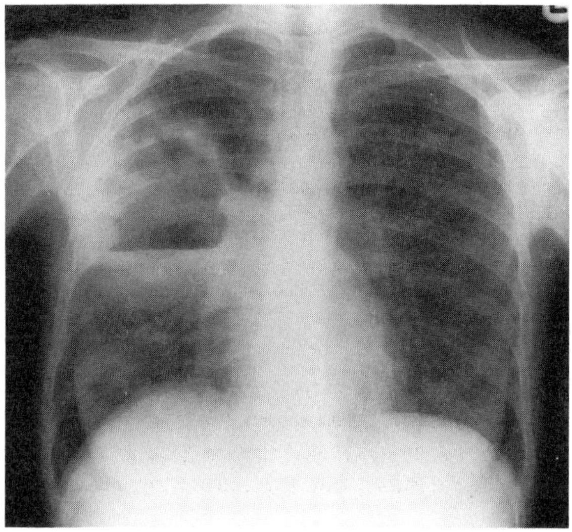

Fig. 45.10 Lung abscess in the right middle lobe, showing the fluid level of contained pus. The X-ray was taken with the patient erect.

Treatment

Chemotherapy

The type of antibiotics used depends on the culture and sensitivity of organisms grown from the sputum.

Postural drainage

This should be planned in order to secure gravitational drainage of the abscess as effectively as possible.

Bronchoscopy

Bronchoscopy is important for both diagnostic and therapeutic purposes (Fig. 45.11). It can be used to diagnose bronchial lesions and also enables the pus to be sucked out.

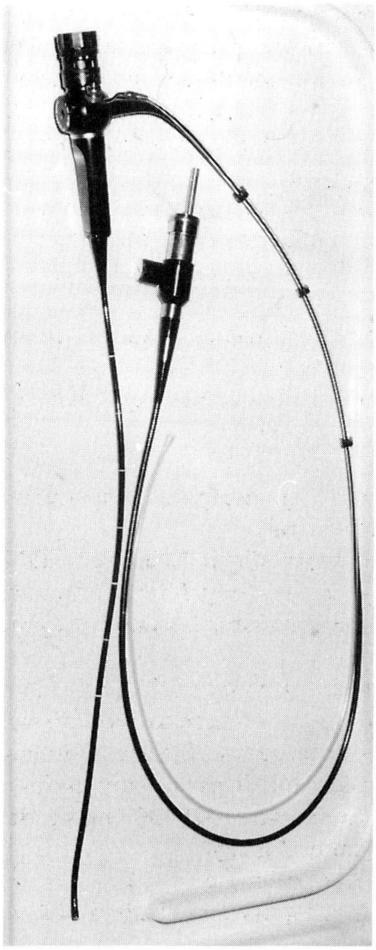

Fig. 45.11 Fibreoptic bronchoscope.

Surgery

Thoracotomy may be carried out to establish the diagnosis if cavitated carcinoma cannot be excluded by other means. Lung abscess due to suppuration distal to bronchial neoplasms must be treated surgically if there are no contraindications to thoracotomy.

SURGICAL MANAGEMENT OF PULMONARY TUBERCULOSIS

Tuberculosis is one of the world's most important communicable diseases. Since the development of new chemotherapeutic agents, the number of patients operated on for tuberculosis has decreased considerably. However, there still remains a number of patients who require surgical consideration.

Bacteriology

Three types of mycobacteria are mainly responsible for the disease in humans:

1. The human type—the vast majority of cases of human tuberculosis is caused by this strain.
2. The bovine type—human infection by bovine bacilli is almost always non-pulmonary and is spread to humans through infected milk.
3. Atypical acid-fast bacilli (anonymous opportunist mycobacteria)—of this group, only two are of major importance. *Mycobacterium kansasii* and *M. intracellulare* (Battey strain). These infections are often resistant to standard chemotherapeutic agents.

Pathology

In the first primary infection with the tubercle bacillus the draining lymph glands are involved in addition to the initial local lesion. The combination of the two lesions is known as the primary Ghon complex. All other tuberculous lesions are regarded as postprimary, and are not accompanied by major involvement of the draining lymph glands.

The classical pathological manifestation of tuberculosis is the tubercle. This consists of a granulomatous lesion containing epithelioid and Langhans giant cells, both derived from macrophages, lymphocytes and varying degrees of fibrosis. Central necrosis in the tubercle is called caseation, and this caseous tissue may later become calcified. If the lesion progresses the caseous material liquefies and discharges into a bronchus so that a cavity forms in the previously necrotic area. In most people the primary Ghon complex will heal and calcify. In a few individuals with lower resistance it may lead to pleural effusion, miliary tuberculosis, tuberculous bronchitis, bronchiectasis, bone, joint, renal or skin lesions.

Postprimary tuberculosis may result from either reactivation of an old focus or reinfection. This usually develops as a pneumonia in a segment or lobe, and is frequently located in the apical or posterior segment of the upper lobes or apex of the lower lobes. In most cases tuberculous pneumonia proceeds to caseation. The disease is almost always bilateral. Pulmonary fibrosis, endobronchial tuberculosis leading to stenosis of bronchus and bronchiectasis are complications of postprimary tuberculosis.

Common modes of presentation of post primary tuberculosis

1. Symptom-free: the tuberculosis is discovered on a routine chest X-ray.
2. Persistent cough, fever and night sweats.
3. Recurrent colds or failure to recover adequately from an attack of flu.
4. Undue tiredness, loss of appetite or loss of weight.
5. Pneumonia.
6. Haemoptysis.
7. Dyspnoea.

Diagnosis

The diagnosis is usually established by a combination of the chest X-ray findings and culture of the bacilli in sputum or gastric aspirate. Lung biopsy—transbronchial or open-lung and mediastinoscopy and lymph node biopsy—may occasionally be the most appropriate way of confirming suspicion of the disease.

Complications

1. Pleural effusion.
2. Tuberculous empyema.
3. Chronic bronchitis.
4. Cor pulmonale.
5. Amyloidosis.
6. Aspergillosis infection in open tuberculous cavities.
7. Haemoptysis.
8. Anaemia.

Treatment

Chemotherapy

Antituberculous chemotherapy is by far the most important measure in the treatment of all forms of tuberculosis, and should be given to every patient with active disease. There are two phases of antituberculous treatment—an initial phase using at least three drugs, and a continuation phase with two drugs. A suitable regime is as follows:

Initial phase.

Rifampicin: 600 mg/day in adults above 50 kg and 450 mg in adults less than 50 kg. In a child a recommended daily dose is 20 mg/kg.

Isoniazid: 300 mg/day in adults; children 5 mg/kg.

Ethambutol: 15 mg/kg per day in adults; children 25 mg/kg.

All three drugs are given concurrently for the first 2 months only.

Continuation phase. Rifampicin and isoniazid are given together for a further 7 months. Other drugs that are available for various regimes are:

Streptomycin: given intramuscularly in a standard dose of 1 g/day, reduced to 500–750 mg in small patients or those over the age of 40 years.

Pyrazinamide: this is particularly useful in tuberculous meningitis—20–30 mg/kg daily to a maximum of 3 g/day.

Sodium aminosalicylate (PAS): adults 10–12 g/day and children 300 mg/kg per day.

Thiacetazone: adults 150 mg and children 2 mg/kg per day.

Surgery

The purpose of surgery in pulmonary tuberculosis is complementary to medical therapy and aims to remove or to assist in the healing of a diseased lung.

The main indications for operations are:

1. An open cavity associated with a positive sputum, beyond 3–6 months after continuous chemotherapy.
2. Persistent positive culture after 6 months of chemotherapy in the presence of bronchiectasis, destroyed lobe or significant bronchial stenosis.
3. The presence of localized infection with atypical organisms, because of the organisms' primary resistance to drugs.

4. Suspected presence of a neoplasm within a tuberculous lesion.
5. Life-threatening haemoptysis.
6. The presence of bronchopleural fistula which has not responded tc closed intercostal drainage.

Prior to surgery nutritional deficits should be corrected and antituberculous treatment should be continued, perhaps with the addition of a fourth drug, preferably streptomycin, for 2 weeks pre-operatively.

HYDATID DISEASE OF THE THORAX (SEE CH. 16)

Hydatid disease is caused by the parasitic tapeworm *Taenia echinococcus*. Twelve different species have been identified but only two of these, *Echinococcus granulosus* and *E. multilocularis*, are known to affect humans. Hydatid disease occurs in nearly all parts of the world, being highly endemic in the Middle East, India, South America and Australia.

Life-cycle of hydatids

Echinococcus granulosus

This is the common variety and is responsible for nearly 95% of all hydatid disease. The adult worm measures 4–6 cm in length and lives in the small bowel of the definitive host, which is usually the dog, although the wolf, the cat or the fox may be infected. Parasites in the alimentary tract of the definitive host shed ova and are excreted in the dog's stool contaminating vegetables, grass or water. The common intermediate host is sheep but cattle, pigs, camels or humans may also be involved. In the intermediate host, hydatid cysts develop in the viscera, including the lung. When infected sheep are slaughtered and the viscera are eaten by the dogs, the life-cycle is completed. Humans are nearly always infected through handling dogs; the hands or food become contaminated with the dog's excreta.

The chitinous coat of the ova is then digested by gastric juice. The embryo is released in the duodenum and activated by bile salts. The parasitic larvae burrow through the mucous membrane of the small bowel and are carried to the liver in the portal circulation. Since the embryo is about 20 mm in length it can block a capillary in many sites. The liver is the first hurdle of the embryo and may become lodged there but about 10–20% pass through the liver and finally obstruct vessels in the lung. It is rare for the embryo to pass both barriers and affect other organs such as bone, kidney, brain, heart muscle and soft tissues.

Echinococcus multilocularis

This very rarely causes lung cysts. The intermediate host is the field mouse and foxes are its natural host. Humans become infected by eating berries contaminated by the foxes' excreta.

Pathology

Echinococcus granulosus

When the embryo lodges in a capillary it begins to form a cyst. A hydatid cyst consists of a double-layered parasitic wall, an inner nucleated germinal layer and an outer non-nucleated hyaline laminated layer. This in turn is surrounded by the ectocyst or pericyst, which is composed of host tissue, both granulation tissue and fibrosis. The cyst contains clear, odourless, slightly alkaline fluid in which there are free scolices and brood capsules. The laminated layer is pure white in colour, resembles the white of a hard-boiled egg and is about 2 mm thick. Daughter cysts develop from the germinal membrane into the fluid-filled cavity. Daughter cysts occur less frequently in cysts in the lung than in the liver. Hydatid cysts in the lungs grow to 1–2 cm in diameter within 6 months. Thereafter the doubling time is from 16 to 20 weeks.

Echinococcus multilocularis

This very rarely affects the lung. The pericyst is not well developed, nor is the laminated membrane. The germinal membrane penetrates the wall of the cyst and grows as protoplasmic masses into the surrounding soft tissue. This growth is like an infiltrative malignancy producing multiple cyst cavities. If the germinal layer penetrates the blood vessels it can metastasize to other organs.

Secondary hydatid disease

Secondary hydatid disease of the thorax results from rupture of a primary lung or hepatic cyst. Rupture of a pulmonary cyst may occur spontaneously or may result from attempts at diagnostic aspiration or as a complication of surgical removal. Secondary pulmonary hydatid disease may also occur from invasion of the diaphragm by hepatic cysts which rupture into the lung.

Clinical features

Pulmonary hydatid cysts may be simple or complicated, unilateral or bilateral. The complications are principally rupture, infection or both. About 20% of pulmonary cysts are bilateral due to multiple primary infection. At least 10% of pulmonary hydatids have coexisting hepatic cysts. The clinical manifestations depend on whether the cyst is intact or has ruptured.

Intact cysts

Over 50% of cysts are diagnosed accidentally on routine chest radiographs. Symptoms and signs are caused by the compression of a large cyst on adjacent structures. Cough and haemoptysis are the two most common symptoms. Dyspnoea is rare in a solitary cyst but more common with multiple ones. Fever and dull chest pain are the other common symptoms. Posterior mediastinal cysts may cause pain by bone erosion, dysphagia due to compression on the oesophagus and even paraplegia due to spinal cord compression. Anterior mediastinal cysts may cause dyspnoea by compressing the trachea, and also superior vena caval obstruction. Middle mediastinal cysts can cause catastrophic haemorrhage by erosion of major vessels. Chylothorax can complicate pleural hydatid disease.

Ruptured cysts

Thirty per cent of pulmonary cysts rupture; this may occur either spontaneously or as a result of coughing, sneezing, muscular effort, trauma to the chest or infection. When intrabronchial rupture occurs symptoms depend on the amount of the leak. A small leak may result in cough and the production of a little watery or blood-stained fluid which has a salty taste. When a large cyst erodes a large area of bronchus, sudden coughing occurs with a gush of blood-stained, salty fluid which may contain pieces of membrane, sometimes large enough to occlude the bronchi or trachea. This results in cyanosis or even death. If the ruptured cyst does not become infected the condition may be spontaneously cured leaving only fibrosis at the site of the original cyst. Infection is a more frequent sequel, however, and the clinical picture then becomes that of lung abscess. Fatal anaphylactic shock has been known to occur after rupture into a large vein or the heart. Rupture of the cyst into the pleural cavity may cause tension pneumothorax, pleural effusion, empyema or secondary pleural hydatid disease.

Diagnosis

Diagnosis depends on radiology, cytological examination of the sputum and immunological testing of the blood.

Radiology

A chest radiograph is the most reliable means of diagnosis; posteroanterior and lateral views are always necessary. Pulmonary hydatid cyst typically appears as a round opacity with a clearcut border, usually located in the mid and lower lung fields. When a cyst grows larger than 2 cm in diameter it becomes oval and may be notched by neighbouring bronchial or vascular structures. Cysts very seldom calcify unless they are dead. On screening, cysts alter in size with respiration—the Escudero Nemerow sign. When air enters between the laminated membrane and the pericyst in a limited rupture, this produces the crescent sign. If the laminated membrane is not completely broken and air enters the laminated membrane as well as the pericyst, an appearance described as double arch may be seen. When the hydatid cyst ruptures, some of the fluid is replaced by air, and a fluid level is formed.

Sputum examination

Microscopic examination of the sputum may show scolices, thus establishing the diagnosis.

Blood count

There is marked eosinophilia: 6–60% of the circulating white cells are eosinophils at the time of rupture. When there is superadded infection a polymorphonuclear response occurs.

Immunological tests

Complement fixation test

This is positive in up to 80% of cases. A titre of more than one in eight is suspicious of infection. After successful removal of the cyst, the titre falls back to normal within 3 months.

Haemagglutination test

This is a sensitive and specific test.

Casoni's intradermal test

When sterile standard hydatid fluid is injected intradermally in a patient with a hydatid cyst, a weal with surrounding erythema develops within 20 min, and is followed by an indurated area which persists for 1–2 days. The test is positive in 90% of infected patients and may persist for several years after cure.

Treatment

Whenever technically feasible hydatid cysts should be removed. This is necessary to prevent the complications already mentioned. The aim of surgery is always to remove the laminated membrane without spilling hydatid fluid into the pleural cavity. The fluid should be rendered harmless by injection of a parasitocidal agent into the cyst. Hypertonic saline (10%), formalin (0.5%), ethyl alcohol (70%), fresh eusol (0.5%) and cetrimide (5%) are some of the agents that have been advocated for this purpose.

Technique of removal

1. Simple cysts up to 2.5 cm in diameter are best removed by segmental or wedge resection of the part of the lung that contains the cyst.
2. Cysts up to 12.5 cm in diameter can often be removed by enucleation of the cyst or excision of the cyst together with the pericyst.
3. Very large cysts are more safely treated by lobectomy.

Medical treatment

Recently, mebendazole (Vermox) has been shown to be active against the larval stages of *Echinococcus granulosus*. It kills the parasite by limiting its glucose uptake and thus depleting its glycogen. Intrahepatic cysts regress over a period of 13 months. Success has also been claimed in the treatment of *E. multilocularis*. Mebendazole has been well tolerated in the high doses used. At present the place of mebendazole appears to be for patients who are unfit for surgery, perhaps preoperatively to reduce postoperative complications, and to deal with residual cysts not amenable to surgery.

The usual regime before surgery is as follows: 300 mg three times a day for 3 days, followed by 400 mg three times a day for 3 days, and then 30–50 mg/kg body weight in three divided doses, continuing until 1 month after successful surgery.

Thoracic amoebiasis (see Ch. 31)

Amoebiasis is due to *Entamoeba histolytica*, which primarily affects the large intestine. Thoracic amoebiasis is usually a complication of an amoebic abscess of the liver. Infection is from one human to another. *E. histolytica* is infective only in the cystic form. Cysts swallowed in food or water are digested by alimentary enzymes which free vegetative amoebae. These grow and invade the colonic mucosa, giving rise to ulceration. Some penetrate intestinal veins and reach the liver, producing hepatic amoebiasis and hepatic abscess. Most commonly affected is the upper part of the right lobe.

The hepatic abscess may erode or rupture through the diaphragm, to create a second abscess called a 'collar-stud' abscess in the right lower or middle lobe of the lung. A hepatobronchial fistula with evacuation of the hepatic abscess, amoebic empyema and effusion may also follow the rupture of a hepatic amoebic abscess. Amoebic abscess of the left lobe of the liver may give rise to left thoracic or pericardial amoebiasis.

Clinical features

A previous history of intestinal amoebiasis is present in 50% of cases. Cough and the expectoration of material, variously described as anchovy sauce or chocolate, are the most classical and dramatic symptoms. The patient is usually fevered, sometimes with rigors. Haemoptysis, and right lower chest pain and dyspnoea are common, and painful enlargement of liver with referred pain in the right shoulder tip may be apparent.

Diagnosis

Radiology

Liver enlargement causes smooth or sometimes localized elevation of the right hemidiaphragm, best seen in the lateral view. Obliteration of the costophrenic angle by a small pleural effusion may occur before rupture through the diaphragm. Right-sided pleural effusion, pneumonia, consolidation or abscess formation, usually in the right lower lung field, complete the picture. Pericardial effusion and pneumopericardium may occur in pericardial amoebiasis.

Serology

E. histolytica is antigenic and produces an immune response in the host. The antibodies usually persist for a long time, making it difficult to differentiate between a previous infection and an existing disease. Positive reactions always indicate invasive amoebiasis and are most useful in extraintestinal disease.

Gel diffusion

This test is simple, reproducible, cheap and quickly and easily carried out by a laboratory. Accuracy of 95% is claimed for hepatic amoebiasis.

Indirect haemagglutination test

There is 95% positive titre in patients with extra-intestinal disease. A titre below 1 : 512 without other evidence does not give proof of a recent infection.

Treatment

Treatment of the pulmonary infection requires treatment of the coexisting liver abscess which may need to be aspirated or drained surgically.

Metronidazole is the drug of choice because it is more effective and less toxic. The dose for an adult is 800 mg three times a day for 5 days, but if the patient is acutely ill, the intravenous administration of up to 500 mg four times a day may be necessary. Thoracic amoebiasis carries a high mortality but combined therapy offers the best chance of cure. Emetine hydrochloride (1 mg/kg body weight) intramuscularly for 10 days and chloroquine phosphate in a daily dose of 500 mg orally for 3 weeks may be combined with metronidazole. When administering emetine hydrochloride, electrocardiogram monitoring will be necessary because of its myocardial toxicity.

Surgery

The indications for operation should be few with effective drug therapy. Intercostal tube drainage together with drug treatment is usually adequate for amoebic empyema. If empyema persists then rib resection or decortication may have to be carried out. If there is persistence of a hepatobronchial fistula, i.e. communication between a bronchus and the abscess cavity as shown on a bronchogram, lung resection may be necessary.

All surgical procedures should be carried out under metronidazole cover.

ASPIRATION AND DRAINAGE OF THE CHEST

Indications

The aim of a chest drain is to enable collapsed or partially collapsed lung to re-expand, thereby improving pulmonary function. The conditions for which it is usually required include pneumothorax, haemothorax, empyema, chylothorax, and after thoracotomy.

The site of insertion of the chest drain depends on the nature of the material to be removed. Except in the emergency situation of a tension pneumothorax, the site of drainage should be checked with reference to the clinical localizing signs and the X-ray appearances.

There are three approaches—anterior, axillary and posterior.

Anterior approach

This is made through the second intercostal space in the mid clavicular line, and is one of the easier sites for access. However, it has the disadvantage of traversing the pectoral muscle, and hence it may limit the amount of possible movement of the arm because of pain.

Axillary approach

The fourth or fifth intercostal space in the mid axillary or anterior axillary line is used. It is easy to insert a drain at this site, and to direct the tube into the apex of the thorax. It is less painful when moving the arm since the tube does not have to pass through the pectoral muscles; only the serratus anterior muscle is traversed. It will not be compressed when the patient is lying flat.

Posterior approach

Through the first intercostal space posteriorly is a third possibility, but is rarely used.

Types of intercostal tube

Of the many different types of tubes used, two are worth considering—a rubber catheter, such as the Malecot catheter, which is inserted by means of an introducer, and the Argyle thoracic catheter, which is a plastic tube supplied with its own introducer, making it relatively easy to insert and position accurately. It is much more robust than the red rubber catheter, and can be left in position much longer.

Technique

The axillary approach is described in detail, and similar principles could be used for other approaches as well. This method avoids the dangerous hazard of damage to underlying lung, heart or major vessels, as can occur when trocar-mounted chest drains are inserted under force. In tension pneumothorax, a number 16 or 18 French needle can be inserted in the second intercostal space in the mid clavicular line to evacuate air in an emergency situation, thus allowing time for the more orderly placement of a chest drain. The insertion of a chest tube should be done with a strict aseptic technique, using gown, gloves and mask.

If the patient can get out of bed he or she should be seated comfortably astride a chair resting the head on pillows on a bed or bed table. The forearm of the affected side should rest on a support in front of the patient.

The fourth or fifth intercostal space in the anterior or mid axillary line is selected, and the site for insertion is cleansed with antiseptic solution.

Anaesthesia

The skin is infiltrated with 1% lignocaine. The subcutaneous tissue and intercostal muscles are also infiltrated, and the anaesthesia is carried down over the upper border of the rib to include the periosteum, the extrapleural tissues and the parietal pleura. About 20 ml of 1% lignocaine will be needed. A few minutes are allowed for the anasethetic to achieve its full effect, and the interval is used to prepare the instruments and sutures and to check that the tubing fits the drain and the underwater seal drainage bottle. Providing the skin, muscle, periosteum and pleura have been adequately anaesthetized, the procedure should be painless, although the patient may experience a pushing sensation.

A 2-cm transverse incision is made at the proposed entry site and dissection with the knife is carried down to the upper border of the rib.

Thereafter an artery forceps is used to spread the intercostal muscle over the upper border of the rib and it is then inserted into the intercostal space. When the thoracic cavity is entered there will usually be a gush of air, fluid or blood, or a combination of these.

Once the artery forceps has entered the thoracic cavity, the index finger can be inserted to be certain that the diagnosis is correct. This will be of great diagnostic importance in posttraumatic chest injuries, as bowel or spleen can be felt in cases of diaphragmatic rupture.

At this stage it is most convenient to insert a mattress suture through the centre of the incision and to tie the ends in a loop. This stitch is to be tied when the tube is ultimately removed. A second suture is placed at the edge of the skin incision for securing the drain in place.

Thereafter an Argyle thoracic catheter of the desired size is introduced via the wound and directed to the apex for pneumothorax and to the base in cases of pleural effusion, empyema or haemothorax. No undue force is needed. Once the catheter is in place it is secured with the previously placed suture, and the drain is connected to the underwater seal drain. It is important that the drain should be held in the chest by the retaining suture, and not just by layers of strapping covering the chest acting as splints.

An erect chest X-ray is taken to verify the correct positioning of the tube and the degree of expansion of the lung.

If the lung fails to expand it may be aided by the application of a vacuum pump to the short tube of the underwater seal bottle. A Vernon-Thompson sucker is more appropriate for large air leaks and a Robert's sucker for small ones. It can be dangerous to attach a low-volume (Robert's) sucker in the presence of a large air leak, as it may impede the release of air from the chest, causing tension pneumothorax.

Underwater seal drainage

The underwater seal drainage bottle is one of the simplest and the most useful devices in draining the chest. The end of the tube is connected to the chest drain and placed underwater and serves as a one-way valve which allows fluid and air to escape from the chest, but effectively prevents any air from entering. Negative pressure from a sucker may be applied to the short tube if more rapid drainage is required. All those responsible for a patient with such a drain in place should be aware of certain risks, and take the following precautions:

1. At no time should any part of the apparatus be dismantled, unless the intercostal drain is securely clamped, or a pneumothorax will result.
2. Great care must be taken to make sure that the bottle is connected correctly.
3. At no time should the bottle be lifted higher than the patient, unless the tubes are clamped, because there is a risk that the water in the bottle may siphon into the chest.
4. When there is a large air leak, the tubing should not be clamped even in transport or a tension pneumothorax may result.

Air leak

Persistent bubbling into the bottle suggests a leak in one of three places:

1. In the apparatus and connections.
2. Between the pleural cavity and the outer air, either a leak alongside the drain, or one of the side-holes in the drain having been exposed by the tube having slipped out of the chest.
3. Between the pleural cavity and the air passages (bronchopleural fistula).

Swing

Alterations in the pleural pressure with normal respiratory movements lead to a fluid column moving a few centimetres up and down the tube that is submerged below water. Absence of this swing in the tube could be due to blockage of the tubing, i.e. either the chest drain or the connecting tube, or the lung being fully expanded and occluding the tube openings within the chest.

Removal of the tubes

Chest drains are removed once the lung has re-expanded and the pleural drainage ceases. The drain site is cleaned. The suture anchoring the drain is cut. The patient is then asked to breathe out and hold at full expiration for a few seconds. During that time the tube is rapidly withdrawn and the original suture is tied down to close the incision.

ASPIRATION OF THE CHEST

This may be required for diagnosis or treatment when an effusion is present in the pleural cavity. The positioning of the patient is similar to that previously described for chest drainage and the procedure is performed under sterile conditions. A careful study of the physical signs plus examination of anterio posterior and lateral radiographs are necessary before the site of aspiration is chosen. For large effusions the seventh intercostal space in the posterior axillary line (just below the angle of the scapula with the patient leaning forward) is usually selected. In the case of a small effusion, it is advisable to insert the needle a space or two below the upper limit of dullness to percussion.

Anaesthesia

The site is infiltrated with 1% lignocaine under the skin with a very fine needle. The needle is then changed to a larger needle, and the deeper tissues are infiltrated, paying particular attention to anaesthetizing the parietal pleura.

Apparatus

An aspirating system consists of a 50 ml plastic syringe, a three-way tap, and a series of aspirating needles. There should always be a three-way tap between the needle and syringe so that the syringe can be emptied without having to disconnect it and run the risk of admitting air into the pleural cavity (see Fig. 45.5).

Technique

Once the local anaesthetic has taken effect, a wide-base aspirating needle with the syringe firmly attached is advanced slowly into the pleural cavity while aspirating on the syringe. Arrival in the pleural cavity is indicated when fluid appears in the syringe. To avoid accidental penetration or tearing of the lung, an artery forcep (Spencer-Wells) should be clamped on the needle at skin level to prevent further advancement. The fluid is aspirated into the syringe and, using the three-way tap, discarded through the connection into a sterile jug.

Failure to find fluid on one aspiration should be followed by further attempts, angling the needle slightly from one side to another and up and down, so that aspiration is attempted either higher or lower (after checking the physical signs and chest X-ray).

Possible complications

1. Removal of too much fluid too quickly. Following the removal of a large quantity of fluid or air, sudden expansion of a lung that has been collapsed for a considerable time either due to a large pleural effusion or a chronic pneumothorax may lead to the development of unilateral pulmonary oedema. This complication, while rare, should be recognized.
2. Air embolism and pleural shock. Tearing of the visceral pleura or puncture of a superficial vessel may allow air to enter the pulmonary venous system through the needle or, commonly, from neighbouring alveoli.
3. Rupture of an intercostal vessel. This should only occur if the aspirating needle has been introduced too high in the intercostal space; the vessels lie just immediately below the rib.

PLEURAL BIOPSY

Pleural biopsy and aspiration can be satisfactorily combined by the use of an Abram's needle. The site of the biopsy is the same as that of pleural aspiration. A 5-mm skin incision is made at the chosen site. Abram's punch is connected to a 20-ml glass syringe and pushed through the pleura in a closed position. During this insertion the needle should be guarded by holding it 4–5 cm from the tip to prevent entry of its whole length. A reference knob on the proximal end of the needle indicates the position of the side-hole. To take a biopsy the whole needle is slightly angulated and withdrawn a little until the side-hole is felt to catch on the edge of the parietal pleura. The inner trocar of the assembly is then rotated sharply clockwise and on its advance it will cut off a small specimen. The whole needle is withdrawn and the specimen for histology is retrieved from within the needle tip.

TUMOURS OF BRONCHUS AND LUNG

Malignant tumours

Carcinoma of the lung

Bronchial carcinoma is by far the most common malignant pulmonary tumour. It is the commonest cause of death from cancer in males, and in females it now ranks second to carcinoma of the breast.

Aetiology

All available evidence incriminates tobacco smoking, especially of cigarettes, as the main cause of lung cancer. For pipe and cigar smokers the risk appears to be less than that of cigarettes, but there is probably still some degree of increased risk. The increased incidence of lung cancer in urban areas suggests that air pollution may be a further aetiological factor and, specifically, exposure to radioactive materials, asbestos, nickel, arsenic and coal gas has been incriminated.

Pathology

Carcinoma of the lung can be classified by the basic cell type of the tumour. The main categories are:

1. Squamous cell (epidermoid) carcinoma (35%).
2. Small cell anaplastic carcinoma, often called oat cell carcinoma (30%).
3. Adenocarcinoma (18%).
4. Large cell carcinoma (17%).

Squamous cell carcinoma

This is the commonest type of lung cancer, arising in respiratory epithelium of the bronchi, usually of the segmental size or larger. These tumours frequently metastasize to the hilar, mediastinal and supraclavicular lymph nodes, and less frequently by the blood stream to the brain, bones and liver.

Small cell (oat cell) carcinoma

This tumour, like squamous cell carcinoma, tends to arise in the larger bronchi. It is particularly rapidly fatal, with early metastasis and rapid invasion of mediastinal and more distant lymph nodes. Often they are widely disseminated before lung symptoms are produced.

Adenocarcinoma

Most of these tumours arise in the periphery of the lung. The metastatic spread of adenocarcinoma is very much like that of oat cell carcinoma. It has a special propensity for the liver, adrenal gland, central nervous system and bone. This pattern of carcinoma is possibly unrelated to smoking. Alveolar cell carcinoma, bronchiolar carcinoma or bronchioloalveolar cell carcinoma is a variant of adenocarcinoma.

Large cell carcinoma

These tumours also occur in the periphery of the lung. Their behaviour is also like that of adenocarcinoma, including a high rate of cerebral metastasis.

Clinical features

The clinical manifestations may be due to the tumour itself, the local mechanical effects of the tumour, secondary infection, metastases, or non-metastatic extrapulmonary symptoms. About 5% of patients are asymptomatic, and the disease is discovered during a routine chest X-ray.

Clinical manifestations of the tumour

Cough and haemoptysis are the two most common symptoms, occurring in about 70% of patients. Haemoptysis is usually blood-staining of the sputum, but occasionally the blood loss is moderate to large. Pleuritic chest pain may arise if there is invasion of the pleura by the carcinoma.

Mechanical effects of the tumour

If a segmental, lobar or main bronchus is partially or completely occluded by the tumour, respiratory function will be impaired. Collapse of lung will give rise to breathlessness (Fig. 45. 12). Occasionally wheeze or stridor due to involvement of a main bronchus or the trachea may be the presenting symptom.

Secondary infection

This may result in recurrent pneumonia, or the classical symptoms of bronchiectasis, lung abscess or empyema. This is because of bronchial occlusion or rigidity of the bronchus interfering with efficient drainage of the affected lung.

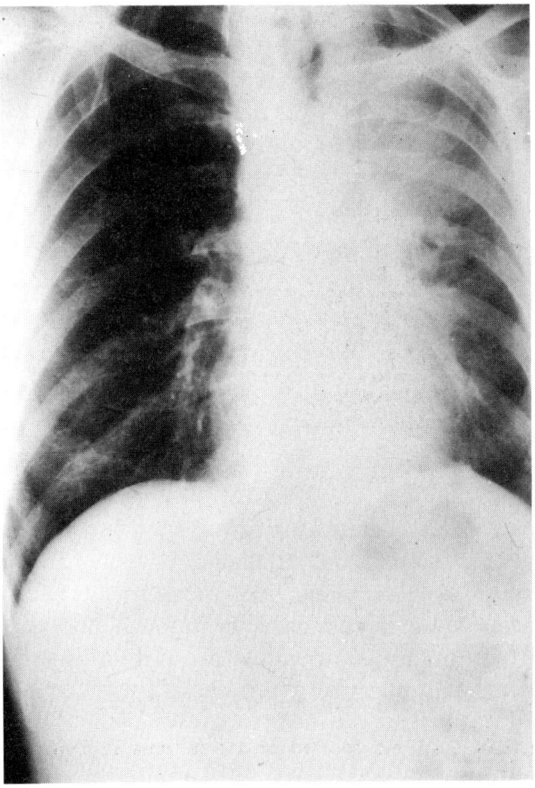

Fig. 45.12 Carcinoma of the bronchus, causing collapse of the left upper lobe.

Metastases

Intrathoracic

A pleural effusion is often due to direct invasion by the tumour, and the effusion is frequently blood-stained. Pericardial effusion may also develop.

Recurrent laryngeal nerve palsy causes hoarseness of the voice. On the left side secondary lymph glands in the hilum may involve the recurrent laryngeal nerve as it hooks around the aorta. Phrenic nerve paralysis, either due to invasion by the primary tumour or secondary lymph glands, causes paralysis of the hemidiaphragm. Horner's syndrome—small pupil, partial ptosis, enophthalamos and lack of sweating on that half of the face—may arise if there is cervical sympathetic involvement. If the brachial plexus is invaded by tumour of an apical region the clinical presentation is referred to as a Pancoast's syndrome.

Superior vena caval obstruction is a complication caused by the tumour or superior mediastinal glands compressing the great veins.

Chest pain may be caused by rib involvement by either direct infiltration or bony metastasis.

Extrathoracic metastatic symptoms

The common sites for metastatic deposits are the supraclavicular lymph nodes, liver, bone, brain, adrenal glands and skin.

Non-metastatic extrapulmonary manifestations

Clubbing of the fingers (hypertrophic pulmonary osteoarthropathy) may occur (Fig. 45.13), and non-specific symptoms are anorexia, loss of weight and weakness.

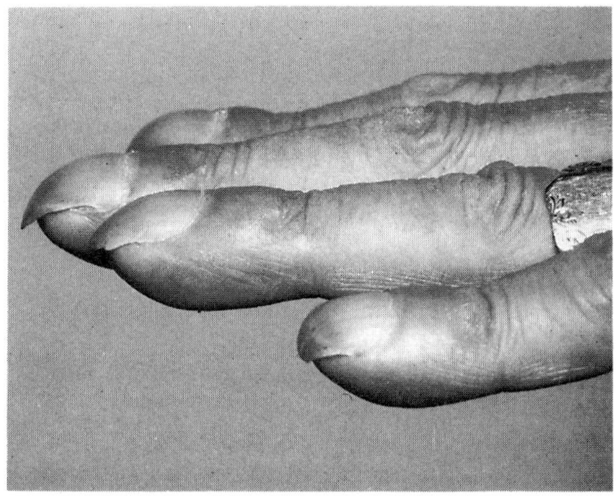

Fig. 45.13 Clubbing of fingers in a patient with carcinoma of the bronchus. The angle between the nail and the skinfold is obliterated, and the nail is curved and the fingertip more rounded than normal.

Endocrine and metabolic complications

Over the years a large number of hormones, mostly polypeptides, have been isolated from extracts of bronchial carcinomas, and the abnormal production and secretion of one or more of these substances may produce the appropriate endocrine effects. Although only a minority of tumours behave clinically in this way, the least uncommon are the adrenocorticosteroids, parathormone, antidiuretic hormone and the gastrointestinal hormones. Thus the patient may present with a Cushing-like syndrome, hypercalcaemia or reduced urine output.

Signs

It follows from the description of the patterns of pathological behaviour of these tumours that a search is made during the examination for any signs of marked weight loss, palpable lymph nodes in the supraclavicular fossae, and the other areas of nodes; hepatomegaly; ascites, and for any swellings or other deformities in the skeleton. In the chest examination localized reduction in breath sounds, added dry or moist sounds on auscultation or dullness to percussion raise the clinical suspicion. More precise information will be obtained from the X-ray and other investigations which should follow.

X-ray

Carcinoma of the lung may assume a variety of radiographic appearances (Figs 45.14 and 45.15). The common ones are unilateral enlargement of the hilum, a large irregular peripheral mass, a lung cavity, or persistence of an area of collapse or pneumonia. A pleural effusion may be present, and there may be evidence of paralysis of the phrenic nerve with an elevated hemidiaphragm. Osteolytic lesions may also be seen in the ribs.

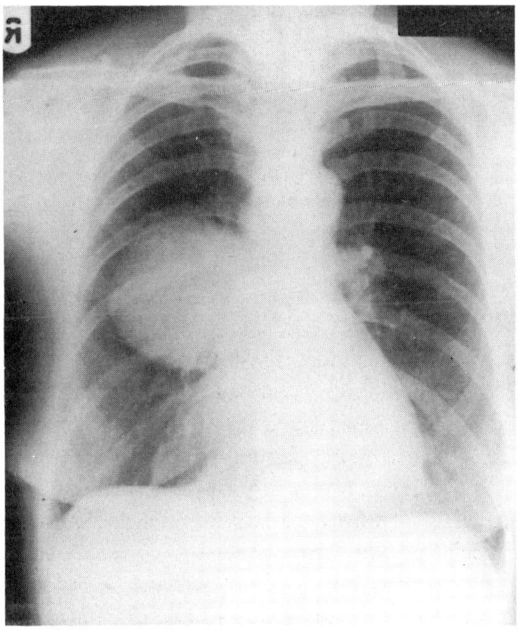

Fig. 45.14 Large rounded carcinoma mass in right mid zone.

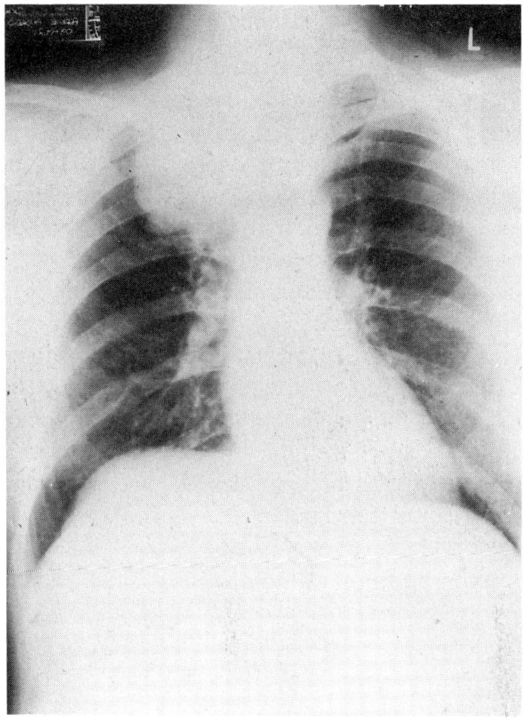

Fig. 45.15 Large rounded carcinoma mass in right upper zone.

Bronchoscopy

If there is any doubt on clinical or radiological grounds, the next step is to perform bronchoscopy. Bronchial biopsy, or the taking of brushings for cytology, will provide material for histological confirmation of the diagnosis. It is also useful to assess the potential operability of the lesion.

Sputum cytology

This is a valuable investigation of a pathologist skilled in interpretation of the material. Not surprisingly, larger and more central lesions yield more positive results than do peripheral lesions.

Biopsy

If cytological methods fail to give a definite diagnosis, percutaneous needle biopsy may be attempted. If there is a secondary pleural effusion or other reason to suspect pleural involvement, pleural biopsy may be performed either using an Abram's needle or under direct vision at thoracoscopy.

Assessment for treatment

When a patient is being considered as a possible candidate for operation the two factors most affecting the operability and prognosis are the cell type, already discussed, and the extent of spread beyond the lung. It is critical to evaluate any involvement of mediastinal structures and the available methods include computerized tomography scan and mediastinoscopy. The former, although it appears especially useful in identifying subcarinal glands, may have a false-negative rate with respect to other areas of the mediastinum of up to one-third. Direct inspection of the mediastinal planes and the opportunity to biopsy through the endoscope requires special expertise and, in skilled hands, can give much helpful information.

If distal metastases are suspected, in bones, liver or brain, appropriate isotope scans may identify these with reasonable accuracy.

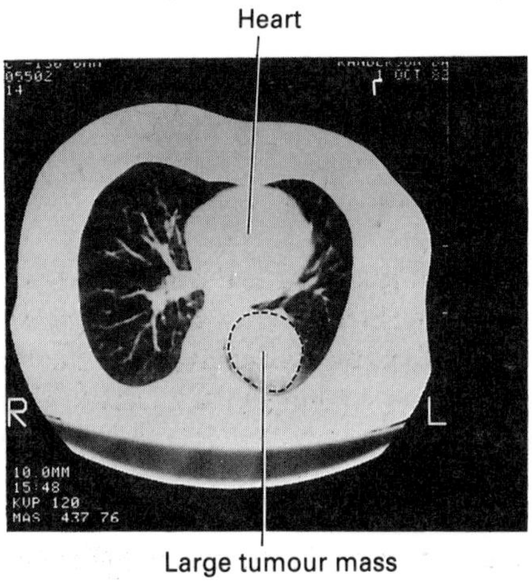

Fig. 45.16 Computerized tomography scan defining tumour mass in left lung.

Treatment

Surgical resection remains the most effective method of treatment for patients with carcinoma of the lung. When the tumour cannot be removed surgically there is, in effect, little or no chance of long-term survival for the patient. Small cell (oat cell) carcinoma, even at presentation, is almost invariably disseminated, and is seldom considered a resectable lesion.

When there is no evidence of distant metastasis or invasion of extrapulmonary structures, surgical exploration is usually indicated. The first consideration is therefore whether the patient is suitable for radical surgery.

Contraindications to surgery

Medical factors

1. Chronic lung disease with poor pulmonary function—preoperative pulmonary function tests should be carried out in all patients who are assessed for thoracotomy.
2. Uncontrolled cardiac failure, arrhythmia or a history of recent myocardial infarction also contraindicates resection.
3. Unstable angina.
4. Advanced age.

Local factors

1. Mediastinal invasion.
2. Recurrent laryngeal nerve or phrenic nerve palsy.
3. Tracheal involvement.
4. Widened tracheal carina and fixation of the main bronchus.
5. Malignant pleural effusion.
6. Pericardial or cardiac involvement.
7. Presence of extrathoracic metastases.

Surgical procedures

1. Wedge resection—removal of a wedge of lung tissue (Fig.45.17).
2. Segmental resection—removal of a bronchopulmonary segment.
3. Lobectomy—removal of a lobe.
4. Pneumonectomy—removal of a whole lung.

Survival rate

The overall 5-year survival rate following resection of part of or the whole lung is about 35% and the 10-year survival rate is 10–15%. For solitary lesions less than 4 cm in diameter there is a 45% 5-year survival rate after resection.

Radiotherapy

An attempt may be made to ablate the tumour—

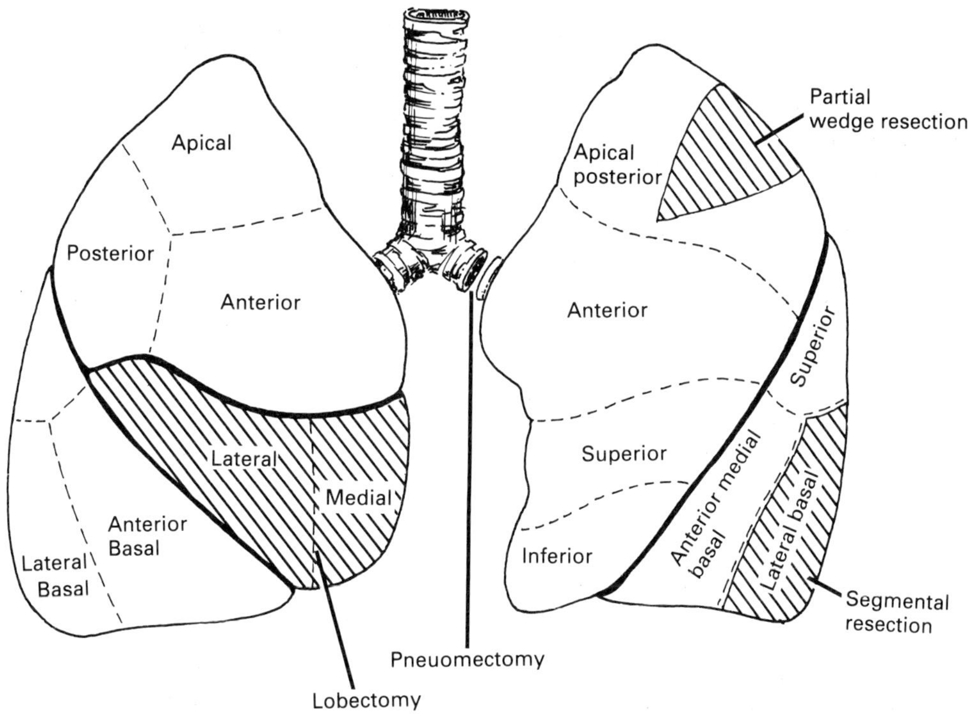

Fig. 45.17 The shaded areas represent different types of lung resection. The various anatomical segments of the lung are marked.

although most types, apart from the small cell variety, are relatively radioresistant—in the following situations:

1. Inoperable tumours.
2. Patients in whom operation is contraindicated for medical reasons, or those who refused to have an operation.
3. Those in whom carcinoma occurs after previous surgical excision.

Some degree of palliation can sometimes be achieved by local radiotherapy, particularly where there are pressure symptoms or pain from a bony metastasis. The amount of relief is, however, unpredictable and often disappointing.

Small cell (oat cell) carcinoma

Surgery has little role in management, and a combination of chemotherapy and radiotherapy is usually given. Any 5-year survival with this type of cancer is unusual.

Small cell lung cancer is the most radiosensitive cell type, but since it is usually a disseminated disease radiotherapy essentially only deals with the localized effects of the primary lesion. The main hope of control probably lies with the chemotherapeutic agents.

There is increasing evidence of the value of combined chemotherapy in the treatment of small cell carcinoma. A combination of at least three drugs is used. Cytotoxic chemotherapy has its own significant side-effects, related primarily to neutropenia and thrombocytopenia.

BENIGN TUMOURS

Benign tumours are uncommon. The least rare are carcinoid and hamartoma.

Carcinoid tumours

Carcinoid tumours usually occur in the large bronchi. Most are found in the right side, almost always within view of the bronchoscope. Occasionally it can show malignant potential, with metastases to the regional lymph nodes, bone and liver. Rarely do bronchial carcinoid tumours give rise to the carcinoid syndrome.

Hamartoma

The term hamartoma is applied to a tumour in which normal components of the organ are combined in a disorganized manner. It is most commonly peripheral, only rarely occurring within a bronchus. Malignant change in these tumours is very rare.

Clinical features

The clinical presentation of a benign tumour depends on whether the tumour is endobronchial or peripheral. Endobronchial tumours cause bronchial obstruction, producing symptoms of dyspnoea, wheezing, haemoptysis, cough or recurrent pneumonia. The clinical diagnosis of an endobronchial tumour is usually obvious and is confirmed by bronchoscopy and biopsy.

In contrast, benign parenchymal tumours are usually asymptomatic and are discovered on a routine chest X-ray. Hamartomas often have a lobulated appearance and may contain punctate calcifications (popcorn calcification).

Treatment

Treatment is surgical excision. The aim of surgical treatment is to alleviate symptoms, obtain a histological diagnosis and rule out malignancy, particularly for parenchymal lesions.

Pulmonary metastases

Many malignant neoplasms produce metastatic deposits in the lungs (Fig. 45.18). Neoplasms that commonly metastasize to the lungs are from the breast, kidney, prostate, testis, colon, rectum, ovary and urinary bladder. They are usually asymptomatic at first, but as they enlarge and erode the normal lung tissues they may cause haemoptysis, cough and signs of respiratory insufficiency. With perhaps the occasional exception of renal carcinoma, in which rarely a truly solitary metastasis may be present, resection of the segment of lung bearing a secondary deposit is not advised.

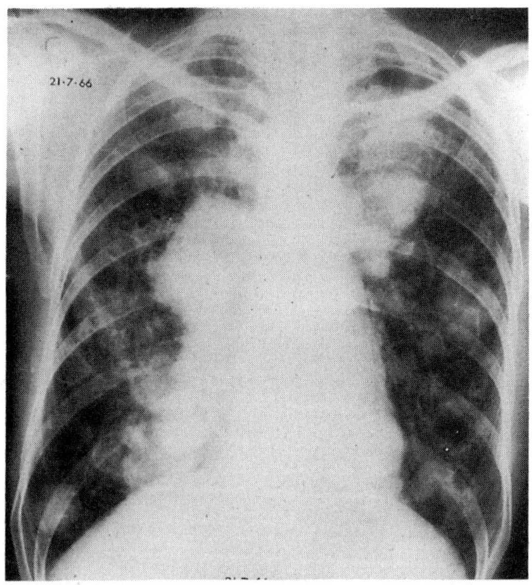

Fig. 45.18 Chest X-ray showing multiple metastases, mostly round in outline—so-called cannonball metastases. These arose from a primary renal carcinoma.

Index